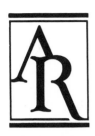

ANNUAL REVIEW OF PHARMACOLOGY AND TOXICOLOGY

ANNUAL REVIEW OF PHARMACOLOGY AND TOXICOLOGY

VOLUME 40, 2000

ARTHUR K. CHO, *Editor*
University of California School of Medicine, Los Angeles

TERRENCE F. BLASCHKE, *Associate Editor*
Stanford University Medical Center, Stanford

ING K. HO, *Associate Editor*
University of Mississippi Medical Center, Jackson

HORACE H. LOH, *Associate Editor*
University of Minnesota Medical School, Minneapolis

www.AnnualReviews.org   science@annurev.org   650-493-4400

ANNUAL REVIEWS
4139 El Camino Way • P.O. Box 10139 • Palo Alto, California 94303-0139

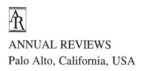

ANNUAL REVIEWS
Palo Alto, California, USA

International Standard Serial Number: 0362-1642
International Standard Book Number: 0-8243-0440-3
Library of Congress Catalog Card Number: 61-5649

Annual Review and publication titles are registered trademarks of Annual Reviews.

⊗ The paper used in this publication meets the minimum requirements of American National Standards for Information Sciences—Permanence of Paper for Printed Library Materials, ANSI Z39.48-1992.

Annual Reviews and the Editors of its publications assume no responsibility for the statements expressed by the contributors to this *Annual Review.*

Typeset by Impressions Book and Journal Services, Inc., Madison, WI
Printed and Bound in the United States of America

PREFACE

This volume includes three prefatory chapters, followed by a section of chapters selected by the Editorial Committee to reflect its views on topics and issues in pharmacology and toxicology that are particularly relevant to the new millennium. The topics by Sheiner et al, Broder et al, White, Nagata et al, Ohlstein et al, Debouck et al, and Holford et al are by no means exclusive but are the result of a selection based on space considerations and the ability of the Committee to identify appropriate authors able to complete the chapters within a narrow time frame.

THE EDITORIAL COMMITTEE

Contents

RELATED ARTICLES

From the *Annual Review of Biochemistry,* Volume 69, 2000:

Apoptosis Signaling, V. Dixit and A. Strasser
Chemical Synthesis of Proteins, S. Kent
Cyclooxygenases: Structural, Cellular and Molecular Biology, W. Smith,
  D. DeWitt, and R. Garavito
Two-Component Signal Transduction, A. Stock, V. Robinson, and
  P. Goudreau

From the *Annual Review of Cell and Developmental Biology,* Volume 15,
  1999:

Biochemical Pathways of Caspases Activation During Apoptosis, Imawati
  Budihardjo, Holt Oliver, Michael Lutter, Xu Luo, and Xiaodong Wang

From the *Annual Review of Medicine,* Volume 51, 2000:

Genetics of Psychiatric Disease, Wade H. Berrettini
Nonsteroidal Anti-Inflammatory Drugs and Cancer Prevention, John A.
  Baron and Robert S. Sandler

From the *Annual Review of Physiology,* Volume 62, 2000:

The Mechanism of Action of Thyroid Hormones, Jinsong Zhang and Mitchell
  A. Lazar
Insights from Mouse Models into the Molecular Basis of Neurodegeneration,
  N. Heintz and H. Y. Zoghbi
*Ligand-Gated Ion Channel Interactions with Cytoskeletal and Signaling
  Proteins,* Morgan Sheng and Daniel T. S. Pak

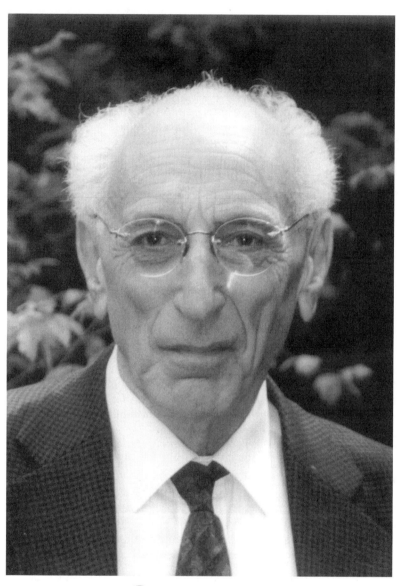

Annu. Rev. Pharmacol. Toxicol. 2000. 40:1–16

TARGETS OF DRUG ACTION

A.S.V. Burgen

Department of Pharmacology, University of Cambridge, Cambridge, CB2 1QJ, United Kingdom; e-mail: asvb@cam.ac.uk

Key Words acetylcholine, botulinum, carbonic anhydrase, conformation, DHFR, drug design, muscarinic, NMR, receptors

■ **Abstract** This article considers early work from the author's laboratory on muscarinic receptor specificity, subtypes, and conformational variability, with the use of nuclear magnetic resonance in pharmacology and the conformational variants of dihydrofolate reductase and general questions of receptors. It also considers some current approaches to drug development and receptor function, particularly as influenced by increasing knowledge of three-dimensional structure of receptors.

A CHANGE OF PLANS

Like many pharmacologists, my original training was in medicine, and I fully expected to spend my career in clinical work, as a pediatrician. However, immediately after graduation in London, I was seriously ill and one of my frequent visitors was my professor of physiology, Samson Wright. He persuaded me not to go straight into clinical work on recovery but to spend some time in a laboratory. What about joining the new pharmacology department at the Middlesex Hospital Medical School that Cyril Keele was just establishing? he asked. I said that I would, for a year only, but then I got hooked. I began attending the monthly meetings of the Physiological Society (in those days there was no separate pharmacological society), and the major topics presented were concerned with the growing evidence that the role of acetylcholine as a transmitter could be extended from the parasympathetic postganglionic endings to the sympathetic ganglia and the neuromuscular junction. The experimental evidence in favor was developed by WS Feldberg, GL Brown, Bernard Katz, and FC MacIntosh under the genial, but critical approval of our doyen, Sir Henry Dale. These developments were strenuously opposed by JC Eccles, who held to the all electrical theory of synaptic transmission and that all the acetylcholine effects people were looking at were "epiphenomena." This in no way discomforted Feldberg, who wrote of the extension of the theory to the central nervous system with great confidence: "The present position of the theory of acetylcholine as central transmitter is all but settled." Later he added a bit of caution: "perhaps not the universal central transmitter." This all made for a very exciting time, and quite naturally I found myself working on cholinergic problems. This was 1945, when news of the wartime work on organophosphorus anticholinesterase compounds became public. They were a fascinating series of compounds producing irreversible inhibition with apparently great specificity, and so, like Avram Goldstein (1), I began to study them. Like Avram, I needed to learn the mysteries of the Warburg and also to tackle kinetic problems. It was proved that the action was due to dialkylphosphorylation of the enzyme at the active site responsible for substrate hydrolysis, and that the inhibition was not totally irreversible but that the stability of the phosphorylation depended on the attached groups. Subsequent evidence obtained by others showed that the phosphorylation was on a serine in the active site. I regret that we failed to realize that the very slow kinetics of eserine and prostigmine inhibition also indicated an acylation of the enzyme.

One day, a colleague in the biochemistry department, Frank Dickens, came by with a problem. He had seen a paper by Torda and Wolff that claimed that botulinum toxin inhibited the synthesis of acetylcholine by cholineacetylase, which excited him, and he and a postdoc, Leonard Zatman, had acquired a grant to study it in detail. They had received a sample of highly purified toxin from the chemical warfare group at Porton, but alas, this sample of toxin had absolutely no effect on acetylcholine synthesis. Evidently, the effect described by the previous authors had been due to impurities. So how did botulinum work and could we help? The isolated phrenic nerve-diaphragm preparation had recently been introduced by Edith Bülbring, so we tried the toxin on that and it produced very reproducible neuromuscular block, which we could analyze. The block was not at all like that produced by curare. The muscle remained completely sensitive to the close intravascular injection of acetylcholine. We found a way of measuring the release of acetylcholine when the phrenic nerve was stimulated and discovered that its release was greatly reduced. Thus, botulinum acted on the release process presynaptically and synthesis was quite unaffected (1a).

MOVING TO MONTREAL

One evening after visiting my wife in hospital, where she had just given birth to our daughter, I got on a bus and encountered FC (Hank) McIntosh, who finding where I had just been, said, "Come home and wet the baby's head." In the course of the evening he told me that he had accepted the chair of physiology at McGill University in Montreal. "What about coming too?" he asked. Thus, shortly after the botulinum work was completed, I moved with him to McGill, where one of my next pharmacological adventures occurred. This adventure concerned the action of acetylcholine on the auricle examined with intracellular electrodes and was carried out with Kathleen Terroux. Acetylcholine increased the resting potential and radically reduced the duration of the action potential by increasing the rate of depolarization. The potassium dependence of the resting potential was also increased. We concluded that the effects on the electrical properties could all be attributed to an increase in potassium permeability, but we had no idea how the negative inotropic action was produced. This was the first demonstration of the mechanism of an inhibitory action of acetylcholine (2). Further development had to be left to others because I succumbed to a recurrence of my illness. When I returned to work, it seemed too disheartening to try and catch up, so I started a new line of work to try and disentangle the effects of parasympathetic stimulation on secretion in the salivary glands. The effects were dramatic enough: The maximum rate of saliva secretion per minute could exceed the weight of the gland. This not being the place to discuss details of the complex processes that have been uncovered in the secretion of water and electrolytes, suffice it to say that it is a sort of neurogenically controlled "kidney" where the fluid is produced by the acini and modified as it travels down the ducts. However, one aspect of the action of acetylcholine was novel. I found that some hydrophilic nonelectrolytes that could not enter the salivary gland cells passed into saliva in rather high concentration, which could best be explained if acetylcholine had opened intercellular channels (3). Later, Konrad Martin and I looked at the influence of sympathetic stimulation and found that this effect was very dramatic—even large nonelectrolytes such as sucrose were secreted—and so the possibility of a paracellular path could not be ignored (4). It has subsequently appeared from other work that a feature of the secretory process is a paracellular equilibration that essentially equilibrates the composition of the primary secretion produced by the acini with that of the plasma. The nature of the receptor-effector system responsible seems poorly defined, but norepinephrine opens up larger channels than acetylcholine does.

In 1957 I had the good fortune to spend the summer at Woods Hole working with that master neurophysiologist, Stephen Kuffler, on the (noncholinergic) nerves that inhibit transmission at the lobster neuromuscular junction (5). We made extracts of lobster nerve cord and muscle and found activity on muscle and the heart. To separate activities, we used paper chromatography with rather crude paper (all the large sheets of filter paper from the MBL stores had yellow marks on them, which on enquiry we found were due to the stores having been flooded the previous winter). Nevertheless, the separation worked all right, and it looked as though the activity might be due to the amino acids in the extracts, notably glutamate and aspartate; these had strong stimulatory activity on the lobster heart (6) and gaba was inhibitory. I should add that when I made alcoholic extracts of lobster muscle, the residual chunks of meat were very popular!

On my return to Montreal, I also ran a research unit at the Montreal General Hospital and had a chance to do some human pharmacology as well as some pharmacokinetics on the folic acid system.

PROFESSOR OF PHARMACOLOGY IN CAMBRIDGE

By 1962, it was becoming clear that the receptor concept was the basis of most, if not all, drug action and that most receptors were likely to be the site of action of endogenous regulators, mostly still unknown and whose role was yet to be defined. So far only the tip of the iceberg had been uncovered. Much of the future of pharmacology thus would be concerned with four problems: (a) defining the receptors, including isolating and characterizing them; (b) finding the endogenous regulators; (c) developing drug analogues; and (d) trying to understand the basis of the specificity of drugs for receptors. I decided that for the near future I wanted to concentrate on the fourth of these objectives, and I drew up a theoretical analysis that provided a protocol of what details we needed to find out about drug-receptor complexes (7). In order to develop such a program, it was necessary to select systems suitable for this kind of evaluation (it will not be surprising that the theme of acetylcholine keeps reappearing!).

My colleagues, Rod King and Palmer Taylor, and I decided first to examine the structure-activity of the aromatic sulphonamides as inhibitors of carbonic anhydrase. Because the binding constant to a site represents the ratio between the association and dissociation constants for a ligand, we thought that examining the rate constants by fast kinetics might give some useful clues. We started with two expectations: that the strength of binding would be mainly reflected in the stability of enzyme-inhibitor complex, and hence in its dissociation rate, and that the association rate would be dependent primarily on the rate of diffusional access to the binding site and would not change much between different sulphonamides. To our surprise, this was not the case. The binding constant correlated well with the association rate and the connection with the dissociation rate was clearly both smaller and less consistent (8). This was seen particularly clearly in a simple homologous series of 4-alkyl benzene sulphonamides, where the binding increased steadily up to C_5. There was only a small change in the off-rate, but the increased binding was reflected mainly in an increase in the association rate, which was in any case far below the limit set by diffusional access. When we looked at a similar series of 3-alkyl esters of benzenesulphonamide, the increased binding showed no dependence at all on the off-rate (9). By examining the pH and ionic strength dependence, as well as the binding to the apoenzyme and cobalt enzyme, we produced evidence that this unexpected behavior could be attributed to the formation of an intermediate hydrophobic complex (not complexed with the zinc in the active site) whose concentration was the rate-limiting step, and which was followed by a unimolecular transformation into the final zinc-coordinated complex. Changes in ligand structure were concerned mainly with determining the concentration of the intermediate complex, which was reflected in the rate of formation of the final complex, and that is why the stability of the complex was so dependent on the on-rate (10). It seems likely that multistep processes in forming drug receptor complexes are common. In this instance, no significant conformational change in the enzyme was involved, but as discussed below, in the formation of many drug complexes conformational changes are present.

We once thought receptors were simple. I began to have doubts when Laurence Spero and I developed an elegant method for following the efflux of potassium from intestinal smooth muscle in response to muscarinic agonists (11). To our suprise, we found that the dose-response relations for this were different from those for muscle contraction. We then played with the possibility that there were distinct receptors for the two responses, but the evidence did not support this. Rather, it led us to conclude that the receptor could be coupled to different responses in different ways (12). With Nigel Birdsall, John Young, Robin Hiley, and Ed Hulme, we went on to make precise measurements of the binding of ligands to muscarinic receptors, initially in the cerebral cortex. The binding of antagonists seemed to obey simple mass action rules and to accord very well with the affinities found by inhibition of contractile responses in smooth muscle (13). The trouble began when we looked at the binding of agonists (14), which was not simple but corresponded to at least two binding sites of very different magnitude. Later we found we could identify three such components, the proportions of which seemed the same for all full agonists, but which were different in different areas of the brain (15). These different forms of the receptor seemed stable because when we inactivated one form, the residual forms did not reestablish the proportions. On the other hand, we could convert the forms with the highest affinity into the lower-affinity forms by simply raising the ionic strength (16). When cardiac receptors were examined, the situation seemed similar, but it was not just high-ionic strength that could convert the higher- into the lower-affinity forms. This change was also dramatically produced by GTP, which converted virtually all of the highest-affinity form into the lowest-affinity form (17)—a further hint at the physiological significance of the multiple forms.

At this point, Rudi Hammer appeared on the scene bearing a new drug, pirenzipine, which in animal and human studies showed selectivity notably toward gastric secretion. Lo and behold, it was an antagonist, which by a factor of approximately 20 was more active against cortical than smooth muscle receptors, and even more surprising, some of the binding curves, those for cortex, hippocampus, and submandibular gland, did not have unitary slopes (18). Our analysis led to the conclusion that we were seeing the presence of at least three subtypes of the receptor; subsequently, a few other ligands were found that also showed discrimination of this kind. It was not long before the cloning of receptors got underway, and soon there was clear evidence of at least five subtypes and of the now-familiar situation found with other receptors: the existence of many subtypes with widely different amino acid sequences. It remains interesting that despite the very different sequences in the subtypes, so few ligands discriminate between them, a fact that needs to be borne in mind in elucidating details of receptor binding sites.

I deal with just one other aspect of muscarinic receptors. In 1951, Riker and Wescoe reported that the neuromuscular blocker, gallamine, acted on cardiac muscarinic receptors, an action shown by Clark and Mitchelson not to be competitive. Stockton, Birdsall, Hulme, and I reexamined the effects of this substance in the binding assay. We found that gallamine reacted with the muscarinic receptors in heart selectively, and although it was not competitive, it acted allosterically, reducing the affinity of both antagonists and agonists, by as much as 250-fold in the case of oxotremorine-M. It also dramatically slowed the reaction of antagonists with the receptor, a reliable indicator of allostery. Evidently, gallamine interacts with a second site in the receptor, distinct from that for the agonists or antagonists producing a changed conformation, which is reflected in different degrees of modification of binding for each ligand; i.e. the new conformation has a different structure activity profile (19). Some other substances have subsequently been found to have this same kind of action. It is interesting that gallamine also acts allosterically on cholinesterase.

The lessons to be drawn from the multiple states in which muscarinic receptors can exist are of general importance for the understanding of drug action. It has long been assumed that the interaction of agonists somehow changed the receptor to bring it into an active state, but the evidence from the kind of results recounted above show that a variety of conformational states are accessible to the receptor, depending both on other components of the receptor complex and on the nature of the drugs reacting with it. Such characteristics have been studied in most detail in the receptors coupled to ion channels, notably bacteriorhodopsin and the nicotinic receptor, which leave no doubt about the complexity of the transient and more-stable states that can exist. It has been pointed out on a number of occasions that the states of a receptor as seen by agonists and antagonists respond differentially to such features of drug structure as stereochemistry, the size and polarity of substituents, and so on. Because of the conformational changes, the "face" of the receptor presented to the ligand is altered, maybe radically, and this has importance in considerations of drug design.

HARVARD

One day in Cambridge I met Oleg Jardetzky, who was on a sabbatical in the biochemistry department, and he interested me in the possibility of using nuclear magnetic resonance (NMR) in pharmacology. The result was that I spent the summer of 1966 in Oleg's lab in the pharmacology department at Harvard. I arrived with an antibody against phenoxycholine, which bound acetylcholine, and with my postdoc, Jim Metcalfe. The NMR machine we used was an early unlocked type, which needed a lot of magnet adjustment and did not have perfect voltage stabilization. This meant that before starting a run, we had to find out whether there was a ballgame going on in Boston. If there was, it precluded an experiment because the mains was too unstable! However, we were able to show that the freedom of motion of tetramethylammonium was reduced by the antibody and that there were differential effects on the motion of groups in choline esters and ethers (20).

The considerable range of possibilities for the study of pharmacological problems by NMR and other physical techniques led to the British Medical Research Council establishing a Molecular Pharmacology Research Unit in the Department of Pharmacology at Cambridge, which provided excellent facilities and staff positions; notably, it enabled us to recruit an NMR specialist, Jim Feeney, from Varian Associates. So what did we find out by NMR? We started to look at conformation problems. We examined the motional characteristics first of small molecules, such as alkyl ammoniums. We were able to show that most of their motion in solution was due to a tumbling of the whole molecule rather than to rotation around bonds. We also showed that such small peptides as TRF, LHRF, and gastrin tetrapeptide were random coils without any evidence of tertiary structure (21). In the normal state, with intact SS bonds, the structures of vasopressin and oxytocin resembled each other, with restricted motional possibilities in the ring, and showing no evidence of either hydrogen bonding or the tail peptide being folded over the ring, as had previously been suggested. When the disulphide was reduced, they showed the same flexibility as the other linear peptides (22). These observations led to a discussion of whether flexible molecules bind to their receptors, by selection from the population of conformers or by conformational adaptation of the first weakly bound complex, the so-called zipper mechanism (23). The latter mechanism implies that a weak interaction of part of the molecule with the receptor occurs initially, with the full interaction developing as a result of rotation of the bonds in the nonbound part of the molecule. This kind of mechanism has been considered extensively for the problem of interaction of DNA in forming the complementary double helix.

A study with Phil Seeman and Jim Metcalfe of the interaction of anaesthetics with cell membranes showed that the mobility of anesthetics was greatly reduced by the membrane and that they were almost certainly confined to the lipid phase of the membrane. As the concentration of anaesthetic increased, the mobility increased, reflecting an increased fluidity of the membrane lipid, and only when the concentration reached levels that were lytic did any evidence of binding to protein emerge (24).

We decided that a combined kinetic and NMR study of a well-defined system of a protein and ligands would be interesting, and our choice fell on bacterial dihydrofolate reductase (from *Lactobacillus casei*), a relatively small, single-subunit enzyme of great importance in relation to chemotherapy. Despite its small size, it has binding sites for rather large molecules, such as the coenzyme NADP (H), and for folates, as well as for such inhibitors as methotrexate and trimethoprim. The detailed studies that followed could not have been achieved without a strong team, which included Jim Feeney, Gordon Roberts, and Berry Birdsall. Binding studies soon showed the complexities we could anticipate. The binding of NADPH together with methotrexate was highly cooperative, increasing by over 700-fold, but on the other hand it was equally negatively cooperative with folinic acid, whose binding was reduced 500-fold, so that the binding of NADPH was changed by a factor of 3.5×10^5 by the binding of these second ligands (25, 26). Another interesting finding came from the realization that the binding site for methotrexate (or folate) was so extensive that we had to consider the possibility it might be occupied by two fragments of the ligand simultaneously. We found that p-aminoglutamate (PABG) bound and so did 2,4-diaminopyrimidine (DAP), and that they could bind simultaneously and did so cooperatively. When we looked at a series of N-alkyl derivatives of PABG, the binding increased with chain length in the binary complex, by two orders of magnitude for the hexyl derivative, but when DAP$_o$ was also bound the effect of chain extension was completely lost (27). We soon found that the complex dependence of binding on the structure of the ligands required the postulation of multiple conformations. This is where NMR showed one of its strengths. Using proton NMR, one could see in the complex of the enzyme with trimethoprim and NADP (*a*) two sets of proton resonances from the nicotinamide end of the NADP—one set shifted upfield and the other shifted downfield—and (*b*) that two of the enzyme histidines were doublets. With ^{31}P NMR, one could see two sets of resonances for the pyrophosphates. It was abundantly clear that two conformations of the enzyme were present in roughly equal amounts, and they interconverted relatively slowly, so that distinct spectroscopic differences could be observed for both the enzyme and the coenzyme; the binding curve had shown only a simple, single binding constant (28). In another study, using NADP on whose carbonyl group ^{13}C replaced the normal ^{12}C, we saw by ^{13}C NMR that in the ternary complex with folate, the carbonyl group was present in three distinct, coexisting conformations whose relative abundance was altered by pH (29); evidence for this had also been found by fast kinetics. How exciting it was to actually have direct evidence of conformational populations, even though binding studies had left no doubt of their existence. In some complexes where the conformation was predominantly in one form, NMR enabled us to pick out aspects of the binding of ligands that put a marker on the conformations involved, but it did not give us a global picture of the binding site or of the overall conformation of the protein. Of course, X-ray structures can do that, but you need structures for many complexes to be able to interpret fully the structure activity problems.

I have said enough, perhaps too much, about how questions of the conformation of receptors absorbed me during this time. To quote from a review I presented in 1981, "drugs essentially interact with regulatory systems and the biological machinery for regulation is predominantly through conformation control."

I should not forget to tell you that in the middle of all this I moved to become the Director of the National Institute for Medical Research in Mill Hill, London in 1971 and I am happy to say that the Molecular Pharmacology group came with me and the work went on.

RETIREMENT

In 1982 I retired from Mill Hill. I went back to live in Cambridge and became the head of Darwin, a graduate college in Cambridge University. I also became responsible for the international activities of the Royal Society, as Foreign Secretary. These activities took up so much of my time and energies that it became impractical to continue in the laboratory. Thus, in 1984, my life as an experimental scientist came to an end. I also had another new interest in the creation of a

European academy of science, the Academia Europaea, which was inaugurated in 1988. For these reasons, what I have written here is essentially ancient history. Any account of the later developments in the fields I have covered must be left to those who are still busy there.

However, I take this opportunity to stand back and look at some of the things happening in pharmacology and to hazard a guess or two as to where it is going. Pharmacology has always been closely interdependent with its related subjects— physiology, biochemistry, pathology, and clinical science—and together with all of these sciences has been hugely influenced by the development of molecular biology. Among other things, this has meant a much greater dependence on instrumentation and the need for larger research teams. The trend is likely to increase further, but it is unlikely to rival what has happened in physics. Academic pharmacology is mainly concerned with understanding how existing drugs act. I return to the question of drugs intervening in regulatory systems. A therapeutic action on a regulatory system implies either that we may be dealing with a disordered regulatory system and that what we seek to achieve with drug action is to restore some component to within normal limits, or alternatively that a therapeutic result can be obtained by shifting the normal level of regulation. A major problem is that because of the parsimony of biological structure, the elements of the system we want to influence are likely to be used in other systems that we do not wish to perturb.

Recent research has yielded a great deal of information about how receptors work and, in some cases, details of their structure. It is now clear that the existence of receptor subtypes is a general condition that offers a prospect of finer discrimination, including differentiation of the effector systems to which they are coupled and which could lead to more selective action of drugs. However, finding drugs selective for individual subtypes is far from a simple matter. Is the effort worth it and how far will this deal with undesirable side actions? A promising way of finding out is to use selective mutagenesis to knock out single subtypes and to establish both what physiological changes result and also the change in reaction to the available nonselective drugs for the sytstem. A recent report on knockout of muscarinic M2 receptors showed the panoply of actions that this subtype is involved in (30). It was no surprise that the delineated actions of the M2 receptor were multiple, involving not only the heart but several central nervous system actions too. Studies of this sort would be especially valuable if carried out over the lifetime and generations of test species. The limitations of simply seeking specificity at the receptor level are highlighted. A really selective M2 antagonist might be a better drug, but it would not attain the ideal of producing only a single physiological change. Further selectivity would have to be dependent on other features of the global activity, such as the criticality of the regulatory system in the various physiological systems, and how the selectivity is influenced by pharmacokinetics and by promoters such as cytokines (31). However, it is to be expected that many knockout studies will be forthcoming and will help to define with greater precision the range of drug actions. Interference with regulatory systems invokes compensatory changes in second-order systems such as receptor down-regulation and changes in transcription, and there is also clear evidence that interference in the regulation of one receptor may secondarily interact with other related, and also not obviously related, systems (32, 33). These are ancillary targets that could be exploited in combination.

A perpetual problem in therapeutics has been those individuals who show atypical sensitivity to a drug or who develop side effects. Many of these cases are likely to be related to genetic differences. Recent studies of single nucleotide polymorphisms in β-adrenergic receptors provide the beginning for understanding some of them and indeed for describing pathology related to variant receptors (34). The question is global in its scope and is likely to define some uncommon new pathological states, but it could have a practical value in therapeutics in the future. A consortium of major drug companies has recently set up a project to map these polymorphisms, with the objective of minimizing side effects by identifying those that might affect drug responses; it is reported that at least one firm has already incorporated a search for polymorphisms in its drug discovery program (35). It is not likely to be long before quick tests for individual gene sequences may be so generally available that it will be feasible to pretest patients before giving them therapy. The mechanisms through which drug receptors are localized to particular types of cells and within cells is also just beginning to be explored (36). Mislocalization is another pathological possibility that could have interesting consequences, and therapeutic alteration to the balance of locations could be another basis for drug action. Developments in cell biology are uncovering an abundance of novel aspects of cell and tissue regulation. Some may reveal possible new targets for drug intervention, which may turn out to have therapeutic implications or to improve our understanding of toxicity. The control of blood vessel growth as an anticancer therapy is one such. The research in this area is so diverse and is changing so rapidly that it is not practical to go into detail here.

In the past, new drug development has followed several paths: the selection of some organ system or disease on which new synthetic compounds can be tested; the examination of the spectrum of activity of a novel compound, either synthesized or found naturally in plants or microorganisms; or the serendipitous observation of an extraneous activity. The latter was, for example, the origin of the antidepressants, following the observation that tuberculosis patients receiving isoniazid or iproniazid experienced a sense of well-being greater than that accounted for by the improvement in their physical state. An interesting recent example has appeared in the attempt to overcome bacterial resistance to vancomycin by chemical modification: Aryl substitution on one of the sugars revealed a different mechanism of action, which could well be the starting point for a new group of antibacterials (37).

When a compound with a novel action has been identified, its subsequent development into an effective agent that ends up in our therapeutics is by no means trivial, and some current developments are directed at improving and accelerating at least the discovery process. These include high-speed, semiautomatic testing of large numbers of compounds on isolated systems, mainly using receptor binding or enzyme activity and combinatorial synthesis to produce large numbers of candidate compounds to put into the high-speed tests. The latter is particularly attractive in peptide synthesis because the synthetic steps are merely repetitive. A good example of both these developments was the search for an analogue of enkephalin composed of d-amino acids. An automated synthesis yielded a set of 52 million acetylhexapeptides with practically all the possible sequences. These were tested in groups for μ-receptor activity on rat brain homogenates by the displacement of labeled DAMGO from the receptor. Iterative selection from the active groups subsequently led to the identification of the best sequence, which bound with the respectable value of 18 nM (38). Combinatorial methods can also be used for other syntheses and could, for instance, produce compounds in which some basic pharmacophor is varied by many substituents. Commercial packages for exploiting these methods are now readily available.

Although these enhanced trial-and-error methods will continue to be exploited, the hope of designing drugs in a more rational way is fundamental. In principle, this is available when the structure of the receptor is known and the area of the surface with which a drug interacts has been identified. Most drug binding sites are on proteins, and the three-dimensional structure of proteins is being determined at an astonishing rate by X-ray diffraction, by electron microscopy, and by NMR, so that several thousand are now known and recorded in the Protein Database. They include a number of important drug sites, such as dihydrofolate reductase and HIV proteases, for which the structure of complexes with inhibitors is also available. These structures give invaluable information about the three-dimensional structure of the effective binding site for that ligand and they yield details of the interatomic interactions involved. There are few surprises about the kinds of interactions identified, except for the discovery that bound water may be an important bridge. Calculations of the binding energy can be made using standard methods for electrostatic, hydrogen-bond, and dispersion interactions. Increasing levels of sophistication can be employed, and in some, though by no means all, cases they can give an encouraging order of magnitude agreement with the experimental figures (39); the energy calculation is very sensitive to the precision with which the groups are apposed.

The attempt can also be made to fit other active molecules presumed to be binding to the same site in the absence of an experimental structure for the complex. This uses computer methods that explore all the mutual dispositions of the ligand with the receptor, that calculate the free energy, and that select the configuration(s) giving the highest binding energy; many programs will also cover the range of conformations available to the ligand in binding if it is not a rigid molecule (40). When the binding of trimethoprim and methotrexate for DHFR was examined in this way, it was found that the optimal fit to the binding site was for conformations different from those found in the crystalline state (41); this was already known for methotrexate from the X-ray data. Note that there will be penalty in energy terms in such a selection, and this is usually ignored in the calculations. Now, the binding area for trimethoprim is smaller than what is known from the X-ray structure to be available for methotrexate, which interacts with an additional area. Thus, trimethoprim by no means exploits all the possibilities of binding to the site, and it is not surprising that when trimethoprim was extended with a carboxylic chain related to the glutamate end of methotrexate, the affinity was increased by up to three orders (42). You will notice how this refers back to the binding of fragments of methotrexate discussed earlier. It means also that if the structure of the binding site is known, a wider range of possible binding subsites may be revealed and alternative combinations of subsites may be identifiable, leading to the proposal of novel drug structures. More generally, it means that visualization of the whole potential binding site as a three-dimensional surface on which hydrophilic and charged areas are displayed is an open playing field on which to start afresh to find molecules that give the optimal match to this surface. Several strategies are available for seeking such a molecule. A structure database can be accessed and used as a source of selected compounds to be tested against the whole site. An alternative approach is to visualize subsites one at a time, to find molecular fragments to fit them, and then to generate a complete molecule by filling in connections between the fragments.

So far in this account we have assumed that the conformation of the receptor site is invariant, but some of the amino acid side chains and even some of the peptide chains may be mobile. The fit to the receptor will then be less precisely prescribed. This has already been noted in inhibitors of HIV protease and adds a complication, but it provides an extra measure of flexibility in choice of structures (43); there is no intrinsic reason why allowance for this cannot be built into fitting programs.

Major conformational changes of the sort we have discussed for antagonist-agonist pairs are a different matter. This is clearly a problem. It might be anticipated that the conformation found in the unoccupied (ground state) would have a good prospect of matching antagonists, although there is no reason to assume that all antagonists combine with the ground state (vide DHFR inhibitors). For agonists the situation is intrinsically more complex, because by definition they are binding to a changed conformation. There remains the possibility that only part of the binding site is transformed in the active conformation and that subsites might therefore still provide guides to lead compounds from which conventional development techniques could be used. Of course, a natural regulator molecule for the site will usually be known and may provide a lead, and another strategy is considered below.

There will be situations where the three-dimensional structural information available is confined to that of the unoccupied receptor. In this case, the binding site first needs to be identified. Of the many binding sites that have been found in proteins, most are situated in clefts or indentations in the protein surface, and these should be sought on the receptor as the most promising areas to be examined. An additional guide comes from knowledge of the effects of mutagenesis giving indications of where residues affecting binding are located in the sequence and, hence, in the folded structure.

The reliance on having a three-dimensional structure for the binding site that has been determined by X-ray or other methods could become less important when methods for predicting the three-dimensional structure of proteins based simply on amino acid sequence become sufficiently advanced. It is beginning to look as though there might be only a limited repertoire of patterns of protein structure; it is perhaps pertinent that in hemoglobin, mutants are known involving practically all the residues, but the three-dimensional structure and function shows little variation. Predictions of structure can thus be modeled on comparison with an experimentally determined structure followed by refinement. This substantially reduces the number of degrees of freedom that need to be considered in the folding program. An example of this is the way the discovery of the transmembrane structure of bacteriorhodopsin was carried over to provide a realistic postulation of a similar set of seven transmembrane helices for adrenergic, muscarinic, and other membrane-located receptors. But note that so far, this has not led to reliable prediction of the three-dimensional structure of the extracellular and intracellular parts of these proteins. This is a disappointment because these are the very areas that constitute the binding sites for the substances we are interested in and that provide the basis for specificity. The need for finding how to fold these peptide loops is vital and, it is hoped, may be possible before long. The problem of the receptor structure complementary to an agonist is one that would be intermediate if the structure of the unoccupied receptor or the complex with an antagonist is known, because this becomes again an exercise, albeit a more complex one, in refinement of trial agonist-receptor complexes.

Another question is how to deal with the new regulatory substances being uncovered. Many of these are proteins or peptides, and therefore they have obvious bioavailability or kinetic limitations as drugs. A great deal of thought has gone into finding nonpeptide equivalents. Although some emphasis has been given to the more conservative approach of replacement of some of the amino acids with novel pseudo–amino acids or on combinations of amino acids with other frameworks, bolder spirits have been encouraged by the existence of morphine as an equivalent for the opioid peptides to treat these receptor sites as similar in principle to those for smaller regulators. Indeed, this has been thoroughly justified because, as a result of conventional screening methods, potent compounds have been found for angiotensin (Losartan and later compounds), oxytocin, gastrin, endothelin, and other peptide receptors among molecules no different in kind from those that would have been developed for small molecule receptors. One of the most obviously desirable peptide equivalents would be for insulin because so much is known about its structure and that of its receptor.

The approaches to new drug development I have outlined are being pursued vigorously and imaginatively in drug companies and in academic medicinal chemistry groups, and they are likely to produce many novel ligands. Despite their promise, it would not be expected that that they would have made any great impact on the appearance of new drugs in therapy as yet, because the total drug development process is a long one and the discovery of new leads, and even the development of good derivatives, is only a small part; poor bioavailability, toxicity, and failures in clinical trials put paid to many hopefuls.

We live in a time when even large pharmaceutical companies feel insecure and amalgamate to become even larger, when they rely on only a few blockbusters to make their profit and have to live with a short period of patent protection. This means that even more than in the past, the targets they will concentrate on are those where a big impact can be made: cancer, AIDS, Alzheimer's, psychoactives, etc. It will be fascinating to see how the new approaches open up possibilities in these fields. Alas, there will be many interesting new compounds that will never merit economic development but would be fascinating experimental tools for the pharmacologist. It is to be hoped that they will not simply molder away in company archives.

Visit the Annual Reviews home page at www.AnnualReviews.org.

LITERATURE CITED

1. Goldstein A. 1997. A rewarding research pathway. *Annu. Rev. Pharmacol. Toxicol.* 37:1–28
1a. Burgen ASV, Dickens F, Zatman LJ. 1949. The action of botulinum toxin on the neuromuscular junction. *J. Physiol.* 109:10–24
2. Burgen ASV, Terroux KG. 1953. On the negative inotropic effect in the cat's auricle. *J. Physiol.* 120:449–64
3. Burgen ASV. 1956. The secretion of non-electrolytes in the parotid saliva. *J. Cell Comp. Physiol.* 48:113–38
4. Martin K, Burgen ASV. 1962. Changes in the permeability of the salivary gland caused by sympathetic stimulation and by catecholamines. *J. Gen. Physiol.* 46:225–43
5. Burgen ASV, Kuffler SW. 1957. Two inhibitory fibres forming synapses with a single nerve cell in the lobster. *Nature* 180:1490–91
6. Enger PES, Burgen ASV. 1957. The effects of some anino acids on the perfused lobster heart. *Biol. Bull.* 113:345–46
7. Burgen ASV. 1966. The drug-receptor complex. *J. Pharm. Pharmacol.* 18:137–49
8. Taylor PW, King RW, Burgen ASV. 1970. Kinetics of complex formation between human carbonic anhydrase and aromatic sulphonamides. *Biochemistry* 9:2638–45
9. King RW, Burgen ASV. 1976. Kinetic aspects of structure-activity relations; the binding of sulphonamides by carbonic anhydrase. *Proc. R. Soc. London Ser. B* 193:107–25
10. Taylor PW, King RW, Burgen ASV. 1970. Inflence of pH on the kinetics of complex formation between sulphonamides and human carbonic anhydrase. *Biochemistry* 9:3894–903
11. Burgen ASV, Spero L. 1968. The action of acetylcholine and other drugs on the efflux of potassium and rubidium from smooth muscle of guinea-pig ileum. *Br. J. Pharmacol.* 34:99–115
12. Burgen ASV, Spero L. 1970. The effects of calcium and magnesium on the response of intestinal smooth muscle to drugs. *Br. J. Pharmacol.* 40:492–500
13. Hulme EC, Birdsall NJM, Burgen ASV,

Mehta P. 1978. The binding of antagonists to brain muscarinic receptors. *Mol. Pharmacol.* 14:737–50

14. Birdsall NJM, Burgen ASV, Hulme EC. 1978. The binding of agonists to brain muscarinic receptors. *Mol. Pharmacol.* 14:723–36

15. Birdsall NJM, Hulme EC, Burgen ASV. 1980. The character of muscarinic receptors in different areas of the brain. *Proc. R. Soc. London Ser. B* 207:1–12

16. Burgen ASV. 1986. The effects of ionic strength on cardiac muscarinic receptors. *Br. J. Pharmacol.* 88:451–55

17. Birdsall NJM, Berrie CP, Burgen ASV, Hulme EC. 1980. Modulation of the binding properties of muscarinic receptors: evidence for receptor-effector coupling. In *Receptors for Neurotransmitters and Peptide Hormones,* ed. G Pepeu, MJ Kuhar, SJ Enna, pp. 107–16. New York: Raven

18. Hammer R, Berrie R, Birdsall NJM, Burgen ASV, Hulme EC. 1980. Pirenzipine distinguishes between different subclasses of muscarinic receptors. *Nature* 283:90–92

19. Stockton JM, Birdsall NJM, Burgen ASV, Hulme EC. 1983. Modification of the binding properties of muscarinic receptors by gallamine. *Mol. Pharmacol.* 23:551–57

20. Burgen ASV, Jardetzky O, Metcalfe JC, Wade-Jardetzky N. 1967. Investigation of a hapten-antibody complex by nuclear magnetic resonance. *Proc. Natl. Acad. Sci. USA* 58:447–53

21. Feeney J, Roberts GCR, Brown JP, Burgen ASV, Gregory H. 1972. Conformational studies of some component peptides of pentagastrin. *J. Chem. Soc.* PII:601–4

22. Feeney J, Roberts GCR, Rockey JH, Burgen ASV. 1971. Conformational studies of oxytocin and lysine vasopressin in aqueous solution using high resolution NMR spectroscopy. *Nat. New Biol.* 232:108–10

23. Burgen ASV, Roberts GCR, Feeney J. 1975. Binding of flexible ligands to macromolecules. *Nature* 253:753–55

24. Metcalfe JC, Seeman P, Burgen ASV. 1968. The proton relaxation of benzyl alcohol in erythrocyte membranes. *Mol. Pharmacol.* 4:87–95

25. Birdsall B, Burgen ASV, Roberts GCR. 1980. Binding of coenzyme analogues to *Lactobacillus casei* dihydrofolate reductase: binary and ternary complexes. *Biochemistry* 19:3723–31

26. Birdsall B, Burgen ASV, Hyde EI, Roberts GCR, Feeney J. 1981. Negative cooperativity between folinic acid and coenzyme in their binding to *Lactobacillus casei* dihydrofolate reductase. *Biochemistry* 20:2186–95

27. Birdsall B, Burgen ASV, Rodrigues de Miranda J, Roberts GCR. 1978. Cooperativity in ligand binding to dihydofolate reductase. *Biochemistry* 17:2102–10

28. Gronenborn A, Birdsall B, Hyde E, Roberts G, Feeney J, Burgen A. 1981. 1H and 31P NMR characterization of two conformations of the trimethoprim-NADP$^+$-dihydrofolate reductase complex. *Mol. Pharmacol.* 20:145–53

29. Birdsall B, Gronenborn A, Clore GM, Roberts GCR, Feeney J, Burgen ASV. 1981. 13C NMR evidence for three slowly interconverting conformations of the dihydrofolate reductase-NADP$^+$-folate complex. *Biochem. Biophys. Res. Commun.* 101:1139–44

30. Gomeza J, Shannon H, Kostenis E, Felder C, Zhang L, et al. 1999. Pronounced pharmacologic deficits in M2 muscarinic receptor knockout mice. *Proc. Natl. Acad. Sci. USA* 96:1692–97

31. Rosoff ML, Wei J, Nathanson NM. 1996. Isolation and characterisation of the chicken m2 acetylcholine promoter region. Induction of gene transcription by leukaemia inhibitory factor and ciliary neurotrophic factor. *Proc. Natl. Acad. Sci. USA* 93:14889–94

32. Haddad E-B, Russell J. 1998. Regulation

of the expression and function of the M2 muscarinic receptor. *Trends Pharmacol. Sci.* 19:322–27

33. Weng G, Bhalla US, Iyengar R. 1999. Complexity in biological signalling systems. *Science* 284:92–96

34. Büscher R, Herrmann V, Insel PA. 1999. Human adrenoreceptor polymorphisms: evolving recognition of clinical importance. *Trends Pharmacol. Sci.* 20:94–99

35. Mahsood E. 1999. A consortium plans free SNP map of human genome. *Nature* 398:545–46

36. Luttrell LM, Ferguson SSG, Daaka Y, Miller WE, Maudsley S, et al. 1999. β-Arrestin-dependent formation of β2 adrenergic receptor-Src protein kinase complexes. *Science* 283:655–61

37. Ge M, Chen Z, Onishi HR, Kohler J, Silver LL, et al. 1999. Vancomycin derivatives that inhibit peptidoglycan biosynthesis without binding d-Ala-d-Ala. *Science* 284:507–11

38. Dooley CT, Chung NN, Wilkes BC, Schiller PW, Bidlack JM, et al. 1994. An all d-amino acid opioid peptide with central analgesic activity from a combinatorial library. *Science* 266:2019–22

39. Hünenberger PH, Helms V, Narayama N, Taylor SS, McCammon JA. 1999. Determinants of ligand binding to cAMP-dependent protein kinase. *Biochemistry* 38:2358–66

40. Koehler KF, Rao SN, Snyder JP. 1996. Modelling drug-receptor interactions. See Ref. 45, pp. 235–36

41. Itai A, Mizutani MY, Nishibata Y, Tomioka N. 1996. Computer-assisted new lead design. See Ref. 45, pp. 107–9

42. Birdsall B, Feeney J, Pascual C, Roberts GCK, Kompis I, et al. 1984. A 1H nmr study of the interactions and conformations of rationally designed brodimoprim analogues in complexes with *Lactobacillus casei* dihydrofolate reductase. *J. Med. Chem.* 23:1672–76

43. Giannis A, Rübsam. 1997. Peptidomimetics in drug design. *Adv. Drug Res.* 29:1–78

44. Cohen NC, ed. 1996. *Guidebook on Moleculer Modelling in Drug Design.* San Diego, CA: Academic

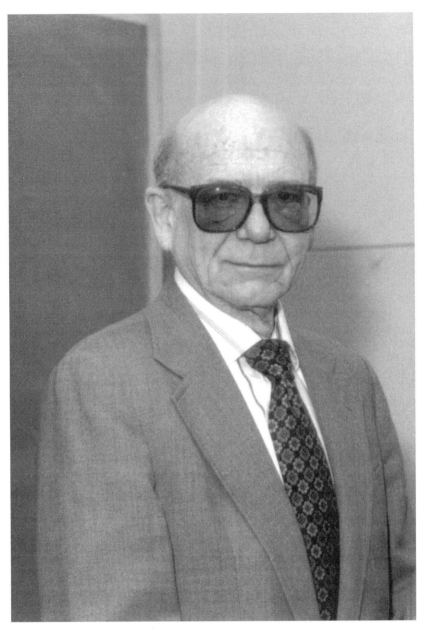

James R. Gillette

Annu. Rev. Pharmacol. Toxicol. 2000. 40:19–41

LABORATORY OF CHEMICAL PHARMACOLOGY, NATIONAL HEART, LUNG, AND BLOOD INSTITUTE, NIH: A Short History

James R. Gillette

5615 Northfield Road, Bethesda, Maryland 20817–6735; e-mail: gillettejrrj@erols.com

Key Words   drug metabolism and disposition, immunology, neuropharmacology, pharmacokinetics, toxic chemically reactive metabolites

■ **Abstract**   The Laboratory of Chemical Pharmacology (LCP) began in 1950 as the Section of Pharmacology within the National Heart Institute, the National Institutes of Health. Its first chief was Bernard B. Brodie, considered by many to be one of the fathers of modern pharmacology. Since its inception, LCP has made many significant contributions to the fields of pharmacology and toxicology. LCP was among the first to study (*a*) the effects of drugs on the turnover of serotonin and norepineprine in brain and other tissues, (*b*) the absorption of drugs from the gastrointestinal tract and their passage across the blood-brain barrier, (*c*) the oxidation and reduction of drugs and other foreign compounds by liver microsomal enzymes (later known as the cytochrome P450 enzymes) and inhibitors and inducers of these enzymes, (*d*) the formation of toxic chemically reactive metabolites of drugs and other foreign compounds, and (*e*) mechanisms of immunological responses. Approximately 300 scientists worked in LCP during its existence, and they and their collaborators published more than 1,300 papers. This is a short history of the people who worked in it and of their contributions to biomedical sciences.

PROLOGUE

The Laboratory of Chemical Pharmacology (LCP) evolved from a small laboratory within the Goldwater Memorial Hospital in New York City during the Second World War. At that time the Japanese Army had overrun Southeast Asia, the principal source of quinine. Clearly, drugs were needed to control malaria in the Allied armies, if they were to perform effectively in malaria-infested regions. A group of scientists recruited and led by a bright young renal physiologist, James Shannon, was asked to solve the problem (1). Through the influence of EK Marshall, Shannon had become convinced that the pharmacological effects of a drug were more closely related to the concentration of the drug in the blood than to any arbitrary dose of the drug. At that time, this was a revolutionary idea. But showing such relationships required analytical methods capable of detecting the parent drug in absence of its metabolites in blood and other tissues.

In approaching the problem, Bernard Brodie, together with his technician, Sidney Udenfriend, developed principles that could be used to develop analytical methods for many drugs. The general approach (2) was to extract unchanged drug into "the least polar solvent" capable of quantitatively extracting the drug, to wash the organic extract to remove polar metabolites, to return the drug to an aqueous buffer, and to detect the unchanged drug either directly by measuring its absorbancy in a spectrophotometer or fluorescence in a fluorometer or indirectly by converting it to a detectable derivative. Using analytical procedures based on these principles, Shannon's group studied many compounds of potential use in the treatment of malaria. They discovered (3), for example, that Atabrine in dogs and volunteers had a very long half-life in the body and that the best way of dosing soldiers was to administer a loading dose followed by smaller maintenance doses. There is no doubt that the Goldwater group played a major role in assuring victory in the Pacific.

After the war, Shannon's Goldwater group dissolved. Shannon became the Director of the Squibb Institute for Medical Research. Others, including Udenfriend, dispersed to academia. But Brodie remained at Goldwater. However, the two principles that guided the anti-malarial program, (*a*) that the pharmacological effects of a drug were more closely related to the concentration of the drug in the blood than to any arbitrary dose of the drug, and (*b*) development of analytical methods based on extraction of drugs into the least polar solvent, guided Brodie's approach to pharmacology for the next several years. Indeed, from 1947 through 1953, Brodie and his associates published more than twenty papers in the *Journal of Pharmacology and Experimental Therapeutics* on the disposition of various drugs, including carbonamide, dicumarol, aminopyrine (Pyramidon), benzazoline (Priscoline), ethyl biscoumacetate (Tromexan), dibenamine, caffeine, pentobarbital, ephredine, and phenybutazone (Butazolidin).

Early Discoveries

While still in New York, Brodie & Julius Axelrod (4) discovered that acetanilide was converted, amongst other things, to both aniline and N-acetylaminophenol. Flinn & Brodie (5) further showed that N-acetylaminophenol, later known as acetaminophen or paracetamol, was a potent analgesic. Moreover, Brodie & Axelrod (6) also found that phenacetin, then a major component of many analgesic preparations, was also converted in the body to N-acetylaminophenol. These studies thus illustrated another principle that was to guide the work of LCP for several years: Pharmacological effects of drugs are frequently mediated in part by metabolites of drugs. Identification of the metabolites might therefore lead to the development of more specific and safer drugs.

Brodie et al also showed that the short action of procaine was due to its short half-life in the body. They suggested that the ester bond in procaine be replaced by an amide bond to form procaine amide, which has a longer half-life (7) and thus was useful in the treatment of cardiac arrhythmias (8).

In another study, Brodie et al discovered that the elimination of the "ultra-short-acting" barbiturate, thiopental, from the body was rather slow; indeed, its short action was due to its rapid distribution into deep pharmacokinetic compartments, such as fat (9). Repeated doses of thiopental thus could result in prolonged narcosis, because the drug would accumulate in the body until the serum levels remained at pharmacologically effective levels even after the redistribution phases were complete.

In still another study, Brodie et al (10) discovered that N-acetyl 4-aminoantipyrine was not significantly bound to blood or organ components but was distributed with body water. The amount of body water thus could be calculated from measurements of the drug in blood at various times.

THE EARLY YEARS

Shannon soon became disenchanted with industry and in 1949 accepted the position of Scientific Director of the National Heart Institute. He immediately started to recruit the best people he could find for his staff. This was not as easy as it might seem. At that time, government laboratories had a poor reputation. But owing to his persistence and persuasive personality, he collected a group of scientists who would become leaders in many biomedical sciences, including pharmacology. He was aided in his recruitment by a quirk in the draft law that permitted young physicians to enlist in the Public Health Service and thereby to work at NIH rather than to serve in M.A.S.H. units in Korea. Among the scientists he recruited were Robert Berliner, James Wyngaarden, Thomas Kennedy, Christian Anfinsen, Robert Bowman, Marjorie and Evan Horning, and later, Donald Frederickson.

Shannon also was able to convince Brodie in 1950 to join him as the head of the Section of Chemical Pharmacology of the National Heart Institute, which became the Laboratory of Chemical Pharmacology (LCP) in 1952. Shannon staffed the section with people such as Drs. Sidney Udenfriend, Bert La Du, and Elwood Titus, and several "technicians," including Julius Axelrod, Lewis Aronow, Herbert Weisbach, Jack Cooper, and Parkhurst Shore. The initial cadre of the National Heart Institute was housed in NIH's Building 3, which was far too small for the group envisioned by Shannon. So the move of Brodie's group from Goldwater to Bethesda was gradual until the new Clinical Center was built in Bethesda. Even after the Clinical Center was built, Brodie still maintained a group at Goldwater, headed by John Burns, whom Brodie had recruited after the war.

Drug-Metabolizing Enzymes

After Brodie became chief of LCP, he was contacted by Glenn Ullott, of Smith Kline and French, who told him of a compound that had some very strange properties. Even at fairly large doses the compound, known as SKF-525A, seemed to exert no obvious action of it own, but it prolonged the action of many barbiturates. This could readily be demonstrated by injecting the compound just prior to the barbiturate into mice and measuring the length of time that they "slept." The question was whether the effect was due to the potentiation of the action of the barbiturate in brain or to a slowing of the metabolism of the barbiturate. Studies by Axelrod et al (11) revealed that the levels of the drug on the awakening were virtually unaffected by SKF-525A, but the half-life of the barbiturate was prolonged. And studies by Cooper et al (12) indicated that SKF-525A inhibited the in vitro as well as in vivo metabolism of many other drugs, suggesting that there may be something in common for the enzymes that metabolized the drugs.

But what were these enzymes? At that time the Spinco ultracentrifuge had just been invented and it became possible to isolate various fractions of liver homogenates. Using fractions separated with this instrument, Axelrod (13) discovered that amphetamine was metabolized to phenylacetone by the 9,000 x g supernatant fraction, but not by either the microsomal fraction or the soluble fraction alone. By brilliant insight he concluded that the enzyme was in the microsomes and that the soluble fraction provided NADPH (then known as TPNH). At about the same time, but unknown to Axelrod, Mueller & Miller at the University of Wisconsin (14) discovered that the N-demethylation of the carcinogen, N-dimethylaminoazobenzene, required liver microsomes, NADP, the soluble fraction, and a substrate for the generation of NADPH.

Subsequently, various members of LCP discovered that many seemingly different reactions were catalyzed by enzymes in liver microsomes in the presence of an NADPH generation system: for example, the O-dealkylation of phenacetin (Axelrod), the N-demethylation of aminopyrine and other alkylamines (Bert La Du, Leo Gaudette, and Natalie Trousof), the oxidation of hexobarbital (Jack Cooper), and the hydroxylation of aromatic compounds (Sidney Udenfriend & Chozo Mitoma). Brodie recognized the implications of these findings, and he and his colleagues published the classic paper on the oxidative microsomal enzymes (15), later to be known collectively as cytochrome P450. Shortly thereafter Axelrod left Brodie and went back to school (part time) to get his Ph.D. degree (1), which he obtained within a year.

In 1954, the Clinical Center of the NIH was completed and LCP moved to its facilities in the eastern wings of the 7th and 8th floors. Sidney Udenfriend became the first Deputy Chief of the Laboratory and had his office on the 8th floor, and Brodie had his on the 7th floor. With the increase in space, there was an increase in the number of scientists and a great increase in the breadth of the studies of biomedical problems.

Drug metabolism remained an active field. James Fouts studied inhibitors of the microsomal enzymes (16, 17) and the reduction of nitro compounds, such as chloramphenicol and ρ-nitrobenzoic acid (18), and azo-compounds, such as Prontosil (19), by liver microsomes. I was assigned by La Du to the problem of solubilizing and purifying the microsomal enzyme, a problem that defied my best efforts. Nevertheless, La Du and I were able to prove that although hydrogen peroxide was formed by liver microsomes, the enzymes were not typical peroxidases, such as horseradish peroxidase, and we obtained the first evidence that TPNH cytochrome c reductase (later known as NADPH cytochrome P450 reductase) might be involved in the reactions (20).

Other Studies During the 1950s and Early 1960s

A major objective of the laboratory at the time was to determine the factors that governed the transfer of drugs across biological membranes. In a series of papers, reviewed in (21), Lewis Schanker et al discovered that the rate of absorption of drugs from the small and large intestines depended on the pKa of the drug, the pH of the medium, and the lipid solubility of the nonionized form of the drug. Moreover, Shore et al (22) studied the absorption of drugs from the stomach and discovered that acidic conditions in the stomach could lead to the accumulation of weak bases. Thus for some drugs there may be an entero-stomachic circulation as well as an entero-hepatic circulation. In other work in the laboratory, Schanker studied mechanisms of biliary secretion (23), and Steven Mayer & Roger Maickel studied the properties of the blood-brain barrier (24, 25).

John Burns and his group in Goldwater continued to study the metabolism of phenylbutazone analogues (26), which led to the development of a new uricosuric drug. But Burns' major interest at the time was the elucidation of the synthesis of ascorbic acid (27).

La Du & Vincent Zannoni (28) became interested in the enzymes that catalyzed the metabolism of tyrosine, a problem that led to La Du's interest in pharmacogenetics. Neil Moran & Marion Cotton (29) and Cotton & Harriet Maling (30) performed studies on the effect of drugs on the cardiac contractile force. Severinghaus began studies on factors that governed the pulmonary dead space (31) and the serum pCO2 and pO2 (32).

But one of the most significant projects of the laboratory resulted from a collaboration of Sidney Udenfriend with Robert Bowman. Udenfriend had become an expert in the theory of the fluorescence of compounds, and recognized the importance of developing ways of determining both the activation and the fluorescence spectra in order to develop more specific and sensitive methods for assaying biochemicals. Bowman became intrigued with the problem and developed a spectrophotofluorometer. With this prototype, Udenfriend and his postdoctoral student, Daniel Duggan (33), began to explore the factors that governed fluorescence, and thus the usefulness of the instrument, later known as the Aminco-Bowman Spectrophotofluorometer.

With this advance in methodology, Udenfriend together with Donald Bogdanski & Herbert Weissbach were able to detect small amounts of serotonin in brain (34). Shore developed techniques for assaying small amounts of catecholamines (35), and together with Alan Burkhalter & Victor Cohn developed a method for histamine (36). These methods provided the basis of numerous papers during the next two decades by LCP and other laboratories throughout the world. For example, the methods led to the discovery by Brodie et al that reserpine caused the release of serotonin (37) and norepinephrine from tissues.

Shortly after this time, Bert La Du left the laboratory and I became head of the Section on Drug Enzyme Interactions. Sidney Udenfriend also left to form his own laboratory, within the National Heart Institute, to which incidentally he attracted the future Nobel laureate, Marshall Nirenberg, from the National Arthritis Institute. John Burns then moved to Bethesda and became the second Deputy Laboratory Chief.

At this time Allan Conney joined Burns to work on an ascorbic acid problem, but he soon convinced Burns and several others in other laboratories of NIH to study the effects of 3-methylcholanthrene pretreatment on the metabolism of different drugs, which led to a classic paper published in *Science* (38). The fact that 3-methylcholanthrene affected different reactions differently provided one of the first indications that there were multiple forms of cytochrome P450. He continued his work by showing that phenobarbital and other compounds (39; reviewed in 40) were able to induce cytochrome P450 enzymes. At about the same time, Remmer (41) in Germany and Kato & Chiesara (42) in Italy were also studying the effects of pretreatment of animals with barbiturates and were also coming to the conclusion that barbiturates could serve as inducers of liver microsomal enzymes. Later, Joan Booth (43) in LCP discovered that anabolic steroids were inducers.

Neuropharmacology

Early in the 1960s John Burns left the laboratory to join Burroughs Wellcome, and Parkhurst Shore served for a short time as the third Deputy Laboratory Chief. However, Shore soon left for the Southwestern Medical School in Dallas, Texas, and then Erminio Costa became the fourth Deputy Laboratory Chief.

During the 1960s, most of LCP focused its attention on various aspects of neuropharmacology. Brodie and Costa and colleagues continued studies on the mechanisms by which drugs affected the synthesis, transport, and storage of norepinephrine and serotonin in various organs of the body. In a series of more than 40 papers they studied the effects of reserpine, tetrabenazine, decarboxylase inhibitors (44), dopamine beta oxidase inhibitors (45), and "false transmitters" (46). In the late 1960s Norton Neff, Thomas Tozer, and colleagues (47) studied the rates of uptake and release of radiolabeled norepinephrine from rat heart and began to apply mathematical expressions for two-compartment systems to analyze the kinetics of these processes.

Marjorie Horning, in the Laboratory of Chemistry of the National Heart Institute, in collaboration with Maling (48), discovered that the source of fatty acids appearing in liver after alcohol administration was adipose tissue, a finding that led Brodie to his interest in lipolysis. After Sutherland made his seminal discoveries of the role of cyclic AMP, Gopal Krishna (49) developed a simple method for the assay of cyclic AMP, which greatly facilitated studies of control mechanisms of lipolysis in adipose tissues. Indeed, this became a major objective of the laboratory during this phase, resulting in more than 30 papers on the mechanism of lipolysis in adipose tissues. Frandsen & Krishna (50) subsequently developed methods for the assay of cyclic GMP and guanylate cyclase activity, which help to elucidate the role of cyclic GMP in the retina (51).

Titus' section also became interested in neuropharmacology. Lewis Ignarro (52) discovered that both alpha and beta adrenergic receptors were present in mouse spleen. Hans Dengler (53) studied the uptake of norepinephrine into isolated brain tissues. Arthur Michaelson & Palmer Taylor (54) studied uptake mechanisms in heart subcellular particles. Subsequently, Titus, with Colin Chignell (55) and later with William Hart, (56) began to purify components of the sodium potassium ATPase. Chignell soon became interested in the development and use of sophisticated analytical methods (57), including circular dichroism measurements (58) and spin-labeled probes for ESR measurements (59), for analyzing protein configurations and protein binding.

Pharmacokinetics of Parent Drugs

Although the general strategy during the 1960s was to attempt to relate either the intensity or the duration of action of a drug to its concentration in the blood, we began to wonder about the effects of reversible binding of drugs to blood components on drug action and drug metabolism. Analysis of the problem revealed that marked differences in the extent of reversible binding of a drug to blood components, especially when the drug is also extensively bound to extravascular components, may result in only trivial differences in its unbound concentration at receptor sites (60), which governs the proportion of receptor sites occupied by the drug. We also found that reversible binding of a drug to blood components may either increase or decrease the half-life of the drug, depending on the hepatic extraction ratio, and devised a nomogram for estimating where the crossover point would occur for given sets of factors (61). In attempts to relate enzyme kinetics to the clearance of drugs by the liver, Sandy Pang (62) developed an approach based on the formation and subsequent metabolism of metabolites in single-pass liver perfusion experiments that would differentiate between the "well stirred" and the "parallel tube" models. Unfortunately, the results indicated that neither model was adequate, and Pang began her life-long quest for understanding the kinetics of drug metabolism in perfused organs.

We used pharmacokinetic studies to determine the extent to which species, sex, and individual differences in drug responses could be explained by differences in metabolism of drugs. In fact, Gertrude Quinn et al (63) had published their classic paper showing that most of the species, strain, and sex differences in the pharmacologic action of barbiturates could be attributed to differences in drug metabolism. Ryuichi Kato in LCP had expanded these studies to other drugs and the effects of various treatments (64, 65). Moreover, Elliot Vesell & John Page (66) in LCP began to demonstrate, using phenylbutazone in human twins, that most of the individual differences in drug metabolism were due to genetic differences.

When attempts to relate plasma levels of drugs to pharmacologic effects failed, we looked for metabolites of the drug that might have pharmacologic activity. Accordingly, James Dingell and I found that the anti-reserpine action of imipramine, discovered by Fridolin Sulser (67), was due to its demethylated metabolite, desipramine, (68) and that species differences in the anti-reserpine action were due to differences in the relative rates of formation and elimination of desipramine (69). In addition, Folke Sjoqvist et al (70) found that desipramine exerted its "anti-tremorine" effect by inhibiting the conversion of tremorine to oxotremorine, its active metabolite, but desipramine actually prolonged the action of oxotremorine by inhibiting its metabolism.

But the strategy failed to explain species differences in the teratogenic effects of thalidomide. We were aware that thalidomide frequently caused teratogenic effects in humans, monkey, and rabbits, but rarely in rats. We were also aware that thalidomide in aqueous solutions is unstable at pH 7 and is converted to many hydrolysis products nonenzymatically (71). It was not surprising, therefore, that Herbert Schumacher & David Blake (72) discovered virtually no species differences in the biological half-life of the drug in rats and rabbits. But we discovered that the drug became covalently bound to proteins in liver.

We were aware of the seminal work in the laboratory of James & Elizabeth Miller (73) at the University of Wisconsin indicating that carcinogenic agents, including polycyclic hydrocarbons, azobenzenes, estradiol, and 2-acetylaminofluene, were converted to chemically reactive agents that became covalently bound to proteins and nucleic acid. Thus our finding that thalidomide could react covalently with protein prompted us to write (72), "The radioactivity bound to the soluble fraction of liver 24 hr after thalidomide administration could not be removed by exhaustive dialysis. It therefore seems possible that after thalidomide enters the fetus it might cause teratogenesis by acylating various components which are essential for normal fetal development." Unfortunately, at that time we were not able to devise an experiment that would provide convincing evidence that covalent binding of the drug to macromolecules actually resulted in teratogenesis.

We were able to demonstrate that other drugs could be converted to metabolites that became covalently bound to macromolecules. But it soon became evident that before we could claim that a substance caused toxicity through the formation of a chemically reactive metabolite, we must determine whether changes in the extent of binding of the reactive metabolite, caused by changes in the metabolism of the parent drug and the reactive metabolite, would result in parallel changes in the incidence or severity of a toxicity.

Since we couldn't think of any easily detected toxicity to explore at the time, my section of the laboratory dropped the project and studied other things.

THE LAST TWENTY-FIVE YEARS

In about 1968, Erminio Costa took a position as chief of a laboratory in the Mental Health Institute, and I became the fifth Deputy Laboratory Chief. Shortly there-after, Brodie had his first heart attack and his health began to deteriorate.

Chemically Reactive Metabolites

Before Brodie went away to recuperate from one of his illnesses, he encouraged Watson Reid, together with Gopal Krishna, Glenn Sipes, and Arthur Cho, to explore the possibility that chemically reactive metabolites could cause toxicities. Their studies of the hepatic toxicity of bromobenzene and other halogenated aromatic compounds led to the publication of the classic paper by Brodie et al (74), showing that the hepatotoxicity of bromobenzene was mediated through a chemically reactive metabolite.

At that time we had a pretty good idea that the reactive metabolites of the halogenated aromatic compounds were epoxides. As early as 1950 Eric Boyland (75) in England had proposed the formation of epoxides of aromatic compounds, which he inferred from the finding of 1,2-dihydronaphthalene-1,2-diol in urine of animals dosed with naphthalene. In 1960 Joan Booth et al (76) in Boyland's laboratory found that 1,2-dihydronaphthalene and 1,2,3,4-tetrahydronaphthalene 1,2-oxide were converted to the same glutathione metabolite when they were incubated with glutathione and either rat liver slices or microsomes. In 1967, Jordan Holtzman et al (77) in LCP found that only one of the oxygen atoms in the 1,2-dihydronaphthalene 1,2-diol formed from naphthalene by mouse liver microsomes originated from atmospheric oxygen. And in 1968 Donald Jerina et al (78) in NIDDK, NIH, were able to trap radiolabeled 1,2-dihydronaphthalene 1,2-oxide formed from radiolabeled naphthalene by rat liver microsomes. But subsequent work by David Jollow et al (79) provided more definitive evidence that bromobenzene 3,4-oxide caused liver necrosis.

Because of deteriorating health, Brodie retired in 1971 and I became acting Chief of the laboratory until 1973, at which time I was confirmed as Chief. The size of the laboratory was reduced to the east wing of the 8th floor of the Clinical Center, and the sections headed by Elwood Titus and Watson Reid were trans-ferred out of the laboratory.

During the 1970s, the laboratory focused most of its efforts on discovering other drugs that might cause toxicities through the formation of chemically reactive metabolites. Indeed, more than 150 papers (cited in reference 80) were published during the following 23 years on toxicities produced by halogenated benzenes, ρ- and o-bromophenols, acetaminophen, ρ-chloroacetanilide, phenacetin, isoniazid, iproniazid, ipomeanol, furosemide, spironolactone, 2-acetylaminofluene, 2-hydroxyestrogens, allyl alcohol, niridazole, nitrofurantoin, nitrobenzene, nitroso compounds, carbon tetrachloride, chloramphenicol, and chloroform and other halogenated anesthetic gases.

Many of these papers were devoted to studying possible reactive metabolites of acetaminophen, which in large doses, causes liver necrosis in humans. These papers, beginning with one by Jerry Mitchell et al (81), showed that acetaminophen caused liver necrosis in animals through the formation of a chemically reactive metabolite. Although it seemed certain that the toxic metabolite was N-acetylimidoquinone, it was not certain how this metabolite was formed. At first it seemed possible that it was formed by way of N-hydroxyacetaminophen, which was known to decompose to the imidoquinone. Indeed, Jack Hinson spent considerable effort in synthesizing and studying the formation of various N-hydroxy aromatic compounds, including N-hydroxyacetyl-ρ-chloroanilide (82) and N-hydroxyphenacetin (83). Gerard Mulder & Hinson (84) demonstrated that N-hydroxyphenacetin was stable for several hours in aqueous solutions, but converting it to its NO-glucuronide or NO-sulfate markedly decreased its stability. In 1979, however, Hinson & Pohl (85) were able to show that N-hydroxyacetaminophen was a metabolite of N-hydroxyphenacetin but not of acetaminophen. Thus the N-acetylimidoquinone was formed directly from acetaminophen and not indirectly through an N-hydroxyacetaminophen. Moreover, it was also shown that phenacetin could be converted to reactive metabolites by several different mechanisms (86), which led me to call it "fascinating phenacetin."

Most of our studies for detecting the formation of chemically reactive metabolites depended on the detection of covalently bound radiolabeled material after the administration of radiolabeled drugs to animals. However, studies with doubly labeled chloramphenicol made us more cautious in our interpretation. These studies revealed that the half-life of the two labels were completely different. In fact, much of the covalently bound C^{14} from the dichloroethylamino group in chloramphenicol appeared in blood plasma and persisted for days. Further studies by Pohl et al (87) revealed that the dichloroethyl amino group was converted to oxamic acid, which entered the two-carbon pool, and served as a precursor of glycine and serine, which were then incorporated into albumin and other proteins. We thus became aware that other pathways of metabolism besides demethylation and deethylation pathways could lead to incorportation of C^{14} into amino acids and thence into proteins.

We became cautious in attempting to determine the mechanism by which a given chemically reactive metabolite caused toxicities. It became obvious that reactive metabolites might cause toxicities through many different mechanisms, not all of which were mediated by the covalent binding of the chemically reactive metabolite to a specific macromolecule. For example, it seemed possible that the chemically reactive metabolite might abstract a hydrogen atom from a lipid and thereby initiate lipid peroxidation, which could lead to toxicities; in this pathway the reactive metabolite would be converted to a stable metabolite, which would not be covalently bound to macromolecules. Moreover, it also seemed likely that a chemically reactive metabolite could react with many different macromolecules, including various proteins, DNA, and RNA. The relative rates would depend on many factors, including the stability of the reactive metabolite in both lipid membranes and water, the location of formation of the metabolite within cells, the amounts of various target macromolecules, the number of target sites on the individual macromolecules, and the rates at which the altered macromolecules are repaired or replaced. To focus attention on the identification of the various altered macromolecules, as many of our friends wished us to do, seemed fruitless as means of identifying the covalently bound material that caused the toxicity. Indeed, even if we had identified several of the altered macromolecules, how were we to determine which one was the crucial altered macromolecule? We also wondered whether the toxicity might not be caused by several different injuries acting in concert. We even came to the conclusion that the magnitude of the amount of covalently bound material would not be particularly useful for predicting toxicities, because many of the altered macromolecules probably would not be essential to the life of the cells.

In an attempt to caution investigators about over-interpreting relationships between covalent bonding and toxicities, I wrote in 1974 (88): "Studies of covalent binding to tissue macromolecules by themselves have little predictive value in determining whether a given compound will evoke a given kind of toxicity. Indeed, without correlative studies, no more emphasis should be placed on the finding that a reactive metabolite becomes covalently bound to tissue macromolecules than would be placed on the finding that a reversibly acting drug is localized in a given tissue in drug disposition studies."

For these reasons, LCP focused on studies to identify reactive metabolites and to elucidate the mechanisms of their formation and inactivation. For example, Sidney Nelson et al (89) found that isoniazid is first acetylated to form N-acetyl isoniazid, which then undergoes hydrolysis to form acetylhydrazine. The acetylhydrazine then is converted to a chemically reactive metabolite that causes necrosis in animals. Similarly, iproniazid (89, 90) undergoes hydrolysis to isopropyl hydrazine, which in turn is converted to a toxic, chemically reactive metabolite. Pohl et al (91) were able to demonstrate that chloroform was converted to phosgene. Although carbon tetrachloride was probably converted to reactive metabolites by several mechanisms, the major pathway (92) appears to be reductive dechlorination to form trichloromethyl radical, which reacts with oxygen to form a peroxy radical, which decomposes to phosgene. Enflurane (93), halothane, and other halogenated alkanes (94) appear to undergo hydroxylation to form hydroxy-halo-intermediates, which decompose to ketones or acyl halides.

Kinetics of Reactive Metabolites

The amount of covalently bound material, measured at different times, can provide an indirect measure of the amount of reactive metabolite entering the organ, whether generated there or carried there by the blood. For convenience, the amount may be expressed as: Amount = Dose ABC (95), where A is the fraction of the dose that is absorbed, B is the fraction of the absorbed material that is converted to the chemically reactive metabolite, and C is the fraction of the chemically reactive metabolite that becomes covalently bound. The purpose of this approach was to emphasize that ratio B could be increased either by increasing the activity of the enzyme that formed the reactive metabolite or by decreasing the activity of enzymes that catalyzed side pathways and that ratio C could be increased by decreasing mechanisms of inactivation of the reactive metabolite.

Several functional categories of reactive metabolites were envisioned based on their various stabilities (96). At one extreme, the reactive metabolite might be so stable that virtually every organ in the body would be exposed to it; indeed, some of it might be excreted into the urine and thereby constitute a potential environmental hazard. At the other extreme, the reactive metabolite might never escape the active site of the enzyme in which it was formed; in this case the precursor would be considered to be a "suicide inhibitor" or a "metabolically activated inhibitor." Intermediate cases would include (a) reactive metabolites that escaped cells in which they were formed and entered other cells in either the same or different organs, where they could cause toxicities, or (b) the formation of stable metabolites that would leave the cells in which they were formed and be carried by the blood to other cells or organs in which the metabolites would be converted to short-lived reactive metabolites. It also seemed possible that a given reactive metabolite might be in one category under some conditions and in another category under other conditions. For example, at low doses of acetaminophen virtually all of the reactive metabolite may react with glutathione and thereby very little if any of it would escape the cells, but at high doses glutathione stores may become depleted and the life of the metabolite may be prolonged sufficiently to permit its escape.

Because the expected effects of inducers and inhibitors on the area under the curve of the reactive metabolite will differ with the category of the reactive metabolite, it seemed useful to devise methods for determining the category of given reactive metabolites. Various kinetic expressions (97) were derived for different in vitro experiments, based on the assumption of a steady-state (pseudo zero order) rate of formation of the reactive metabolite and its inactivation by a combination of a first-order reaction to form a stable metabolite and a bimolecular reaction with a nucleophile, such as a protein or glutathione. The mathematical expressions for such systems may be rearranged to provide straight-line plots of the effects of different concentrations of the nucleophile.

By using variations of this approach, Hinson & Larry Andrews (98) were able to elucidate the mechanisms of decomposition of the N-O-glucuronide and the N-O-sulfate of phenacetin; Henry Sasame et al (99) were able to demonstrate that not all phenolic metabolites of propranolol were formed from presumptive arene oxides; Terrence Monks and Serrine Lau (100, 101) were able to show that bromobenzene oxide escapes hepatocytes both in vitro and in vivo.

Renal Toxicity

Studies by Lau and Monks revealed that the bromobenzene-induced renal toxicity, discovered by Reid (102), followed a complicated series of events. Because pretreatment of animals with 3-methylcholanthrene decreased the severity of the hepatic necrosis caused by bromobenzene (103) and increased the formation of *o*-bromophenol, we had begun to view the formation of *o*-bromophenol as a protective mechanism. But Lau & Monks (104) showed that *o*-bromophenol was a more potent renal toxicant than bromobenzene. In a series of papers, they also showed that bromohydroquinone was more toxic and diglutathionyl bromohydroquinone was still more toxic to the kidney than bromobenzene. They (105) further showed that acivicin, a selective inhibitor of γ-glutathionyl transpeptidase present on the brush border cells of the kidney, prevented the toxicity. Thus it seems likely that diglutathionyl bromohydroquinone is formed predominately in the liver and is carried to the kidney where it enters brush border cells by the γ-glutathionyl transpeptidase mechanism, and is then converted to a toxic metabolite in the renal brush border cells. Since leaving LCP, Lau & Monks have greatly extended their studies to include many other hydroquinone and quinone compounds.

Suicide Enzyme Inhibitors

The major contributions of LCP to the field of "suicide inhibitors" of cytochrome P450 enzymes have been relatively recent. Indeed, our first experience with "suicide inhibitors" arose during the early 1970s when we were attempting to explain the feminizing effects of spironolactone. Although it was subsequently shown that this effect at low doses of the drug is probably due to its interaction with dihydrotestosterone receptors (106), Raymond Menard et al (107–109) found that spironolactone at high doses caused the destruction of 17 α-hydroxylase in testes and adrenals.

During the mid-1980s, Pohl became interested in mechanisms by which cytochrome P450 and other hemoproteins might be inactivated by various drugs. Clearly, reactive metabolites might react with hemoproteins in several different ways. They might react solely with the heme to form various heme derivatives; they might react solely with the protein portion of the enzyme; they might form a bridge between the heme and the protein of the enzyme; or they might react with the heme to form a heme radical that reacted with the protein. Helen Davies et al (110, 111) obtained support for the covalent binding of heme to protein by producing cytochrome P450s labeled with radioactive heme in vivo, and demonstrating that some of the radioactivity was covalently bound after treatment of tissue preparations and intact animals with various drugs. After joining Pohl, Yoichi Osawa became interested in studying the mechanisms by which heme became covalently bound to protein. As a model he studied the reaction of monobromotrichloromethane with reduced myoglobin. In these reactions, he (112) discovered that a dichloromethyl group reacted with the heme, which in turn reacted with histidine 93 of myoglobin. Similar studies (113) revealed that the reaction of monobromotrichloromethane with hemoglobin resulted in the binding of heme to cysteine 93 of the beta chain via the ring I vinyl group.

Deuterium Isotope Effects

During the course of our studies to elucidate mechanisms of cytochrome P450 enzymes, Kiyoshi Nagata et al (114) discovered that rat liver microsomes catalyzed the conversion of testosterone to Δ^6-testosterone. After excluding the possibility that the double bond was formed by dehydration of the hydroxylated metabolites, we proposed that it was formed by a double hydrogen abstraction mechanism. At that time we were unable to devise an experiment that would prove our hypothesis. But Nagata had discovered that purified 7-α hydroxylase (CYPIIA1) could also convert testosterone to Δ^6-testosterone and its epoxide in addition to 7-α hydroxytestosterone. This finding suggested to Kenneth Korzekwa that studies of various deuterated forms of testosterone might provide the information necessary to confirm the double hydrogen extraction mechanism and even to provide clues to which hydrogen was abstracted first. After developing the appropriate mathematical equations and performing the necessary experiments with Nagata's enzyme preparation, he (115) established not only that the double extraction mechanism was valid, but also that the 6-α hydrogen was abstracted before the 7-α hydrogen.

These studies prompted my desire to understand the theory of isotope effects as applied to cytochrome P450 enzymes in the hope that many questions about the mechanisms of these enzymes might be resolved. I especially wondered about the mechanisms by which the cytochrome P450 enzymes were able to form several metabolites from the same substrate. Three general mechanisms seemed plausible. In the first mechanism (which I called the parallel pathway mechanism), the substrate combines with the ferric form of the enzyme in different orientations, and the orientations do not change during the enzymatic cycle; thus each orientation leads to a different metabolite. In the second mechanism (which I called the nondissociative mechanism), the substrate combines with ferric form of the enzyme in different orientations, but the binding site is sufficiently large that the substrate may change orientations during the enzymatic cycle. In the third mechanism (which I called the dissociative mechanism), first postulated by Gerald Miwa & Anthony Lu (116), the substrate combines with the ferric form of the enzyme, but it may also dissociate from the enzyme during the enzymatic cycle, equilibrate with the substrate in the aqueous medium, and recombine with the activated enzyme in either the same or different orientations.

Derivation (117) of the appropriate equations for these mechanisms with nondeuterated and deuterated substrates suggested experiments that would differentiate between them. Using these concepts, John Darbyshire & Katsumi Sugiyama (118) studied the mechanism by which CYP2C11 metabolizes testosterone to

2α-hydroxytestosterone, 16α-hydroxytestosterone, and androstenedione. The results clearly showed that the mechanism could not be the nondissociative mechanism, but whether it was by the parallel pathway mechanism or by the dissociative mechanism was unclear. One experiment supported the parallel pathway mechanism, but two other experiments supported the dissociative mechanism.

We also wondered about the mechanism by which testosterone was converted to 16α-hydroxyandrostenedione. Clearly, it required two enzymatic cycles to achieve its oxidation state. But does the presumptive androstenedione intermediate dissociate from the active site, equilibrate with that in the medium, and then recombine with the enzyme, or does the intermediate never leave the active site of the enzyme before it undergoes the second cycle? Although it is rather easy to evaluate the extreme cases for the formation of secondary metabolites by determining the effects of increasing concentrations of the substrate on the formation of a secondary metabolite, there was no obvious way at the time for evaluating intermediate cases. Using the relevant mathematical expressions for such cases, Sugiyama & Darbyshire studied the conversion of testosterone to 16α-hydroxyandrostenedione by P450 2C11 and found that about 15% of the 16α-hydroxyandrostenedione was formed directly from testosterone (119).

Immunology

As early as 1971 (74) we recognized that immune responses might be caused by chemically reactive metabolites. For many years, however, there seemed to be no obvious way of approaching the problem. In the mid-1980s, however, Hiroko Satoh in LCP developed an antibody that recognized the trifluoroacetyl group derived from halothane and used it to show that proteins containing the group were present on the surface of hepatocytes of animals treated with halothane (120). Pohl later learned that scientists in England (121, 122) had found that patients recovering from halothane toxicity had developed antibodies that reacted with liver proteins from animals receiving the drug. Since it seemed possible that these antibodies might play a role in the development of immune reactions, Gerald Kenna came to LCP with the patients' sera to work with Pohl. Studies by him and other members of Pohl's section revealed that the antibodies recognized several liver neoantigens, most of which contained the trifluoroacetyl group derived from halothane (123). The identification of these proteins was reported in more than thirty papers and summarized in (124).

During the mid-1960s, Michael Beaven (125) became interested in studying factors that affected levels of histamine in various organs, including the stomach (126), and retained that interest after he left LCP to join another laboratory within the National Heart Institute. His group rejoined LCP in the early 1980s, and he took a sabbatical to work in the laboratory of James C. Metcalfe in England. There he learned to measure free intracellular Ca^{++} using quin-2 (127). After returning to LCP, he and his colleagues embarked on a major program of the laboratory to study the cascade of events that occur following the reaction of antigens with antibodies, including IgE, attached to membranes of 2H3 basophil leukemic cells (128). From the 1980s through 1994, his section published more than 70 papers that showed the involvement of the phosphatidylinositol cascade in causing increases in free intracellular Ca^{++}, phosphorylation of proteins (such as myosin) by protein kinase C, and the release of granules containing histamine and other inflammatory mediators (reviewed in 129, 130).

EPILOGUE

Because the major interests of LCP at the time of my retirement in 1994 were in various aspects of immunology, Edward Korn, the Scientific Director of NHLBI, decided to combine LCP with the group of Warren Leonard to form the Laboratory of Molecular Immunology. LCP, as such, thus ceased to exist after my retirement.

The outstanding talents of the scientists in LCP and its support staff, including our secretaries, Helen Balaguer and Bonnie (Farley) Chambers, made the achievements of LCP possible. Space does not permit a listing of all of the honors and awards received by various alumni of LCP, but the following may be noteworthy. Julius Axelrod and Lewis Ignarro are Noble Laureates. Bernard Brodie and Julius Axelrod have been Lasker awardees. The American Society for Pharmacology and Therapeutics has elected John Burns, Steven Mayer, Bert La Du, Sydney Spector, Allan Conney, Palmer Taylor, and Jerry Mitchell as presidents; The Society's award in Drug Metabolism is in the honor of Bernard B. Brodie; Bernard Brodie, Julius Axelrod, and Sidney Udenfriend have won the Sollman Award; Parkhurst Shore, Steven Mayer, James Fouts, Lewis Schanker, Ronald Kuntzman, Colin Chignell, Jerry Mitchell, and Sidney Nelson won the Abel Award; Elliott Vesell, Allan Conney, and Sydney Spector won the ASPET Award for Experimental Therapeutics; Harvey Kupferberg won the Epilepsy Research Award; John Burns won the Weiker Memorial Award; Elliott Vesell won the Gold Award; I won the first Brodie Award. Glenn Sipes has served as president of the Society of Toxicology; Allan Conney, Michael Boyd, and Alan Buckpitt have received the SOT Achievement Award; Allan Conney received the Arnold J. Lehman Award; Erik Dybing and Sidney Nelson received the Frank R. Blood Award. Robert Smith and Ryuichi Kato have served as presidents of the International Society for the Study of Xenobiotics, which has selected Ryuichi Kato and me as honorary members.

Visit the Annual Reviews home page at www.AnnualReviews.org.

LITERATURE CITED

1. Kanigel R. 1986. *Apprentice to Genius: The Making of a Scientific Dynasty.* New York: Macmillan. 271 pp.
2. Brodie BB, Udenfriend S, Baer JE. 1947. The estimation of basic organic compounds in biological materials: I. general principles. *J. Biol. Chem.* 168:299–309
3. Shannon JA, Earle DP, Brodie BB, Taggart JV, Berliner RW. 1944. The pharmacological basis for the rational use of Atabrine in the treatment of malaria. *J. Pharmacol. Exp. Ther.* 81:307–30
4. Brodie BB, Axelrod J. 1948. The estimation of acetanilide and its metabolic products, aniline, N- acetyl p-aminophenol and p-aminophenol (free and total conjugated) in biological fluids and tissues. *J. Pharmacol. Exp. Ther.* 94:22–28
5. Flinn F, Brodie BB. 1948. The effect on the pain threshold of N-acetyl p-aminophenol, a product derived in the body from acetanilide. *J. Pharmacol. Exp. Ther.* 94:76–77
6. Brodie BB, Axelrod J. 1949. The fate of acetophenetidin (Phenacetin) and method for the estimation of acetophenetidin and its metabolites in man in biological material. *J. Pharmacol. Exp. Ther.* 97:58–67
7. Mark LC, Kayden HJ, Steele JM, Cooper JR, Berlin I, et al. 1951. The physiological disposition and cardiac effects of procaine amide. *J. Pharmacol. Exp. Ther.* 102:5–15
8. Kayden HJ, Steele JM, Mark LC, Brodie BB. 1951. The use of procaine amide in cardiac arrhythmias. *Circulation* 4:13–22
9. Brodie BB, Bernstein E, Mark LC. 1952. The role of body fat in limiting the duration of action of thiopental. *J. Pharmacol. Exp. Ther.* 105:421–26
10. Brodie BB, Berger EY, Axelrod J, Dunning MF, Porosowska Y, Steele JM. 1951. Use of N-acetyl 4-aminoantipyrine (NAAP) in measurement of total body water. *Proc. Soc. Exp. Biol. Med.* 77:794–98
11. Axelrod J, Reichenthal J, Brodie BB. 1954. Mechanism of the potentiating action of beta-diethylaminoethyl diphenylpropylacetate. *J. Pharmacol. Exp. Ther.* 112:49–54
12. Cooper JR, Axelrod J, Brodie BB. 1954. Inhibitory effects of beta-diethylaminoethyl diphenylpropylacetate on a variety of drug metabolic pathways in vitro. *J. Pharmacol. Exp. Ther.* 112:55–63
13. Axelrod J. 1955. The enzymatic deamination of amphetamine (benzedrine). *J. Biol. Chem.* 214:753–63
14. Mueller DC, Miller JA. 1953. The metabolism of methylated amioazo dyes. II. Oxidative demethylation of rat liver microsomes. *J. Biol. Chem.* 202:579–87
15. Brodie BB, Axelrod J, Cooper JR, Gaudette L, La Du BN, et al. 1955. Detoxication of drugs and other foreign compounds by liver microsomes. *Science* 121:603–4
16. Fouts JR, Brodie BB. 1955. Inhibition of drug metabolic pathways by the potentiating agent, 2,4- dichloro-6-phenylphenoxyethyl diethylamine. *J. Pharmacol. Exp. Ther.* 115:68–73
17. Fouts JR, Brodie BB. 1956. On the mechanism of drug potentiation by iproniazid (2-isopropyl-l-isonicotinyl hydrazine). *J. Pharmacol. Exp. Ther.* 116:480–85
18. Fouts JR, Brodie BB. 1957. The enzymatic reduction of chloramphenicol, p-nitrobenzoic acid and other aromatic nitro compounds in mammals. *J. Pharmacol. Exp. Ther.* 119:197–207
19. Fouts JR, Kamm JJ, Brodie BB. 1957. Enzymatic reduction of prontosil and other azo dyes. *J. Pharmacol. Exp. Ther.* 120:291–300
20. Gillette JR, Brodie BB, La Du BN. 1957. The oxidation of drugs by liver microsomes: on the role of TPNH and oxygen. *J. Pharmacol. Exp. Ther.* 119:532–40
21. Schanker LS. 1962. Passage of drugs

across body membranes. *Pharmacol. Rev.* 14:501–30

22. Shore PA, Brodie BB, Hogben CAM. 1957. The gastric secretion of drugs: a pH partition hypothesis. *J. Pharmacol. Exp. Ther.* 119:361–69

23. Schanker LS. 1968. Secretion of organic compounds in bile. In *Handbook of Physiology. Section 6: Alimentary Canal: Bile; Digestion; Ruminal Physiology,* ed. CF Code. 5:2433–49. Washington, DC: Am. Physiol. Soc.

24. Mayer S, Maickel RP, Brodie BB. 1959. Kinetics of penetration of drugs and other foreign compounds into cerebrospinal fluid and brain. *J. Pharmacol. Exp. Ther.* 127:205–11

25. Mayer SE, Maickel RP, Brodie BB. 1960. Disappearance of various drugs from the cerebrospinal fluid. *J. Pharmacol. Exp. Ther.* 128:41–43

26. Burns JJ, Yu TF, Ritterband A, Perel JM, Gutman AB, Brodie BB. 1957. A potent new uricosuric agent, the sulfoxide metabolite of the phenylbutazone analogue, G-25671. *J. Pharmacol. Exp. Ther.* 119:418–26

27. Burns JJ, Ashwell G. 1960. L-ascorbic acid. In *The Enzymes,* ed. P Boyers et al, 3:387–406. 2nd ed.

28. La Du BN, Zannoni VG. 1956. The tyrosine oxidation system of liver. III. Further studies on the oxidation of p-hydroxyphenylpyruvic acid. *J. Biol. Chem.* 219:273–81

29. Cotten M, Moran NC. 1957. Effects of increased reflex sympathetic activity on contractile force of the heart. *Am. J. Physiol.* 191:461–63

30. Cotten M, Maling HM. 1957. Relationships among stroke work, contractile force and fiber length during changes in ventricular function. *Am. J. Physiol.* 189:580–86

31. Severinghaus JW, Stupfel M. 1955. Respiratory dead space increase following atropine in man, and atropine, vagal or ganglionic blockade and hypothermia in dogs. *J. Appl. Physiol.* 8:81–87

32. Bradley AF, Stupfel M, Severinghaus JW. 1956. Effect of temperature on PC02 and P02 of blood in vitro. *J. Appl. Physiol.* 9:201–4

33. Duggan DE, Bowman RL, Brodie BB, Udenfriend S. 1957. A spectrophotofluorometric study of compounds of biological interest. *Arch. Biochem. Biophys.* 68:1–14

34. Udenfriend S, Bogdanski DF, Weissbach H. 1955. Fluorescence characteristics of 5-hydroxytryptamine (serotonin). *Science* 122:972

35. Shore PA. 1959. A simple technique involving solvent extraction for the estimation of norepinephrine and epinephrine in tissues. *Pharmacol. Rev.* 11: 276–77

36. Shore PA, Burkhalter A, Cohn VH Jr. 1959. A method for the fluorometric assay of histamine in tissues. *J. Pharmacol. Exp. Ther.* 127:182–86

37. Brodie BB, Tomich EG, Kuntzman R, Shore PA. 1957. On the mechanism of action of reserpine: effect of reserpine on capacity of tissues to bind serotonin. *J. Pharmacol. Exp. Ther.* 119:461–67

38. Conney AH, Gillette JR, Inscoe JK, Trams ER, Posner HS. 1959. Induced synthesis of liver microsomal enzymes which metabolize foreign compounds. *Science* 130:1478–79

39. Conney AH, Burns J. 1959. Stimulatory effect of foreign compounds on ascorbic acid biosynthesis and on drug-metabolizing enzymes. *Nature* 184:363–64

40. Conney AH. 1967. Pharmacological implications of microsomal enzyme induction. *Pharmacol. Rev.* 19:317–66

41. Remmer H. 1958. Die Beschleunigung des Evipanabbaues unter der Wirkung von Barbituraten. *Naturwissenschaften* 45:189

42. Kato R, Chiesara E. 1962. Increase of pentobarbitone metabolism induced in rats pretreated with some centrally acting compounds. *Br. J. Pharmacol.* 18:29–38

43. Booth J, Gillette JR. 1962. The effect of anabolic steroids on drug metabolism by

microsomal enzymes in rat liver. *J. Pharmacol. Exp. Ther.* 137:374–79

44. Brodie BB, Kuntzman R, Hirsch CW, Costa E. 1962. Effects of decarboxylase inhibition on the biosynthesis of brain monoamines. *Life Sci.* 1:81–84

45. Kuntzman R, Costa E, Creveling C, Hirsch CW, Brodie BB. 1962. Inhibition of norepinephrine synthesis in mouse brain by blockade of dopamine beta-oxidase. *Life Sci.* 1:85–92

46. Boullin DJ, Costa E, Brodie BB. 1966. Discharge of tritium-labeled guanethidine by sympathetic nerve stimulation as evidence that guanethidine is a false transmitter. *Life Sci.* 5:803–8

47. Neff NH, Tozer TN, Hammer W, Costa E, Brodie BB. 1968. Application of steady-state kinetics to the uptake and decline of H3-NE in the rat heart. *J. Pharmacol. Exp. Ther.* 160:48–52

48. Horning MG, Williams EA, Maling HM, Brodie BB. 1960. Depot fat as source of increased liver triglycerides after ethanol. *Biochem. Biophys. Res. Commun.* 3:635–40

49. Krishna G, Birnbaumer L. 1970. On the assay of adenyl cyclase. *Anal. Biochem.* 35:393–97

50. Frandsen EK, Krishna G. 1976. A simple ultrasensitive method for the assay of cyclic AMP and cyclic GMP in tissues. *Life Sci.* 18:529–41

51. Chader GJ, Fletcher RT, O'Brien PJ, Krishna G. 1976. Differential phosphorylation by GTP and ATP in isolated rod outer segments of the retina. *Biochemistry* 15:1615–20

52. Ignarro LJ, Titus E. 1968. The presence of antagonistically acting alpha and beta adrenergic receptors in the mouse spleen. *J. Pharmacol. Exp. Ther.* 160:72–80

53. Dengler H, Spiegel HE, Titus EO. 1961. Uptake of tritium-labeled norepinephrine in brain and other tissues of cat in vitro. *Science* 133:1072–73

54. Michaelson IA, Taylor PW Jr, Richardson KC, Titus E. 1968. Uptake and metabolism of dl-norepinephrine by sub-cellular particles of rat heart. *J. Pharmacol. Exp. Ther.* 160:277–91

55. Chignell CF, Titus E. 1969. Identification of components of (Na + plus K +)-adenosine triphosphatase by double isotopic labeling and electrophoresis. *Proc. Natl. Acad. Sci. USA* 64:324–29

56. Hart WM Jr, Titus EO. 1973. Isolation of a protein component of sodium-potassium transport adenosine triphosphatase containing ligand-protected sulfhydryl groups. *J. Biol. Chem.* 248:1365–71

57. Chignell CF. 1972. Application of physicochemical and analytical techniques to the study of drug interactions with biological systems. *Crit. Rev. Toxicol.* 1:413–65

58. Chignell CF. 1970. Circular dichroism as a tool for studying the interaction of drugs with biomolecules. In *Proc. 4th Int. Cong. Pharmacol.* 1:217–26. Basel: Schwabe

59. Chignell CF. 1971. The interaction of a spin-labeled sulfonamide with bovine carbonic anhydrase B. *Life Sci.* 10:699–706

60. Gillette JR. 1968. Problems associated with the extrapolation of data from in vitro experiments to experiments in intact animals. In *Fund. Prin. Drug Eval. Am. Pharm. Assoc.,* May 8–10, 1968, ed. DH Tedeshi, RE Tedeshi, pp. 69–84. New York: Raven

61. Gillette JR, Pang KS. 1977. Theoretic aspects of pharmacokinetic drug interactions. *Clin. Pharmacol. Ther.* 22:623–39

62. Pang KS, Gillette JR. 1978. Kinetics of metabolite formation and elimination in the perfused rat liver preparation: differences between the elimination of preformed acetaminophen and acetaminophen formed from phenacetin. *J. Pharmacol. Exp. Ther.* 207:178–94

63. Quinn GP, Axelrod J, Brodie BB. 1958. Species, strain and sex differences in metabolism of hexobarbitone, amidopyrine, antipyrine, and aniline. *Biochem. Pharmacol.* 1:152–59

64. Kato R, Gillette JR. 1965. Effect of star-

vation on NADPH-dependent enzymes in liver microsomes of male and female rats. *J. Pharmacol. Exp. Ther.* 150:279–84

65. Kato R, Gillette JR. 1965. Sex differences in the effects of abnormal physiological states on the metabolism of drugs by rat liver microsomes. *J. Pharmacol. Exp. Ther.* 150:285–91

66. Vesell ES, Page JG. 1968. Genetic control of drug levels in man: phenylbutazone. *Science* 159:1479–80

67. Sulser F, Watts J. 1961. On the anti-reserpine actions of imipramine (Tofranil). In *Techniques for the Study of Psychotropic Drugs,* ed. G Tonini, pp. 1–3. Modena, Italy: Soc. Tipogr. Modenese

68. Gillette JR, Dingell JV, Sulser F, Kuntzman R, Brodie BB. 1961. Isolation from rat brain of a metabolic product, desmethylimipramine, that mediates the antidepressant activity of imipramine (Tofranil). *Experientia* 17:417–20

69. Dingell JV, Sulser F, Gillette JR. 1964. Species differences in the metabolism of imipramine and desmethylimipramine (DMI). *J. Pharmacol. Exp. Ther.* 143:14–22

70. Sjoqvist F, Hammer W, Schumacher H, Gillette J. 1968. The effect of desmethylimipramine and other "anti-tremorine" drugs on the metabolism of tremorine and oxotremorine in rats and mice. *Biochem. Pharmacol.* 17:915–34

71. Schumacher H, Smith RL, Williams RT. 1965. The metabolism of thalidomide: the spontaneous hydrolysis of thalidomide in solution. *Br. J. Pharmacol.* 25:324–37

72. Schumacher H, Blake DA, Gillette JR. 1968. Disposition of thalidomide in rabbits and rats. *J. Pharmacol. Exp. Ther.* 160:201–11

73. Miller EC, Miller JA. 1952. In vivo combination between carcinogens and tissue constituents and their possible role in carcinogenesis. *Cancer Res.* 12:547–56

74. Brodie BB, Reid WD, Cho AK, Sipes G, Krishna G, Gillette JR. 1971. Possible mechanism of liver necrosis caused by aromatic organic compounds. *Proc. Natl. Acad. Sci. USA* 68:160–64

75. Boyland E. 1950. Biological significance of the metabolism of hydrocarbons. *Sym. Biochem. Soc.* 5:40–54

76. Booth J, Boyland E, Sato T, Sims P. 1960. Metabolism of polycyclic hydrocarbons. 17. The reaction of 1:2-dihydronaphthalene and 1:2-epoxy 1,2,3,4-tetrahydronaphthalene with glutathione catalyzed by tissue preparations. *Biochem. J.* 77:182–86

77. Holtzman JL, Gillette JR, Milne GWA. 1967. The incorporation of 18-O into naphthalene in the enzymatic formation of 1,2-dihydronaphthalene-1,2-diol. *J. Biol. Chem.* 242:4386–87

78. Jerina DM, Daly JW, Witkop B. Zaltzman-Nirenberg P, Udenfriend S. 1968. The role of arene oxide-oxepin systems in the metabolism of aromatic substrates. 3. Formation of 1,2-naphthalene oxide from naphthalene by liver microsomes. *J. Am. Chem. Soc.* 90:6525–27

79. Jollow DJ, Mitchell JR, Zampaglione N, Gillette JR. 1974. Bromobenzene-induced liver necrosis. Protective role of glutathione and evidence for 3,4-bromobenzene oxide as the hepatotoxic metabolite. *Pharmacology* 11:151–69

80. Gillette JR. 1995. Keynote address: man, mice, microsomes, metabolites, and mathematics 40 years after the revolution. *Drug Metab. Rev.* 27:1–44

81. Mitchell JR, Jollow DJ, Potter WZ, Davis DC, Gillette JR, Brodie BB. 1973. Acetaminophen-induced hepatic necrosis. I. Role of drug metabolism. *J. Pharmacol. Exp. Ther.* 187:185–94

82. Hinson JA, Mitchell JR, Jollow DJ. 1975. Microsomal N-hydroxylation of p-chloroacetanilide. *Mol. Pharmacol.* 11:462–69

83. Hinson JA, Mitchell JR. 1976. N-hydroxylation of phenacetin by hamster liver microsomes. *Drug Metab. Dispos.* 4:430–35

84. Mulder GJ, Hinson JA, Gillette JR. 1977. Generation of reactive metabolites of N-hydroxy-phenacetin by glucoronidation and sulfation. *Biochem. Pharmacol.* 26: 189–96

85. Hinson JA, Pohl LR, Gillette JR. 1979. N-hydroxyacetaminophen: a microsomal metabolite of N-hydroxyphenacetin but apparently not of acetaminophen. *Life Sci.* 24:2133–38

86. Gillette JR, Nelson SD, Mulder GJ, Jollow DJ, Mitchell JR, Pohl LR, Hinson JA. 1981. Formation of chemically reactive metabolites of phenacetin and acetaminophen. *Adv. Exp. Med. Biol.* 136 Part B:931–50

87. Pohl LR, Reddy GB, Krishna G. 1979. A new pathway of metabolism of chloramphenicol which influences the interpretation of its irreversible binding to protein in vivo. *Biochem. Pharmacol.* 28:2433–40

88. Gillette JR. 1974. Commentary. A perspective on the role of chemically reactive metabolites of foreign compounds in toxicity. I. Correlation of changes in covalent binding of reactivity metabolites with changes in the incidence and severity of toxicity. *Biochem. Pharmacol.* 23:2785–94

89. Nelson SD, Mitchell JR, Timbrell JA, Snodgrass WR, Corcoran GB. 1976. Isoniazid and iproniazid: activation of metabolites to toxic intermediates in man and rat. *Science* 193:901–3

90. Nelson SD, Mitchell JR, Snodgrass WR, Timbrell JA. 1978. Hepatotoxicity and metabolism of iproniazid and isopropylhydrazine. *J. Pharmacol. Exp. Ther.* 206: 574–85

91. Pohl LR, Bhooshan B, Whittaker NF, Krishna G. 1977. Phosgene: a metabolite of chloroform. *Biochem. Biophys. Res. Commun.* 79:684–91

92. Mico BA, Pohl LR. 1983. Reductive oxygenation of carbon tetrachloride: trichloromethylperoxyl radical as a possible intermediate in the conversion of

carbon tetrachloride to electrophilic chlorine. *Arch. Biochem. Biophys.* 225:596–609

93. Burke TR Jr, Branchflower RV, Lees DE, Pohl LR. 1981. Mechanism of defluorination of enflurane. Identification of an organic metabolite in rat and man. *Drug Metab. Dispos.* 9:19–24

94. Anders MW, Pohl LR. 1985. Halogenated alkanes. In *Bioactivation of Foreign Compounds,* pp. 283–312. New York: Academic

95. Gillette JR. 1974. Formation of reactive metabolites as a cause of drug toxicity. In *Ciba Found. Symp. 26 on The Poisoned Patient. The Role of the Laboratory,* pp. 29–55. Amsterdam: Assoc. Sci.

96. Gillette JR. 1986. Significance of covalent binding of chemically reactive metabolites of foreign compounds to proteins and lipids. *Adv. Exp. Med. Biol.* 197: 63–82

97. Gillette JR. 1980. Kinetics of decomposition of chemically unstable metabolites in the presence of nucleophiles: derivation of equations used in graphical analyses. *Pharmacology* 20:64–86

98. Hinson JA, Andrews LS, Gillette JR. 1979. Kinetic evidence for multiple chemically reactive intermediates in the breakdown of phenacetin N-O-glucuronide. *Pharmacology* 19:237–48

99. Sasame HA, Liberato DJ, Gillette JR. 1987. The formation of glutathione conjugate derived from propranolol. *Drug Metab. Dispos.* 15:349–55

100. Monks TJ, Lau SS, Gillette JR. 1984. Diffusion of reactive metabolites out of hepatocytes: studies with bromobenzene. *J. Pharmacol. Exp. Ther.* 228:393–99

101. Lau SS, Monks TJ, Greene KE, Gillette JR. 1984. Detection and half-life of bromobenzene-3,4-oxide in blood. *Xenobiotica* 14:539–43

102. Reid WD. 1973. Mechanism of renal necrosis induced by bromobenzene or chlorobenzene. *Exp. Mol. Pathol.* 19: 197–214

103. Reid WD, Christie B, Eichelbaum M, Krishna G. 1971. 3-methylcholanthrene blocks hepatic necrosis induced by administration of bromobenzene or carbon tetrachloride. *Exp. Mol. Pathol.* 15:362–72
104. Lau SS, Monks TJ, Greene KE, Gillette JR. 1984. The role of ortho-bromophenol in the nephrotoxicity of bromobenzene in rats. *Toxicol. Appl. Pharmacol.* 72:539–49
105. Monks TJ, Lau SS, Highet RJ, Gillette JR. 1985. Glutathione conjugates of 2-bromohydroquinone are nephrotoxic. *Drug Metab. Dispos.* 13:553–59
106. Cutler GB Jr, Pita JC Jr, Rifka SM, Menard RH, Sauer MA, Loriaux DL. 1978. SC 25152: a potent mineralocorticoid antagonist with reduced affinity for the 5 alpha-dihydrotestosterone receptor of human and rat prostate. *J. Clin. Endocrinol. Metab.* 47:171–75
107. Menard RH, Stripp B, Gillette JR. 1974. Spironolactone and testicular cytochrome P-450: decreased testosterone formation in several species and changes in hepatic drug metabolism. *Endocrinology* 94:1628–36
108. Menard RH, Martin HF, Stripp B, Gillette JR, Bartter FC. 1974. Spironolactone and cytochrome P-450: impairment of steroid hydroxylation in the adrenal cortex. *Life Sci.* 15:1639–48
109. Menard RH, Guenthner TM, Taburet AM, Kon H, Pohl LR, et al. 1979. Specificity of the in vitro destruction of adrenal and hepatic microsomal steroid hydroxylases by thiosteroids. *Mol. Pharmacol.* 16: 997–1010
110. Davies HW, Britt SG, Pohl LR. 1986. Carbon tetrachloride and 2-isopropyl-4-pentanamide-induced inactivation of cytochrome P-450 leads to heme-derived protein adducts. *Arch. Biochem. Biophys.* 244:387–92
111. Davies HW, Britt SG, Pohl LR. 1986. Inactivation of cytochrome P-450 by 2-isopropyl-4-pentanamide and other xeno-

biotics leads to heme-derived protein adducts. *Chem. Biol. Interact.* 58:345–52
112. Osawa Y, Martin BM, Griffin PR, Yates JR, Shabanowitz J, et al. 1990. Metabolism-based covalent bonding of the heme prosthetic group to its apoprotein during the reductive debromination of BrCCl3 by myoglobin. *J. Biol. Chem.* 265: 10340–46
113. Kindt JT, Woods A, Martin BM, Cotter RJ, Osawa Y. 1992. Covalent alteration of the prosthetic heme of human hemoglobin by BrCCl3. Cross-linking of heme to cysteine residue 93. *J. Biol. Chem.* 267:8739–43
114. Nagata K, Liberato DJ, Gillette JR, Sasame HA. 1986. An unusual metabolite of testosterone. 17 beta-hydroxy-4,6-androstadiene-3-one. *Drug Metab. Dispos.* 14:559–65
115. Korzekwa KR, Trager WF, Nagata K, Parkinson A, Gillette JR. 1990. Isotope effect studies on the mechanism of the cytochrome P-450IIA1-catalyzed formation of delta 6-testosterone from testosterone. *Drug Metab. Dispos.* 18:974–79
116. Harada N, Miwa GT, Walsh JR, Lu AYH. 1984. Kinetic isotope effects on cytochrome P-450-catalyzed oxidation reactions. Evidence for the irreversible formation of an active oxygen intermediate of cytochrome P-448. *J. Biol. Chem.* 259:3005–10
117. Gillette JR, Darbyshire JF, Sugiyama K. 1994. Theory for the observed isotope effects on the formation of multiple products by different kinetic mechanisms of cytochrome P450 enzymes. *Biochemistry* 33:2927–37
118. Darbyshire JF, Gillette JR, Nagata K, Sugiyama K. 1994. Deuterium isotope effects on A-ring and D-ring metabolism of testosterone by CYP2C11: evidence for dissociation of activated enzyme-substrate complexes. *Biochemistry* 33: 2938–44
119. Sugiyama K, Nagata K, Gillette JR, Dar-

byshire JF. 1994. Theoretical kinetics of sequential metabolism in vitro. Study of the formation of 16 alpha-hydroxyandrostenedione from testosterone by purified rat P450 2C11. *Drug Metab. Disp.* 22: 584–91

120. Satoh H, Fukuda Y, Anderson DK, Ferrans VJ, Gillette JR, Pohl LR. 1985. Immunological studies on the mechanism of halothane-induced hepatotoxicity: immunohistochemical evidence of trifluoroacetylated hepatocytes. *J. Pharmacol. Exp. Ther.* 233:857–62

121. Vargani D, Nieli-Verganmi G, Alberti A, Neuberger J, Eddlston ALWF, Davis M, Williams R. 1980. Antibodies to the surface of halothane-altered rabbit hepatocytes in patients with severe halothane-hepatitis. *N. Engl. J. Med.* 303:66–71

122. Kenna JG, Neuberger J, Williams R. 1984. An enzyme linked immunosorbent assay for detection of antibodies against halothane-altered hepatocyte antigens. *J. Immunol. Methods* 75:3–14

123. Kenna JG, Satoh H, Christ DD, Pohl LR. 1988. Metabolic basis for a drug hypersensitivity: antibodies in sera from patients with halothane hepatitis recognize liver neoantigens that contain the trifluoroacetyl group derived from halothane. *J. Pharmacol. Exp. Ther.* 245:1103–9

124. Pohl LR, Pumford NR, Martin JL. 1996. Mechanisms, chemical structures and drug metabolism. *Eur. J. Haematol.* 57: 98–104

125. Brodie BB, Beaven MA, Erjavec F, Johnson HL. 1966. Uptake and release of H3-histamine. Mechanisms of release of biogenic amines. *Proc. Int. Wenner-Gren Symp., Stockholm, Feb. 1965,* pp 401–15. Oxford: Pergamon

126. Beaven MA, Horakova Z, Johnson HL, Erjavec F, Brodie BB. 1967. Selective labeling of histamine in rat gastric mucosa. *Fed. Proc.* 26:233–36

127. Rogers J, Hesketh TR, Smith GA, Beaven MA, Metcalfe JC, Johnson P, Garland PB. 1983. Intracellular pH and free calcium changes in single cells using quene 1 and quin 2 probes and fluorescence microscopy. *FEBS Lett.* 161:21–27

128. Beaven MA, Rogers J, Moore JP, Hesketh TR, Smith GA, Metcalfe JC. 1984. The mechanism of the calcium signal and correlation with histamine release in 2H3 cells. *J. Biol. Chem.* 259:7129–36

129. Beaven MA, Baumgartner RA. 1996. Downstream signal initiated in mast cells by Fc epsilon RI and other receptors. *Curr. Opin. Immunol.* 89:766–72

130. Beaven MA. 1996. Calcium signalling: sphingosine kinase versus phospholipase c? *Curr. Biol.* 6:798–801

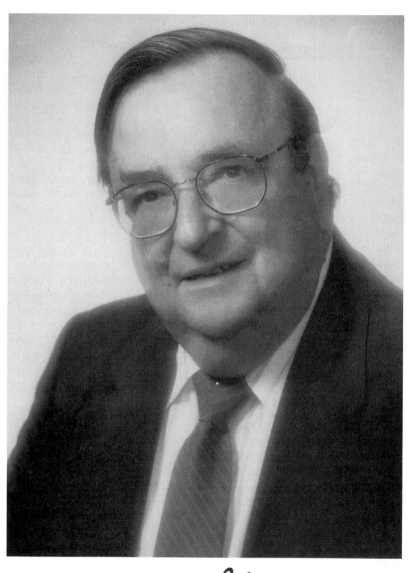

Annu. Rev. Pharmacol. Toxicol. 2000. 40:43–65

CHLORINATED METHANES AND LIVER INJURY: Highlights of the Past 50 Years

Gabriel L. Plaa

Département de Pharmacologie, Faculté de Médecine, Université de Montréal, CP 6128, Succursale Centre-ville, Montréal, Québec, Canada H3C 3J7; e-mail: plaag@magellan.umontreal.ca

Key Words   carbon tetrachloride, chloroform, ketones, lipid peroxidation, regeneration

■ **Abstract**   The chlorinated methanes, particularly carbon tetrachloride and chloroform, are classic models of liver injury and have developed into important experimental hepatotoxicants over the past 50 years. Hepatocellular steatosis and necrosis are features of the acute lesion. Mitochondria and the endoplasmic reticulum as target sites are discussed. The sympathetic nervous system, hepatic hemodynamic alterations, and role of free radicals and biotransformation are considered. With carbon tetrachloride, lipid peroxidation and covalent binding to hepatic constituents have been dominant themes over the years. Potentiation of chlorinated methane-induced liver injury by alcohols, aliphatic ketones, ketogenic compounds, and the pesticide chlordecone is discussed. A search for explanations for the potentiation phenomenon has led to the discovery of the role of tissue repair in the overall outcome of liver injury. Some final thoughts about future research are also presented.

INTRODUCTION

My interest in the chlorinated methane hepatotoxicants began during my graduate training at the University of California, San Francisco campus. My master's work dealt with a chemical analytical problem in forensic toxicology. In 1956, immediately after my master's work, however, my mentor, the late Dr. Charles H. Hine, provided me with a graduate student stipend and a very modest research fund to study the halogenated hydrocarbons. So, my PhD dissertation dealt with certain aspects of this subject. Later, during my own academic career, my research programs always involved these agents (1).

According to Drill (2), the hepatotoxic properties of chloroform and carbon tetrachloride were recognized about 100 years ago. These chlorinated methanes are classic models of liver injury and have developed into important experimental hepatotoxicants. Other hepatotoxicants are often compared with these agents.

This describes how knowledge about chlorinated methane-induced liver injury evolved over the past five decades. An exhaustive discussion of the subject is not

0362–1642/00/0415–0043$14.00

presented. Only selected aspects were chosen to highlight some important concepts. Complete coverage of the subject, particularly carbon tetrachloride, prior to 1973 can be found elsewhere (3–6).

EARLY CONCEPTS OF LIVER INJURY

Most of the research interest in chemical-induced liver injury in the early part of the twentieth century focused on the morphological development of the different lesions, based on histological evaluation by light microscopy. The descriptions still serve as the basis of our current understanding of the morphological aspects of liver lesions. The dominant research theme during this period was how dietary conditions or individual dietary components (diets high or low in fats, carbohydrates, or proteins; the presence of choline, methionine, or cystine) could modify the hepatotoxic response (2). By midcentury, scientists turned to explaining various morphological events in terms of altered physiological or biochemical function (7). In the past 50 years, research has largely dealt with mechanisms of action, not only in terms of the target organ itself but in terms of the aggressor toxicant as well.

In 1954, Himsworth (8) published a monograph on liver injury that serves as a wonderful reservoir of the knowledge available at the time. He identified two factors—vascular and nutritional—as playing influential roles in the development of liver injury in its various forms. The so-called vascular factors, believed to reflect circulatory abnormalities, were thought to be responsible for the acute zonal necrotic lesions (centrilobular, periportal, and midzonal) observed in animals following exposure to different hepatotoxicants and a cause of the massive hepatic necrosis seen with other agents. The idea of nutritional factors arose mainly from studies where deficiencies in diets were investigated; the hepatic lesions included were largely chronic, rather than acute, in form. Finally, Himsworth put forth the concept that hepatic necrosis of parenchymal cells could be produced in one of two ways—"by the presence of noxious agents or by the absence of some factor essential to cellular life."

MITOCHONDRIA AND THE ENDOPLASMIC RETICULUM AS SITES

With the advances made in biochemistry, particularly the isolation and functional characterization of subcellular organelles, researchers began to search for biochemical explanations for the development of liver lesions. The principal model studied was the zonal hepatocellular lesion produced after acute exposure to carbon tetrachloride; the primary pathological events of interest were the accumulation of lipids within the hepatocyte (steatosis) and the appearance of hepatocellular death (necrosis), two independent events (9). A relatively complete histological, histochemical, and biochemical study by Wahi et al (10) in rats showed that the earliest histological evidence of derangement (necrosis and inflammatory cell infiltration) occurred 6 h after administration of carbon tetrachloride.

In 1956, Christie & Judah (11) proposed that the mechanism of action of carbon tetrachloride was one of altered mitochondrial permeability, leading to loss of essential cofactors and disruption of cellular metabolism. Mitochondrial respiration was depressed 10 h after intoxication of rats with lethal doses; after 15 h, the oxidation of octanoate, pyruvate, citrate, hydroxybutyrate, and malate was markedly reduced. Histologically, however, necrosis began at 5 h, and by 18 h massive necrosis was observed; all animals died within 36 h. This hypothesis received support from Heim et al (12), who found a decrease in coenzyme A content in guinea pig livers treated with lethal doses of carbon tetrachloride. The alterations observed in these studies, however, might well have been a result of the presence of necrotic tissue rather than the cause of the necrosis.

In theory, a biochemical lesion responsible for initiation of such severe lesions should be reflected as a functional change before extensive damage becomes evident histologically. Other investigators, who were interested in mechanisms responsible for steatosis, also looked at mitochondrial function but discounted the effects as causal events. Calvert & Brody (13) were unable to show consistent mitochondrial biochemical changes sooner than 20 h after in vivo haloalkane intoxication; no temporal correlation between the histological findings present at 5 h and the biochemical events was obtained. Recknagel & Anthony (14) observed a lag of 14–20 h between intoxication of the animal and the appearance of mitochondrial changes, whereas increased hepatic lipids were already prominent by 3 h. Both groups showed that the mitochondrial changes could be divorced from the changes in hepatic lipids. Later, the membranes of the endoplasmic reticulum were identified as the site of origin of the triglycerides (5), and triglyceride secretion into plasma was markedly reduced by 2 h (15). Recknagel & Lombardi (16) observed that changes in endoplasmic reticular function (reduced glucose-6-phosphatase activity, increased cytochrome c reductase activity) were evident by 2 h after carbon tetrachloride administration, well before the changes seen in mitochondria. Other investigators (5, 6, 9) showed that depressed protein synthesis in the endoplasmic reticulum occurred in rats within 3 h after carbon tetrachloride exposure, accompanied by dispersion of polyribosomes. Also, a rapid decline in liver microsomal cytochrome P450 content was observed. Moore et al (17) showed that the activity of the microsomal calcium pump was markedly reduced 0.5 h after carbon tetrachloride administration in rats. Calcium homeostasis, which involves mitochondrial, endoplasmic reticular, and cytosolic calcium pools, is markedly perturbed after carbon tetrachloride, chloroform, bromotrichloromethane, and 1,1-dichloroethylene intoxication (18–20). Thus, the endoplasmic reticulum appeared as a more likely site of action.

THE SYMPATHETIC NERVOUS SYSTEM AND LIVER INJURY

Altered sinusoidal circulation following carbon tetrachloride intoxication in rats was proposed by several investigators (7). In 1960, Calvert & Brody (21) proposed that carbon tetrachloride exerted its necrotic effect, not by acting on the liver parenchyma directly, but by causing a persistent sympathetic discharge resulting in diminished hepatic blood flow and cellular hypoxia. In contrast to Himsworth (8), who envisioned an action of the hepatotoxicant on hepatic cells and a tissue response leading to mechanical modification of sinusoidal blood flow, the concept of Calvert & Brody centered on the central nervous system as the site of action of carbon tetrachloride. The new provocative hypothesis was based on indirect evidence (no measurements of hepatic blood flow or of tissue hypoxia were performed) using adrenergic- and ganglionic-blocking agents as well as spinal cord transection (21–24) to modify or block the usual hepatotoxic responses to carbon tetrachloride (centrilobular necrosis, lipid accumulation). By far, the best protection was afforded by cervical cordotomy at the level of C-6 or C-7.

Because cervical cordotomy could theoretically affect a number of physiological systems, a series of studies was undertaken in my laboratory to unravel the remarkable protection afforded by this procedure. The possibility of decreased absorption of carbon tetrachloride was eliminated (25). We observed, however, that the rats undergoing cordotomy became poikilothermic. By 10 h after surgical interruption, the rectal temperature of animals transected at C-7 approached that of the room. The severity of the hypothermic response was dependent on the level of the cord transection in a pattern that paralleled the degree of protection afforded by cordotomy. Also, it was shown that if cord-transected (C-6 or C-7) rats were placed in an incubator to maintain normal body temperature, carbon tetrachloride exerted its necrotic effect (26, 27). Furthermore, with animals maintained under hypothermic conditions, one could produce carbon tetrachloride-induced liver necrosis, if the agent was administered three times, every 12 h, and the rats killed 24 h after the last treatment. Finally, hypothermia induced by immersion of normal rats in cold water also resulted in a protective effect comparable to that of cordotomy (27). We showed that the oxygen consumption of cord-sectioned rats maintained at room temperature decreased to 50% of that of normal rats by 1 h and to 30% of that of normal rats by 5 h. Our explanation for the protective effect of cervical cordotomy was that in hypothermia, the metabolic activity of the liver was diminished, and this would reduce the bioactivation of carbon tetrachloride into its hepatotoxic intermediates. We further showed that large infusions of norepinephrine, epinephrine, or mixtures of these catecholamines did not result in lesions similar to those produced by carbon tetrachloride (27). We also found that rats subjected to immunological sympathectomy after birth (injection of antisympathetic nerve growth factor) and later adrenal demedullated were not protected against carbon tetrachloride (28). Thus, these experiments showed that from all points of view, a vascular role attributed to carbon tetrachloride via release of catecholamines should be rejected as a primary cause of injury.

Regarding steatosis, the Calvert & Brody hypothesis (21) proposed that a persistent sympathetic discharge due to an action of carbon tetrachloride on the central nervous system resulted in an oversupply of fatty acids from adipose tissue to the liver. The events by which carbon tetrachloride causes steatosis are reasonably well understood in terms of pathogenesis and biochemical sequences (5, 29, 30). Generally, the evidence points to a failure of the hepatic triglyceride secretory mechanism as the causal event of major importance in the case of carbon tetrachloride, not enhanced supply of fatty acids from peripheral stores (5). There is agreement that fatty acids must be available from adipose tissue for the liver to synthesize triglycerides, and that interruption of the pituitary-adrenal axis diminishes plasma free fatty acids. This leads to a block in the accumulation of triglycerides. The peripheral stores, however, play a permissive role in this situation, rather than one of initiation.

Although the original sympathetic nervous system explanation for the hepatotoxic action of carbon tetrachloride is no longer tenable, there are acute hepatic hemodynamic consequences following exposure to carbon tetrachloride that justify consideration. Using the isolated perfused rat liver, we demonstrated (31–33) that the circulatory action of carbon tetrachloride was actually biphasic. In these experiments the animals received the haloalkane in vivo; the livers were removed and perfused in vitro at various times after its administration. During the initial phase (1–6 h after treatment), there was a moderate increase in hepatic resistance (evident by perfusate flow/portal pressure curves) that returned to normal by 6 h; this was followed by a more prolonged increase in resistance that persisted for several days (96 h after treatment). The biphasic cycle observed was quite reproducible. To determine the causal relationships involved in the phenomenon, a variety of protective measures were investigated (promethazine, dimethoxy-propyltrimethylammonium chloride, ethylenediaminetetraacetic acid, hypophysectomy, cordotomy, hypothermia), as well as comparisons to the hepatic effects of ethionine (steatosis present but no necrosis) and thioacetamide (necrosis present but no steatosis). These experiments allowed us to conclude that the initial phase (first 6 h) of increased hepatic resistance was due to the accumulation of triglycerides, whereas the later phase (after 6 h) was associated with the appearance of hepatic necrosis.

Although the primary hepatotoxic action of carbon tetrachloride does not involve the catecholamines, adrenoreceptor agonists can affect the progression of the lesion. In mice, epinephrine or norepinephrine administered subcutaneously was shown to potentiate the hepatotoxic properties of a small dose of the chlorinated methane in a dose-related fashion (34). Electrical stimulation of the ventromedial hypothalamus in rats was reported (35) to enhance markedly carbon tetrachloride- or dimethylnitrosamine-induced liver injury, and this effect was attenuated by surgical sympathetic denervation of the liver. The authors suggested that the hypothalamus seemed to be involved in the progression of the lesion, but attributed the sympathetic effect to one on hepatic metabolism rather than on blood flow. More recently, Roberts and collaborators (36–40) observed that phenylpropylamine and methamphetamine can potentiate carbon tetrachloride- and acetaminophen-induced hepatotoxicity in rodents, but that the temporal aspects of each type of potentiation differ, which suggests that the pathways involved are also different. With carbon tetrachloride, both central and peripheral (hepatic microcirculation) adrenoreceptor components are put forth as possibilities, whereas with acetaminophen the evidence suggests an adrenoreceptor-related effect on liver glutathione (40).

FREE-RADICALS, BIOTRANSFORMATION, AND LIVER INJURY

It is commonly held that in most instances, chemical-induced hepatotoxicity is the result of biochemical disruptions caused by reactive metabolites arising from biotransformation (41–43). The putative chemical species in most cases, however, has not necessarily been identified, but the cascade of events leading to hepatic dysfunction is usually reasonably well described based on in vitro and in vivo studies. Examples where bioactivation becomes the initiating event include such necrogenic hepatotoxicants as carbon tetrachloride, bromotrichloromethane, chloroform, halothane, bromobenzene, acetaminophen, furosemide, isoniazid, thioacetamide, dimethylnitrosamine, allyl formate, and aflatoxin. The bioactivation characteristics of aliphatic organohalogens (including the chlorinated methanes), their detection, and relevance were reviewed by Sipes & Gandolfi (44).

In a seminal article published in 1961, Butler (45) showed that carbon tetrachloride administered to dogs was reduced to chloroform; he postulated the homolytic fission of the carbon-chlorine bond as a possible mechanism, leading to the formation of a free radical as the ultimate toxic moiety. Both Slater (46) and Recknagel (5) proposed, independently, that the putative carbon tetrachloride-derived free radical could attack membranes, leading to peroxidation and resulting in necrosis or steatosis. The trichloromethyl free radical ($\cdot CCl_3$) was eventually identified by spin trapping in rat liver microsomes incubated with carbon tetrachloride and in livers from animals treated with the haloalkane (47). The free radical reacts very rapidly with oxygen to yield a highly reactive trichloromethylperoxy free radical ($\cdot CCl_3O_2$), which is said to be the initiator of lipid peroxidation (47). Furthermore, a carbon dioxide anion radical has been described and its adduct identified in the urine of rats treated with the haloalkane, but its role in the hepatotoxic process, if any, is still not established (48, 49). The biotransformation of carbon tetrachloride occurs in the endoplasmic reticulum and is mediated by cytochrome P450; the principal isoform implicated as the catalyst is CYP2E1, but evidence for CYP2B1/2 exists as well (50–53).

LIPID PEROXIDATION, COVALENT BINDING, AND LIVER INJURY

The carbon tetrachloride-derived free radical(s) can bind irreversibly to hepatic proteins and lipids and can initiate a process of autocatalytic lipid peroxidation by attacking the methylene bridges of unsaturated fatty acid side chains of microsomal lipids. Recknagel & Ghoshal (54) demonstrated that conjugated dienes, typical of peroxidized polyenoic fatty acids, appeared in hepatic microsomal lipids 1.5 h after rats were exposed to nonlethal doses of carbon tetrachloride. The peroxidative process is thought to result in early morphologic alteration of the endoplasmic reticulum, loss of cytochrome P450 activity, loss of glucose-6-phosphatase activity, depressed protein synthesis, loss of the capacity of the liver to form and excrete very-low-density lipoproteins, and eventually cell death (6, 47, 55). Bromotrichloromethane, the bond dissociation energy of which is lower than that of carbon tetrachloride and more reactive to homolytic cleavage (6, 47, 56), is more potent than carbon tetrachloride in terms of hepatotoxicity and lipid peroxidative properties (6, 18, 20, 56). Chloroform, the bond dissociation energy of which is higher than that of bromotrichloromethane or carbon tetrachloride, is also bioactivated by cytochrome P450 but not to a free radical (47); the highly reactive electrophilic metabolite phosgene was demonstrated in phenobarbital-pretreated rats subsequently given chloroform (57, 58).

Lipid peroxidation is not the only process associated with the formation of free radicals after carbon tetrachloride intoxication. The reactive products also bind covalently to hepatic macromolecules; binding to lipids, proteins, and nucleic acids has been demonstrated (59). Binding to cytochrome P450, which leads to its destruction, occurs rapidly in vivo and in some instances can be shown to be independent of lipid peroxidation (60–63). Castro (59) has been a proponent of covalent binding of carbon tetrachloride–derived products as an important element of the hepatotoxic mechanism of this agent. In 1973, Recknagel & Glende (6), as strong supporters of the lipid peroxidation hypothesis, were critical of those advocating a "toxic metabolite"–based theory. However, 10 years later, after recognizing the difficulties brought on by some of the artificial conditions used in vitro for following lipid peroxidation, Recknagel et al (18) also put lipid peroxidation into perspective; they pointed out that the covalent binding of carbon tetrachloride–derived products could provoke secondary mechanisms that finally resulted in important pathological consequences.

Lipid peroxidation, however, need not always appear after exposure to hepatotoxicants, even if reactive metabolites are formed (64, 65). 1,1-Dichloroethylene, trichloroethylene, ethylene dibromide, dimethylnitrosamine, and thioacetamide serve as examples. Klaassen & Plaa (66) found no evidence of the presence of conjugated dienes (a sensitive in vivo indicator of lipid peroxidation) after administration of chloroform in rats with dosages that resulted in steatosis and necrosis; depression of hepatic glucose-6-phosphatase activity (associated with peroxidation in the endoplasmic reticulum) was also absent. Brown et al (67) found that rats pretreated with phenobarbital, but not untreated animals, produce conjugated dienes during chloroform exposure; depression of glucose-6-phosphatase activity was also reported to occur after chloroform only in phenobarbital-pretreated rats (68). Because chloroform-induced liver injury is more severe in phenobarbital-pretreated rats, the possibility exists that the initial lesion induced by chloroform in these animals is merely aggravated by the additional appearance of lipid peroxidation. It is interesting to note that Wang et al (69) recently compared the time courses of carbon tetrachloride and chloroform hepatotoxic responses and found that cellular degeneration and necrosis appear sooner following carbon tetrachloride intoxication in rats. Previously, we had established dose-response curves for hepatotoxicity with several haloalkanes (70–72) and demonstrated in mice and dogs that the potency of carbon tetrachloride as an hepatotoxicant was much greater than chloroform. Perhaps the presence of lipid peroxidation with carbon tetrachloride accounts for the differences in potency between these two chlorinated methanes. These findings and others cast doubt on the general applicability of lipid peroxidation as a mechanism of action for hepatotoxicants (73, 74).

Normal cellular metabolism itself can lead to reactive oxygen species (superoxide, hydrogen peroxide, singlet oxygen, and hydroxyl radical), and all cells contain defense systems to prevent or limit damage; glutathione is the major element, but α-tocopherol and ascorbic acid play important roles (75). An imbalance between prooxidants and antioxidants is known as oxidative stress; redox cycling can cause oxidative stress in cells. Calcium-induced permeability transition of the mitochondrial inner membrane may initiate cell death in oxidative stress; morphological and functional changes in mitochondria are features of oxidative stress-induced cell injury (76–78). It is now established that nonparenchymal cells can be involved in oxidative stress leading to hepatotoxicity (79). Reactive oxygen intermediates are generated by macrophages, as well as by endothelial cells and stellate cells (Ito cells), but under physiological conditions, cellular antioxidants normally present prevent the intermediates from producing cytotoxicity. Enhanced formation of oxygen intermediates has been demonstrated with carbon tetrachloride, galactosamine, and 1,2-dichlorobenzene. With the latter agent, recent evidence indicates that Kupffer cell–derived oxygen species are largely responsible for lipid peroxidation (80) Also, Kupffer cell activation and inflammatory cells have been implicated in the potentiation of carbon tetrachloride liver injury by retinol (81, 82).

POTENTIATION OF LIVER INJURY

The potentiation of liver injury caused by one agent because of the simultaneous or sequential exposure to another chemical is not a recent discovery. Anecdotal clinical evidence and experimental laboratory evidence of interactions between ethanol and carbon tetrachloride or chloroform appeared in the literature before

1930 (see 2, 3), but experiments designed to explain this interesting phenomenon did not appear until much later. With the development of the pentobarbital sleeping time assay for quantifying liver injury (70), an experimental tool was available to assess this phenomenon in rodents. In 1962 Kutob & Plaa (83) demonstrated that administration of a nonlethal dose of ethanol to mice prior to their subsequent exposure to a small dose of chloroform resulted in potentiation of the haloalkane-induced liver injury. Later these findings were extended to carbon tetrachloride in experiments where elevations in plasma aminotransferase activity to quantify liver injury were employed (71, 72, 84). As an explanation for the potentiation of chloroform toxicity, we proposed that the elevation in hepatic triglycerides resulting from the ethanol pretreatment might cause enhanced hepatic retention of chloroform, thus increasing the hepatic internal "dose" of toxicant. Some evidence supporting the hypothesis was presented (83), but the issue was never investigated in depth and remains unresolved.

Aliphatic alcohols other than ethanol can enhance the hepatotoxic properties of carbon tetrachloride (85). We studied the potentiating characteristics of isopropanol (86–90) and showed that the potency of isopropanol exceeds that of ethanol; the severity of the hepatotoxic response is also more extensive with isopropanol potentiation. Isopropanol is rapidly biotransformed to acetone; comprehensive dose-effect and time-effect studies (87, 91), as well as various scenarios of altered metabolism, demonstrated that acetone, the major metabolite of isopropanol, is responsible for the potentiating properties of isopropanol. Finally, it was postulated that the isopropanol-carbon tetrachloride interaction observed in rodents might present itself in humans during occupational exposures (90). Later two industrial accidents did occur, one in the United States (92) and the other in Taiwan (93); they mimicked the potentiation phenomenon we first observed in rodents.

Other aliphatic ketones have been shown to potentiate the hepatotoxic properties of carbon tetrachloride and chloroform. These include the following: 2-butanone (methyl ethyl ketone), 2-pentanone (methyl propyl ketone), 2-hexanone [methyl n-butyl ketone (MnBK)], 2,5-hexanedione (metabolite of MnBK), 4-methyl-2-pentanone [methyl isobutyl ketone (MiBK)], 1-hydroxy-4-methyl-2-pentanone (metabolite of MiBK), and 2-heptanone (methyl amyl ketone) (94–99). Also, certain chemicals are biotransformed to ketones ("ketogenic" chemicals), like n-hexane, 2-butanol, or 4-methyl-3-pentanol, and are effective potentiators (100–103). The metabolic ketosis produced by 1,3-butanediol (biotransformed to β-hydroxybutyrate) is responsible for the potentiating properties of this agent, as an excellent correlation exists between the plasma concentrations of β-hydroxybutyrate and the severity of the potentiation (101). Furthermore, the potentiating properties of this ketone body probably accounts for the potentiation of carbon tetrachloride liver injury observed in acute alloxan- or streptozotocin-induced diabetic rats (104–107), as well as the differences in chloroform toxicity observed in fed and fasting rats (108).

Carbon tetrachloride and chloroform are not the only chlorinated hydrocarbon solvents whose hepatotoxic properties are enhanced by ketones. The others consist of 1,1,2-trichloroethane, 1,1-dichlorethylene, bromoform, bromodichloromethane, and dibromochloromethane, but not 1,1,1-trichloroethane, 1,1,2,2,-tetrachloroethane, trichloroethylene, or tetrachloroethylene (103, 109–111). There is a strong suggestion that weak hepatotoxic chlorinated alkanes are not converted into potent hepatotoxicants by a previous exposure to ketones. With the brominated methane derivatives, however, this conclusion does not appear to be applicable because potent hepatotoxic combinations are produced by ketone potentiation (103, 109, 111).

Pessayre et al (112) showed that trichloroethylene can aggravate the hepatotoxic response to carbon tetrachloride in rats and that mixtures of these two agents are more potent hepatotoxicants than either given singly; the interaction was confirmed by others (113–115). Acetone potentiates the hepatotoxicity of trichloroethylene-carbon tetrachloride mixtures and has variable effects on the hepatotoxic effects of other chlorinated hydrocarbon mixtures composed of chloroform, carbon tetrachloride, 1,1,1-trichloroethane, 1,1,2-trichloroethane, tetrachloroethylene, 1,1,2,2-tetrachloroethane, or 1,1-dichloroethylene (113, 116). Furthermore, multiple exposures of acetone to rats receiving concurrently repetitive administrations of carbon tetrachloride were shown to enhance the appearance of liver fibrosis (117). Thus, the potentiation of halogenated hydrocarbon hepatotoxicants by ketones and ketogenic substances is extensive and covers both acute and chronic aspects of the injury.

Chlordecone (Kepone), a cyclic organochlorine pesticide containing a carbonyl group, is a remarkable potentiator of chlorinated methane liver injury, in contrast to its nonketonic analog mirex. We were the first to describe the potentiating properties of chlordecone on chloroform hepatotoxicity in mice (118) and continued to study the chlordecone-chloroform combination later in rats. Shortly thereafter, Mehendale and his colleagues published their first chlordecone-potentiation experiments with carbon tetrachloride in rats (119); later they demonstrated that bromotrichloromethane hepatotoxicity was also potentiated (120). Mehendale's group has published extensively on the carbon tetrachloride potentiation model and has made some important observations, including the role of tissue repair on the overall outcome of the potentiation (121). The acute effects of chlordecone on chloroform toxicity persist because the agent is poorly metabolized and is very lipophilic (122, 123); a threshold chlordecone liver concentration appears to exist. The potentiation of chloroform can still be elicited 20 days after exposure to a single dose of chlordecone, coinciding with the presence of enhanced covalent binding of chloroform-derived reactive metabolites and persistent chlordecone liver residues (122).

Regarding mechanisms involved in the potentiations observed with ethanol, isopropanol, 1,3-butanediol, various aliphatic ketones, and chlordecone, increased production of haloalkane-derived reactive metabolites (via cytochrome P450) is certainly of major importance (51, 100, 122, 124–132). The induction of CYP2E1 by ethanol and acetone is well established. Methyl n-alkyl ketones were shown to induce CYP2E1 and CYP2B1/2 (133) and chlordecone was shown to induce CYP2B1/2 (134–136). Experiments where the irreversible (covalent) binding of chloroform-derived or carbon tetrachloride–derived radioactivity to liver constituents (usually microsomal proteins or lipids) was followed in vivo or in vitro have consistently shown increased binding in treatment regimens with the various potentiators. One exception is a study reported by Davis & Mehendale (137) with chlordecone, where enhanced covalent binding of carbon tetrachloride–derived radiolabel was not observed; in this experiment, however, the dosage of chlordecone employed (5 mg/kg) was below the threshold dose of chlordecone (10 mg/kg) determined by Plaa et al (123). Later, Britton et al (131) used 15 mg of chlordecone/kg and demonstrated a 67% increase in cytochrome P450 content and an increase in the covalent binding of carbon tetrachloride–derived radioactivity to microsomal protein and lipids in vivo. In another study from Mehendale's group (138), the authors report that increased covalent binding after chlordecone was not found, but on this occasion the authors apparently measured radiolabel bound to total liver proteins. All things considered, enhanced bioactivation of the haloalkane hepatotoxicant (likely due to induction of cytochrome P450) appears to be the major mechanism of action.

Nevertheless, there are indications that other mechanisms may also be involved in these potentiations. With isopropanol potentiation, mitochondrial and lysosomal damage following carbon tetrachloride appears more severe than that produced by a larger dose of carbon tetrachloride given alone (139). The lesion observed in animals treated with chlordecone and carbon tetrachloride or chloroform differs from that seen with carbon tetrachloride or chloroform given alone (118, 119). More severe hepatobiliary dysfunction (possibly due to altered membranes) was reported with the combination of chlordecone-carbon tetrachloride (119, 140). Lysosomal fragility to osmotic stress in vitro was enhanced when the hepatic organelles were obtained from rats treated in vivo with the combination of chlordecone-chloroform or acetone-chloroform (130). In the same study, morphological evaluation suggested mitochondria respond differently to chloroform in chlordecone- or 2-hexanone–pretreated animals compared with vehicle-pretreated rats; the mitochondria appeared to have reached a terminal stage of damage earlier than the cell in general. Finally, Mehendale and his colleagues (121, 141–143) postulate that in chlordecone-potentiated carbon tetrachloride hepatotoxicity, early tissue repair processes are markedly disrupted; the greater severity of the lesion observed and its consequences appear due to the absence of this protective mechanism. Thus it is clear that a complete explanation for the potentiation phenomenon remains unresolved.

TISSUE REPAIR AND RECOVERY

Although various aspects of chemical-induced liver injury have been studied for over 50 years, interest generally has focused on the early initiating events leading to hepatocellular dysfunction, rather than on the later recovery phase of the lesion.

Searching for the "biochemical lesion" has dominated research in this area. However, repair is an important component of the lesion. Hepatocellular regeneration begins within 6 h after administration of a small dose of carbon tetrachloride in rats; yet the centrilobular necrosis is just becoming evident (144, 145). With the combination of carbon tetrachloride and several potentiating agents (n-hexane, 2-hexanone, 2,5-hexanedione, isopropanol, and acetone), recovery time was assessed using biochemical indices (activities of serum enzymes) and morphological patterns (quantitative histology) of liver injury; appropriate dose-response curves were established from the percentage of animals affected (146). Recovery time was shown to be related to the maximal severity of the lesion, regardless of the potentiating combination. Although pretreatment with the potentiator resulted in an enhanced hepatotoxic response from a small dose of carbon tetrachloride, the dose-response curve for the enhanced response was no different than that produced by a larger, but equitoxic, dose of the haloalkane given alone. These data were interpreted as indicating that the five potentiators did not alter the temporal progression of carbon tetrachloride-induced liver injury.

Mehendale and his collaborators have performed an extensive series of experiments to assess the role of tissue repair in potentiated liver injury (142, 147–150). The studies originated from the observation that chlordecone-potentiated carbon tetrachloride hepatotoxicity in rats was quantitatively quite remarkable and resulted in greatly enhanced lethality when compared with the results obtained in animals not pretreated with the pesticide. Normally, two tissue repair processes are observed after exposure to a small dose of the haloalkane (121, 142); the early phase regeneration (EPR) response (arrested G_2 hepatocytes activated to proceed through mitosis) occurs quickly (peaks at about 6 h) and is followed (at about 24 h) by the secondary phase regeneration (SPR) response (hepatocytes mobilized from G_0/G_1 to proceed through mitosis). During chlordecone potentiation of carbon tetrachloride liver injury, EPR is thought to be eliminated and SPR decreased; thus the progression of the severe injury is facilitated and leads to lethality. There is evidence that induction of EPR may accelerate SPR. It is interesting to note that a large dose of carbon tetrachloride given alone also results in a regeneration response similar to that obtained with chlordecone and a small dose of haloalkane. Experiments performed with colchicine, partial hepatectomy, carbon tetrachloride autoprotection, nutritional factors, and different animal species have provided data consistent with the purported roles attributed to EPR, SPR, and liver injury (121, 142, 143).

The role of tissue repair has been assessed with other hepatotoxicants (143). The data indicate that thioacetamide, o-dichlorobenzene, and trichloroethylene when given alone affect hepatic tissue regeneration in a manner not unlike that observed with carbon tetrachloride. Increased lethality, however, was not observed with isopropanol- or ethanol-potentiated carbon tetrachloride–induced liver injury (151, 152). Mehendale (141) and Soni & Mehendale (143) have proposed a two-stage model for chemical-induced hepatotoxicity. Stage one would involve initiation and infliction of injury; stage two would lead to recovery or progression to massive injury, depending on the effects of the toxicant on cellular regeneration (enhanced regeneration would lead to recovery; inhibition would lead to massive injury). Although various aspects of the repair-recovery process are still hypothetical and speculative, the concept itself is thought-provoking and certainly an important contribution to the understanding of chemical-induced liver injury. It will be interesting to see how it evolves with time.

SOME FINAL THOUGHTS

The amount of knowledge acquired over the past 50 years about the liver injury produced by chlorinated methanes, particularly carbon tetrachloride, is truly remarkable. One can wonder, however, what might have happened if chloroform, instead of carbon tetrachloride, had been the gold standard for studying the biochemistry of chemical-induced acute necrogenic liver injury. Certainly the free-radical picture and the phenomenon of lipid peroxidation as we know it today might have been very different because each one seems to play a different role with chloroform. Acquired knowledge about carbon tetrachloride has had a great influence on research approaches designed to understand other types of chemical-induced hepatotoxicity. In drug-induced liver disease, the acetaminophen and halothane models, however, have now attained their own distinct identities. Also, the chlorinated methanes are not very useful for understanding the idiosyncratic liver injury that may occur in an unpredictable fashion with some therapeutic agents.

The steatosis observed after the acute administration of chlorinated methanes is largely attributed to a failure of the triglyceride secretory mechanism of the hepatocyte. Yet, the possible effects of these agents on the more recently described molecular events involved in triglyceride secretion (153–156) remain to be investigated. This area of research should be brought up-to-date, in line with more current concepts.

Unfortunately, the perception of altered mitochondria as only a late event in the temporal development of the liver injury produced by the chlorinated methanes might have contributed to an apparently lessened interest in the role of this organelle in other forms of chemical-induced liver injury. Yet, the importance of mitochondrial function in oxidative stress-related aspects of hepatotoxicity is now evident. Also, early mitochondrial dysfunction has been proposed as an important element in bromobenzene toxicity (157), and inhibition of mitochondrial β-oxidation has been associated with the microvesicular steatosis observed in rats following valproic acid intoxication (158). This biochemical lesion is now considered of major importance in other forms of liver injury in humans and animals (159, 160). It would be worthwhile that in the future, mitochondrial function be revisited even for chlorinated methane–induced liver injury, possibly as a contributory lesion.

Despite all the advances made with chemical-induced liver injury, we still cannot establish which of the changes observed lead to cell death and which are secondary disturbances. We know what can be done to a liver cell and yet not destroy it. Judah's words published in 1970 (9) are still appropriate 30 years later: "Necrosis is a histologist's conception. The dead cell is recognized by changes that are the consequences of cell death. . . . These signs take some time to develop, hence one is ignorant of the precise moment of cell death." It is likely that the fervent search for the "biochemical lesion" pursued over the past 40 years has distorted our ability to recognize what the necrotic process actually represents. In this regard, the two-stage model of toxicity proposed by Mehendale (141) from chlordecone-carbon tetrachloride interactions is a novel way of looking at chemical-induced liver injury. Cohen & Khairallah (161) discussed an analogous situation with acetaminophen hepatotoxicity (a field largely influenced by prior experience acquired with carbon tetrachloride). They came to the conclusion that multiple independent insults to cells may be involved in toxicity and proposed the concept of a multistage process as being appropriate for acetaminophen; collectively, a number of cellular events set in motion and perpetuate the processes that determine outcome. Such ideas should become stimulating influences and should be pursued in future hepatotoxic research.

The discovery by Mehendale and his colleagues (121, 142, 143) of the consequences of early-phase–regeneration and secondary-phase–regeneration tissue repair processes, and their interactions, on the outcome of carbon tetrachloride–induced hepatotoxicity (with or without chlordecone potentiation) is an exciting and intriguing development. It expands our conception of the overall process of liver injury in a significant manner. The fact that elements of the processes are applicable to other hepatotoxicants appears to be quantifiable and follows dose-dependent criteria (including the appearance of a threshold) contributes greatly to their importance. The pursuit of the biochemical and molecular aspects of these phenomena in much greater depth, including genetic expression, should undoubtedly have a marked influence on our better understanding of chemical-induced hepatotoxicity. The next 15 years or so should be really interesting.

Visit the Annual Reviews home page at www.AnnualReviews.org.

LITERATURE CITED

1. Plaa GL. 1997. A four-decade adventure in experimental liver injury. *Drug Metab. Rev.* 29:1–37
2. Drill VA. 1952. Hepatotoxic agents: mechanism of action and dietary interelationship. *Pharmacol. Rev.* 4:1–42
3. von Oettingen WF. 1955. The Halogenated Aliphatic, Olefinic, Cyclic, Aromatic, and Aliphatic-Aromatic Hydrocarbons Including the Halogenated Insecticides, Their Toxicity and Potential Dangers. Public Health Serv. Publ. no. 414. Washington, DC: US Gov. Print. Off. 430 pp.
4. Popper H, Schaffner F. 1957. *Liver: Structure and Function.* New York: McGraw-Hill. 777 pp.
5. Recknagel RO. 1967. Carbon tetrachloride hepatotoxicity. *Pharmacol. Rev.* 19: 145–208
6. Recknagel RO, Glende EA Jr. 1973. Car-

bon tetrachloride hepatotoxicity: an example of lethal cleavage. *CRC Crit. Rev. Toxicol.* 2:263–97

7. Stoner HB, Magee PN. 1957. Experimental studies on toxic liver injury. *Br. Med. Bull.* 13:102–7

8. Himsworth HP. 1954. *The Liver and Its Diseases.* Cambridge, MA: Harvard Univ. Press. 222 pp.

9. Judah JD, McLean AEM, McLean EK. 1970. Biochemical mechanisms of liver injury. *Am. J. Med.* 49:609–16

10. Wahi PN, Tandon HD, Bharadwai TP. 1955. Acute carbon tetrachloride hepatic injury, parts I and II. *Acta Pathol. Microbiol. Scand.* 37:305–15

11. Christie GS, Judah JD. 1954. Mechanism of action of carbon tetrachloride on liver cells. *Proc. R. Soc. London Ser. B* 142:241–57

12. Heim F, Leuschner F, Ott A. 1956. Der Einfluss von Tetrachlorkohlenstoff auf die Ferment- und Co-enzym-A Aktivität der Leber. *Arch. exp. Pathol. Pharmakol.* 229:360–65

13. Calvert DN, Brody TM. 1958. Biochemical alterations of liver function by halogenated hydrocarbons. I. In vitro and in vivo changes and their modification by ethylenediamine tetracetate. *J. Pharmacol. Exp. Ther.* 124:273–81

14. Recknagel RO, Anthony DD. 1959. Biochemical changes in carbon tetrachloride fatty liver: separation of fatty changes from mitochondrial degeneration. *J. Biol. Chem.* 234:1052–59

15. Recknagel RO, Lombardi B, Schotz MC. 1960. New insight into pathogenesis of carbon tetrachloride fat infiltration. *Proc. Soc. Exp. Biol. Med.* 104:608–10

16. Recknagel RO, Lombardi B. 1961. Studies of biochemical changes in subcellular particles of rat liver and their relationship to a new hypothesis regarding the pathogenesis of carbon tetrachloride fat accumulation. *J. Biol. Chem.* 236:564–69

17. Moore L, Davenport GR, Landon EJ. 1976. Calcium uptake of a rat liver microsomal subcellular fraction in

response to in vivo administration of carbon tetrachloride. *J. Biol. Chem.* 251:1197–201

18. Recknagel RO, Glende EA Jr, Waller RL, Lowrey K. 1982. Lipid peroxidation: biochemistry, measurement, and significance in liver cell injury. See Ref. 162, pp. 213–41

19. Plaa GL, Hewitt WR 1989. Detection and evaluation of chemically induced liver injury. In *Principles and Methods of Toxicology,* ed. AW Hayes, pp. 599–628. New York: Raven. 2nd ed.

20. Comporti M. 1998. Lipid peroxidation as a mediator of chemical-induced hepatocyte death. See Ref. 163, pp. 221–57

21. Calvert DN, Brody TM. 1960. Role of the sympathetic nervous system in CCl_4 hepatotoxicity. *Am. J. Physiol.* 198:669–76

22. Brody TM, Calvert DN. 1960. Release of catechol amines from the adrenal medulla by CCl_4. *Am. J. Physiol.* 198:682–85

23. Brody TM, Calvert DN, Schneider AF. 1961. Alterations of carbon tetrachloride-induced pathologic changes in rat by spinal transection, adrenalectomy, and adrenergic blocking agents. *J. Pharmacol. Exp. Ther.* 131:341–45

24. Stern PH, Brody TM. 1963. Catecholamine excretion following carbon tetrachloride administration. *J. Pharmacol. Exp. Ther.* 141:65–73

25. Larson RE, Plaa GL, Crews LM. 1964. Effect of spinal cord transection on carbon tetrachloride hepatotoxicity. *Toxicol. Appl. Pharmacol.* 6:154–62

26. Larson RE, Plaa GL. 1963. Spinal cord transection and CCl_4 toxicity. *Experientia* 19:604–6

27. Larson RE, Plaa GL. 1965. A correlation of the effects of cervical cordotomy, hypothermia, and catecholamines on carbon tetrachloride-induced hepatic necrosis. *J. Pharmacol. Exp. Ther.* 147:103–11

28. Larson RE, Plaa GL, Brody MJ. 1964. Immunological sympathectomy and

CCl$_4$ hepatotoxicity. *Proc. Soc. Exp. Biol. Med.* 116:557–60

29. Plaa GL, Larson RE. 1964. CCl$_4$-induced liver damage. *Arch. Environ. Health* 9:536–43

30. Lombardi B. 1966. Considerations on the pathogenesis of fatty liver. *Lab. Invest.* 15:1–20

31. Rice AJ, Roberts RJ, Plaa GL. 1967. The effect of carbon tetrachloride, administered in vivo, on the hemodynamics of the isolated perfused rat liver. *Toxicol. Appl. Pharmacol.* 11:422–31

32. Rice AJ, Plaa GL. 1968. Effect of hypophysectomy and spinal cord transection on carbon tetrachloride-induced changes in the hemodynamics of the isolated perfused rat liver. *Toxicol. Appl. Pharmacol.* 12:194–201

33. Rice AJ, Plaa GL. 1969. The role of triglyceride accumulation and of necrosis in the hemodynamic responses of the isolated perfused rat liver after administration of carbon tetrachloride. *Toxicol. Appl. Pharmacol.* 14:151–62

34. Schwetz BA, Plaa GL. 1969. Catecholamine potentiation of carbon tetrachloride-induced hepatotoxicity in mice. *Toxicol. Appl. Pharmacol.* 14:495–509

35. Iwai M, Shimazu T. 1988. Effects of ventromedial and lateral hypothalamic stimulation on chemically-induced liver injury in rats. *Life Sci.* 42:1833–40

36. Roberts SM, Harbison RD, Seng JE, James RC. 1991. Potentiation of carbon tetrachloride hepatotoxicity by phenylpropanolamine. *Toxicol. Appl. Pharmacol.* 111:175–88

37. Roberts SM, Harbison RD, James RC. 1994. Methamphetamine potentiation of carbon tetrachloride hepatotoxicity in mice. *J. Pharmacol. Exp. Ther.* 271: 1051–57

38. Roberts SM, Harbison RD, James RC. 1995. Mechanistic studies on the potentiation of carbon tetrachloride hepatotoxicity by methamphetamine. *Toxicology* 97:49–57

39. Roberts SM, Harbison RD, Westhouse RA, James RC. 1995. Exacerbation of carbon tetrachloride-induced liver injury in the rat by methamphetamine. *Toxicol. Lett.* 76:77–83

40. Roberts SM, DeMott RP, James RC. 1997. Adrenergic modulation of hepatotoxicity. *Drug Metab. Rev.* 29:329–53

41. Plaa GL, Hewitt WR. 1982. Biotransformation products and cholestasis. In *Progess in Liver Diseases,* ed. H Popper, F Schaffner, pp. 179–94. New York: Grune & Stratton

42. Plaa GL. 1991. Toxic responses of the liver. In *Casarett and Doull's Toxicology,* ed. MO Amdur, J Doull, CD Klaassen, pp. 334–53. New York: Pergamon. 4th ed.

43. Plaa GL. 1997. Free-radical-mediated liver injury. See Ref. 164, pp. 175–84

44. Sipes IG, Gandolfi AJ. 1982. Bioactivation of aliphatic organohalogens: formation, detection, and relevance. See Ref. 162, pp. 181–212

45. Butler TC. 1961. Reduction of carbon tetrachloride in vivo and reduction of carbon tetrachloride and chloroform in vitro by tissues and tissue constituents. *J. Pharmacol. Exp. Ther.* 134:311–19

46. Slater TF. 1966. Necrogenic action of carbon tetrachloride in the rat: a speculative mechanism based on activation. *Nature* 209:36–40

47. Cheeseman KH, Albano EF, Tomasi A, Slater TF. 1985. Biochemical studies on the metabolic activity of halogenated alkanes. *Environ. Health Perspect.* 64: 85–101

48. Connor HD, Thurman RG, Galizi MD, Mason RP. 1986. The formation of a novel free radical metabolite from CCl$_4$ in the perfused rat liver and in vivo. *J. Biol. Chem.* 261:4542–48

49. LaCagnin LB, Connor HD, Mason RP, Thurmond RD. 1988. The carbon dioxide anion radical adduct in the perfused rat liver: relationship to halocarbon-

induced toxicity. *Mol. Pharmacol.* 33: 351–57

50. Raucy JL, Kraner JC, Lasker JM. 1993. Bioactivation of halogenated hydrocarbons by cytochrome P4502E1. *Crit. Rev. Toxicol.* 23:1–20

51. Raymond P, Plaa GL. 1995. Ketone potentiation of haloalkane-induced hepato- and nephrotoxicity. II. Implication of monooxygenases. *J. Toxicol. Environ. Health* 46:317–28

52. Kim SG, Chung HC, Cho JY. 1996. Molecular mechanism for alkyl sulfide-modulated carbon tetrachloride-induced hepatotoxicity: the role of cytochrome P450 2E1, P450 2B and glutathione-S-transferase expression. *J. Pharmacol. Exp. Ther.* 277:1058–66

53. Gruebele A, Zawaski K, Kaplan D, Novak RF. 1996. Cytochrome P4502E1- and cytochrome P4501B1/2B2-catalyzed carbon tetrachloride metabolism: effects on signal transduction as demonstrated by altered immediate-early (c-Fos and c-Jun) gene expression and nuclear AP-1 and NF-kappa B transcription factor levels. *Drug Metab. Disp.* 24:15–22

54. Recknagel RO, Ghoshal AK. 1966. Lipid peroxidation as a vector in carbon tetrachloride hepatotoxicity. *Lab. Invest.* 15:132–48

55. Comporti M. 1985. Lipid peroxidation and cellular damage in toxic liver injury. *Lab. Invest.* 53:599–623

56. Koch RR, Glende EA Jr, Recknagel RO. 1974. Hepatotoxicity of bromotrichloromethane—bond dissociation energy and lipoperoxidation. *Biochem. Pharmacol.* 23:2907–15

57. Mansuy D, Beaune P, Cresteil T, Lange M, Leroux JP. 1977. Evidence for phosgene formation during liver microsomal oxidation of chloroform. *Biochem. Biophys. Res. Commun.* 79:513–17

58. Pohl LR, Bhooshan B, Whittaker NF, Krishna G. 1977. Phosgene: a metabolite of chloroform. *Biochem. Biophys. Res. Commun.* 79:684–91

59. Castro JA. 1984. Mechanistical studies and prevention of free radical cell injury. In *IUPHAR 9th Int. Congr. Pharmacol., Proc.*, ed. W Paton, J Mitchell, P Turner, 2:243–50. London: Macmillan

60. Manno M, DeMatteis F, King IJ. 1988. The mechanism of the suicidal, reductive inactivation of microsomal cytochrome P-450 by carbon tetrachloride. *Biochem. Pharmacol.* 37:1981–90

61. Tierney DJ, Haas AL, Koop DR. 1992. Degradation of cytochrome P450 2E1: selective loss after labilization of the enzyme. *Arch. Biochem. Biophys.* 293: 9–16

62. Moody DE. 1992. Effect of phenobarbital treatment on carbon tetrachloride-mediated cytochrome P-450 loss and diene conjugate formation. *Toxicol. Lett.* 61:213–24

63. Fujii K. 1997. Preventive effect of isoflurane on destruction of cytochrome P450 during reductive dehalogenation of carbon tetrachloride in guinea-pig microsomes. *Drug Metab. Drug Interact.* 14: 99–107

64. Plaa GL, Witschi HP. 1976. Chemicals, drugs, and lipid peroxidation. *Annu. Rev. Pharmacol. Toxicol.* 16:125–41

65. Cluet J-L, Boisset M, Boudene C. 1986. Effect of pretreatment with cimetidine or phenobarbital on lipoperoxidation in carbon tetrachloride- and trichloroethylene-dosed rats. *Toxicology* 38:91–102

66. Klaassen CD, Plaa GL. 1969. Comparison of the biochemical alterations elicited in livers from rats treated with carbon tetrachloride, chloroform, 1,1,2-trichlorethane and 1,1,1-trichloroethane. *Biochem. Pharmacol.* 18:2019–27

67. Brown BB Jr, Sipes IG, Sagalyn AM. 1974. Mechanisms of acute hepatic toxicity: chloroform, halothane, and glutathione. *Anesthesiology* 41:554–61

68. Lavigne JG, Marchand C. 1974. The role of metabolism in chloroform hepatotoxicity. *Toxicol. Appl. Pharmacol.* 29:312–26

69. Wang PV, Kaneko T, Tsukada H, Nakano M, Nakajima T, Sato A. 1997. Time courses of hepatic injuries induced by chloroform and by carbon tetrachloride: comparison of biochemical and histopathological changes. *Arch. Toxicol.* 71: 638–45

70. Plaa GL, Evans EA, Hine CH. 1958. Relative hepatotoxicity of seven halogenated hydrocarbons. *J. Pharmacol. Exp. Ther.* 123:224–29

71. Klaassen CD, Plaa GL. 1966. The relative effects of various chlorinated hydrocarbons on liver and kidney function in mice. *Toxicol. Appl. Pharmacol.* 9:139–51

72. Klaassen CD, Plaa GL. 1967. The relative effects of various chlorinated hydrocarbons on liver and kidney function in dogs. *Toxicol. Appl. Pharmacol.* 10:119–31

73. Anders MW. 1988. Bioactivation mechanisms and hepatocellular damage. See Ref. 165, pp. 389–400

74. Popper H. 1988. Hepatocellular degeneration and death. See Ref. 165, pp. 1087–103

75. Liebler DC, Reed DJ. 1997. Free-radical defense and repair mechanisms. See Ref. 164, pp. 141–71

76. Farber JL. 1990. The role of calcium ions in toxic cell injury. *Environ. Health Perspect.* 84:107–11

77. Rosser BG, Gores GJ. 1995. Liver cell necrosis: cellular mechanisms and clinical implications. *Gastroenterology* 108: 252–75

78. Reed DJ. 1998. Evaluation of chemical-induced oxidative stress as a mechanism of hepatocyte death. See Ref. 163, pp. 187–220

79. Laskin DL, Gardner CR. 1998. The role of nonparenchymal cells and inflammatory macrophages in hepatotoxicity. See Ref. 163, pp. 297–320

80. Hoglen NC, Younis HS, Hartley DP, Gunawardhana L, Lantz RC, Sipes IG. 1998. 1,2-Dichlorobenzene-induced lipid peroxidation in male Fischer 344 rats is Kupffer cell dependent. *Toxicol. Sci.* 45: 376–85

81. Hooser SB, Rosengren RJ, Hill DA, Mobley SA, Sipes IG. 1994. Vitamin A modulation of xenobiotic-induced hepatotoxicity in rodents. *Environ. Health Perspect.* 102(Suppl. 9):39–43

82. Badger DA, Sauer JM, Hoglen NC, Jolley CS, Sipes IG. 1996. The role of inflammatory cells and cytochrome P450 in the potentiation of CCl_4-induced liver injury by a single dose of retinol. *Toxicol. Appl. Pharmacol.* 141:507–19

83. Kutob SD, Plaa GL. 1962. The effect of acute ethanol intoxication on chloroform-induced liver damage. *J. Pharmacol. Exp. Ther.* 135:245–52

84. Strubelt O, Obermeier F, Siegers CP. 1978. The influence of ethanol pretreatment on the effects of nine hepatotoxic agents. *Acta Pharmacol. Toxicol.* 43: 211–18

85. Cornish HH, Adefuin J. 1967. Potentiation of carbon tetrachloride toxicity by aliphatic alcohols. *Arch. Environ. Health* 14:237–40

86. Traiger GJ, Plaa GL. 1971. Differences in the potentiation of carbon tetrachloride in rats by ethanol and isopropanol pretreatment. *Toxicol. Appl. Pharmacol.* 20:105–12

87. Traiger GJ, Plaa GL. 1972. Relationship of alcohol metabolism to the potentiation of CCl_4 hepatotoxicity induced by aliphatic alcohols. *J. Pharmacol. Exp. Ther.* 183:481–88

88. Traiger GJ, Plaa GL. 1973. Effect of isopropanol on CCl_4-induced changes in perfused rat liver hemodynamics. *Arch. Int. Pharmacodyn. Thér.* 202:102–5

89. Traiger GJ, Plaa GL. 1973. Effect of aminotriazole on isopropanol- and acetone-induced potentiation of CCl_4 hepatotoxicity. *Can. J. Physiol. Pharmacol.* 51:291–96

90. Traiger GJ, Plaa GL. 1974. Chlorinated hydrocarbon toxicity: potentiation by

isopropyl alcohol and acetone. *Arch. Environ. Health* 28:276–78

91. Plaa GL, Traiger GJ. 1973. Mechanism of potentiation of CCl₄-induced hepatotoxicity. In *Pharmacology and the Future of Man—Proc. 5th Congr. Pharmacol.*, ed. T Loomis, 2:100–13. Basel: Karger

92. Folland DS, Schaffner W, Grinn HE, Crofford OB, McMurray DR. 1976. Carbon tetrachloride toxicity potentiated by isopropyl alcohol. *J. Am. Med. Assoc.* 236:1853–56

93. Deng JG, Wang JD, Shih TS, Lan FL. 1987. Outbreak of carbon tetrachloride poisoning in a color printing factory related to the use of isopropyl alcohol and an air conditioning system in Taiwan. *Am. J. Ind. Med.* 12:11–19

94. Traiger GJ, Bruckner JV. 1976. The participation of 2-butanone in 2-butanol-induced potentiation of carbon tetrachloride hepatotoxicity. *J. Pharmacol. Exp. Ther.* 196:493–500

95. Hewitt WR, Miyajima H, Côté MG, Plaa GL. 1980. Acute alteration of chloroform-induced hepato- and nephrotoxicity by n-hexane, methyl n-butyl ketone, and 2,5-hexanedione. *Toxicol. Appl. Pharmacol.* 53:230–48

96. Hewitt WR, Brown EM, Plaa GL. 1983. Relationship between the carbon skeleton length of ketonic solvents and potentiation of chloroform-induced hepatotoxicity in rats. *Toxicol. Lett.* 16: 297–304

97. Raisbeck MF, Brown EM, Hewitt WR. 1986. Renal and hepatic interactions between 2-hexanone and carbon tetrachloride in F-344 rats. *Toxicol. Lett.* 31: 15–21

98. Vézina M, Kobusch AB, du Souich P, Greselin E, Plaa GL. 1990. Potentiation of chloroform-induced hepatotoxicity by methyl isobutyl ketone and two metabolites. *Can. J. Physiol. Pharmacol.* 68: 1055–61

99. Raymond P, Plaa GL. 1995. Ketone potentiation of haloalkane-induced hepato- and nephrotoxicity. I. Dose-response relationships. *J. Toxicol. Environ. Health* 45:465–80

100. Hewitt WR, Miyajima H, Côté MG, Hewitt LA, Cianflone DJ, Plaa GL. 1982. Dose-response relationships in 1,3-butanediol-induced potentiation of carbon tetrachloride toxicity. *Toxicol. Appl. Pharmacol.* 64:529–40

101. Pilon D, Brodeur J, Plaa GL. 1986. 1,3-Butanediol-induced increases in ketone bodies and potentiation of CCl₄ hepatotoxicity. *Toxicology* 40:165–80

102. Pilon D, Charbonneau M, Brodeur J, Plaa GL. 1986. Metabolites and ketone body production following methyl n-butyl ketone exposure as possible indices of MnBK potentiation of carbon tetrachloride hepatotoxicity. *Toxicol. Appl. Pharmacol.* 85:49–59

103. Plaa GL. 1988. Experimental evaluation of haloalkanes and liver injury. *Fundam. Appl. Toxicol.* 10:563–70

104. Hanasono GK, Côté MG, Plaa GL. 1975. Potentiation of carbon tetrachloride-induced hepatotoxicity in alloxan- or streptozotocin-diabetic rats. *J. Pharmacol. Exp. Ther.* 192:592–604

105. Hanasono GK, Witschi HP, Plaa GL. 1975. Potentiation of the hepatotoxic responses to chemicals in alloxan-diabetic rats. *Proc. Soc. Exp. Biol. Med.* 149:903–7

106. Villarruel M, Fernández G, de Ferreyra EC, de Fenos OM, Castro JA. 1982. Studies on the mechanism of alloxan-diabetes potentiation of carbon tetrachloride-induced liver necrosis. *Br. J. Exp. Pathol.* 63:388–93

107. Watkins JB, Sanders RA, Beck LV. 1988. The effect of long-term streptozotocin-induced diabetes on the hepatotoxicity of bromobenzene and carbon tetrachloride and hepatic biotransformation in rats. *Toxicol. Appl. Pharmacol.* 93:329–38

108. Wang PV, Kaneko T, Sato A, Charbonneau M, Plaa GL. 1995. Dose- and route-dependent alteration of metabolism and toxicity of chloroform in fed and fasting

rats. *Toxicol. Appl. Pharmacol.* 135:19–26

109. Plaa GL, Hewitt WR. 1982. Potentiation of liver and kidney injury by ketones and ketogenic substances. In *Advances in Pharmacology and Therapeutics II,* ed. H Yoshida, Y Hagihara, S Ebashi, 5:65–75. Oxford, UK: Pergamon

110. MacDonald JR, Gandolfi AJ, Sipes IG. 1982. Acetone potentiation of 1,1,2-trichloroethane hepatotoxicity. *Toxicol. Lett.* 13:57–69

111. Hewitt WR, Brown EM, Plaa GL. 1983. Acetone-induced potentiation of trihalomethane toxicity in male rats. *Toxicol. Lett.* 16:385–96

112. Pessayre D, Cobert B, Descatoire V, Degott C, Babany G, et al. 1982. Hepatotoxicity of trichloroethylene-carbon tetrachloride mixtures in rats. *Gastroenterology* 83:761–72

113. Charbonneau M, Oleskevich A, Brodeur J, Plaa GL. 1986. Acetone potentiation of rat liver injury induced by trichloroethylene-carbon tetrachloride mixtures. *Fundam. Appl. Toxicol.* 6:654–61

114. Borzelleca JR, O'Hara TM, Gennings C, Granger RH, Sheppard MA, Condie LW Jr. 1990. Interactions of water contaminants. I. Plasma enzyme activity and response surface methodology following gavage administration of CCl$_4$ and CHCl$_3$ or TCE singly and in combination in the rat. *Fundam. Appl. Toxicol.* 14:477–90

115. Steup DR, Wiersma D, McMillan DA, Sipes IG. 1991. Pretreatment with drinking water solutions containing trichloroethylene or chloroform enhances the hepatotoxicity of carbon tetrachloride in Fischer 344 rats. *Fundam. Appl. Toxicol.* 16:798–809

116. Charbonneau M, Greselin E, Brodeur J, Plaa GL. 1991. Influence of acetone on the severity of the liver injury induced by haloalkane mixtures. *Can. J. Physiol. Pharmacol.* 69:1901–7

117. Charbonneau M, Tuchweber B, Plaa GL. 1986. Acetone potentiation of chronic liver injury induced by repetitive administration of carbon tetrachloride. *Hepatology* 6:694–700

118. Hewitt WR, Miyajima H, Côté MG, Plaa GL. 1979. Acute alteration of chloroform-induced hepato- and nephrotoxicity by mirex and Kepone. *Toxicol. Appl. Pharmacol.* 48:509–27

119. Curtis LR, Williams WL, Mehendale HM. 1979. Potentiation of the hepatotoxicity of carbon tetrachloride following preexposure to chlordecone (Kepone) in the male rat. *Toxicol. Appl. Pharmacol.* 51:283–93

120. Agarwal AK, Mehendale HM. 1982. Potentiation of bromotrichloromethane hepatotoxicity and lethality by chlordecone preexposure in the rat. *Fundam. Appl. Toxicol.* 2:161–67

121. Calabrese EJ, Mehendale HM. 1996. A review of the role of tissue repair as an adaptive strategy: why low doses are often non-toxic and why high doses can be fatal. *Food Chem. Toxicol.* 34:301–11

122. Hewitt LA, Caillé G, Plaa GL. 1986. Temporal relationships between biotransformation, detoxication and chlordecone potentiation of chloroform-induced hepatotoxicity. *Can. J. Physiol. Pharmacol.* 64:477–82

123. Plaa GL, Caillé G, Vézina M, Iijima M, Côté MG. 1987. Chloroform interaction with chlordecone and mirex: correlation between biochemical and histological indices of toxicity and quantitative tissue levels. *Fundam. Appl. Toxicol.* 9:198–207

124. Sipes IG, Stripp B, Krishna G, Maling HM, Gillette JR. 1973. Enhanced hepatic microsomal activity to pretreatment of rats with acetone or isopropanol. *Proc. Soc. Exp Biol. Med.* 142:237–40

125. Maling HM, Stripp B, Sipes IG, Highman B, Saul W, Williams MA. 1975. Enhanced hepatotoxicity of carbon tetrachloride, thioacetamide, and dimethylnitrosamine by pretreatment of rats with

ethanol and some comparisons with potentiation by isopropanol. *Toxicol. Appl. Pharmacol.* 33:291–308

126. Cianflone DJ, Hewitt WR, Villeneuve DC, Plaa GL. 1980. Role of biotransformation in the alterations of chloroform hepatotoxicity produced by Kepone and mirex. *Toxicol. Appl. Pharmacol.* 53:140–49

127. Branchflower RV, Pohl LR. 1981. Investigation of the mechanism of the potentiation of chloroform-induced hepatotoxicity and nephrotoxicity by methyl n-butyl ketone. *Toxicol. Appl. Pharmacol.* 61:407–13

128. Hewitt LA, Hewitt WR, Plaa GL. 1983. Fractional hepatic localization of $^{14}CHCl_3$ in mice and rats treated with chlordecone or mirex. *Fundam. Appl. Toxicol.* 3:489–95

129. Hewitt LA, Valiquette C, Plaa GL. 1987. The role of biotransformation-detoxication in acetone-, 2-butanone-, and 2-hexanone-potentiated chloroform-induced hepatotoxicity. *Can. J. Physiol. Pharmacol.* 65:2313–18

130. Hewitt LA, Palmason C, Masson S, Plaa GL. 1990. Evidence for the involvement of organelles in the mechanism of ketone-potentiated chloroform-induced hepatotoxicity. *Liver* 10:35–48

131. Britton RS, Dolak JA, Glende EA Jr, Recknagel RO. 1987. Potentiation of carbon tetrachloride hepatotoxicity by chlordecone: dose-response relationships and increased covalent binding in vivo. *J. Biochem. Toxicol.* 2:43–55

132. Wang PV, Kaneko T, Tsukada H, Nakano M, Sato A. 1997. Dose- and route-dependent alterations in metabolism and toxicity of chemical compounds in ethanol-treated rats: difference between highly (chloroform) and poorly (carbon tetrachloride) metabolized hepatotoxic compounds. *Toxicol. Appl. Pharmacol.* 142:13–21

133. Imaoka S, Funae Y. 1991. Induction of cytochrome P450 isozymes in rat liver by methyl n-alkyl ketones and n-alkylbenzenes. Effects of hydrophobicity of inducers on inducibility of cytochrome P450. *Biochem. Pharmacol.* 42(Suppl.): S143–50

134. Lewandowski M, Levi P, Hodgson E. 1989. Induction of cytochrome P-450 isozymes by mirex and chlordecone. *J. Biochem. Toxicol.* 4:195–99

135. Kocarek TA, Schuetz EG, Guzelian PS. 1991. Selective induction of cytochrome P450e by Kepone (chlordecone) in primary cultures of adult rat hepatocytes. *Mol. Pharmacol.* 40:203–10

136. Kocarek TA, Schuetz EG, Guzelian PS. 1994. Regulation of cytochrome P450 2B1/2 mRNAs by Kepone (chlordecone) and potent estrogens in primary cultures of adult rat hepatocytes on Matrigel. *Toxicol. Lett.* 71:183–96

137. Davis ME, Mehendale HM. 1980. Functional and biochemical correlates of chlordecone exposure and its enhancement of CCl_4 hepatotoxicity. *Toxicology* 15:91–103

138. Young RA, Mehendale HM. 1989. Carbon tetrachloride metabolism in partially hepatectomized and sham-operated rats pre-exposed to chlordecone (Kepone). *J. Biochem. Toxicol.* 4:211–19

139. Côté MG, Traiger GJ, Plaa GL. 1974. Effect of isopropanol-induced potentiation of carbon tetrachloride on rat hepatic ultrastructure. *Toxicol. Appl. Pharmacol.* 30:14–25

140. Curtis LR, Mehendale HM. 1981. Hepatobiliary dysfunction and inhibition of adenosine triphosphatase activity of bile canaliculi-enriched fractions following in vivo mirex, photomirex, and chlordecone exposures. *Toxicol. Appl. Pharmacol.* 61:429–40

141. Mehendale HM. 1991. Role of hepatocellular regeneration and hepatolobular healing in the final outcome of liver injury—a two-stage model of toxicity. *Biochem. Pharmacol.* 42:1155–62

142. Mehendale HM. 1994. Mechanism of the

interactive amplification of halomethane hepatotoxicity and lethality by other chemicals. In *Toxicology of Chemical Mixtures,* ed. RSH Yang, pp. 299–334. San Diego: Academic

143. Soni MG, Mehendale HM. 1998. Role of tissue repair in toxicologic interactions among hepatotoxic organics. *Environ. Health Perspect.* 106(Suppl. 6):1307–17

144. Lockard VG, Mehendale HM, O'Neal RM. 1983. Chlordecone-induced potentiation of carbon tetrachloride hepatotoxicity: a light and electron microscopic study. *Exp. Mol. Pathol.* 39:230–45

145. Lockard VG, Mehendale HM, O'Neal RM. 1983. Chlordecone-induced potentiation of carbon tetrachloride hepatotoxicity: a morphometric and biochemical study. *Exp. Mol. Pathol.* 39:246–56

146. Charbonneau M, Iijima M, Côté MG, Plaa GL. 1985. Temporal analysis of rat liver injury following potentiation of carbon tetrachloride hepatotoxicity with ketonic or ketogenic compounds. *Toxicology* 35:95–112

147. Bell AN, Young RA, Lockard VG, Mehendale HM. 1988. Protection of chlordecone-potentiated carbon tetrachloride hepatotoxicity and lethality by partial hepatectomy. *Arch. Toxicol.* 61:392–405

148. Mehendale HM, Purushotam KR, Lockard VG. 1989. The time course of liver injury and [^{3}H]thymidine incorporation in chlordecone-potentiated CHCl$_3$ hepatotoxicity. *Exp. Mol. Pathol.* 51:31–47

149. Mehendale HM, Thakore KN, Rao CV. 1994. Autoprotection: stimulated tissue repair permits recovery from injury. *J. Biochem. Toxicol.* 9:131–39

150. Soni MG, Mehendale HM. 1991. Protection from chlordecone-amplified carbon tetrachloride toxicity by cyanidanol: regeneration studies. *Toxicol. Appl. Pharmacol.* 108:58–66

151. Ray SD, Mehendale HM. 1990. Potentiation of CCl$_4$ and CHCl$_3$ hepatotoxicity and lethality by various alcohols. *Fundam. Appl. Toxicol.* 15:429–40

152. Rao PS, Dalu A, Kulkarni SG, Mehendale HM. 1996. Stimulated tissue repair prevents lethality in isopropanol-induced potentiation of carbon tetrachloride hepatotoxicity. *Toxicol. Appl. Pharmacol.* 140:235–44

153. Vance JE, Vance DE. 1990. Lipoprotein assembly and secretion by hepatocytes. *Annu. Rev. Nutr.* 10:337–56

154. Rusinol A, Verkade H, Vance JE. 1990. Assembly of rat hepatic very low density lipoproteins in the endoplasmic reticulum. *J. Biol. Chem.* 268:3555–62

155. Kuipers F, Jong MC, Lin Y, Eck M, Havinga R, et al. 1997. Impaired secretion of very low density lipoprotein-triglycerides by apolipoprotein E-deficient mouse hepatocytes. *J. Clin. Invest.* 100:2915–22

156. Yamauchi T, Iwai M, Kobayashi N, Shimazu T. 1998. Noradrenaline and ATP decrease the secretion of triglyceride and apoprotein B from perfused rat liver. *Eur. J. Physiol.* 435:368–74

157. Maellaro E, Del Bello B, Casini AF, Comporti M, Ceccarelli D, et al. 1990. Early mitochondrial disfunction in bromobenzene treated mice: a possible factor of liver injury. *Biochem. Pharmacol.* 40:1491–97

158. Tang W, Borel AG, Fujimiya T, Abbott FS. 1995. Fluorinated analogues as mechanistic probes in valproic acid hepatotoxicity: hepatic microvesicular steatosis and glutathione status. *Chem. Res. Toxicol.* 8:671–82

159. Fromenty B, Pessayre D. 1995. Inhibition of mitochondrial beta-oxidation as a mechanism of hepatotoxicity. *Pharmacol. Ther.* 67:101–54

160. Tennant BC, Baldwin BH, Graham LA, Ascenzi MA, Hornbuckle WE, et al. 1998. Antiviral activity and toxicity of fialuridine in the woodchuck model of hepatitis B virus infection. *Hepatology* 28:179–91

161. Cohen SD, Khairallah A. 1997. Selective protein arylation and acetaminophen-

induced hepatotoxicity. *Drug Metab. Rev.* 29:59–77

162. Plaa GL, Hewitt WR, eds. 1982. *Toxicology of the Liver.* New York: Raven

163. Plaa GL, Hewitt WR, eds. 1998. *Toxicology of the Liver.* Washington, DC: Taylor & Francis. 2nd ed.

164. Wallace KB, ed. 1997. *Free Radical Toxicology.* Washington, DC: Taylor & Francis

165. Arias IM, Jakoby WB, Popper H, Schachter D, Shafritzs DA, eds. 1988. *The Liver: Biology and Pathobiology.* New York: Raven. 2nd ed.

Annu. Rev. Pharmacol. Toxicol. 2000. 40:67–95

PHARMACOKINETIC/PHARMACODYNAMIC MODELING IN DRUG DEVELOPMENT

L. B. Sheiner[1] and J-L. Steimer[2]

[1]Departments of Laboratory Medicine, Biopharmaceutical Sciences, and Medicine, University of California San Francisco, San Francisco, California 94143; e-mail: lbs@c255.ucsf.edu; [2]F. Hoffmann-La Roche Ltd, Pharmaceutical Development/Biostatistics, CH-4070 Basel, Switzerland; e-mail: jean-louis.steimer@roche.com

Key Words   mechanistic models, learning, confirming, empirical models, predictive models, statistical modeling

■ **Abstract**   We propose a framework for considering the role of pharmacokinetic/pharmacodynamic modeling in drug development and an appraisal of its current and potential impact on that activity. After some introduction, definitions, and background information on drug development, we discuss subject-matter models that underlie pharmacokinetic/pharmacodynamic modeling and show how they determine appropriate statistical models. We discuss the broad role modeling can play in drug development, enhancing primarily the "learning" steps, i.e. acquiring the information needed for the label and for planning efficient confirmatory clinical trials. Examples of past applications of modeling to drug development are presented in tabular form, followed by a discussion of some practical issues in application. Modeling will not reach its potential utility until it is manifest as a visible and separate work unit within a drug development program. We suggest that that work unit is the "in numero" study: a protocol-driven exercise designed to extract additional information, and/or answer a specific drug-development question, through an integrated model-based (meta-) analysis of existent raw data, often pooled across separate (clinical) studies.

INTRODUCTION

In this paper, we propose a framework for considering the role of pharmacokinetic/pharmacodynamic (PK/PD) modeling in drug development and an appraisal of its current and potential impact on that activity. We take a broad view herein of the dose-exposure-effect relationship, one in which (*a*) "exposure" can be the concentration vs time profile, or a summary measure such as area under the concentration curve or C_{max} (maximum concentration), and (*b*) "effect" may be a pharmacological marker, an index of efficacy, or a measure of safety.

In an effort to reconcile the sometimes conflicting views of "models" held by clinical pharmacologists and clinical trial statisticians, we are at some pains to elucidate the separate but interdependent roles of the models of each discipline:

0362–1642/00/0415–0067$14.00

subject-matter–specific PK/PD models for the former, and more-general statistical models for the latter.

The paper discusses first theory and then practice. After this introduction and sections on definitions, background information on drug development, and fixing notation, we define first estimation and inference and then the types of subject-matter models that underlie PK/PD modeling. Following that, we show how the subject-matter models determine the statistical models and then conclude the theoretical development by discussing what role modeling might play in drug development. We then present some examples of the application of modeling to drug development and some practical issues in such application. The paper concludes with some speculation on the future of modeling in drug development.

To maintain focus within the space allotment available, we do not attempt an exhaustive literature review. Rather we focus on key ideas and cite supporting literature as appropriate. We also omit the following topics, all of which are relevant to our subject but which are either somewhat peripheral to it or either more specific or more general than appropriate to the level of abstraction we have chosen: detailed discussion of specific PK/PD models [see Holford & Sheiner (1, 2) and Derendorf & Meibohm (3) for review]; design and analysis of traditional dose-response clinical trials [for example, see Senn (4)]; PK/PD in early (preclinical) phases and transition from animal to man (see 5–10); and the application of modeling to pharmacoeconomics or public-policy decisions [for example, see e.g. Blower et al (11)]. Such modeling is expanding, and PK/PD models are part of a hierarchy of models useful for this purpose.

DEFINITIONS

We offer the following possibly idiosyncratic definitions of terms that are used extensively in this paper: drug development, the information-gathering activities that begin when a lead compound is first introduced into man and that end when the accumulated information is summarized and presented to a regulatory agency for a market-access decision; model (data model; model for data), a mathematical form specifying the probability distribution of random variables representing observations [here drug concentration(s) and effect(s)] in a subject-matter domain, and which may be the composition of several submodels (e.g. one for PK, another for PD), including ones for the distribution of unobservable conceptual entities (called latent variables in certain domains), e.g. drug clearance in the population; pharmacokinetics (PK), the relationship between drug inflow (a more-general view than dose) and drug concentration(s) at various body sites, notably the so-called biophase(s), or site(s), of drug action, and for which subprocesses (submodels) for drug absorption, distribution, metabolism, and elimination determine the relationship; pharmacodynamics (PD), the relationship between drug concentrations and pharmacological effects (sometimes called surrogate effects, but more properly called bioresponses), and the relationship, in turn, of these responses to clinical outcomes; parameter, a fixed constant serving to quantify some aspect of a model; mechanistic model, a model whose parameters correspond to physical or conceptual entities in the subject-matter domain of the model, e.g. a model of drug distribution to an organ that is parameterized in organ blood flow, volume, and drug diffusivity; empirical model, a nonmechanistic model (a semimechanistic model is the composition of two or more submodels, at least one of which is mechanistic and one empirical); descriptive model, a model that is a priori applicable only to a restricted set of circumstances (designs, patient groups) because values of some or all important design or baseline variables that affect outcomes do not appear explicitly; and predictive model, a model that explicitly incorporates variables quantifying important design and baseline features so that the model can predict outcomes conditional upon arbitrary (and perhaps untested) values of those variables.

DRUG DEVELOPMENT

As discussed previously (12), drug development is an information-gathering process that can be thought of as two successive learn-confirm cycles. The first cycle (traditional phase 1 and phase 2a) addresses the question of whether benefit over existing therapies (in terms of efficacy/safety) can reasonably be expected. It involves learning (phase 1) what is the largest short-term dose that can be administered to humans without causing harm, and then testing (phase 2a) whether that dose induces some measurable short-term benefit in patients for whom the drug is intended to be therapeutic. An affirmative answer at this first stage provides the justification for a more-elaborate second cycle. This next cycle (traditional phase 2b and phase 3) attempts to learn (phase 2b) what is a good (if not optimal) drug regimen to achieve useful clinical value (acceptable benefit/risk) and ends with several [or, for the future, perhaps just one (13)] formal clinical (phase 3) trials of that regimen versus a comparator. If the trial(s) reject the null hypothesis of no incremental benefit of the new drug over the comparator (or occasionally no less benefit), the drug is approvable. Although models are used to assign probability values in the confirmatory analysis of clinical trials, the most credible of such analyses rely on a special class of statistical models, those that make essentially no untestable assumptions. This is a desirable feature, as the fewer the untested assumptions on which a conclusion rests, the less vulnerable to criticism is the conclusion. The independence from assumptions is achieved by focusing inference on the value of a simple statistic whose distribution (the model) depends on controllable study design and not on the origin of the data (i.e. not on a model for the data). An example is when the number of beneficial outcomes in a group randomly assigned to new drug treatment is compared with the number of such in a group randomly assigned to control treatment. The probability that the observed difference in frequencies would arise by chance under the null hypothesis can be assessed using Fisher's exact test, which depends for its validity only on the validity of the randomization and not on the biology underlying the outcomes.

Occasionally, the connection between observed outcomes and conclusions is less direct than in the above example, and inference requires a more-sophisticated model, a data model. For example, when the difference in mean outcomes between drug and control groups is to be compared using a t test, the validity of the inference depends not only on the validity of the randomization, but also on the validity of the assumption that the distribution of outcomes in each group is described by a normal probability law, with identical variances. (In fact, this dependence is weak: The test performs well even when this assumption is not strictly true.) Even in such cases, however, the model is of a particularly simple type: It is a descriptive model of the distribution of the data (or a statistic) under the null hypothesis.

In contrast to the confirming phases of drug development, the learning phases entail so-called explanatory analyses, i.e. analyses that estimate the quantitative relationship between inputs and outcomes according to some mechanistic view of the relationship (see below). What we call inputs are such things as drug dose and timing, patient characteristics, disease stage, etc, and the outcomes are observable clinical results, such as the time between starting treatment and the first occurrence of an untoward event (such as recurrence of neoplasm). Although one might try to view learning as an exercise in confirming (for example, one might test the null hypothesis of no difference between outcomes of small versus large doses), it is far more natural to view learning as the task of constructing a model of the input-outcome relationship itself. This relationship is usually expected to be far more complex than the null hypothesis, which states, with respect to drug inflow at least, that outcome is unrelated to it. A crucial distinction is not only what is being modeled (the drug action, or alternative hypothesis versus the null), but also that the model sought is a predictive one, not a descriptive one. A goal of phase 2b is to predict the best dose for each patient type—old, young, fat, thin, etc—which is a broader objective than to assess the relative value of only those particular doses that happened to be used in the phase 2 trials. Thus, a model suited to learning must interpolate between, and extrapolate beyond, the value of the conditions of the actual study or studies available. The need for a predictive model directly drives the types of models that can be considered as useful learning model candidates—most important, they must be mechanistic as opposed to empirical. That is, they must (*a*) extrapolate beyond the bounds of the design on which they are defined (models must explicitly express the values of those bounds), and (*b*) provide credible extrapolations (models must incorporate the current scientific understanding of their subject matter field).

Empirical models do neither. A mechanistic model, in turn, must be causal: It may not predict outcomes at a given time conditional on events that have not yet occurred. These requirements, as shown below, determine the types of statistical models that are candidates for learning models.

Much has been written about inference for hypothesis testing. There is no need for a review article in a pharmacology journal on this essentially statistical topic. Rather, this article focuses on the uses of scientific predictive models in drug development and on their application primarily to learning, although we also consider their (more controversial) use for confirmation. A companion article (13a) goes into greater detail on a particular new use of predictive models, the activity of designing confirmatory (and learning) trials using computer simulation of predictive models of those trials.

NOTATION

Before proceeding further, it is useful to introduce some notation so that the ideas presented above, and to be elaborated on further below, can be stated with sufficient precision. We consider the unit information-gathering activity in drug development to be the clinical trial and therefore offer notation for this context. In a clinical trial, individuals are chosen for study, are observed for baseline covariates such as sex and age, denoted $\mathbf{X}$ (boldface indicates vectors and matrices), are assigned to treatments, and are treated and observed for outcomes $\mathbf{Y}$, according to a plan, or nominal design, denoted $\mathbf{D}$. Nominal design includes all ostensibly controllable factors affecting the conduct of the trial, e.g. the types and number of subjects, the treatments to be administered, the outcome measurements to be made (and the schedule of those measurements), and the type of data analyses to be performed. It thus defines all the procedures to be followed, all the data to be gathered, and, not to be neglected, the manner in which conclusions (inferences) are to be drawn from those data, including how to deal with missing data (see below). Nominal design depends, therefore, on $\mathbf{X}$, which may be indicated by the notation $\mathbf{D^n} = \mathbf{D^n|X}$.

Nominal design is an abstract ideal. In fact, in any real study, deviations from nominal design are inevitable (e.g. some patients will not follow treatment instructions faithfully). The actual design, i.e. the realized value of the controllable variables, number of individuals, treatments, etc, is denoted $\mathbf{D}$. Technically, one distinguishes between the random variable, say $\mathbf{X}$, i.e. the potential baseline covariate values of an individual, and $\mathbf{x}$, the particular realized value of $\mathbf{X}$ for a given individual. In an abuse of notation, we use the symbol $\mathbf{X}$ (and similarly $\mathbf{D}$, $\mathbf{Y}$) to refer to both of these quantities and hope that the context will make clear which is meant.

The symbol [$\mathbf{A}$] denotes, generically, the probability distribution function for $\mathbf{A}$, if it is a continuous random variable, or probability mass function, if it is discrete. For two (or more) random variables $\mathbf{A}$ and $\mathbf{B}$, the symbol [$\mathbf{A},\mathbf{B}$] denotes their joint probability distribution, [$\mathbf{A}$] denotes the marginal distribution of $\mathbf{A}$ ($\int[\mathbf{A},\mathbf{B}]d\mathbf{B}$), and [$\mathbf{A}|\mathbf{B}$] denotes the conditional distribution of $\mathbf{A}$ given the value of variable $\mathbf{B}$ ([$\mathbf{A},\mathbf{B}$]/[$\mathbf{B}$]). Implicit in this paper is that the models we discuss are parametric models, i.e. they have definite mathematical forms, quantified by a finite (small) number of fixed parameters. We denote the parameters of a distribution generically as θ, and where we wish to draw attention to these, we write, for example, $[A; \theta]$.

ESTIMATION AND INFERENCE FOR PROBABILITY MODELS

Estimation and inference for full probability models is almost always based either on likelihood or on Bayes theory [for a general discussion of these methods as applied to the types of models usually encountered in PK/PD, see Davidian & Giltinan (14); for additional emphasis on Bayesian methods, see Gelman et al (15)]. These two modes of inference are similar; indeed, under the latter view, the former is simply a special case.

With the likelihood approach, a point estimate of the parameter of a model is the parameter value that maximizes the data probability under that model (the estimate is called the maximum likelihood estimate). This amounts to choosing to believe that the true state of nature is, given the chosen form of the model, the instance of that form under which the data that were actually seen are most probable. Likelihood theory also provides a means of assessing the degree to which other states of nature (parameter values) are compatible with the data and, hence, provides a plausible interval or set of parameter values, as those values not contradicted by the data at a certain fixed level of probability.

Bayes theory goes a step further by providing a coherent method of modifying a current view of the state of nature in light of newly acquired data. It does so by regarding the model parameter as an unknown random quantity with a prior distribution that expresses one's current belief as to its likely value (distribution). Bayes theorem is then used to combine this prior distribution with the data likelihood to yield a posterior distribution that represents an updated view of the parameter value, incorporating both prior knowledge and new evidence. The updating procedure involves integration, rather than maximization, a numerically more-challenging problem. The posterior distribution expresses the probability of every possible parameter value; a plausibility region, such as that provided by the likelihood procedure, should it be desired, is then an immediate consequence.

For the purposes of this paper, it makes little difference which of these two methods is contemplated. The central point is that they share the requirement for a probability model for the data. Both are to be distinguished from frequentist theory, which provides no general procedure for estimating complex data models, although certain ad hoc frequentist methods of inference have well-established desirable properties for certain such models.

The past several decades have witnessed major advances in our ability to actually provide maximum likelihood or Bayes estimates of complex models for data. At this point, feasible procedures exist to provide either type of estimate for at least moderately complex models with moderate-to-large (but not very large) data sets (for example, see 14).

MODELS

Once a nominal design is chosen, a clinical trial can be thought of as a series of three steps, each generated by a different model (or submodel). First, a study population is drawn from the model [X]. Given a population and a nominal design, the study can be executed. An actual design (**D**) arises from the model [**D**|**D**^{n},**X**] and ultimately results in outcomes, according to the model [**Y**|**D**,**X**]. (Note the assumption that given the actual design **D**, the nominal design **D**^{n} does not influence the outcomes.)

The above is not quite correct. Strictly speaking, [**D**|**D**^{n},**X**] should be written [**D**|**D**^{n},**X**,**Y**], where (in an abuse of notation) causality demands that the dependence on **Y** of any elements of **D** associated with time t be limited to those elements of **Y** associated with times $s < t$. Likewise, [**Y**|**D**,**X**] is written [**Y**|**D**,**X**,**Y**], where again the dependence of elements of **Y** on elements of **D** or other elements of **Y** is understood to obey the requirements of causality. We now discuss in some further detail the three models defined above.

Covariate Model: [X]

A great deal of data has been accumulated on baseline covariate values in populations as part of clinical trials and also by health care organizations. One may hope to use these empirical distributions for [X] and thereby avoid formal modeling. Models [X] are important for simulating clinical trials (see below) (see also 13a). They are less important for other uses of modeling in drug development, as the particular pattern of covariates of the subjects in a given study can be regarded as fixed and the analysis conditioned on them.

Predictive models of drug action (see below) will usually depend on covariates, and it may be of interest to discover this dependence, for example to determine optimal dosing for a population subgroup such as the elderly. However, the frequency of the elderly in the population (i.e. [X]) is not of central importance; what matters is the relationship between outcomes and being elderly (i.e. [Y|X]).

Deviation from Protocol Model: [D|D^n,X,Y]

Following the conceptualization of Urquhart (16), deviations from protocol can be divided into three types: (a) initiation deviations, e.g. certain types of individuals may selectively refuse to enter the study; (b) compliance (execution) deviations, e.g. some individuals who enter the study may not comply fully with instructions, (missing doses, clinic visits, etc); and (c) termination deviations, i.e. individuals may drop out of the study prematurely for many possible reasons.

Scientific models are unlikely here, as deviations may often depend on such nondeterministic things as personal preference, forgetting, and the like. As for [**X**], one may hope to use empirical probability distributions based on accumulated experience with deviations from protocol in past clinical trials. Parametric models for compliance deviations have also been discussed in the literature (e.g. 17, 18). For reasons discussed more fully below, the model [**D**], unlike the model [**X**], is important not only for simulation, but also for clinical trial interpretation.

Outcome Model: [Y|X,D,Y]

The predictive models of greatest immediate relevance to drug development, and those of greatest relevance to this article, are input-outcome models that relate drug inflow (part of **D**) to clinically important outcomes (part of **Y**), conditional on other inputs, **X**. These models are often referred to as pharmacokinetic/pharmacodynamic (PK/PD) models, as they tend to incorporate submodels for these processes.

Causality is assumed to flow from drug doses through PK processes to concentrations, and thence to pharmacological effects and ultimately to clinical outcomes. This notion involves the intuitively obvious but powerful assumption of conditional independence: Any entity on this causal path is completely determined, given full knowledge of the immediately preceding entity. Thus, given full knowledge of drug concentrations, knowledge of drug inflow contributes nothing to knowledge of pharmacological effects.

This causal view allows one to consider exposure as the conditioning variable for a PD analysis, i.e. when **Y** is restricted to PD observations, one may use the model [**Y**|**X**,E,**Y**], where E is exposure. E may denote any of the entities on the causal path from drug to pharmacological effect: drug inflow rate, plasma drug concentration versus time, biophase drug concentration versus time, the hypothetical level of some signaling or bioeffector substance versus time, or some integrated measure of systemic exposure such as area under the concentration curve (see 19).

Which exposure variable to use is determined by where the rate-limiting step between drug input and PD effect lies. If all processes preceding the PD process are rapid relative to it, a simple nonlinear transformation of drug inflow versus time will serve as well as any more-elaborate exposure measure to drive the PD model. In contrast, if drug distribution to the biophase is rate limiting, then a model for this dynamic process will be indicated. In essence, the concept of exposure allows the explicit appearance of time in the model [**Y**|**X**,E,**Y**] to be eliminated, relegating it to the model [E|**X**,**D**] (or perhaps the more elaborate [E|**X**,**D**,**Y**]).

The deviation from protocol model and the outcome model have thus far been presented as models for generic individuals. But these two models must, like the model for **X**, deal with the variability from individual to individual and within an individual over time. This is discussed below.

STATISTICAL ISSUES IN MODELING

Although it is not always the case, modeling the distribution of a random variable can generally be regarded as two distinct tasks: modeling its mean or expected value (or some other natural "location" parameter), and modeling its variability around that mean (variance, or some other natural "scale" parameter). The model for the expected value generally captures most, if not all, of the mechanistic subject-matter science and is usually the province of the subject-matter expert. In contrast, statisticians are generally most familiar with and expert in modeling random variability. To some extent this separation is unfortunate, as the modeling choices made for each subtask are interdependent. We take the opportunity here to remark on the interaction between them, primarily to point out how the need for mechanistic models limits the options for statistical modeling. Because subtle statistical issues do not arise for [$\mathbf{X}$], for concreteness and clarity of presentation, we limit our discussion in this section to a particular submodel of the outcome model, the PK submodel, but the points made apply equally well to the other parts of the outcome model and to the deviation from protocol model.

Exchangeability and Conditional Independence

The idea of exchangeability is a statistical concept, important to modeling in general and to the issue of predictive versus descriptive models in particular. Data are exchangeable if the joint probability model for all of them is unchanged under a permutation of data indices, i.e. exchanging the position of one datum for that of another. It is usually appropriate to model exchangeable data as independent and identically distributed. Thus, if one can make data exchangeable by appropriate use of covariates and/or subject-specific parameters (see below), the modeling task is made much easier, as one need model only a generic instance of the data (as indeed we have been doing thus far). The joint distribution then becomes simply the product of instances of the generic distribution. In particular, it will almost always be reasonable, introducing the subscript i to distinguish among individuals, to assume that given $\mathbf{X}$ and population parameters $\boldsymbol{\theta}$, observations from different individuals are independent, i.e.

$$[\mathbf{Y}_1, \mathbf{Y}_2, \ldots, \mathbf{Y}_i, \ldots \mid \mathbf{X}_1, \mathbf{X}_2, \ldots, \mathbf{X}_i, \ldots]$$
$$= [\mathbf{Y}_1|\mathbf{X}_1] \, [\mathbf{Y}_2|\mathbf{X}_2] \, .. \, [\mathbf{Y}_i|\mathbf{X}_i]. \ldots \quad 1.$$

Explicit reference to covariates is crucial to establishing exchangeability. Consider, for example, two observed drug concentrations, Y_j and Y_k, drawn from the same individual. A possible model for the distribution of either one might be [Y] = $N(\mu, \sigma^2)$, a normal distribution with mean μ and variance σ^2. For Y_j and Y_k to be exchangeable and independent, then at least the following two assertions must hold. Both concentrations are (a) drawn after a dose of the same magnitude and (b) drawn at the same time after the dose.

If both assertions hold, then the model is an adequate descriptive model of either observation, and the joint distribution of the two observations is $N(\mu,\sigma^2)$ $\times$ $N(\mu,\sigma^2)$. However, if the assertions do not hold, then the observations are not exchangeable and may not be independent, i.e. the above model cannot be used. In contrast, if the model $[Y] = N\{(D_s/V)\exp[-(Cl/V)t_s], \sigma^2\}$ were used instead, where $\mathbf{X}_s = (D_s,t_s)$ and $\boldsymbol{\theta} = (V,Cl)$ for $s = j,k$, then the data would become exchangeable, and independent conditional on $\mathbf{X}$ and $\boldsymbol{\theta}$, and the joint density of Y_j and Y_k would be the product of two instances of the model. This latter model qualifies as a predictive model, as it allows prediction (at least within the individual to whom it applies) of concentrations at other times than (t_j, t_k) after doses other than (D_j, D_k), i.e. predictions of outcomes of experiments not yet performed.

Marginal Models Versus Conditional Models

Although exchangeability simplifies things enormously, as one need consider only a model for $\mathbf{Y}_i$ to have a model for $(\mathbf{Y}_1,\mathbf{Y}_2, \ldots)$, $\mathbf{Y}_i$ itself—considered as a set of observations from an individual on a given occasion—is still multivariate, and its elements are not independent, as they all arise from a common design that is administered to a single "system," the subject i. A so-called marginal model attempts to deal with this intraclass correlation by positing an empirical model for the correlation between the elements of $\mathbf{Y}_i$. Thus, if each individual had five PK measurements, a saturated empirical marginal model would posit a 5×5 covariance matrix for each $\mathbf{Y}_i$, which might be regarded as constant across individuals, thereby introducing $5 \times 6/2 = 15$ so-called nuisance parameters into $\boldsymbol{\theta}$, in addition to the more-interesting population parameters, such as population average (marginal) drug clearance (CL) and volume (V).

The great advantage of this approach is that it allows the modeler to focus on the issues of concern (population average physiology) and allows simple empirical models to handle the statistical complication of intraindividual correlation, which may be of little intrinsic scientific interest. Unfortunately, the price of this convenience can be high. First, how can one be certain that intraindividual variability is not of scientific interest? Avoiding explicit modeling of certain data features runs the risk of hiding important insights. More important, however, this approach provides only a descriptive, not a predictive, model, thus restricting its applicability. In particular, in this example, each person must have five (or fewer) PK observations. Second, for these observations to share a common correlation matrix, they must at least all be taken according to the same time schedule after the same dosage regimen. The approach will fail if each individual receives a different regimen (as is inevitable if medications are self-administered) and/or is observed according to different schedules (inevitable for outpatient studies).

Because of this failing, an alternative, so-called hierarchical model approach has gained currency among PK/PD modelers. This approach establishes within-individual exchangeability, independence, and predictiveness, by conditioning on individual-specific $\mathbf{X}$ and $\mathbf{D}$ and individual-specific parameters. Thus, a minimal hierarchical model for $\mathbf{Y}_i$ is

$$[\mathbf{Y}_i|\mathbf{X}_i, \mathbf{D}_i; \boldsymbol{\theta}] = \int [\mathbf{Y}_i, \boldsymbol{\phi}_i|\mathbf{X}_i, \mathbf{D}_i; \boldsymbol{\theta}] \, d\boldsymbol{\phi}_i = \int [\mathbf{Y}_i|\mathbf{D}_i; \boldsymbol{\phi}_i] \, [\boldsymbol{\phi}_i|\mathbf{X}_i; \boldsymbol{\theta}] \, d\boldsymbol{\phi}_i, \quad 2.$$

where $\boldsymbol{\phi}_i$ is the set of PK parameters of individual i's PK model (for example, volume of distribution and clearance), and $\boldsymbol{\theta}$ consists not only of the population mean values of $\boldsymbol{\phi}_i$, but also of parameters quantifying the extent of their interindividual variability and of others quantifying the magnitude of errors in measurement of the PK observations in $\mathbf{Y}_i$. The model is called hierarchical because at a first level, the distribution of individual elements of $\mathbf{Y}$ depends on parameters $\boldsymbol{\phi}_i$ and design $\mathbf{D}$ (e.g. dose, time), whereas at a second level of the hierarchy, the distribution of $\boldsymbol{\phi}_i$ depends on population parameters $\boldsymbol{\theta}$ and baseline covariates $\mathbf{X}$. A Bayesian approach adds a third level to the hierarchy: a prior distribution on $\boldsymbol{\theta}$, entailing its own hyperparameters.

Note that under the hierarchical formulation (Equation 2), the only PK model that is required (it appears as an expression for the expected value of the conditional model of the first level) is the one that is most familiar to PK modelers: a PK model for the disposition of a drug in a single individual. This is not simply a fortunate accident, it is a direct consequence of the suitability (and hence the reason this form is chosen) of the hierarchical model formulation for the scientific mechanistic view: Physiology (and pharmacology) operates at the level of individuals, not populations; scientific models are available for the former, not the latter.

Informative Missingness

Of particular concern for data analysis is the possibility that $\mathbf{D}$ differs from $\mathbf{D}^n$ in a way that depends on the parameters of the model for $\mathbf{Y}$ (in contrast to the observed $\mathbf{Y}$; dependence on the latter is not a problem) (see below). Such so-called informative deviations may occur, for example, if those dropping out of a study of new drug versus placebo do so because they are not improving. If analysis is made conditional on $\mathbf{D}$, without taking into account its informativeness, the result is not simply that useful information is lost, but also that bias may result: Even if drug is far more effective than placebo, comparison of outcomes only in protocol completers may well show no group difference, as the only individuals remaining to the end in either treatment group are those who improve. This issue has received much attention in the recent statistical literature (for example, see 20, 21).

In the above example, let T denote the time at which an individual drops out and after which no further data are gathered (T can be set to infinity for study completers). Let $\mathbf{Y}$ denote the outcome variable of primary interest, the severity of illness at fixed times after study treatment begins. The data from an individual is $(\mathbf{Y},T)$, where $\mathbf{Y}$ consists only of observations scheduled before time T.

The standard approach to a dropout problem such as this is somehow to impute the missing data ("last observation carried forward" is one such imputation scheme) and analyze the now "complete" data using the analysis procedure proposed by the nominal design. This approach has many problems, but it may sometimes suffice for a (conservative) confirmatory analysis (but see 21). It is clearly inappropriate, however, to invent data and treat it as real when the goal is a predictive model.

A possibly better approach to dealing with the informativeness of T is to subdivide the patients into those with like values of T and to perform separate comparative analyses in each group (20). This is tantamount to factoring $[\mathbf{Y},T]$ as $[\mathbf{Y}|T][T]$, a so-called pattern mixture model (22), and estimating the first and more-interesting factor only.

The problem with the pattern mixture model approach is that it is neither mechanistic nor predictive. It is not mechanistic because it defies causality: T depends on $\mathbf{Y}$ at T (or before), not the other way around. It cannot be predictive because we cannot know an individual's T beforehand, and thus cannot know which of the several $[\mathbf{Y}|T]$ models to apply to his data. Note, however, that the model may serve well as a descriptive one for a confirmatory analysis, e.g. of whether benefit is greater in the drug-treated group than in the placebo group at any given level of duration of study participation.

A mechanistic approach factors $[\mathbf{Y},T]$ as $[T|\mathbf{Y}][\mathbf{Y}]$, a so-called selection model. This model is causal, and the second factor is the model of true interest: the nondropout treatment-response model. The problem with this approach is that one may be forced to make assumptions about the form of $[\mathbf{Y}]$ that are not testable on the data at hand because key observations are missing, i.e. $[\mathbf{Y}]$ may not be fully identifiable on the current data. Assumptions based on the subject-matter science (i.e. prior knowledge) and use of a fully Bayesian framework may allow credible inference nonetheless. The use of a selection model formulation becomes both easier and more credible when the additional assumption can be made that $[T|\mathbf{Y}]$ depends not on "true" $\mathbf{Y}$ but only on the actually observed values of $\mathbf{Y}$. In this case, T is said to be ignorable, as it contains no information about $[\mathbf{Y}]$ not already available in the observed $\mathbf{Y}$ itself. If this assumption can be made, one may fit $[\mathbf{Y}]$ to $\mathbf{Y}$ and not bother with $[T|\mathbf{Y}]$ if it is not of interest [for recent examples of analyses of the same type of study, an analgesic trial, using selection models with and without the ignorability assumption, see Sheiner et al (23) and Pulkstenis et al (24)].

USES OF MODELING IN DRUG DEVELOPMENT

From the producer's or sponsor's point of view, the goal of (commercial) drug development is market-access approval so profits can be made. From the consumer's point of view, the goal is useful remedies. The producer's profit incentive is constrained to serve the consumer's needs by regulation, which tries to insure that market access is granted only to products that are likely to produce net benefit when used in the approved manner for the approved class of individuals. For regulation to work as intended, the final regulatory hurdle prior to market entry must be relatively objective. Confirmatory trials and analyses fulfill this criterion, as discussed above, whereas explanatory ones do not. Thus, in theory, modeling can only prove useful to those activities in drug development where great objectivity is not essential (Table 1).

Development decisions—i.e. which molecules will be carried forward, what studies will be done in what order, the design of specific studies on which go/no-go decisions will be based, etc—influence essentially only the producer's risk. Here the consumer's and producer's motivations coincide, and regulation need not be invoked, except to protect the safety of human subjects. Modeling can be useful here by providing credible simulations of studies and development plans (see 13a) that allow their relative merits to be quantified.

The labeling items noted in Table 1 all provide details on the conditions of use required to extract net benefit. If the physician can be assured of adequate safety of an initial regimen, he or she can usually titrate an individual to a useful dosage schedule, making suggested dosage and individualized adjustments merely guidelines, rather than essential. Likewise, cautioning use of a drug in a subpopulation is prudent and does not enhance consumer risk.

The usual intention-to-treat analysis of a confirmatory trial provides estimates of the outcome difference attributable to the prescription of the drug, not of the actual taking of it (25). Yet some indication of the actual benefit to be gained

TABLE 1   Modeling in drug development: activities for which great objectivity is not required

Development decisions
    Development Planning
    Study design
Labeling
    Dosage regimens
    Dosage adjustments for special populations
    Safety restrictions
    Quantifying benefit
Market-access testing
    Great potential benefit
    High prior presumption of positive benefit/risk
    Excessive "cost" of objective evidence
    More powerful statistical tests

when a drug is taken as instructed is useful and, using current confirmatory trial designs, can be obtained only through model-based explanatory analyses. Such information, even if somewhat uncertain, can only benefit consumers.

Given the discussions above, it is surprising there are any circumstances under which modeling is admissible in testing for the market access decision. Yet where there is great potential benefit, lesser objectivity may be allowed for market access, with appropriate follow-up requirements. This is the basis of the accelerated approval policy of 1992 by the Food and Drug Administration (FDA) (26), used so effectively to allow anti-HIV treatments to be marketed only shortly after preliminary indications of efficacy and safety were available. One may take the recent FDA mandate (13) to consider a single study plus "confirmatory evidence" (an unfortunate choice of words, as their "confirmatory" is synonymous with our "explanatory") as adequate for approval as another step toward blending strictly objective evidence with evidence more sensitive to assumptions, even where great potential benefit is not an issue.

Where benefit/risk appears well known from prior data, market access may be granted based on less-objective evidence. This is the basis for granting ANDA (Abbreviated New Drug Application) approval to generic preparations based on bioequivalence measures. High prior presumption of favorable benefit/risk, combined with the fear that obtaining objective data will either be excessively costly or present unacceptable ethical risks, presumably underlies the recent proposal to grant approval for drugs approved for adults to be used in the pediatric population, based largely on the use of PK/PD modeling to bridge adult and pediatric data (27).

A final, more-technical application of modeling to market-access decisions is its use to assure that confirmatory analyses invoking complex but more-powerful statistical tests do not increase consumer risk. A nice approach is provided by Rubin and coworkers (28, 29). These authors show how the analysis of a clinical trial marred by noncompliance, but fulfilling certain assumptions (such as that access to the experimental treatment is impossible for those not assigned to it), can test the null hypothesis of no drug effect against the (powerful) alternative that a drug acts beneficially among those assigned to it only in those who actually receive it. This alternative contrasts with the usual (less powerful) intention-to-treat alternative, that benefit accrues from assignment, regardless of receipt. In this example, simulation, and hence a model, essentially for noncompliance is needed to assign a P value to the more-powerful "instrumental variables analysis" statistic. All assumptions are explicit, so that regulators can decide whether they are credible.

EXAMPLES OF MODELING IN DRUG DEVELOPMENT

Table 2, organized to reflect the categories of Table 1 but expanding on it somewhat, cites conditions for the use of modeling in drug development and provides public-domain examples. Table 2 also specifies which types of models and what sources of experimental data are required for the particular use. The types of experimental data are categorized and denoted as follows: S1, preclinical, in vitro, or in vivo animal; S2, normal human subjects; and S3, diseased human subjects. Note in particular that most of the analyses in Table 2 at least allow, if they do not positively benefit from, pooling of data from multiple sources and studies. The explicit recognition of variation in **X** and **D** by mechanistic models allows such synthesis, which is difficult if not impossible with the empirical models used for confirmatory analyses. This represents perhaps the greatest single virtue of the model-based approach.

The examples listed and discussed in Table 2, and those discussed above, confirm that mathematical modeling has achieved a degree of maturity that allows it to make a useful contribution to drug development. This point has also been made from various perspectives in several recent survey papers (for example, see 30–35).

PRACTICAL ISSUES FOR MODELING

Despite the overwhelming evidence of utility, as provided above, modeling is not yet in the mainstream of drug development. This is partly because, despite repeated claims that PK and PD principles should guide drug development (5, 30, 74–76), the potential of the approach is still underestimated. Among the prominent factors preventing full application of PK/PD modeling, Reigner et al (32) cite the variable understanding of PK/PD concepts among the members of the (project) teams in charge of development within pharmaceutical companies. Notwithstanding, the key problem, in our opinion, is that the potential rewards of PK/PD modeling (as defined in this paper) cannot be realized without a substantial investment of time and resources, and any additional investment of time in development is perceived nowadays as a delay.

Indeed, modeling will delay development if it is not adequately planned for and integrated into the clinical development program. Until modeling gains the same recognition, sponsorship, and stature as other drug developmental activities, such as in vitro or animal in vivo studies, it cannot deliver on its promise to increase efficiency and comprehensiveness of knowledge. How this might be accomplished is discussed further in the next section.

In contrast, we do not believe that regulatory attitudes toward modeling are important factors impeding its greater application. Indeed, regulatory attitudes toward using model-based analyses as part of a submission for approval for market access seem generally in line with the theoretical positions presented herein (see above). Use of explanatory analyses for labeling have been encouraged for years [e.g. use of the so-called pharmacokinetic screen (54, 77)]. Several ICH (International Conference on Harmonization) guidelines [e.g. ICH4 on dose-response information (78)] make explicit reference to modeling for such purposes as dose ranging, and the US FDA has issued a *Guidance for Industry* on popu-

TABLE 2 Pharmacokinetic/pharmacodynamic (PK/PD) modeling in drug development: examples and features[a]

Area	Goal	Data source	Pool data[b]	Add'l models[c]	Examples (References)
General	Improve methodology for drug-effect assessment, evaluate value of pharmacological surrogates	S1—S3	+	—	One major task of (and opportunity for) clinical pharmacology is to help identify and validate PD surrogates (36). As recent examples in the cardiovascular (37) and CNS (38, 39) areas illustrate, mechanistic PK/PD understanding (and appropriate modeling procedures) will be needed in order to ascertain the degree of validity of surrogates for efficacy determination.
	Use observational data	S2, S3	+ +	[D|X]	A Markov mixed effect model was proposed to describe and quantify observational compliance data (collected via electronic medication monitor systems) in HIV-positive patients taking zidovudine (18, 40). The model is likely to have broad validity in other therapeutic areas, and to serve as a useful tool for simulation and model-based analysis of clinical trial data. The use of observational data on drug systemic exposure from a clinical trial with primary therapeutic objectives provides additional insight into the dose-effect relationship (30), as it also does in complex situations such as anti-HIV combination therapy (41).
Preclinical	Explore implications of data/models	S2, S3	+ + +	[X], [D|D[n],X]	Based on a model of infectious and noninfectious HIV virions, model-based analysis of existing data showed that direct measurement of infectious viral load provided sufficient information to estimate antiretroviral drug efficacy (42).

	Screen lead compounds	S1	—	Physiologically based PK/PD modeling helped select the short-acting intravenous sedatives that were most likely to improve on midazolam (32).
	Develop PK/PD models	S1	+ +	A variety of effect measurements and mathematical modeling techniques were developed using animal experiments with psychotropics (7), opioids (9), anti-convulsants (10), and cardiovascular agents (8).
	Animal-man scale-up	S1	+ + +	Evidence that reliable predictions of clearance, PK parameters and Conc × time & Effect × time profiles in man can be made from animal data is accumulating (32, 43). (For a review, see 6.)
Drug development (plan)	Guide dose-escalation in entry into human studies	S1	—	Successful PK/PD-based choices of dose range and regimen have been reported in such diverse therapeutic areas as oncology, anticoagulant therapy, and infectious disease (32).
	Select lead compound	S1	—	Mechanistic mathematical modeling offers a way to determine the relative potencies of compounds with similar modes of action, e.g. 5alpha-reductase inhibitors (44) and benzodiazepines (45).
	Discontinue indication	S3	+	Model-based predictions were corroborated by clinical trial results, and provided a rationale for stopping development of a new formulation of interferon with improved PK. PK/PD modeling revealed that increasing the circulating half-life of interferon 2a twofold was of limited therapeutic benefit (32, 46).

(continued)

TABLE 2 *Continued*

Area	Goal	Data source	Pool data[b]	Add'l models[c]	Examples (References)
	Which drug/drug interactions require study	S1–S3	+	—	Assessment of drug/drug interactions in vivo may be achieved through "many" interaction studies, as for ciprofloxacin (47). Mechanistic model-based PK analyses (48, 49) help assess which interactions are likely and provides novel quantitative tools for study design and analyses.
	Select dosage and/or regimen for phase 2 and/or phase 3	S1, S2	+ +	[X]	Several drug companies found that dual modeling of exposure-efficacy and exposure-safety relationships in phases 1 and 2a allows more reliable and sometimes earlier determination of the correct dose for pivotal therapeutic trials (32, 50).
	Design phase 3 trial	S1–S3	+ + +	[X], [DID^n,X]	Model-based study design has been used in transplantation (51), Alzheimer's disease (52), and HIV therapy (42). Clinical trial simulation is currently an area of active research (13a).
	Design trial for special populations	S2, S3	+ + +	[X], [DID^n,X]	Studies in special populations (e.g. the very young or the very old) impose severe restrictions on data collection (e.g. sparse blood sampling for PK) (53, 54), which imply model-based data analysis. This also applies to studies of diseases with high prevalence only in developing countries [e.g. malaria (55)].

Special objectives	S3	+	[X]	Applications of modeling include the evaluation of impact of dosing omissions of a dopaminomimetic on prolactin suppression (56), the description of change in action of levodopa in presence of an inhibitor of its metabolism (57), and the measurement of in vivo parameters (e.g. insulin sensitivity) in provocation tests (e.g. intravenous glucose tolerance test) (58, 59).
Labeling				
Dosage regimen	S2, S3	+ + +	[X]	The recommended initial dose of ketorolac for postoperative pain was based on the model-based relationship between dose, time postdose, and percentage of patients with adequate pain relief (60).
Assess new formulation	S2, S3	−	−	Assessing the value of a new formulation through model-based prediction of concentration and/or effect time courses can provide a rationale for, e.g., a long-acting PEG-interferon (61) or against further development [e.g. an early formulation of PEG-interferon (46) or lithium in manic-depressive disorders (62)].
Assess need for specific population study	S2, S3	+ + +	−	Integrated model-based analysis of existing data (i.e. in numero investigations; see below) can provide a rationale for dosage adjustment in special patient populations, e.g. remifentanil (63), ondansetron (64), S12024 (52). Model-based evidence, if convincing, may obviate the need for specific experimental studies, e.g. in renal insufficiency.
Safety restriction	S3	+ +	−	A population PK analysis helped to delineate the risk of the anti-cancer agent docetaxel in patients with liver insufficiency (65, 66).

(continued)

85

TABLE 2 *Continued*

Area	Goal	Data source	Pool data[b]	Add'l models[c]	Examples (References)
	Quantify benefit "confirmatory"	S3	+ +	[DID[n],X]	Variable compliance affects the mean outcome in the treated group: A model-based "instrumental variables" analysis was shown to provide an unbiased estimate of the fully compliant response, with minimal assumptions (29).
	Integrated summary of PK and PD	S2, S3	+ + +	[X], [DID[n],X]	The Dose-AUC relationship of saquinavir was characterized over a broad range of doses, conditions, and formulations, using data from 23 human studies (67). An ambitious development would be the integrated model-based analysis of all pre-ANDA PK (or PD) data for a new drug, as part of the regulatory dossier. We do not know of any such example.
Market-access testing	Bridging (ethnic groups)	S2, S3	+ + +	–	PK/PD modeling has been used to bridge clinical data (and adjust dosage) across races (e.g. Caucasian and Japanese) (68). This provides an opportunity for making global development plans "leaner" and less demanding of patient populations.
	Extended or meta-analysis of prior studies for "confirmatory" evidence	S2, S3	+ + +	[DID[n],X]	Model-based meta-analysis of pooled PD data from multiple clinical studies with different designs helped strengthen the claim for efficacy and provided quantitative estimates of type and magnitude of action [e.g. for tacrine's action on disease progression in Alzheimer's disease (69, 70) and felodipine in hypertension (71)].

Extension to new population (e.g. pediatrics)	S1–S3	+ + +	—	Mechanistic modeling, e.g. for valproic acid (72) and erythropoietin (73), provided a framework for extrapolating PK and PD from adults to pediatrics, with substantial improvement over empirical allometric scaling.
Model-based tests of efficacy	—	—	[X], [DID^n,X]	The power of a test of the null hypothesis *vs* the instrumental variables alternative (drug acts only in those who take it) is greater than that of the conventional ITT approach (drug acts in all assigned to it, regardless of whether it is taken or not) (29; see text).

[a] CNS, Central nervous system; PEG, polyethylene glycol; AUC, area under the concentration; ANDA, Abbreviated New Drug Application; ITT, Intention-To-Treat.

[b] +, The degree to which the analyses will profit from pooling data from several studies.

[c] Models needed in addition to input-outcome model, [YID,X].

87

lation pharmacokinetics (79), which opens the door to widespread application of mixed-effects predictive models. The guidance stresses the need for high standards of quality for both data and modeling methodology. A similar initiative was recently taken by the Australian authorities (35). We have already referred to the FDA *Modernization Act* (13) and the recent FDA guidance on pediatrics (27) as evidence that the FDA will accept scientific model–based evidence for efficacy where there is high prior presumption of same, and/or where strong empirical evidence is difficult or impossible to obtain.

PERSPECTIVES

We view future developments in the following areas as crucial to progress.

Good Practices

The paper by Peck et al (13a) largely reflects the consensus of a recent conference (80) (see also http://www.dml.georgetown.edu/depts/pharmacology/cdds/SDDGP .html), where good practices in modeling and simulation of clinical trials are discussed and summarized in a consensus paper. Improved practices for simulation will have major positive impact on other modeling activities in drug development, because the essential requirements for good practice are the same: transparency, clarity, completeness of documentation, and parsimony.

Legitimacy of Modeling

Modeling will not reach its potential utility until it is recognized as a visible and separate work unit within a drug development program. We propose to call that unit an in numero study, i.e. a protocol-driven exercise designed to extract additional information, and/or answer a specific drug-development question, through an integrated model-based (meta-) analysis of existent raw data, often pooled across (clinical) studies. For the in numero study to be recognized as a separate work unit, at least the following changes in the organization of the development process will be required: (*a*) greater continuity of scientific personnel between phase 1 and phase 2; (*b*) increasing involvement of scientists with modeling backgrounds at the beginning of and during clinical development; and (*c*) participation of pharmacometricians (individuals specifically skilled in mathematical modeling and the subject matter of PK/PD) on pivotal team decisions (e.g. through provision of key model-based computer simulations) (see 13a).

Modeling Databases

An impressive variety of PK/PD models have already been defined and applied to numerous drugs. If such modeling is to become even more useful and efficient, a database of accumulated experience (models and results) will be indispensable.

Needless to say, developing, maintaining, and updating such a database is a formidable task; drug-development scientists do not yet have even a common vocabulary (witness our need to define notation in this article).

Increasingly, drugs are being developed that exhibit high-affinity interaction only for specific receptors. Quantitative signals of such specific interaction ("biomarkers") will undoubtedly be forthcoming and will serve as surrogates for clinical efficacy. Thus, we may expect the future to bring richer and more-detailed PK/PD data, and hence greater opportunity for informative modeling. Yet such modeling faces the following difficulty: Most of the (new) data on drug kinetics and dynamics is generated by the pharmaceutical industry, whereas most of the aggregated (and cleaned) data across compounds within a given class resides in regulatory agencies (e.g. FDA), and much of the talent and time required for developing models is to be found within academia. A cooperative model-building effort is therefore necessary and will be facilitated by the evolution of information technology. Even if technical difficulties are surmounted, however, collaboration implies the sharing in the public domain of new and potentially valuable information, and business practices designed to impede leakage of such information will present barriers to progress.

Methodology

Advances in measurement, modeling, and computation are likely to further expand the spectrum of application of PK/PD modeling in drug development. In the past decades, major progress has been made in developing chemical assays of drugs and metabolites in multiple body fluids, and most notably in developing reliable, sensitive, reproducible, quickly responsive, and noninvasive in vivo measurements of drug effects in man (81–83).

Progress in modeling goes hand-in-hand with progress in measurement. The first steps in the pathway from dose to (clinical) effect (concentration in blood, concentration in biophase, mass-action effect on receptors, and thence on the dynamics of a signaling molecule) are relatively well understood in principle, if not in detail in every case, and prototype-model schemas exist that can be elaborated parametrically or nonparametrically to suit the circumstances (19, 45). However, models in several key generic areas are missing or need considerable improvement.To discuss this only briefly:

1. $[X]$: Systematic differences may exist between patients recruited to studies and those in the population ultimately to be treated.
2. $[D|D^n,X,Y]$: Compliance and dropout are receiving increasing attention in the statistics literature (17, 18, 23, 84), as analyses conditioned on these become observational studies, subject to confounding (25). Standard remedies (e.g. intention to treat, last observation carried forward) even in the pure confirmatory context can be shown not always to be conservative (21). Analyses incorporating compliance will have to deal with missing data (not all compli-

ance is observed), and for this a model for compliance is needed. A Markov mixed-effects model (18) is a start but requires further validation and improvement.

3. **[Y|D,X,Y]**: Mechanistic physiological models are high dimensional. They can be made practical by limiting the degrees of freedom through informative prior distributions in a full Bayesian analysis (for example, see 85). Models for chronic-disease progress are often simple (e.g. linear with time), especially in cases where the timescale of a clinical trial is short relative to that of the progression of disease. Nonetheless, in any real trial, disease progress is confounded with placebo effect for all patients, and thus sorting out progress/ placebo from progress/placebo/drug can be a difficult exercise in identifiability (for an interesting example, see 69, 70). Mechanistic models for circadian variation in PK/PD (for example, see 37, 86) or the link between exposure and adverse effects (for example, see 87) are not yet well developed and require further work.

Essential to increased application of PK/PD modeling techniques has been and may remain the spectacular increase in computational power of the past decade. This has made practical such computationally intensive numerical techniques as (*a*) Markov Chain Monte-Carlo methods for estimation of full (Bayesian) probability models of data (88), (*b*) bootstrap and other sample-reuse methods for honest inference from complex-model analyses (89, 90) [use of this approach has also been suggested in a recent draft by the FDA guidance on bioequivalence for determining confidence bounds (91)], and (*c*) simulation of complex models for experimental design (see 13a).

The view that modeling merits increased application to clinical investigation appears to be shared by others; for example, recent papers appearing in the statistics literature (92, 93) emphasize the value of model-based approaches to clinical biostatistics, the key role that the biostatistician can play as a modeler (in the sense used herein), and, if he is to do so, the fact that he will need increased understanding of the subject-matter science (here, PK/PD).

In our view, the future is bright for increased application of modeling in drug development, as such application is simply a means to, and manifestation of, the transformation of the intellectual basis of drug development from empiricism to science. Such transformations in other domains have inevitably entailed uncomfortable change, but just as inevitably they have brought rapid and spectacular progress.

ACKNOWLEDGMENTS

This work was supported in part by (LBS) NIH grant GM26676.

Visit the Annual Reviews home page at www.AnnualReviews.org.

LITERATURE CITED

1. Holford N, Sheiner L. 1981. Understanding the dose-effect relationship: clinical applications of pharmacokinetic/pharmacodynamic models. *Clin. Pharmacokinet.* 6:429–53
2. Holford N, Sheiner L. 1981. Pharmacokinetic and pharmacodynamic modelling in vivo. *CRC Crit. Rev. Bioeng.* 5:273
3. Derendorf H, Meibohm B. 1999. Modeling of pharmacokinetic/pharmacodynamic (PK/PD) relationships: concepts and perspectives. *Pharm. Res.* 16:176–85
4. Senn S. 1997. *Statistical Issues in Drug Development. Statistics in Practice.* New York: Wiley
5. Campbell D. 1990. The use of kinetic-dynamic interactions in the evaluation of drugs. *Psychopharmacology* 100:433–50
6. Lave T, Coassolo P, Reigner B. 1999. Prediction of hepatic metabolism clearance based on interspecies allometric scaling techniques and in vitro-in vivo correlations. *Clin. Pharmacokinet.* 36: 211–31
7. Mandema J. 1991. *EEG effect measures and relationships between pharmacokinetics and pharmacodynamics of psychotropic drugs.* PhD thesis. Leiden Univ., Leiden, The Netherlands. 318 pp.
8. Mathot R. 1995. *Preclinical pharmacokinetic-pharmacodynamic modelling of the cardiovascular effects of adenosine receptor ligands.* PhD thesis. Leiden Univ., Leiden, The Netherlands. 306 pp.
9. Cox E. 1997. *Preclinical pharmacokinetic-pharmacodynamic relationships of synthetic opioids.* PhD thesis. Leiden Univ., Leiden, The Netherlands. 207 pp.
10. Della Paschoa O. 1998. *Preclinical pharmacokinetic-pharmacodynamic modelling of the anticonvulsant effect.* PhD thesis. Leiden Univ., Leiden, The Netherlands. 237 pp.
11. Blower S, Porco T, Darby G. 1998. Predicting and preventing the emergence of antiviral drug resistance in HSV-2. *Nat. Med.* 4:673–78
12. Sheiner L. 1997. Learning versus confirming in clinical drug development. *Clin. Pharmacol. Ther.* 61:275–91
13. Food Drug Admin. 1997. *Food Drug Mod. Act 1997.* Subsect. 115: *Food Drug Cosmet. Act,* Sect. 505D. Washington, DC: US Gov. Print. Off.
13a. Holford NHG, Kimko HC, Monteleone JPR, Peck CC. 2000. Simulation of Clinical Trials. *Annu. Rev. Pharm. Tox.* 40:209–34.
14. Davidian M, Giltinan D. 1995. *Nonlinear Models for Repeated Measurement Data.* London: Chapman & Hall
15. Gelman A, Carlin J, Stern H, Rubin D. 1995. *Bayesian Data Analysis.* London: Chapman & Hall
16. Urquhart J. 1999. Variable patient compliance as a source of variability in drug response. *Estave Found. Conf. Var. Hum. Drug Response, 1998, Sitges, Spain. Excerpta Med. Congr. Ser.,* Vol. 1178. In press
17. De Klerk E, Van der Linden S, Van der Heijde D, Urquhart J. 1997. Facilitated analysis of data on drug regimen compliance. *Stat. Med.* 16:1653–64
18. Girard P, Blaschke T, Kastrissios H, Sheiner L. 1998. A Markov mixed-effect regression model for drug compliance. *Stat. Med.* 17:2313–33
19. Verotta D, Sheiner L. 1995. A general conceptual model for non-steady-state pharmacokinetic/pharmacodynamic data (plus response and rejoinder). *J. Pharmacokinet. Biopharmcol.* 23:1–10
20. Wu M, Bailey K. 1989. Estimation and comparison of changes in the presence of informative right censoring: conditional linear model. *Biometrics* 45:939–55
21. Frangakis C, Rubin D. 1999. Addressing complications of intention-to-treat analysis in the combined presence of all-

or-none treatment-noncompliance and subsequent missing outcomes. *Biometrika* 86:365–79

22. Little R. 1993. Pattern-mixture models for multivariate incomplete data. *J. Am. Stat. Assoc.* 88:125–34

23. Sheiner L, Beal S, Dunne A. 1997. Analysis of non-randomly censored ordered categorical longitudinal data from analgesic trials (with comment & rejoinder). *J. Am. Stat. Assoc.* 92:1235–55

24. Pulkstenis E, Ten Have T, Landis J. 1998. Model for the analysis of binary longitudinal pain data subject to informative dropout through remediation. *J. Am. Stat. Assoc.* 93:438–50

25. Sheiner L, Rubin D. 1995. Intention-to-treat analysis and the goals of clinical trials. *Clin. Pharmacol. Ther.* 57:6–15

26. Food and Drug Admin. 1992. New Drug, Antibiotic, and Biological Product Regulations; Accelerated Approval; Final Rule. Washington, DC: US Gov. Print. Off.

27. Food and Drug Admin. 1996. *Content and Format for Pediatric Use Supplement.* Washington DC: Cent. Drug Eval. Res., FDA

28. Angrist J, Imbens G, Rubin D. 1996. Identification of causal effects using instrumental variables. *J. Am. Stat. Assoc.* 91:444–72

29. Rubin D. 1998. More powerful randomization-based p-values in double-blind trials with non-compliance. *Stat. Med.* 17:371–85

30. Steimer J, Ebelin M, Van Bree J. 1993. Pharmacokinetic and pharmacodynamic data and models in clinical trials. *Eur. J. Drug Metab. Pharmacokinet.* 18:61–76

31. Vozeh S, Steimer J, Rowland M, Morselli P, Mentre F, et al. 1996. The use of population pharmacokinetics in drug development. *Clin. Pharmacokinet.* 30:81–93

32. Reigner B, Williams P, Patel I, Steimer J, Peck C, et al. 1997. An evaluation of the integration of pharmacokinetic and pharmacodynamic principles in clinical drug development. Experience within

Hoffmann La Roche. *Clin. Pharmacokinet.* 33:142–52

33. Samara E, Granneman R. 1997. Role of population pharmacokinetics in drug development: a pharmaceutical industry perspective. *Clin. Pharmacokinet.* 32: 294–312

34. Minto C, Schnider T. 1998. Expanding clinical applications of population pharmacodynamic modeling. *Br. J. Clin. Pharmacol.* 46:321–33

35. Tett S, Holford N, McLachlan A. 1998. Population pharmacokinetics and pharmacodynamics: an underutilized resource. *Drug Inf. J.* 32:693–710

36. Rolan P. 1997. The contribution of clinical pharmacology surrogates and models to drug development—a critical appraisal. *Br. J. Clin. Pharmacol.* 44:219–25

37. Hempel G, Karlsson M, De Alwis D, Toublanc N, Mc Nay J, et al. 1998. Population pharmacokinetic-pharmacodynamic modeling of moxonidine using 24-hour ambulatory blood pressure measurements. *Clin. Pharmacol. Ther.* 64:622–35

38. Billard V, Gambus P, Chamoun N, Stanski D, Shafer S. 1997. A comparison of spectral edge, delta power, and bispectral index as EEG measures of alfentanil, propofol, and midazolam drug effect. *Clin. Pharmacol. Ther.* 61:45–58

39. Mahmood I, Tammara V, Baweja R. 1998. Does percent reduction in seizure frequency correlate with plasma concentration of anticonvulsant drugs? Experience with four anticonvulsant drugs. *Clin. Pharm. Ther.* 64:547–52

40. Vanhove G, Schapiro J, Winters M, Merigan T, Blaschke T. 1996. Patient compliance and drug failure in protease inhibitor monotherapy. *JAMA* 276: 1955–56

41. Vanhove G, Gries J, Verotta D, Sheiner L, Coombs R, et al. 1997. Exposure-response relationships for saquinavir, zidovudine and zalcitabine in combination therapy. *Antimicrob. Agents Chemother.* 41:2433–38

42. Wu H, Ding A, De Gruttola V. 1998.

Estimation of HIV dynamic parameters. *Stat. Med.* 17:2463–85

43. Mahmood I, Balian J. 1999. The pharmacokinetic principles behind scaling from preclinical results to phase I protocols. *Clin. Pharmacokinet.* 36:1–11

44. Olsson Gisleskog P, Hermann D, Hammarlund-Udenaes M, Karlsson M. 1998. A model for the turnover of dihydrotestosterone in the presence of the irreversible 5?-reductase inhibitors GI198745 and finasteride. *Clin. Pharmacol. Ther.* 64:636–47

45. Tuk B, Danhof M, Mandema J. 1998. *In vivo modeling of mechanisms of receptor mediated pharmacological responses.* PhD thesis. Leiden Univ., Leiden, The Netherlands. 204 pp.

46. Nieforth K, Nadeau R, Patel I, Mould D. 1996. Use of an indirect pharmacodynamic stimulation model of MX protein induction to compare in vivo activity of interferon alfa-2a and a polyethylene glycol-modified derivative in healthy subjects. *Clin. Pharmacol. Ther.* 59:636–46

47. Schaefer H, Ahr G, Kuhlmann J. 1995. Pharmacokinetic development of quinolone antibiotics. *Int. J. Clin. Pharmacol. Ther. Toxicol.* 33:266–76

48. Tucker G. 1992. The rational selection of drug interaction studies: implications of recent advances in drug metabolism. *Int. J. Clin. Pharmacol. Ther. Toxicol.* 30:550–53

49. Ludden T. 1997. Evaluation of potential drug-drug interactions using the population approach. See Ref. 94, pp. 41–45

50. Nichols D, Milligan P, Jonsson E, Karlsson M. 1997. Application of population analysis in phase I/II clinical drug development. See Ref. 94, pp. 215–25

51. Hale M, Nicholls A, Bullingham R, Hene R, Hoitsma A, et al. 1998. The pharmacokinetic-pharmacodynamic relationship for mycophenolate mofetil in renal transplantation. *Clin. Pharm. Ther.* 64:672–83

52. Laveille C, Lachaud-Pettiti V, Neuman E, Jochemsen R. 1998. Application of population pharmacokinetics to the phase II development of an anti-Alzheimer's disease compound, S12024. *J. Clin. Pharmacol.* 38:315–23

53. Collart L, Blaschke T, Boucher F, Prober C. 1992. Potential of population pharmacokinetics to reduce the frequency of blood sampling required for estimating kinetic parameters in neonates. *Dev. Pharmacol. Ther.* 18:71–80

54. Temple R. 1983. The Testing of Drugs in the Elderly. Memo. Sept. 30. Washington, DC: FDA

55. Ezzet F, Mull R, Karbwang J. 1998. Population pharmacokinetics and therapeutic response of CGP 56697 (artemether + benflumetol) in malaria patients. *Br. J. Clin. Pharmacol.* 46:553–61

56. Grevel J, Brownell J, Steimer J, Gaillard R, Rosenthaler J. 1986. Description of the time-course of the prolactin suppressant effect of the dopamine agonist CQP201–403 by an integrated pharmacokinetic-pharmacodynamic model. *Br. J. Clin. Pharmacol.* 22:1–13

57. Troconiz I, Naukkarinen T, Ruottinen H, Rinne U, Gordin A, et al. 1998. Population pharmacodynamic modeling of levodopa in patients with Parkinson's disease receiving entacapone. *Clin. Pharm. Ther.* 64:106–16

58. Bergman R, Cobelli C. 1980. Minimal modeling, partition analysis, and the estimation of insulin sensitivity. *Fed. Proc.* 39:110–15

59. Bergman RN, Prager R, Volund A, Olefsky JM. 1987. Equivalence of the insulin sensitivity index in man derived by the minimal model method and the euglycemic glucose clamp. *J. Clin. Invest.* 79:790–800

60. Mandema J, Stanski D. 1996. Population pharmacodynamic model for ketorolac analgesia. *Clin. Pharmacol. Ther.* 60:619–35

61. Xu R, Rakhit A, Patel I, van Brummelen P. 1998. PK/PD modeling approach to support clinical development of a long-acting interferon (Ro 25–3036) for the

treatment of chronic hepatitis. *Clin. Pharmacol. Ther.* 63:162

62. Gaillot J, Steimer J, Mallet A, Thebault J, Bieder A. 1979. A priori lithium dosage regimen using population characteristics of pharmacokinetic parameters. *J. Pharmacokinet. Biopharmcol.* 7:579–628

63. Minto C, Schnider T, Egan T, Youngs E, Lemmens H, et al. 1997. Influence of age and gender on the pharmacokinetics and pharmacodynamics of remifentanil. I. Model development. *Anesthesiology* 86:10–23

64. De Alwis D, Aarons L, Palmer J. 1998. Population pharmacokinetics of ondansetron: a covariate analysis. *Br. J. Clin. Pharmacol.* 46:117–25

65. Bruno R, Vivler N, Vergniol J, De Phillips S, Montay G, et al. 1996. A population pharmacokinetic model for docetaxel (Taxotere): model building and validation. *J. Pharmacokinet. Biopharmcol.* 24:153–72

66. Bruno R, Hille D, Riva A, Vivier N, ten Bokkel-Huinnink W, et al. 1998. Population pharmacokinetics/pharmacodynamics of docetaxel in phase II studies in patients with cancer. *J. Clin. Oncol.* 16:187–96

67. Steimer J, Fotteler B, Gieschke R, Wiltshire H, Buss N. 1998. Predicting optimal dose of saquinavir via modelling of dose-exposure and exposure-effect relationships. See Ref. 83, pp. 79–86

68. Tanigawara Y. 1997. Recent applications of the population pharmacokinetic approach: pre-marketing and post-marketing. See Ref. 94, pp. 25–37

69. Holford N, Peace K. 1992. Results and validation of a population pharmacodynamic model for cognitive effects in Alzheimer patients treated with tacrine. *Proc. Natl. Acad. Sci. USA* 98:11471–75

70. Holford N, Peace K. 1994. The effect of tacrine and lecithin in Alzheimer's disease. A population pharmacodynamic analysis of five clinical trials. *Eur. J. Clin. Pharmacol.* 47:17–23

71. Wade J, Sambol N. 1995. Felodipine population dose-response and concentration-response relationships in patients with essential hypertension. *Clin. Pharmacol. Ther.* 57:569–81

72. Yukawa E, To H, Ohdo S, Higuchi S, Aoyama T. 1997. Population-based investigation of valproic acid relative clearance using nonlinear mixed effects modeling: influence of drug-drug interaction and patient characteristics. *J. Clin. Pharmacol.* 37:1160–67

73. Port R, Ding R, Fies T, Schaerer K. 1998. Predicting the time course of hemoglobin in children treated with erythropoietin for renal anaemia. *Br. J. Clin. Pharmacol.* 46:461–66

74. Kroboth P, Schmith V, Smith R. 1991. Pharmacodynamic modelling. Application to new drug development. *Clin. Pharmacokinet.* 20:91–98

75. Peck C, Barr W, Benet L, Collins J, Desjardins R, et al. 1994. Opportunities for integration of pharmacokinetics, pharmacodynamics, and toxicokinetics in rational drug development. *J. Clin. Pharmacol.* 34:111–19

76. Holford N. 1995. The target concentration approach to clinical drug development. *Clin. Pharmacokinet.* 29:287–91

77. Temple R. 1987. The clinical investigation of drugs for use by the elderly: food and drug guidelines. *Clin. Pharmacol. Ther.* 42:681–85

78. Int. Conf. Harmonisation. 1994. *Dose Response Information to Support Drug Registration.* Washington, DC: Cent. Drug Eval. Res., FDA

79. Food and Drug Admin. 1999. *Guidance for Industry: Population Pharmacokinetics.* Washington, DC: Cent. Drug Eval. Res., FDA

80. Cent. Drug Dev. Sci. 1999. *Modeling & Simulation of Clinical Trials: Best Practices Workshop.* Arlington VA: Georgetown Univ. Med. Cent.

81. Breimer D, Danhof M, eds. 1990. *Measurement and Kinetics of In Vivo Drug*

Effects. Advances in Simultaneous Pharmacokinetic/Pharmacodynamic Modelling. Leiden, The Netherlands: Leiden/ Amsterdam Cent. Drug Res.

82. Danhof M, Peck C, eds. 1994. *Measurement and Kinetics of In Vivo Drug Effects. Advances in Simultaneous Pharmacokinetic/Pharmacodynamic Modelling.* Leiden, The Netherlands: Leiden/ Amsterdam Cent. Drug Res.

83. Danhof M, Steimer J, eds. 1998. *Measurement and Kinetics of In Vivo Drug Effects. Advances in Simultaneous Pharmacokinetic/Pharmacodynamic Modelling.* Leiden, The Netherlands: Leiden/ Amsterdam Cent. Drug Res.

84. Goetghebeur E, Lapp K. 1997. The effect of treatment compliance in a placebo-controlled trial: regression with unpaired data. *Appl. Stat.* 46:351–64

85. Gelman A, Bois F, Jiang J. 1996. Physiological pharmacokinetic analysis using population modeling and informative prior distributions. *J. Am. Stat. Assoc.* 91:1400–12

86. Francheteau P, Steimer J, Dubray C, Lavene D. 1991. Mathematical model for in vivo pharmacodynamics integrating fluctuation of the response: application to the prolactin suppressant effect of the dopaminomimetic drug DCN 203–922. *J. Pharmacokinet. Biopharmcol.* 19:287–309

87. Gieschke R, Reigner B, Steimer J. 1997. Exploring clinical study design by computer simulation based on pharmacokinetic/pharmacodynamic modelling. *Int. J. Clin. Pharmacol. Ther.* 35:469–74

88. Racine-Poon A, Wakefield J. 1998. Statistical methods for population pharmacokinetic modelling. *Stat. Methods Med. Res.* 7:63–84

89. Yafune A, Ishiguro M. 1999. Bootstrap approach for constructing confidence intervals for population pharmacokinetic parameters. I: A use of bootstrap standard error. *Stat. Med.* 18:581–99

90. Yafune A, Ishiguro M. 1999. Bootstrap approach for constructing confidence intervals for population pharmacokinetic parameters. II: A bootstrap modification of Standard Two-Stage (STS) method for phase I trial. *Stat. Med.* 18:601–12

91. Food and Drug Admin. 1997. *Draft Guidance for Industry: In Vivo Bioequivalence Studies Based on Population and Individual Bioequivalence Approaches, October 1997.* Washington, DC: Cent. Drug Eval. Res., FDA

92. van Houwelingen H. 1997. The future of biostatistics: expecting the unexpected. *Stat. Med.* 16:2773–84

93. Foulkes M. 1998. Advances in HIV/ AIDS statistical methodology over the past decade. *Stat. Med.* 17:1–25

94. Aarons L, Balant L, Danhof M, Gex-Fabry M, Gundert-Remy U, et al, eds. 1997. *The Population Approach: Measuring and Managing Variability in Response, Concentration and Dose.* Luxembourg: Off. Official Publ. Eur. Communities

Annu. Rev. Pharmacol. Toxicol. 2000. 40:97–132

Sequencing the Entire Genomes of Free-Living Organisms: The Foundation of Pharmacology in the New Millennium

Samuel Broder and J. Craig Venter

Celera Genomics, Rockville, Maryland 20850; e-mail: BroderSE@celera.com, jcventer@celera.com

Key Words   human genomics, comparative genomics, shotgun sequencing, single nucleotide polymorphism (SNP), DNA variation, pharmacogenetics

■ **Abstract**   The power and effectiveness of clinical pharmacology are about to be transformed with a speed that earlier in this decade could not have been foreseen even by the most astute visionaries. In the very near future, we will have at our disposal the reference DNA sequence for the entire human genome, estimated to contain approximately 3.5 billion bp. At the same time, the science of whole genome sequencing is fostering the computational science of bioinformatics needed to develop practical applications for pharmacology and toxicology. Indeed, it is likely that pharmacology, toxicology, bioinformatics, and genomics will merge into a new branch of medical science for studying and developing pharmaceuticals from molecule to bedside.

THE IMPENDING AVAILABILITY OF A COMPLETE REFERENCE SEQUENCE FOR THE HUMAN GENOME

Our DNA sequence and its variation provide a special record of human evolution and the migration of populations (1–14). We will learn how this sequence varies among populations and among individuals, including the role of such variation in the pathogenesis of important illnesses and responses to pharmaceuticals. We will localize and annotate every human gene and the regulatory elements that control the timing, tissue-site specificity, and extent of gene expression. For any given physiologic process, we will have a new paradigm for addressing its evolution, its development, its function, and its mechanism. This will revitalize medicine by identifying important new targets for prevention, diagnosis, and therapy. Clinical pharmacologists will be able to approach issues of rational candidate drug design and the reduction of serious side effects by using bioinformatics to analyze the relevant genes and gene variations (polymorphisms), including the promoters and the enhancers, involved. Knowledge regarding the alleles that gov-

0362–1642/00/0415–0097$14.00

97

ern the safety and efficacy of pharmaceutical agents (including comparative genomics) will make it possible to streamline the preclinical and clinical development of new drugs and customize interventions to the specific genotypes of patients. Medical progress will be driven more by knowledge of gene structure and function and less by empiricism and intuition.

It is important to recall that the first complete genome of any free-living organism (*Haemophilus influenzae*) was published by scientists at the Institute for Genomic Research roughly 5 years ago (15). During the past 5 years, the sequences of the entire genomes of 23 organisms have been published (Table 1; see also http://www.tigr.org/tdb/mdb/mdb.html) (15–37). What was, a few short years ago, thought to be impossible has become not merely possible but inevitable.

WHOLE GENOME SEQUENCING

What has led us to such a future? The development of advanced automation, robotics, and computer software for industrial-scale DNA sequencing has proceeded at a remarkable pace. With the successful sequencing of the *H. influenzae* genome in its entirety, it became clear that the DNA of entire complex organisms many megabases in size could be accurately and rapidly sequenced by using a "shotgun" sequencing strategy (14).

In this strategy, a single random DNA-fragment library is prepared following mechanical or sonic shearing of entire genomic DNA and inserted in suitable vector systems (e.g. plasmids). The ends of a large number of randomly selected fragments are sequenced from both insert ends until every part of the genome has been sequenced several times on average. For any given average sequence read length, the number of end sequences needed can be determined by the Lander and Waterman application of Poisson statistics. This number will depend on the goals of the sequencing project and particularly the degree of tolerance for a small number of gaps in the sequence results (i.e. if the tolerance for gaps is low, the number of end sequences must be high). The sequences are then computationally "reassembled" to provide the complete genome. For higher organisms, which contain one genome from the mother and one genome from the father, this approach yields an important dividend: Points of common DNA variation such as single nucleotide polymorphisms (to which we return at several points in this chapter) become evident.

This overall strategy, coupled with the advent of completely automated DNA sequencing machines such as the new ABI Prism 3700 DNA Analyzer (manufactured by PE Biosystems, PE Corp.), will make it possible for a single center to undertake the determination of the reference sequence of the human genome. Indeed, it gives one pause to consider that every organism of pharmacologic or toxicologic interest is now plausibly a candidate for whole genome sequencing.

TABLE 1   Published free-living organism genomes

Genome	Strain	Domain	Size (MB)	Institution	Ref.
Haemophilus influenzae Rd	KW20	B	1.83	Inst. Genomic Res.	15
Mycoplasma genitalium	G-37	B	0.58	Inst. Genomic Res.	16
Methanococcus jannaschii	DSM 2661	A	1.66	Inst. Genomic Res.	17
Synechocystis sp.	PCC 6803	B	3.57	Kazusa DNA Res. Inst.	18
Mycoplasma pneumoniae	M129	B	0.81	Univ. Heidelberg	19
Saccharomyces cerevisiae	S288C	E	13	Int. Consort.	20
Helicobacter pylori	26695	B	1.66	Inst. Genomic Res.	21
Escherichia coli	K-12	B	4.60	Univ. Wisc.	22
Methanobacterium thermoautotrophicum	Delta H	A	1.75	Genome Ther. & Ohio State Univ.	23
Bacillus subtilis	168	B	4.20	Int. Consort	24
Archaeoglobus fulgidus	DSM4304	A	2.18	Inst. Genomic Res.	25
Borrelia burgdorferi	B31	B	1.44	Inst. Genomic Res.	26
Aquifex aeolicus	VF5	B	1.50	Diversa	27
Pyrcoccus horikoshii	OT3	A	1.80	Natl. Inst. of Tech. and Eval. (Japan)	28
Mycobacterium tuberculosis	H37Rv (lab strain)	B	4.40	Sanger Cent.	29
Treponema pallidum	Nichols	B	1.14	Inst. Genomic Res./Univ. Texas	30
Chlamydia trachomatis	Serovar D (D/UW-3/ Cx)	B	1.05	Univ. Calif. Berkeley/Stanford	31
Rickettsia prowazekii	Madrid E	B	1.10	Univ. Uppsala	32
Caenorhabditis elegans			100	Wash. Univ./Sanger Cent.	33
Helicobacter pylori	J99	B	1.64	Astra Res. Cent. Boston/Genome Ther.	34
Chlamydia pneumoniae	CWL029	B	1.23	Univ. Calif. Berkeley/Stanford	35
Thermotoga maritima	MSB8	B	1.80	Inst. Genomic Res.	36
Aeropyrum pernix	K1	A	1.67	Natl. Inst. of Tech. and Eval. (Japan)	37

This is not a vision for the future or a promissory note as to what science may someday bring. The science and supporting technology are here now.

THE CHALLENGE OF MICROBIAL PATHOGENS

Microbial pathogens (e.g. tuberculosis, cholera, and malaria) are a source of great suffering and death in many developing countries. Moreover, even in nations with advanced health-care technologies and mature research-based pharmaceutical industries, the emergence of multidrug-resistant pathogens is a serious problem. Indeed, some have argued that we are not too far removed from a return to the prepenicillin era in the fight against infectious disease. The problem for research pharmacologists is formidable and getting worse. The evolving field of genomic sequencing allows unique opportunities for understanding microbial pathogenesis and control by having simultaneously at hand the genomes of the pathogen and host.

Knowing the complete genome of microbial pathogens will open up exciting opportunities to develop novel pharmaceuticals and biologics. We will know how many genes are contained in each pathogen, where they are located within that pathogen's genome, and when two or more similar genes (paralogs) exist in a single microbial genome, thereby creating the potential to confound the research pharmacologist's search for an Achilles heel. By simultaneously analyzing the microbial genome and the host genome, it will become possible to define which genes are critical for microbial survival and which are optional; why a given pathogen is virulent in the context of a specific host; how and when toxic cytokines are activated within a host; whether a given pathogen has evolved proteins with molecular mimicry capable of frustrating host immunity or inducing auto-immunity; and how a pathogen (e.g. the tubercle bacillus) is able to survive in a state of latency or dormancy, impervious to the host's immune system. The sum total of this information will make it possible to define vaccines that induce specific and effective immunity against the pathogen while minimizing untoward or toxic side effects in the host.

Malaria provides a model for the challenges and research opportunities, and Wahlgren (38) has provided an elegant perspective on this topic. Falciparum malaria is a leading killer in the African countryside, and multidrug-resistant forms of the disease have emerged on a wide scale. The disease is caused by a protozoan (*Plasmodium falciparum*), whose life cycle involves infecting human erythrocytes, which in turn causes a fulminant hemolytic anemia. One consequence is cerebral malaria, a process facilitated by the patient's own cytokines, which promote adhesion of malarial organisms or their detritus to the inside walls of blood vessels. The resulting cerebral ischemia is often lethal, and perhaps one million people, many of them children, die from this infectious kind of stroke every year.

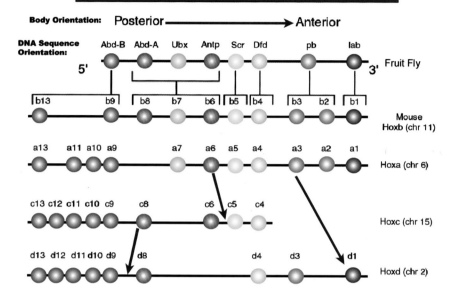

Figure 1 Synteny of homeobox (*Hox*) genes. (*Color coding*) Shows evolutionary relationships of orthologs. *Abd-B*, Abdominal B; *Abd-A*, abdominal A; *Ubx*, ultrabiothorax; *Antp*, antennapedia; *Scr*, sex combs reduced; *Dfd*, deformed; *Pb*, proboscipedia; *Lab*, labial.

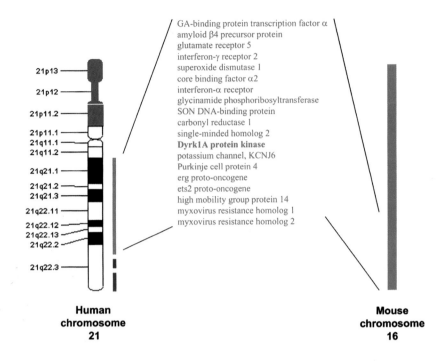

Figure 2 Synteny (*red*) between human chromosome 21 and mouse chromosome 16. *Dyrk1A* protein kinase is in a Down's syndrome critical region and is a candidate gene for causation. (See also http://www.ncbi.nlm.nih.gov/Homology/.)

The best known genes for malarial protection are those for which resistance alleles (nucleotide substitutions) in people in endemic regions exist in a state of balanced polymorphism. Thus, people with one copy of the S allele of the beta subunit of hemoglobin have a selective advantage living in malaria-endemic zones compared with individuals with two wild-type alleles, or with two copies of the mutant allele (in which case they would exhibit sickle cell anemia). The α- and β-thalassemias and glucose-6-phosphate dehydrogenase deficiencies are other examples of genotype polymorphisms whose evolution was driven by the selective advantage conferred on account of resistance to malaria.

More recently, certain cytokines, most notably tumor necrosis factor (TNF), have been implicated in the pathogenesis of malaria. TNF also probably plays a significant role in leishmaniasis, listeriosis, and other infectious diseases of the developing world. High circulating levels of TNF have been found in patients with cerebral malaria, particularly those whose disease runs a lethal course. TNF, among its many activities, up-regulates endothelial adhesion molecules and thereby increases the tendency of infected red cells to stick to the walls of blood vessels and interrupt blood flow. Knight et al (39) recently found that three polymorphisms in the promoter region of the *TNF* gene contribute to malarial pathogenesis and poor outcome through a complex dynamic of increased risk and counterbalancing protective effects. One such polymorphism, *TNF$_{-376A}$*, increases the secretion of TNF most likely by causing the helix-turn-helix transcription factor OCT-1 to bind to a novel region of complex protein-DNA interactions and alter gene expression in human monocytes. These workers found that a single nucleotide $G \rightarrow A$ polymorphism at position 376 upstream of the *TNF* transcriptional initiation site (the OCT-1 binding phenotype) is linked to unfavorable outcome from malarial infection in two ethnically distinct groups of people, one from the Gambia (western African) and the other from Kenya (eastern African). The results underscore the potential to link molecular events to clinical outcomes using the emerging knowledge of whole organism genomics. They are likely to influence future research into the prevention and treatment of malaria and many other diseases.

The *P. falciparum* genome is roughly 30 Mb in size and contains 14 chromosomes. Recently, after overcoming a number of theoretical and practical obstacles owing to the adenine plus thymine richness of its genome, it became possible to obtain the entire genomic DNA sequence of chromosome 2 in *P. falciparum* (40). Thus, one can expect that in the foreseeable future, the technologies for whole genome sequencing of microbial agents will make it possible to sequence the remaining 13 chromosomes and add this pathogen to the list in Table 1. The coupling of whole genome information from *P. falciparum* with whole genome information from its human host is likely to initiate an entire range of new approaches for dealing with the problem of malaria. (It is also possible that DNA sequencing of the intermediary host mosquito or a related insect genome may add still another set of strategic targets for attacking malaria.) The development of knowledge useful in turning the tide against multidrug-resistant malaria is a crucial goal for the science of whole genome sequencing.

DNA SEQUENCE VARIATION

We all evolved in an African savanna, and we all share >99.9% of the nucleotide sequence in our genome, so it is remarkable that the extraordinary diversity of human beings is encoded by only 0.1% variation in our DNA. We are predisposed to different diseases, we respond to the environment in variable ways, we metabolize pharmaceutical agents differently, we may show differences in dose-response relationships for common drugs, and we have a range of susceptibilities to adverse side effects from therapeutic agents (even when there is no discernible difference in individual pharmacokinetics or biochemical pharmacology). Despite the overwhelming similarity in sequence, there are millions of points of DNA variation between any two randomly selected individuals.

The most common form of DNA variation is single nucleotide polymorphism (SNP) (1–14, 41), and in our discussion of malaria above we encountered the enormous implications of SNPs for pharmacology and toxicology. Put simply, a SNP is the substitution of one purine or pyrimidine nucleotide at a given location in a strand of DNA for another purine or pyrimidine nucleotide. Such substitutions can affect gene function, or they can be neutral. Neutrality is generally inferred if a SNP does not alter protein coding. In practice, this inference can be wrong. The most common substitution is a transition in which a pyrimidine is substituted for another pyrimidine, and likewise a purine is substituted for a purine. However, transversions (replacement of a purine for a pyrimidine or vice versa) can occur.

The nomenclature defining a mutation (a disease-causing change) versus a SNP is arbitrary and relative. By convention, when a substitution is present in more that 1% of a target population, it is called a variant or polymorphism. When a substitution is present in less than 1%, and especially when one can assign a clear phenotype (i.e. a disease or clinical condition), it is called a mutation. SNPs may occur across widely separated populations, or they may be relatively specific for a given population. They are virtually always biallelic. Within populations, in both human and model organisms such as *Drosophila,* essentially every SNP is in Hardy-Weinberg equilibrium proportions (A Clark, personal communication).

SNPs may occur inside or outside of a gene. If they occur within a gene, they may reside in an exon (coding region) or intron (noncoding) region. SNPs in a coding region (sometimes called cSNPs) can be either synonymous (no amino acid–altering effect) or nonsynonymous (amino acid altering). There is some level of natural selection against amino acid–altering changes (12, 13). The average person would be expected to be heterozygous for roughly 40,000 nonsynonymous (amino acid-altering) alleles (12).

As we have seen in the case of the TNF_{-376} allele, SNPs can profoundly affect gene function even if they are at a significant distance upstream of the initiation site for gene transcription. One needs to keep in mind that enhancers (i.e. the tissue-specific control sequences on which certain regulatory substances act) may operate over at least 3 kb in either orientation ($5' \rightarrow 3'$ or $3' \rightarrow 5'$) from the start point of transcription.

It has been proposed that those SNPs that are of keenest interest in the pathophysiology of disease are nonsynonymous cSNPs, which alter the sequence of an encoded protein (12). Coding sequences comprise roughly 3% of the human genome, and therefore, it has been suggested that priority be given to shotgun sequencing of ccDNA libraries from many donors, possibly with an emphasis on specific candidate genes by direct amplification of target sequences. A word of caution is in order. It may not be appropriate to discount synonymous SNPs in the pathogenesis of important illnesses. Correlations between SNPs and clinical phenotypes are in their infancy, and it is critical that we do not assume that we know more than we do. A SNP that is "synonymous" for a protein coding point of view might be "antonymous" with respect to the folding of mRNA, the enzymatic activity on certain RNA molecules (e.g. adenosine to inosine conversion), and the function of small nucleolar RNA(snoRNA). This also applies to the set of genes involved in antisense RNA regulation, such as *Tsix,* a gene that performs antisense regulatory functions against *Xist* at the X-inactivation center (42). It is important to recall that splicing variants can also be significantly affected by DNA variation seen only at a genomic level. Moreover, the genes that may be of greatest interest in understanding the pathogenesis of common illnesses or in the development of important new drugs (particularly those that bring about true paradigmatic shifts in therapy) may be dramatically underrepresented (or undetectable) in cDNA libraries. Rarely expressed genes, or genes expressed in an extremely limited range of cells, may be poor candidates for cDNA-based detection systems. Looking for SNPs solely within or near known candidate genes may well result in missed SNPs that would be of great interest to pharmacologists and toxicologists, and scientists generally, in the long run.

Any two sets of chromosomes taken at random will differ roughly at one site per 500–1000 bp. There can be up to one potential variable site per 100 bp in an average segment of contiguous DNA if one examines DNA sequence variation among various populations (1, 5). This is one reason why the whole genome shotgun sequencing strategy discussed earlier is so powerful. Any normal individual will have two sets of chromosomes, all of which will be sequenced in their entirety. Thus, providing the full genome sequence from small numbers of normal donors, indeed from even one individual, will yield millions of SNPs for further study. However, correlations between genotypes and phenotypes (clinical conditions) will require association studies with appropriate levels of statistical power (see below).

The classic Mendelian model, in which a specific mutation in one gene produces a recognizable disease, may not apply to most common illnesses in our society. It is thought that many common illnesses have a polygenic origin, with several genes (to be more precise, gene variants) playing a comparatively small role individually, but with a cumulative effect that leads to a detectable clinical condition or disease. There is considerable interest in using whole genome association studies, as a tool for identifying genes involved in these common disorders, to detect differences in the frequency of DNA sequence variations between unrelated affected individuals and a control group (43).

Genetic association strategies may be direct or indirect (8, 43). The direct-association strategy focuses on common variants in coding or regulatory regions. (The identification of the latter is still problematic and will be greatly facilitated by comparative genomics, which is discussed further below.) Frequencies of these variants in patients and control groups are analyzed statistically, with the goal of identifying alleles that serve as morbidity or mortality risk indicators. The indirect strategy relies on a statistical association between an illness or clinical condition. This occurs when an "innocent" variant is linked to the actual risk-producing variant on a stretch of DNA. The probability of a recombinatorial event occurring between any two points of DNA in a chromosome is related to the distance between the two points. If the distance is comparatively small, the two points (variants) are said to be in linkage disequilibrium. During meiosis, they are likely to share a finite journey through time, and in an individual, the presence of one marker would then predict the other. A "neutral" variant can then be used to detect or uncover a disease-causing variant because they are linked together in a shared haplotype (genomic segment), which is longer for new variants in a population and shorter for ancient variants. The length of the shared haplotype determines whether there is a strong or weak level of linkage disequilibrium. Thus, the indirect strategy employs a dense map of anonymous or random polymorphic markers to search the genome for statistical associations with disease. This can provide a unique tool for new gene discovery, and it does not require the investigator to intuit candidate genes or regulatory elements in advance. In some cases, one can identify a marker with a sufficiently strong predictive power for development as a diagnostic test in its own right. This approach can identify the location of genes even when they would not be considered good candidates for a disease association by first principles. Indeed, we expect the availability of the complete sequence for the human genome to yield any number of surprises in terms of assigning function and disease association to gene loci.

Although both such approaches have been used on a comparatively small scale to study genes in diseases, we will soon have unprecedented opportunities to apply such studies to the entire genome. It is widely viewed that SNPs provide the key to such approaches because of their high frequency, biallelic nature, low mutation rate, and suitability for industrial-scale automation. The precise number of SNPs necessary is still a matter for debate. Kruglyak (43) has recently proposed that roughly 500,000 evenly spaced SNPs will be required for optimal indirect whole genome association studies. This estimate is at the upper limit of various suggested numbers, and yet it is still easily within the range of SNPs that will emerge as part of the whole human genome shotgun sequencing strategy discussed earlier.

A SURVEY OF SNPS

Single base changes may directly cause gross alterations in gene function, but they may also be responsible for subtle correlations with disease. Such SNPs have been linked to a variety of cardiovascular, respiratory, allergic, neurologic, psychiatric, metabolic, bacterial, and neoplastic diseases. Some brief examples of DNA variations that pertain to cancer risk (44–53), infectious disease (38, 39, 54–62), asthma (63–71), and neuropsychiatric diseases (72–81) are summarized in Tables 2–5. In some of the tables areas of controversy are included, as a reminder of the need for more clinical research. A summary of certain alleles associated with drug metabolism is shown in Table 6 (82–100). In some cases, there is an overlap of definitions. Thus, an allele can affect cancer risk (Table 2) but it could also fit in drug metabolism (Table 6).

Sometimes, detection of a functional polymorphism leads to unexpected and dramatic biological insights. Thus, apolipoprotein E has been known for many years to play an important role in lipoprotein metabolism. The *APOE* gene provides an interesting example of genetic polymorphisms, with substantial variation in different groups. This gene affects cholesterol levels. It is surprising that one allelic variant of this gene (*APOE4*) is a significant risk factor in Alzheimer's disease (101, 102). *APOE4* appears to be directly involved in some way because the protein is seen on immunohistochemical staining in the amyloid plaques, amyloid deposits, and neurofibrillary tangles that characterize the brain lesions of Alzheimer's disease.

In this sense, SNPs offer new opportunities for prevention, diagnosis, and treatment strategies. In the not-too-distant future, physicians may be able to use advanced, miniaturized technologies in their clinics or offices to define a patient's SNP profile in order to customize a diagnosis and therapy to the specific patient's needs. We return to a discussion of pharmacogenetics further below, but several recent practical examples of these ideas are worth noting here. The thiopurine methyltransferase gene, which regulates the metabolic inactivation of azathioprine, is a good model for discussion. Substantial hematologic toxicity may accompany the use of this drug in the therapy of rheumatic diseases or transplantation rejection. Patients with a variant allele for thiopurine methyltransferase (TPMT*3A) are at substantially higher risk of hematologic toxicity compared with those with the wild-type allele (100). In another example, dealing with schizophrenia therapy, the best response to the important but potentially toxic drug clozapine was found in patients with two defined genetic polymorphisms in 5-HT_{2A} receptors (80). In another example, polymorphisms of a genetic factor expressed on platelets (*PlA2*) might determine whether use of aspirin can prevent myocardial infarctions in patients (103). Perhaps even the DNA from a buccal swab would be informative in selecting the right pharmaceutical for the right patient.

In functional terms, an SNP can be either good, bad, or neutral, depending on the selective pressures or circumstances faced by the individuals in a population.

TABLE 2 Sequence polymorphisms and cancer risk

Gene	Polymorphism(s)	Allele frequency	Clinical correlation	Reference
BRCA1	185delAG 5382insC	0.5% in Ashkenazi Jews 0.1% in Ashkenazi Jews Rare in other populations	Associated with increased risk of breast and ovarian cancer. Risk of developing cancer by age 70 is 56% for breast cancer and 16% for ovarian cancer. Male carriers have increased risk of developing prostate cancer, with 16% of carriers developing prostatic cancer by age 70.	44
BRCA2	6174delT	0.5% in Ashkenazi Jews; rare in other populations	Associated with increased risk of breast and ovarian cancer. Risk of developing cancer by age 70 is 56% for breast cancer and 16% for ovarian cancer. Male breast cancer appears to be more common in BRCA2 mutation carriers than in BRCA1 carriers.	44
APC	I1307K; Ile to Lys change at residue 1307.	3.5% in Ashkenazi Jews; rare in other populations	Carriage of the I1307K allele is associated with somatic instability in genomic APC DNA and can result in loss of APC expression and the development of cancer. Risk of colorectal and breast cancer are approximately 1.5-fold higher in I1307K carriers than in noncarriers.	45
NAT2 (N-acetyl-transferase 2)	Multiple sequence variant combinations in NAT2 form 11 haplotypes. Subjects carrying the NAT2*4 haplotype (in either the homozygous or hetero-zygous states) are rapid acetylators; subjects with other haplotypes are slow acetylators.	In a set of 556 German volunteers, 23.4% of alleles were of the NAT2*4 haplotype.	Individuals who were homozygous for the rapid acetylation types NAT2*4/NAT2*4 were overrepresented in lung cancer patients compared with control patients; odds ratio, 2.36 (95% confidence interval 1.05–5.32). See also discussion of NAT1 and NAT2 in Table 6.	46

Gene	Polymorphism	Allele distribution	Comments	Ref.
MTHFR (methylene-tetraydro-folate reductase)	677C→T, results in a change from alanine to valine	677C = 0.58, 677T = 0.42 in Caucasian populations	The 677T allele of MTHFR is heat labile and results in reduced enzyme activity leading to lower levels of 5-methyltetrahydrofolate. In men with adequate folate levels, homozygosity for the 677T allele reduced the risk of colorectal cancer, but in men with folate deficiency or those drinking more than 10 g of alcohol/day, 677T did not reduce cancer risk.	47, 48
AR (androgen receptor)	Highly polymorphic CAG repeat present in the first exon of the X-linked androreceptor.	Continuous distribution of CAG repeat length ranging from 12–32 repeats. Modal length of 21 CAG repeats present in 30–40% of women.	Length of the AR CAG repeat is inversely correlated with the transcriptional activity of the AR. AR CAG re-repeat length was found to modify breast cancer risk in women with BRCA1 mutations. Women carrying AR-CAG alleles of >28, >29, or >30 repeats were diagnosed with breast cancer 0.8, 1.8, or 6.3 years earlier than women with BRCA1 mutations with shorter AR-CAG alleles.	49
p53	R72P; Arg to Pro change at residue 72	Allele frequencies have been reported to vary in different study populations. In the largest single normal group studied, 626 control patients from Sweden: R72 = 0.69, P72 = 0.31	The form of p53 carrying an arginine residue at codon 72 is significantly more susceptible to degradation by the HPV E6 protein than is the variant with proline at this position. In one study (50), 72R homozygotes were seven times more likely to develop HPV-associated cancers than were 72R/72P heterozygotes (numbers of 72P homozygotes being too small to analyze separately). This result proved to be controversial, however, and could not be replicated by three subsequent studies examining the effect of the p53 R72P polymorphism on HPV-associated cervical cancer risk.	50–53

TABLE 3 Sequence polymorphisms and infectious disease

Gene	Polymorphism(s)	Allele frequencies	Clinical correlation	Reference
Chemokine receptor 2 (CCR2)	Valine at position 64 is replaced by isoleucine (V64I).	V64, 90; I64, 10%; n = 248	In a study of 3003 HIV-positive patients, individuals carrying the I64 allele progressed to AIDS 2 to 4 years later.	54
Chemokine receptor 5 (CCR5)	32-bp deletion (Δ32)	+ 32 bp, 90.8%, Δ32, 9.2%; n = 1408 Caucasians The Δ32 allele is absent in Western and Central African and Japanese populations.	Carriers of the 32-bp deletion are protected from transmission of HIV.	55, 56
β-Globin	Glycine at position 6 is replaced by valine (G6V).	G6, 92%; V6, 8%; American Blacks G6, 60–80%; V6, 20–40%; African Blacks	The prevalence of malaria infection (42%) was significantly lower in individuals with the sickle-cell trait compared with their normal-hemoglobin counterparts (68%).	57, 58
Human leukocyte antigen (HLA)	HLA-B*35 haplotype HLA-C*w04 haplotype		The HLA-B*35 haplotype is associated with rapid development of AIDS in HIV-infected Caucasians. The HLS-C*w04 haplotype is associated with rapid development of AIDS in HIV-infected Caucasians.	59
Intercellular adhesion molecule 1 (ICAM-1)	Lysine at position 29 is replaced by methionine (K29M).	L29, 67%; M29, 33%; n = 287 Kenyans (controls) L29, 56%; M29, 44%; n = 157 Kenyans (cerebral malaria) L29, 76%; M29, 24%; n = 422 Gambians (controls)	In a case-control study of 547 subjects in Kenya, a single ICAM-1 mutation was present at high frequency. Genotypes at this locus from samples in this case-control study indicated an association of the polymorphism with the severity of clinical malaria such that individuals homozygous for the mutation (M29/M29) have increased susceptibility to cerebral malaria with a relative risk of two.	60, 61

			Ref.
		L29, 76%; M29, 24%; $n = 367$ Gambians (cerebral malaria)	Over 1200 children in The Gambia were typed for polymorphisms of the ICAM-1, gene. None of the polymorphisms typed was significantly associated with severe disease. These data differed significantly from the results of a previous study (Chi 2 = 8.81; $P = 0.003$) in which the ICAM-1 gene polymorphism was shown to be significantly associated with cerebral malaria. This suggests that there may be heterogeneity in genetic susceptibility to this condition between these two African populations.	62
Natural resistance-associated macrophage protein 1 (NRAMP1)	There is a $(CA)_n$ repeat variation in the 5' untranslated region.	CA repeat (201 bp), 84%	Four NRAMP1 polymorphisms were each significantly associated with tuberculosis. Subjects who were heterozygous for two NRAMP1 polymorphisms in intron 4 and the 3' untranslated region of the gene were particularly overrepresented among those with tuberculosis, as compared with those with the most common NRAMP1 genotype (odds ratio, 4.07; 95% confidence interval, 1.86–9.12; chi-square = 14.58; $P = 0.001$).	
	There is a G to C transversion in intron 4 (469 + 14 G/C).	469 + 14G, 92%; 469 + 14C, 8%		
	Aspartic acid at position 543 is replaced by asparagine (D543N).	D543, 93% N543, 7%;		
	There is a 4-bp deletion in the 3' untranslated region (1749 + 55 ΔTGTG).	1749 + 55 (TGTG), 81%; 1749 + 55 (ΔTGTG), 19%; $n = 827$ Gambians		
	The D543 allele is always associated with ΔTGTG in the 3'UTR.			
Tumor necrosis factor (TNF)	There are 3 polymorphisms located in the promoter region of this gene: − 238 G/A, − 308 G/A, − 376 G/A.	− 376 G, 98.5%; − 376 A, 1.5%; $n = 371$ Gambians (controls)	The -376 polymorphism is located in the OCT-1 binding site of the TNF promoter. Only the − 376 A allele binds OCT-1 and it is associated with a fourfold increased susceptibility to cerebral malaria.	39
	The − 376 A allele always occurs along with the − 238 A allele.	− 376 G, 96.9%; − 376 A, 3.1; $n = 384$ Gambians (cerebral malaria)		

TABLE 4 Sequence polymorphisms and asthma

Gene	Polymorphism(s)	Allele frequencies	Clinical correlation	Reference
Beta$_2$-adrenoceptor (B2AR)	Glycine at position 16 is replaced by arginine (G16R). Glutamine at position 27 is replaced by glutamic acid (Q27E). Arginine at position 16 was associated with glutamine at position 27 in 97.8% of the haplotypes determined.	G16, 62%; R16, 38%; n = 269 Americans Q27, 64%; E27, 36%; n = 269 Americans	To assess if different genotypes of these two polymorphisms would show differential responses to inhaled B2AR agonists, 269 children who were participants in a longitudinal study of asthma were genotyped. When compared with homozygotes for G16, homozygotes for R16 were 5.3 times (95% confidence interval, 1.6–17.7) and heterozygotes (G16/R16) were 2.3 times (1.3–4.2) more likely to respond to albuterol, respectively. No association was found between the Q27E polymorphism and response to albuterol.	63
Cystic fibrosis transmembrane regulator (CFTR)	Phenylalanine at position 508 is deleted (ΔF508).	F508, 97.3%; ΔF508, 2.7%; n = 9141 Danes	The CFTR gene encodes a chloride channel found in epithelial cells. Individuals with mutations in both copies of this gene are affected with the chronic lung disease cystic fibrosis. Of the 250 ΔF408 mutation carriers identified in this study, 9% reported having asthma compared with 6% of the noncarriers. The odds ratio for asthma for carriers of the ΔF508 mutation was 2.0 (1.2–3.5, P = 0.02).	64

| Fc(epsilon)RI, beta subunit (high-affinity receptor for immunoglobulin E) | Isoleucine at position 181 is replaced by leucine (I181L). Valine at position 183 is replaced by leucine (V183L). Glutamic acid at position 237 is replaced by glycine (E237G). | I181, 97%; L181, 3% (Caucasians) I181, 84%; L181, 16% (African Blacks) I181, 38%; L181, 72%; n = 221 Kuwaitis V183, 38%; L183, 72%; n = 221 Kuwaitis E237, 80%; G237, 20% (African Blacks) E237, 94.7%; G237, 5.3%; n = 1004 Australians | A sample of black and white asthmatic and control subjects in South Africa was studied to determine whether these variants contribute to the enhanced immunoglobulin E responses in these groups. There was a significant difference in the frequency of L181 between white asthmatics (28%) and white control subjects (3%) (P = 0.00001), but no difference in the frequency of I181L was observed between black asthmatics (22%) and black control subjects (16%). I181L might predispose to atopy in the white population but not in the black population. The Fc(epsilon)RIbeta polymorphism (181/183) was investigated in Kuwaiti asthmatic patients and controls. The variant sequence (L181/L183) was detected in 72% (320/442) of chromosomes analyzed. Homozygous LL genotype was detected in 48% (46/96) asthmatic subjects compared with 31% (39/125) in nonasthmatics. G237 positive subjects had a significantly elevated skin test response to grass (P = 0.0004) and house dust mites (P = 0.04), RAST to grass (P = 0.002), and bronchial reactivity to methacholine (P = 0.0009). The relative risk of individuals with G237 having asthma compared with subjects without the variant was 2.3 (95% confidence interval, 1.26–4.19; P = 0.005). | 65–67 |

(continued)

TABLE 4 *Continued*

Gene	Polymorphism(s)	Allele frequencies	Clinical correlation	Reference
Human leukocyte antigen (HLA)	HLA-B8; HLAS-A10 haplotype; HLA-DQ2 haplotype		In a study of 76 Greek asthmatic patients (35 children/41 adults), increased frequency of HLA-B8 was found in the adults and an increased frequency of HLA-A10 was found in the children. The HLA-DQ2 allele is found more frequently in asthmatic children than in control subjects (60% vs 34%, $P = 0.013$) with a relative risk of 2.8.	68, 69
5-Lipoxygenase (ALOX5)	$(GGGCGG)_{3-6}$ repeat variation in the promoter region	3 repeats, 3.8%; 4 repeats, 172.%; 5 repeats, 77.2%; 6 repeats, 1.8%; $n = 221$ Americans	Individuals with asthma carrying the 5-repeat allele respond to treatment targeted at this enzyme (18–23% improvement in FEV). Individuals without the 5-repeat allele showed no response.	70
Platelet-activating factor; acetylhydrolase (PAFA)	Valine at position 279 is replaced by phenylalanine (V279F).	V279, 82%; F279, 18%; $n = 263$ Japanese (controls); V279, 77%; F279, 23%; $n = 266$ Japanese (asthmatics)	A missense mutation (V279F) in the PAF acetylhydrolase gene results in the complete loss of activity. The prevalence of PAF acetylhydrolase deficiency is higher in Japanese asthmatics than in healthy subjects and the severity of this syndrome is highest in homozygous-deficient subjects. PAF acetylhydrolase gene is a modulating locus for the severity of asthma.	71

TABLE 5 Sequence polymorphisms and drug response—central nervous system

Gene	Polymorphism(s)	Allele frequencies	Clinical correlation	Reference
D$_2$ dopamine receptor	−241 A/G in 3' UTR −141 C ins/del in the promoter region Valine at position 96 is placed by alanine (V96A) Proline at position 310 is replaced by serine (P310S) Serine at position 311 is replaced by cysteine (S311C)	0.004 Caucasians 0.16 Southwestern American Indians; 0.03 Caucasian; 0.23 Japanese	The polymorphism in the promoter region (−141 C) does not affect clozapine response. The serine 310 variant has been reported to be associated with the adverse drug reaction of neuroleptic malignant syndrome. In an in vitro study, the A96 variant showed a reduction of ~50% in the binding of dopamine, chlorpromazine, and clozapine. The binding of other neuroleptic drugs (haloperidol, thioridazine, thiothixene, and risperidone) was not affected. Sequence variation at positions 310 and 311 did not affect drug binding.	72–74
D$_4$ dopamine receptor	A null mutation occurs in ~2% of the general population Exon 1 contains a 12-bp duplication and a 13-bp deletion Exon 3 contains a 48-bp repeat (2–10 copies) and a G194V polymorphism	0.64 4-repeat, 0.20 7-repeat, 0.08 2-repeat alleles	Binding site of atypical neuroleptics clozapine and olanzapine. The 7-repeat allele of the exon 3 VNTR is associated with dependence on opiate drugs. The effect of other polymorphisms on drug efficacy is not yet known.	75–77

(continued)

TABLE 5 *Continued*

Gene	Polymorphism(s)	Allele frequencies	Clinical correlation	Reference
D_5 dopamine receptor	Leucine at position 88 is replaced by phenylalanine (L88F).		In an in vitro study, the N351D polymorphism resulted in a ten-fold decrease in dopamine binding affinity, and a three-fold decrease in R(=)-SKF-38393 binding. The L88F polymorphism showed a slight decrease in the binding of SCH-23390 and risperidone, and a small increase in dopamine binding.	78
	Alanine at position 269 is replaced by valine (A269V).	0.008 Caucasians		
	Proline at position 330 is replaced by glutamine (P330Q).	0.1 Asians		
	Asparagine at position 351 is replaced by aspartic acid (N351D).	0.008 Caucasians		
	Serine at position 453 is replaced by cysteine (S453C).	0.008 Caucasians		
Dopamine transporter (DAT1)	VNTR in 3' UTR		480-bp allele has been associated with attention-deficit hyperactivity disorder.	79
5-HT$_{2A}$ serotonin receptor	Thymine at position 102 is replaced by cytosine (102 T/C).	C allele 0.5 in Caucasians	Receptor target of antipsychotics risperidone, ketanserin, clozapine, and olanzapine. Retrospective analysis of studies showed an association between the 102 T/C and H452Y polymorphisms and clozapine response.	80
	Threonine 25 replaced by asparagine (Thr452Asn).	0.02 Caucasians		
	Alanine 447 replaced by valine (Ala447Val)	0.01 Caucasians		
	Histidine at position 452 is replaced by tyrosine (H452Y).	0.09 Caucasians		
Serotonin transporter (5-HTT)	44-bp insertion/deletion in promoter region	S allele 0.43 in Caucasians	s allele: reduced transcriptional efficiency, associated with anxiety-related traits.	81

TABLE 6 Sequence polymorphisms and drug metabolism

Gene	Polymorphism(s)	Allele frequencies	Clinical correlation	Reference
Cytochrome P-450 2D6 (CYP2D6)	There are 48 positions in the CYP2D6 gene where sequence variations have been reported, resulting in 53 different haplotypes. The allele frequencies for the most common polymorphisms are listed in the next column.	V11, 93.3%; M11, 6.7% P34, 81.6%; S34, 18.4% L91, 84.2%; M91, 15.8% H94, 84.2%; R94, 15.8% 1085 C 84.1%; 1085 G 15.9% 1127 C 97.5%; 1127 T, 2.5% 1749 G 47.4%; 1749 C 52.6% 1935 G 82.9%; 1935 A 17.1% 2637 A 98.3%; 2637 ΔA 1.7% K281, 97.3%; ΔK281, 2.7% R296, 65.7%; C296, 34.3% 3916 G 98.8%; 3916 A, 1.2% S486, 47.1%; T486, 52.9% Null allele 6.9%; n = 1344 Europeans	More than 25 commonly prescribed drugs are metabolized by CYP2D6, including codeine, debrisoquine, indoramin, phenformin, and a number of antiarrythmics, antidepressants, beta-blockers, and neuroleptics. Sequence changes in CYP2D6 can either increase or decrease the rate at which the enzyme functions. Extensive metabolizers need lower doses to achieve therapeutic response, and may suffer adverse effects if a normal dose is given. Poor metabolizers require greatly elevated doses to achieve response and may not respond to some drugs at all.	82–84
Cytochrome P-450 2C9 (CYP2C9)	The wild-type sequence is designated CYP2C9*1. Arginine at position 144 is replaced by cysteine (R144C). This variant allele is designated CYP2C9*2. Isoleucine at position 359 is replaced by leucine (I359L). This variant allele is designated CYP2C9*3.	CYP2C9*1, 79%; CYP2C9*2, 12.5% CYP2C9*3, 8.5%; n = 100 Caucasians	Cytochrome P-450 CYP2C9 is responsible for the metabolism of S-warfarin. The CYP2C9*2 and CYP2C9*3 allelic variants are associated with impaired hydroxylation of S-warfarin. These patients have difficulty at induction of warfarin therapy and are potentially at a higher risk of bleeding complications. The V_{max} values for phenytoin in patients who are heterozygous for the I359/L359 allele are 40% lower than those in patients with the wild-type CYP2C9 allele (I359/I359 homozygotes).	85–87

(continued)

TABLE 6 *Continued*

Gene	Polymorphism(s)	Allele frequencies	Clinical correlation	Reference
Cytochrome P-450 2C19 (CYP2C19)	M1 allele: 1-bp mutation in exon 5 splice site M2 allele: G636A transition in exon 4	M1 allele: 30.7%, $n = 39$ Japanese; 16.7%, $n = 45$ Caucasians M2 allele: 8.9%, $n = 39$ Japanese; 0%, $n = 45$ Caucasians	CYP2C19 catalyzes the 4-hydroxylation of S-phenytoin, hexobarbitone, diazepam, omeprazole, proguanil, and R-warfarin. The M1 1-bp mutation lacks the heme binding domain and is catalytically inactive. It is associated with the poor metabolizer phenotype. The A636 transition in exon 4 creates a stop codon and is also associated with the poor metabolizer phenotype.	86, 88, 89
Glutathine S-transferase Mu (GSTMI)	The presence of a null allele results in decreased total GST activity.	Normal, 46.5%; null, 53.5%; $n = 213$ whites normal, 72.4%; null, 27.6%; $n = 203$ blacks	GSTM1 is a detoxification enzyme with high specificity for epoxides. Individuals who are homozygous for the null allele demonstrated a slightly increased risk for prostate cancer, and smokers who carry the null allele are at increased risk for bladder cancer.	90, 91
N-acetyl transferase 1 (NAT1)	There are 29 positions in the NAT1 gene where sequence variations have been reported, resulting in 24 different haplotypes.	R64, 95%; W64, 5%; $n = 85$ Caucasians R187, 96%; Q187, 4%; $n = 85$ Caucasians	NAT1 can further metabolize hydroxylamine metabolites to N-acetoxy derivatives. Normal NAT-1/fast NAT-2 genotype may be protective for susceptibility to smoking-induced bladder cancer.	92–94
N-acetyl transferase 2 (NAT2)	There are 11 position in the NAT2 gene where sequence variations have been reported, resulting in 26 different haplotypes.	I114T: 55:45, $n = 968$ Caucasians; 76:33, $N = 61$ Indians; 70:30, $N = 214$ African Americans; 72:28, $n = 148$ Hispanics; 99:1, a $n = 224$ Japanese; 95:5, $n = 254$ Chinese R197Q: 55:45, $n = 968$ Caucasians; 67:33, $n = 61$ Indians; 70:30, $n = 214$ African Americans; 72:28, $n = 148$ Hispanics; 99:1, $n = 224$ Japanese; 95:5, $n = 254$ Chinese	NAT2 polymorphisms are associated with higher incidence or severity of adverse drug reactions to isoniazid, hydralazine, procainamide, and sulfamethazole. Slow acetylators {NAT2*5B (I114T), and NAT2*6A [C282T(Y94Y), R197Q]} who smoke may have an eightfold higher risk of bladder and lung cancer due to their inability to detoxify aromatic amines in tobacco smoke. Rapid acetylators (NAT2*4) are at increased risk of colon cancer from acetylation of heterocyclic amines found in cooked meats.	93–95

Paraoxonase (PON1)	Methionine at position 55 is replaced by leucine (M55L). Glutamine at position 192 is replaced by arginine (Q192R).	Q192, 84.5%; R192, 15.5%; n = 166 Indians. Q192, 63.2%; R192, 36.8%; n = 105 Turks. Q192, 73%; R192, 27%; n = 248 Saudis	High serum paraoxonase levels protect against the neurotoxic effects of organophosphate insecticides as well as the nerve agents soman and sarin. The R192 allele specifies high enzymatic activity, whereas the Q192 variant specifies low activity. The M55L polymorphism affects the level of mRNA, with M55L heterozygotes showing an excess of the L55 allele.	96, 97
Thiopurine S-methyl transferase (TPMT)	TMPT has several mutant alleles that exhibit low enzyme activity compared with the wild-type enzyme (TPMT*1). Alanine at position 80 is replaced by proline (A80P). This variant allele is designated TPMT*2. Alanine at position 154 is replaced by threonine (A154T). This variant allele is designated TPMT*3B. Tyrosine at position 240 is replaced by cysteine (Y240C). This variant allele is designated TPMT*3C. Variant TPMT*3A contains both the T154 and C240 amino acid changes.	Haplotype frequencies: TPMT*1, 94.5%; TPMT*2, 0.18%; TPMT*3A, 3%; TPMT*3B, 0.35%; TPMT*3C, 0.71%; TPMT*3D, 0.18%; TPMT*4, 0%; TPMT*5, 0.18%; all other, 0.88%; n = 283 (mixed ethnic groups)	Prevention of transplant rejection and therapy of rheumatoid arthritis by the immunosuppressive drug azathioprine is limited by hemotologic toxicity (leucopenia or agranulosis). This toxicity is a particular problem in patients with low TPMTase activity (homozygotes for variant alleles; ~1% of the population). Other drugs affected by variation in TPMT include mercaptopurine and thioguanine.	98-100

Evolution affects the phenotypes encoded by genotypes, but it cannot operate through the genotype directly (11). Phenotypes that confer a selective advantage at one point in a population's history may at a different point do the opposite. Thus, there is an increased risk for deep venous thrombosis in carriers of the prothrombin G → A^{20210} gene variant (polymorphism). The A allele is deleterious because it is associated with increased prothrombin levels and an approximately threefold increased risk for deep venous thrombosis compared with individuals homozygous for the G allele (104). The median age at the time of the first thrombotic episode is 38 years. Deep venous thrombosis is a serious and potentially life-threatening condition for human beings in western society today. But there was likely a time in human history in which the life expectancy of an individual was well under 38 years. The capacity to undergo blood coagulation quickly and decisively might well have been a selective advantage if wounds from predatory animals or human combatants were a common event in everyday life. Indeed, even as the twentieth century draws to a close, current events do not necessarily support the lack of a selective advantage for the A allele.

PHARMACOGENETICS

Research pharmacologists and toxicologists have begun applying the lessons of modern genetics and molecular biology at perhaps a much faster pace than many other medical sciences. This is clear in the rapid practical applications of pharmacogenetics and supporting technology (83, 84, 105). Yet, as with any genetics testing, there are a number of regulatory and policy issues that require further dialogue (106, 107). Pharmacogenetics, a term originally coined in the 1950s, may now be viewed as the study of correlations between an individual's genotype and that same individual's ability to metabolize an administered drug or compound. Genotypic variation, often in the form of SNPs, exists for many of the enzymes that metabolize important drugs. Extensive metabolism of a drug is a general characteristic of the normal population. Poor metabolism, which typically is associated with excess accumulation of specific drugs or active metabolic products, is generally an autosomal recessive trait requiring a functional change, such as a frameshift or splicing defect in both copies of the relevant gene. Ultraextensive metabolism, which may have the effect of diminishing a drug's apparent efficacy in a given individual, is generally an autosomal dominant state derived from a gene duplication or amplification. Some representative examples of genetic polymorphisms that affect drug metabolism are shown in Table 6. For some fields, such as cancer chemotherapy, several common drugs show wide polymorphism-related metabolic varations, with 30-fold or greater interindividual variability reported (108).

Drug metabolism is often divided into two components: phase I (oxidative) and phase II (conjugative). The cardinal phase I enzymes belong to the cytochrome P-450 (CYP) superfamily of inducible mixed-function monooxygenases located within hepatic endoplasmic reticulum. Thirty or more forms of P-450 enzymes have been identified, each with distinct enzymatic activity. It is difficult to overstate the importance of these enzymes in clinical practice. More than 25 prescription drugs are metabolized by one member of the family, the CYP2D6, alone. It has been estimated that genetic polymorphisms of the *CYP2D6* gene alter clinical care and outcome of nearly one fifth of patients in some ethnic groups. In the case of certain drugs or carcinogens, the P-450 enzymes play a role in generating active moieties from otherwise inactive or poorly active starting compounds (pro-drugs or pro-carcinogens), which may add a layer of complexity in any global overview of these enzymes. Phase II enzymes include the glutathione transferases, N-acetyltransferases, UDP-glucuronyl-transferases, and the sulfotransferases. Genetic polymorphisms in these enzymes can also have important pharmacologic and clinical sequelae. They may also participate in relative cancer risk and causation, depending on their effectiveness in eliminating certain carcinogens (109) (see also Tables 2 and 6). However, with our current state of knowledge, there may be complex or counter-intuitive relationships between cancer and certain polymorphisms, such as those seen in the N-acetyltransferases.

In a sense, every clinical pharmacologist already relies on the tools of medical genetics and genotyping. The common technologies for determining alleles of pharmacogenetic interest are readily adaptable to most reference labs. There are two commonly used techniques. The first is amplification of a specific genetic region by polymerase chain reaction, followed by an analysis of restriction fragment length polymorphism (which reflects alterations in nucleotide sequence). The second involves allele-specific polymerase chain reaction, which depends on oligonucleotides capable of hybridization with common or variant alleles. Only a successful (i.e. precise) hybridization to the known target sequence yields an amplification product, which can in turn be detected on agarose gels. However, it is expected that improvements in microfluidic and chip-based technologies will make it even easier and more convenient, and thus more important, to assess genotypes of important metabolic enzymes. These technologies may also eventually make it possible to address the metabolic pathways for biologic response modifiers, for which very little is known.

The availability of the complete sequence for the human genome, including new knowledge regarding DNA variation, will alter the scope and definition of pharmacogenetics. New genomic knowledge will make it possible to examine families of drug efflux pump genes (e.g. P-glycoprotein) in the gut epithelium and central nervous system for their effects on oral bioavailability and central nervous protective effects, particularly with respect to xenobiotic agents (110). This knowledge may make it possible to clearly predict important pharmacokinetic parameters of certain drugs well in advance of empirical testing. In addition to the possibility of identifying new genes (and new alleles) from known metabolic gene families, pharmacologists will gain unprecedented ways of analyzing polymorphisms in the target receptors of important drugs, as well as in genes involved in the metabolic pathways affected by new agents. As an example, about

6% of patients with asthma do not carry a wild-type allele at the 5-lipoxygenase (*ALOX5*) core promoter locus (see Table 4). In such patients, the *ALOX5* pathway agents (i.e. leukotrienes) do not make a major contribution to their small airway disease, and these asthmatics do not improve with a drug whose mechanism is to inhibit this pathway (70). Also, a common polymorphism of the leukotriene C_4 synthase promoter appears to be a risk factor for aspirin-induced asthma (111). This clearly illustrates the principle that variants in the promoter region of a therapeutic target gene can predict clinical response. This concept is a significant expansion of pharmacogenetics beyond polymorphisms in drug-metabolizing enzymes.

Thus, on several fronts, pharmacologists and toxicologists will be able to address issues of efficacy and safety not reflected in the traditional pharmacokinetic or pharmacodynamic profiles of drugs. Even when patients have identical pharmacokinetic profiles for a given drug, we currently have no way of knowing that there will be comparable interpatient efficacy or safety because the science of pharmacogenetics can now only look at one part of the picture, and even that picture generally excludes important classes of therapeutics, such as biologic-response modifiers and monoclonal antibodies. Some examples of polymorphisms in a target receptor, with important pharmacologic consequences, are shown in Tables 4 and 5. In the future, the growing knowledge, based on the foundation of the complete human genome, will make it possible for pharmaceutical developers to select therapeutic agents according to the individual allele profiles of the intended patient. Said another way, patients will someday get only the drugs they need, and no other. But what is certain now is that pharmacology and toxicology will become dependent on the emerging bioinformatics and computational sciences linked to genomics. Data acquisition and management across multiple disciplines will require new tools and skill sets, necessitating changes in the curricula of pharmacology teaching centers toward a much more computational orientation. It will also be necessary for new cross-relational databases to emerge to serve the needs of pharmacologists and toxicologists in the new genomics era.

COMPARATIVE GENOMICS

The availability of whole genome sequence information in the human is important in its own right, but the full power of this knowledge requires the additional availability of whole genome sequence information from model organisms, especially *Drosophila melanogaster* (common fruit flies) and mice. *Drosophila* has been at the forefront of genetics research for nearly 80 years. This species is an important model for combining genetics, electrophysiology, and molecular biology. A brief listing of some medically important fruit fly genes is shown in Table 7. We expect that our group, in collaboration with the Berkeley Drosophila Genome Project, will publish the complete sequence of *Drosophila* in the near future. Many gene families, ranging literally from A to Z (aldolases to zinc finger

TABLE 7 Model organisms, gene names, and human disease

Fruit flies[a]	Mice	Humans
Congenital heart defects Tinman	Csx/NKx2.5	Csx/NKx2.5
Huntington's polyglutamine repeats cause neural degeneration	Polyglutamine repeats	Polyglutamine repeats
Alzheimer's APPL	APP	APP
Amyotrophic lateral sclerosis SOD	SOD1	SOD1
Cancer Cdx(2) caudal	cdx2	cdx2
Diabetes insulin receptor	Insulin receptor (knockout mice)	Insulin receptor
Retinitis pigmentosa rhodopsin	Rhodopsin	Rhodopsin
NF MERLIN	NF2	NF2
Ataxia telangiectasia mei-41	ATM	ATM

[a]Human disease. APP, amyloid precursor protein; SOD, superoxide dismutase, NF, neurofibromatosis.

transcription factors), suggest that a single invertebrate gene corresponds to a handful of equally related vertebrate genes on different chromosomes. Thus, gene duplication is the engine that drove vertebrate evolution (112).

In the case of vertebrate organisms, not only does homology to human genes exist, there is also something more meaningful called synteny. This means there are related genes arrayed on chromosomes with an evolutionary history common to human counterparts, in a comparable order in terms of exons and gene regulatory elements. Thus, a mouse chromosomal region with such a common evolutionary history and genetic arrangement is said to be syntenic, and the relevant mouse and human genes are said to be orthologs. Synteny and the capacity to overlay complete human and mammalian genome sequences (especially mouse) will affect gene discovery and our understanding of gene structure and function in ways without precedent. We expect the completion of other genomes with importance to pharmacology and toxicology, e.g. rat and canine genomes, not too far behind those of humans and mice. These advances will allow an integration of information from transgenic animals and gene knockout models in far-reaching ways and will stimulate novel strategies for currently intractable therapeutic problems.

The implications of these advances can perhaps be illustrated with a few examples. The homeobox genes are an interesting case. An excellent website by Gaunt can be consulted (http://www.bi.bbsrc.ac.uk/world/sci4Alll/gaunt/dud/gaunt.html). We can examine homeobox (*Hox*) genes (113), a family of genes that are conserved in evolution in detail. These genes direct the development of the body plan and body parts of many morphologically distinct species. The homeobox is a highly conserved 180-bp nucleotide sequence shared by this family of transcription factors. The homeobox in turn encodes the DNA binding region, called the homeodomain, a DNA binding motif.

Homeobox genes are found in clusters, as shown at the top of Figure 1 (see color insert). The $5' \rightarrow 3'$ order is reflected in the spatial correspondence of the genes along the posterior $\rightarrow$ anterior axis in *D. melanogaster,* and this is likewise conserved in other species. There is a rigid correspondence between the order of *Hox* genes within their clusters and that of their expression domains along the body of the embryo. Homeobox genes have a high degree of sequence similarity (denoted by color coding) in Figure 1 and can be found throughout the animal kingdom at the same positions in the cluster. Shown below *Drosophila* in Figure 1 are the corresponding clusters of orthologs in mice, demonstrating a general preservation of these genes, along with the expected pattern of gene duplication in vertebrates in different chromosomes. Verterbrates have four Hox clusters, called *Hoxa, Hoxb, Hoxc,* and *Hoxd.* A more complete understanding of these genes will offer the pharmacologist many new strategies for preventing and treating birth defects and possibly organ or even limb repair.

Cross-species homologues can show similar function, even in organisms separated by hundreds of millions of years of evolution. Thus, dysfunction of the homeotic gene *Pax-6* can cause an eyeless phenotype in *Drosophila* and small eye syndrome in mice, whereas in children, mutations in *Pax-6* results in a complete loss of the iris and also in disturbances of the lens, cornea, and retina, which can contribute to blindness (114, 115). One must use caution in extrapolating these observations too broadly, but they serve as a reminder of the remarkable power of comparative genomics from fruit fly to human.

Knowledge from comparative genomics may make it possible to rethink therapeutic strategies for currently untreatable disorders, including those that arise from cytogenetic abnormalities. For example, is it possible that if an appropriate intervention were made early enough, Down's syndrome (trisomy, critical region chromosome 21q22.2–q22.3) might not inevitably lead to mental retardation? Asked another way, do the models of phenylketonuria and congenital hypothyroidism apply? Is there a way of testing whether an extra dose of a gene causes mental retardation, and could a pharmaceutical agent somehow neutralize the effects of such an extra dose if given early enough? One could note, with some justification, the futility of such hypotheticals in the absence of knowledge of the genes responsible for the disorder, and this underscores the importance of completing the human genome sequence effort quickly.

By utilizing available knowledge of synteny and comparative genomics, a novel family of protein kinases, called Dyrk, was found to represent interesting candidates for a role in this syndrome (116). Human chromosome 21 and the syntenic region of mouse chromosome 16 are shown in Figure 2 (see color insert) (117, 118). The gene *Dyrk1A* is located in the Down's syndrome critical region of chromosome 21. *Dyrk1A* reveals homologies with *minibrain,* a gene in *Drosophila* whose mutations yield reduced neuronal number and defective learning behavior. Mouse models of Down's syndrome, which involve a partial trisomy 16, have been created (119, 120). And perhaps most interesting, mice transgenic for a 180-kb DNA segment derived from the human Down's syndrome critical region had defects in learning and memory (121, 122). Thus, it may soon be possible to identify both the gene(s) responsible for the most significant feature of the syndrome and in vivo systems for designing and testing interventions. These types of research opportunities will be multiplied thousands of times with the completion of the reference human genome program.

THE CHIMPANZEE GENOME

Approximately 5 million years ago, humans and chimpanzees shared a common ancestor. At the nucleotide sequence level, humans and chimpanzees differ by approximately 1.5% (50 Mb), on average. It has been argued that portions of human and chimpanzee genes are sometimes so similar that differences may fall within the range of normal DNA sequence variation (123). The overlapping synteny between humans and chimpanzees means that the completion of a reference human genome will greatly simplify the tasks of sequencing and assembling a reference genome for chimps.

Chimp DNA variation casts light on human DNA variation. Of nearly all human SNPs studied, one or another of the nucleotide allele set is shared with chimpanzees, thus making it possible to differentiate between ancestral and more recent alleles. Hacia et al (124) found that at the vast majority of SNP sites scored, all three nonhuman primates (chimps, pygmy chimps, and gorillas) exhibited one or the other of the human nucleotides, and roughly 75% of the time, the more common allele in humans was the ancestral form.

On the basis of considerable DNA sequence information (especially from the noncoding sequences of the genomic region called the beta-globin gene cluster), Goodman (125) has proposed creating a new phylogenetic classification of primates. In this proposed classification, humans would share their genus with chimpanzees and bonobos (pygmy chimpanzees). Thus, the subtribe *Homina* would contain *Homo* (*Homo*), humans, and *Homo* (*Pan*), chimpanzees and bonobos.

The science of comparative primate genomics can yield a number of interesting insights into the molecular events that contributed to human evolution (125–129). For example, mutations in *cis*-regulatory control elements changed γ-globin gene expression from strictly embryonic to fetal in profile, and there is evidence that natural selection favored such a distinct fetal hemoglobin during the evolution of the anthropoid primates. There were also amino acid–changing substitutions, including those in codons specifying 2,3-diphosphoglycerate–binding sites. A noteworthy consequence at the protein level was a loss of 2,3-diphosphoglycerate–binding capacity, yielding a fetal hemoglobin molecule that binds oxygen with increased affinity. Such a change facilitates the transfer of oxygen from mother to fetus. These changes, taken together, made a prolonged gestation and extensive prenatal brain development possible in anthropoid primates.

The changes in both regulatory elements and coding exons that permitted a prolonged fetal gestation provide but a glimpse of what can be learned when complete genomic information becomes available. These changes are particularly instructive because they are not in any immediate or obvious way associated with brain structure or related anatomical development, and yet these differences in hemoglobin structure and kinetics of expression enabled the evolution of intelligence in primates.

Two questions emerge at this point. What are the genes that define human beings as a unique primate species and how can we apply this knowledge to medical science? McConkey & Goodman (130) have suggested that the first priority would be to identify genes that are situated in close proximity to the archaic chromosomal rearrangements occurring in human evolution after the divergence of humans and chimps from their last common ancestor. The fusion of two ape chromosomes to form human chromosome 2 and a small pericentric inversion in human chromosomes 1 and 18 might be excellent clues about where to search for candidate genes and regulatory elements that uniquely facilitated human evolution (131, 132). In any event, there will be exceptional opportunities to study the genes and pathways involved in affect and emotion; cognition and memory; language, speech, and gesticulation; and attention span, sexuality, craniofacial and neurodevelopment, gait, aging, and resistance to infectious agents (notably retroviruses). The implications for pharmaceutical sciences and such disciplines as rehabilitative medicine are profound.

SOCIETAL RESPONSIBILITY

It is worth discussing the limits of genomics. Understanding the human genome will change science and medicine in profound ways. It will, however, not solve or explain every important problem of the public health. Other components of society will need to express determination and commit resources for solutions. One such problem is the need to respect patient privacy. Another is racism in whatever guise, which is invariably an enemy of science. In our efforts to provide a reference sequence for the human genome, we believe there is neither "good" nor "bad" DNA, only human DNA. Every individual will have a finite number of genetic flaws in his or her genome. Our task is to use the modern tools of pharmacology and genomics to ameliorate these flaws or undo their consequences. There is very good reason for optimism on this front, as we have tried to convey in this chapter. Yet many societies, including our own, have at various times embraced eugenics and other irrational genetic theories of race or ethnicity as the justification for neglect, oppression, or worse. However, the embrace of these negative philosophies is not inevitable. Opening incomparable opportunities for preventing and curing illnesses through genomic science is one way of refuting these pseudoscientific viewpoints. We believe that various governmental and private agencies, especially the National Institutes of Health, need to redouble their efforts to provide resources in the arena of ethics, education, and genomic research. Furthermore, some illnesses have their roots in certain external environmental factors for which genes may not affect outcomes in practical terms. Poverty may be viewed as one such factor. It is, therefore, important for society at large to recognize that advances in science alone, including the reference human genome project, will need to be coupled with programs to address these larger societal issues.

ACKNOWLEDGMENTS

We wish to thank Mary Whiteley, Trevor Woodage, Anibal Cravchik, and Emily Winn-Deen for their helpful scientific input, and Beth Hoyle for her excellent editorial assistance in preparing this manuscript.

Visit the Annual Reviews home page at www.AnnualReviews.org.

LITERATURE CITED

1. Clark AG, Weiss KM, Nickerson DA, Taylor SL, Buchanan A, et al. 1998. Haplotype structure and population genetic inferences from nucleotide-sequence variation in human lipoprotein lipase. *Am. J. Hum. Genet.* 63(2):595–612

2. Kittles RA, Long JC, Bergen AW, Eggert M, Virkkunen M, et al. 1999. Cladistic association analysis of Y chromosome effects on alcohol dependence and related personality traits. *Proc. Natl. Acad. Sci. USA* 96(7):4204–9

3. Kittles RA, Perola M, Peltonen L, Bergen AW, Aragon RA, et al. 1998. Dual origins of Finns revealed by Y chromosome haplotype variation. *Am. J. Hum. Genet.* 62(5):1171–79

4. Harris EE, Hey J. 1999. X chromosome evidence for ancient human histories. *Proc. Natl. Acad. Sci. USA* 96:3320–24

5. Nickerson DA, Taylor SL, Weiss KM, Clark AG, Hutchinson RG, et al. 1998. DNA sequence diversity in a 9.7-kb region of the human lipoprotein lipase gene. *Nat. Genet.* 19(3):233–40

6. Hästabacka J, de la Chapelle A, Kaitila I, Sistonen P, Weaver A, Lander E. 1992. Linkage disequilibrium mapping in isolated founder populations: diastrophic dysplasia in Finland. *Nat. Genet.* 2:204–11

7. Kruglyak L. 1997. The use of a genetic map of biallelic markers in linkage studies. *Nat. Genet.* 17:21–24

8. Risch N, Merikangas K. 1996. The future of genetic studies of complex human diseases. *Science* 273(5281):1516–17

9. Shaw SH, Carrasquillo MM, Kashuk C, Puffenberger EG, Chakravarti A. 1998. Allele frequency distributions in pooled DNA samples: applications to mapping complex disease genes. *Genome Res.* 8:111–23

10. McKeigue PM. 1998. Mapping genes that underlie ethnic differences in disease risk: methods for detecting linkage in admixed populations, by conditioning or parental admixture. *Am. J. Hum. Genet.* 63:241–51

11. Weiss KM. 1998. In search of human variation. *Genome Res.* 8(7):691–97

12. Cargill M, Altshuler D, Ireland J, Sklar P, Ardlie K, et al. 1999. Characterization of single-nucleotide polymorphisms in coding regions of human genes. *Nat. Genet.* 22:231–38

13. Halushka MK, Fan J-B, Bentley K, Hsie L, Shen N, et al. 1999. Patterns of single-nucleotide polymorphisms in candidate

genes for blood-pressure homeostasis. *Nat. Genet.* 22:239–47

14. Venter JC, Adams MD, Sutton GG, Kerlavage AR, Smith HO, Hunkapiller M. 1998. Shotgun sequencing of the human genome. *Science* 280:1540–42

15. Fleischmann RD, Adams MD, White O, Clayton RA, Kirkness EF, et al. 1995. Whole-genome random sequencing and assembly of *Haemophilus influenzae* Rd. *Science* 269:496–512

16. Fraser CM, Gocayne JD, White O, Adams MD, Clayton RA, et al. 1995. The minimal gene complement of *Mycoplasma genitalium. Science* 270:397–403

17. Bult CJ, White O, Olsen GJ, Zhou L, Fleischmann RD, et al. 1996. Complete genome sequence of the methanogenic archaeon, *Methanococcus jannaschii. Science* 273:1058–73

18. Kaneko T, Sato S, Kotani H, Tanaka A, Asamizu E, et al. 1996. Sequence analysis of the genome of the unicellular cyanobacterium *Synechocystis* sp. strain PCC6803. II. Sequence determination of the entire genome and assignment of potential protein-coding regions. *DNA Res.* 3:109–36

19. Himmelreich R, Hilbert H, Plagens H, Pirkl E, Li BC, Herrmann R. 1996. Complete sequence analysis of the genome of the bacterium *Mycoplasma pneumoniae. Nucleic Acids Res.* 24:4420–49

20. The yeast genome directory. 1997. *Nature* 387(Suppl.):5

21. Tomb J-F, White O, Kerlavage AR, Clayton RA, Sutton GG, et al. 1997. The complete genome sequence of the gastric pathogen *Helicobacter pylori. Nature* 388:539–47

22. Blattner FR, Plunkett G III, Bloch CA, Perna NT, Burland V, et al. 1997. The complete genome sequence of *Escherichia coli* K-12. *Science* 277:1453–74

23. Smith DR, Doucette-Stamm LA, Deloughery C, Lee H, Dubois J, et al. 1997. Complete genome sequence of *Methanobacterium thermoautotrophi-* cum DH: functional analysis and comparative genomics. *J. Bacteriol.* 179: 7135–55

24. Kunst F, Ogasawara N, Moszer I, Albertini AM, Alloni G, et al. 1997. The complete genome sequence of the gram-positive bacterium *Bacillus subtilis. Nature* 390:249–56

25. Klenk H-P, Clayton RA, Tomb J-F, White O, Nelson KE, et al. 1997. The complete genome sequence of the hyperthermophilic, sulfate-reducing archeon *Archaeoglobus fulgidus. Nature* 390: 364–70

26. Fraser CM, Casjens S, Huang WM, Sutton GG, Clayton R, et al. 1997. Genomic sequence of a Lyme disease spirochaete, *Borrelia burgdorferi. Nature* 390:580–86

27. Deckert G, Warren PV, Gaasterland T, Young WG, Lenox AL, et al. 1998. The complete genome of the hyperthermophilic bacterium *Aquifex aeolicus. Nature* 392:353–58

28. Kawarabayasi Y, Sawada M, Horikawa H, Haikawa Y, Hino Y, et al. 1998. Complete sequence and gene organization of the genome of a hyper-thermophilic archaebacterium, *Pyrococcus horikoshii* OT3. *DNA Res.* 5:147–55

29. Cole ST, Brosch R, Parkhill J, Garnier T, Churcher C, et al. 1998. Deciphering the biology of *Mycobacterium tuberculosis* from the complete genome sequence. *Nature* 393:537–44

30. Fraser CM, Norris SJ, Weinstock GM, White O, Sutton GG, et al. 1998. Complete genome sequence of *Treponema pallidum,* the syphilis spirochete. *Science* 281:375–88

31. Stephens RS, Kalman S, Lammel CJ, Fan J, Marathe R, et al. 1998. Genome sequence of an obligate intracellular pathogen of humans: *Chlamydia trachomatis. Science* 282:754–59

32. Andersson SGE, Zomorodipour A, Andersson JO, Sicheritz-Ponten T, Alsmark UCM, et al. 1998. The genome sequence of *Rickettsia prowazekii* and

the origin of mitochondria. *Nature* 396:133–40

33. The *C. elegans* Sequencing Consortium. 1998. Genome sequence of the nematode *C. elegans:* a platform for investigating biology. *Science* 282:2012–18

34. Alm RA, Ling L-SL, Moir DT, King BL, Brown ED, et al. 1999. Genomic-sequence comparison of two unrelated isolates of the human gastric pathogen *Helicobacter pylori. Nature* 397:176–80

35. Kalman S, Mitchell W, Marathe R, Lammel C, Fan J, et al. 1999. Comparative genomes of *Chlamydia pneumoniae* and *C. trachomatis. Nat. Genet.* 21:385–89

36. Nelson KE, Clayton RA, Gill SR, Gwinn ML, Dodson RJ, et al. 1999. Evidence for lateral gene transfer between Archaea and bacteria from genome sequence of *Thermotoga maritima. Nature* 399:323–29

37. Kawarabayasi Y, Hino Y, Horikawa H, Yamazaki S, Haikawa Y, et al. 1999. Complete genome sequence of an aerobic hyper-thermophilic crenarchaeon, *Aeropyrum pernix* K1. *DNA Res.* 6:83–101

38. Wahlgren M. 1999. Creating deaths from malaria. *Nat. Genet.* 22(2):120–21

39. Knight JC, Udalova I, Hill AV, Greenwood BM, Peshu N, et al. 1999. A polymorphism that affects OCT-1 binding to the TNF promoter region is associated with severe malaria. *Nat. Genet.* 22(2):145–50

40. Gardner MJ, Tettelin H, Carucci DJ, Cummings LM, Aravind L, et al. 1998. Chromosome 2 sequence of the human malaria parasite *Plasmodium falciparum. Science* 282:1126–32

41. Landegren U, Nilsson M, Kwok PY. 1998. Reading bits of genetic information: methods for single-nucleotide polymorphism analysis. *Genome Res.* 8(8):769–76

42. Lee JT, Davidow LS, Warshawsky D. 1999. Tsix, a gene antisense to Xist at

the X-inactivation centre. *Nat. Genet.* 21(4):400–4

43. Kruglyak L. 1999. Prospects for whole-genome linkage disequilibrium mapping of common disease genes. *Nat. Genet.* 22(2):139–44

44. Struewing JP, Hartge P, Wacholder S, Baker SM, Berlin M, et al. 1997. The risk of cancer associated with specific mutations of BRCA1 and BRCA2 among Ashkenazi Jews. *N. Engl. J. Med.* 336:1401–8

45. Woodage T, King SM, Wacholder S, Hartge P, Struewing JP, et al. 1998. The APCI1307K allele and cancer risk in a community-based study of Ashkenazi Jews. *Nat. Genet.* 20:62–65

46. Cascorbi I, Brockmoller J, Mrozikiewicz PM, Bauer S, Loddenkemper R, Roots I. 1996. Homozygous rapid arylamine N-acetyltransferase (NAT2) genotype as a susceptibility factor for lung cancer. *Cancer Res.* 56:3961–66

47. Chen J, Giovannucci E, Kelsey K, Rimm EB, Stampfer MJ, et al. 1996. A methylenetetrahydrofolate reductase polymorphism and the risk of colorectal cancer. *Cancer Res.* 56:4862–64

48. Ma J, Stampfer MJ, Giovannucci E, Artigas C, Hunter DJ, et al. 1997. Methylenetetrahydrofolate reductase polymorphism, dietary interactions and risk of colorectal cancer. *Cancer Res.* 57:1098–102

49. Rebbeck TR, Kantoff PW, Krithivas K, Neuhausen S, Blackwood MA, et al. 1999. Modification of BRCA1-associated breast cancer risk by the polymorphic androgen-receptor CAG repeat. *Am. J. Hum. Genet.* 64:1371–77

50. Storey A, Thomas M, Kalita A, Harwood C, Gardiol D, et al. 1998. Role of a p53 polymorphism in the development of human papilloma-virus-associated cancer. *Nature* 393:229–34

51. Helland A, Langerod A, Johnsen H, Olsen AO, Skovlund E, Borresen-Dale

AL. 1998. p53 polymorphism and risk of cervical cancer. *Nature* 396:530–32

52. Josefsson AM, Magnusson PKE, Ylitalo N, Quarforth-Tubbin P, Ponten J, et al. 1998. p53 polymorphism and risk of cervical cancer. *Nature* 396:530–32

53. Hildesheim A, Schiffman M, Brinton LA, Fraumeni JF Jr, Herrero R, et al. 1998. p53 polymorphism and risk of cervical cancer. *Nature* 396:530–32

54. Smith MW, Dean M, Carrington M, Winkler C, Huttley GA, et al. 1997. Contrasting genetic influence of CCR2 and CCR5 variants on HIV-1 infection and disease progression. Hemophilia Growth and Development Study (HGDS), Multicenter AIDS Cohort Study (MACS), Multicenter Hemophilia Cohort Study (MHCS), San Francisco City Cohort (SFCC), ALIVE Study. *Science* 277: 959–65

55. Samson M, Libert F, Doranz BJ, Rucker J, Liesnard C, et al. 1996. Resistance to HIV-1 infection in Caucasian individuals bearing mutant alleles of the CCR-5 chemokine receptor gene. *Nature* 382:722–25

56. Wilkinson DA, Operskalski EA, Busch MP, Mosley JW, Koup RA. 1998. A 32-bp deletion within the CCR5 locus protects against transmission of parenterally acquired human immunodeficiency virus but does not affect progression to AIDS-defining illness. *J. Infect. Dis.* 178:1163–66

57. Ntoumi F, Mercereau-Puijalon O, Ossari S, Luty A, Reltien J, et al. 1997. *Plasmodium falciparum:* sickle-cell trait is associated with higher prevalence of multiple infections in Gabonese children with asymptomatic infections. *Exp. Parasitol.* 87:39–46

58. Lawrenz DR. 1999. Sickle cell disease: a review and update of current therapy. *J. Oral. Maxillofac. Surg.* 57:171–78

59. Carrington M, Nelson GW, Martin MP, Kissner T, Vlahov D, et al. 1999. HLA and HIV-1: heterozygote advantage and B35-Cw04 disadvantage. *Science* 283: 1748–52

60. Fernandez-Reyes D, Craig AG, Kyes SA, Peshu N, Snow RW, et al. 1997. A high frequency African coding polymorphism in the N-terminal domain of ICAM-1 predisposing to cerebral malaria in Kenya. *Hum. Mol. Genet.* 6:1357–60

61. Bellamy R, Kwiatkowski D, Hill AV. 1998. Absence of an association between intercellular adhesion molecule 1, complement receptor 1 and interleukin 1 receptor antagonist gene polymorphisms and severe malaria in a West African population. *Trans. R. Soc. Trop. Med. Hyg.* 92:312–16

62. Bellamy R, Ruwende C, Corrah T, McAdam KP, Whittle HC, Hill AV. 1998. Variations in the NRAMP1 gene and susceptibility to tuberculosis in West Africans. *N. Engl. J. Med.* 338:640–44

63. Martinez FD, Graves PE, Baldini M, Solomon S, Erickson R. 1997. Association between genetic polymorphisms of the beta2-adrenoceptor and response to albuterol in children with and without a history of wheezing. *J. Clin. Invest.* 100:3184–88

64. Dahl M, Tybjaerg-Hansen A, Lange P, Nordestgaard BG. 1998. F508 heterozygosity in cystic fibrosis and susceptibility to asthma. *Lancet* 351:1911–13

65. Green SL, Gaillard MC, Song E, Dewar JB, Halkas A. 1998. Polymorphisms of the beta chain of the high-affinity immunoglobulin E receptor (Fc epsilon RI-beta) in South African black and white asthmatic and nonasthmatic individuals. *Am. J. Respir. Crit. Care Med.* 158:1487–92

66. Hijazi Z, Haider MZ, Khan MR, Al-Dowaisan AA. 1998. High frequency of IgE receptor Fc epsilon RI-beta variant (Leu181/Leu183) in Kuwaiti Arabs and its association with asthma. *Clin. Genet.* 53:149–52

67. Hill MR, Cookson WOCM. 1996. A new variant of the beta subunit of the high-

affinity receptor for immunoglobulin E (Fc epsilon RI-beta E237G): associations with measures of atopy and bronchial hyperresponsiveness. *Hum. Mol. Genet.* 5:959–62

68. Apostolakis J, Toumbis M, Konstantopoulos K, Kamaroulias D, Anagnostakis V, et al. 1996. HLA antigens and asthma in Greeks. *Respir. Med.* 90:201–4

69. Gerbase-DeLima M, Gallo CA, Daher S, Sole D, Naspitz CK. 1997. HLA antigens in asthmatic children. *Pediatr. Allergy Immunol.* 8:150–52

70. Drazen JM, Yandava CN, Dube L, Szczerback N, Hippensteel R, et al. 1999. Pharmacogenetic association between *ALOX5* promoter genotype and the response to anti-asthma treatment. *Nat. Genet.* 22:168–70

71. Stafforini DM, Numao T, Tsodikov A, Vaitkus D, Fukuda T, et al. 1999. Deficiency of platelet-activating factor acetylhydrolase is a severity factor for asthma. *J. Clin. Invest.* 103:989–97

72. Arranz MJ, Li T, Munro J, Liu X, Murray R, et al. 1998. Lack of association between a polymorphism in the promoter region of the dopamine-2 receptor gene and clozapine response. *Pharmacogenetics* 8:481–84

73. Ram A, Cao Q, Keck PE Jr, Pope HG Jr, Otani K, et al. 1995. Structural change in dopamine D2 receptor gene in a patient with neuroleptic malignant syndrome. *Am. J. Med. Genet.* 60:228–30

74. Cravchik A, Sibley DR, Gejman PV. 1999. Analysis of neuroleptic binding affinities and potencies for the different human D2 dopamine receptor missense variants. *Pharmacogenetics* 9:17–23

75. Nothen MM, Chicon S, Hemmer S, Hebebrand J, Remschmidt H, et al. 1994. Human dopamine D4 receptor gene: frequent occurrence of a null allele and observation of homozygosity. *Hum. Mol. Genet.* 3:2207–12

76. Gelernter J, Kranzler H, Coccaro E, Siever L, New A, Mulgrew CL. 1997. D4

dopamine-receptor (DRD4) alleles and novelty seeking in substance-dependent, personality-disorder, and control subjects. *Am. J. Hum. Genet.* 61:1144–52

77. Kotler M, Cohen H, Segman R, Gritsenko I, Nermanov L, et al. 1997. Excess dopamine D4 receptor (D4DR) exon III seven repeat allele in opioid-dependent subjects. *Mol. Psychiatry* 2:251–54

78. Cravchik A, Gejman PV. 1999. Functional analysis of the human D5 dopamine receptor missense and nonsense variants: differences in dopamine binding affinities. *Pharmacogenetics* 9:199–206

79. Cook EH Jr, Stein MA, Krasowski MD, Cox NJ, Olkon DM, et al. 1995. Association of attention-deficit disorder and the dopamine transporter gene. *Am. J. Hum. Genet.* 56:993–98

80. Arranz MJ, Munro J, Sham P, Kirov G, Murray RM, et al. 1998. Meta-analysis of studies on genetic variation in 5-HT2A receptors and clozapine response. *Schizophr. Res.* 32:93–99

81. Lesch KP, Bengel D, Heils A, Sabol SZ, Greenberg BD, et al. 1996. Association of anxiety-related traits with a polymorphism in the seratonin transporter gene regulatory region. *Science* 274:1527–31

82. Marez D, Legrand M, Sabbagh N, Guidice JM, Spire C, et al. 1997. Polymorphism of the cytochrome P450 CYP2D6 gene in a European population: characterization of 48 mutations and 53 alleles. *Pharmacogenetics* 7:193–202

83. May DG. 1994. Genetic differences in drug disposition. *J. Clin. Pharmacol.* 34:881–97

84. Linder MW, Prough RA, Valdes R Jr. 1997. Pharmacogenetics: a laboratory tool for optimizing therapeutic efficiency. *Clin. Chem.* 43:254–66

85. Aithal GP, Day CP, Kesteven PJ, Daly AK. 1999. Association of polymorphisms in the cytochrome P450 CYP2C9 gene with warfarin dose requirement and

risk of bleeding complications. *Lancet* 353:717–19

86. Hashimoto Y, Otsuki Y, Odani A, Takano M, Hattori H, et al. 1996. Effect of CYP2C polymorphisms on the pharmacokinetics of phenytoin in Japanese patients with epilepsy. *Biol. Pharm. Bull.* 19:1103–5

87. Stubbins MJ, Harries LW, Smith G, Tarbit MH, Wolf CR. 1996. Genetic analysis of the cytochrome P450 PYP2C9 locus. *Pharmacogenetics* 6:429–39

88. Karam WG, Goldstein JA, Lasker JM, Ghanayem BI. 1996. Human CYP2C19 is a major omeprazole 5-hydroxylase, as demonstrated with recombinant cytochrome P450 enzymes. *Drug Metab. Dispos.* 24:1081–87

89. Inoue K, Yamazaki H, Shimada T. 1998. Linkage between the distribution of mutations in the CYP2C18 and CYP2C19 genes in the Japanese and Caucasian. *Xenobiotica* 28:403–11

90. Murata M, Shiraishi T, Fukutome K, Watanabe M, Nagao M, et al. 1998. Cytochrome P4501A1 and glutathione S-transferase M1 genotypes as risk factors for prostate cancer in Japan. *Jpn. J. Clin. Oncol.* 28:657–60

91. Bell DA, Taylor JA, Paulson DF, Robertson CN, Mohler JL, Lucier GW. 1993. Genetic risk and carcinogen exposure: a common inherited defect of the carcinogen metabolism gene glutathione S-transferase M1 (GST M1) that increases susceptibility to bladder cancer. *J. Natl. Cancer Inst.* 85:1159–63

92. Okkels H, Sigsgaard T, Wolf H, Autrup H. 1997. Arylamine N-acetyltransferase 1 (NAT1) and 2 (NAT2) polymorphisms in susceptibility to bladder cancer: the influence of smoking. *Cancer Epidemiol. Biomarkers Prev.* 6:225–31

93. Spielberg SP. 1996. N-acetyltransferases: pharmacogenetics and clinical consequences of polymorphic drug metabolism. *J. Pharmacokinet. Biopharm.* 24:509–19

94. Butcher NJ, Ilett KF, Mincnin RF. 1998. Functional polymorphism of the human arylamine N-acetyltransferase type 1 gene caused by C190T and G560A mutations. *Pharmacogenetics* 8:67–72

95. Grant DM, Hughes NC, Janezic SA, Goodfellow GH, Chen HJ, et al. 1997. Human acyltransferase polymorphisms. *Mutat. Res.* 376:61–70

96. Davies HG, Richter RJ, Keifer M, Broomfield CA, Sowalla J, Furlong CE. 1996. The effect of the human serum paraoxonase polymorphism is reversed with diazoxon, soman and sarin. *Nat. Genet.* 14:334–36

97. Furlong CE, Li WF, Costa LG, Richter RJ, Shih DM, et al. 1998. Genetically determined susceptibility to organophosphorus insecticides and nerve agents: developing a mouse model for the human PON1 polymorphism. *Neurotoxicology* 19:645–50

98. Otterness D, Szumlanski C, Lennard L, Klemetsdal B, Aarbakke J, et al. 1997. Human thiopurine methyltransferase pharmacogenetics: gene sequence polymorphisms. *Clin. Pharmacol. Ther.* 62:60–73

99. Escousse A, Guedon F, Mounie J, Rifle G, Mousson C, D'Athis P. 1998. 6-Mercaptopurine pharmacokinetics after use of azathioprine in renal transplant recipients with intermediate or high thiopurine methyl transferase activity phenotype. *J. Pharm. Pharmacol.* 50:1261–66

100. Black AJ, McLeod HL, Capell HA, Powrie RH, Matowe LK, et al. 1998. Thiopurine methyltransferase genotype predicts therapy-limiting severe toxicity from azathioprine. *Ann. Intern. Med.* 129(9):716–18

101. Kamboh MI. 1995. Apolipoprotein E polymorphism and susceptibility to Alzheimer's disease. *Hum. Biol.* 67(2):195–215

102. Roses AD. 1996. Apolipoprotein E alleles as risk factors in Alzheimer's disease. *Annu. Rev. Med.* 47:387–400

103. Cooke GE, Bray PF, Hamlington JD, Pham DM, Goldschmidt-Clermont PS. 1998. PlA2 polymorphism and efficacy of aspirin. *Lancet* 351(9111):1253

104. Margaglione M, Brancaccio V, Giuliani N, D'Andrea G, Cappucci G, et al. 1998. Increased risk for venous thrombosis in carriers of the prothrombin G → A^{20210} gene variant. *Ann. Intern. Med.* 129(2):89–93

105. Daly AK. 1995. Molecular basis of polymorphic drug metabolism. *J. Mol. Med.* 73:539–53

106. Gutman S. 1999. The role of Food and Drug Administration regulation of in vitro diagnostic devices—applications to genetics testing. *Clin. Chem.* 45(5):746–49

107. Holtzman NA. 1999. Promoting safe and effective genetic tests in the United States: work of the task force on genetic testing. *Clin. Chem.* 45(5):732–38

108. Krynetski EY, Evans WE. 1998. Pharmacogenetics of cancer therapy: getting personal. *Am. J. Hum. Genet.* 63:11–16

109. Nebert DW, McKinnon RA, Puga A. 1996. Human drug metabolizing enzyme polymorphisms: effects on risk of toxicity and cancer. *DNA Cell Biol.* 15:273–80

110. Sparreboom A, van Asperen J, Mayer U, Schinkel AH, Smit JW, et al. 1997. Limited oral bioavailability and active epithelial excretion of paclitaxel (Taxol) caused by P-glycoprotein in the intestine. *Proc. Natl. Acad. Sci. USA* 94(5):2031–35

111. Sanak M, Simon HU, Szczeklik A. 1997. Leukotriene C4 synthase promoter polymorphism and risk of aspirin-induced asthma. *Lancet* 350:1599–600

112. Spring J. 1997. Vertebrate evolution by interspecific hybridisation—are we polyploid? *FEBS Lett.* 400(1):2–8

113. Burglin TR. 1996. Homeodomain proteins. In *Encyclopedia of Molecular Biology and Molecular Medicine,* ed. RA Meyers, 3:55–76. Weinheim, Ger.: VCH Verlagsgesellschaft

114. Glaser T, Walton DS, Maas RL. 1992. Genomic structure, evolutionary conservation and aniridia mutations in the human PAX6 gene. *Nat. Genet.* 2(3):232–39

115. Quiring R, Walldorf U, Kloter U, Gehring WJ. 1994. Homology of the *eyeless* gene of Drosophila to the *Small eye* gene in mice and Aniridia in humans. *Science* 265(5173):785–89

116. Becker W, Joost HG. 1999. Structural and functional characteristics of Dyrk, a novel subfamily of protein kinases with dual specificity. *Prog. Nucleic Acid Res. Mol. Biol.* 62:1–17

117. Ohira M, Seki N, Nagase T, Suzuki E, Nomura N, et al. 1997. Gene identification in 1.6-Mb region of the Down syndrome region on chromosome 21. *Genome Res.* 7(1):47–58

118. Guimera J, Casas C, Pucharcos C, Solans A, Domenech A, et al. 1996. A human homologue of Drosophila minibrain (MNB) is expressed in the neuronal regions affected in Down syndrome and maps to the critical region. *Hum. Mol. Genet.* 5(9):1305–10

119. Reeves RH, Gearhart JD, Littlefield JW. 1986. Genetic basis for a mouse model of Down syndrome. *Brain Res. Bull.* 16(6):803–14

120. Haydar TF, Blue ME, Molliver ME, Krueger BK, Yarowsky PJ. 1996. Consequences of trisomy 16 for mouse brain development: corticogenesis in a model of Down syndrome. *J. Neurosci.* 16(19):6175–82

121. Smith DJ, Rubin EM. 1997. Functional screening and complex traits: human 21q22.2 sequences affecting learning in mice. *Hum. Mol. Genet.* 6(10):1729–33

122. Smith DJ, Stevens ME, Sudagunta SP, Bronson RT, Makhinson M, et al. 1997. Functional screening of 2 Mb of human chromosome 21q22.2 in transgenic mice implicates minibrain in learning defects

associated with Down syndrome. *Nat. Genet.* 16(1):28–36

123. Clark AG. 1999. Chips for chimps. *Nat. Genet.* 22(2):119–20

124. Hacia JC, Fan J-B, Ryder O, Jin L, Edgemon K, et al. 1999. Determination of ancestral alleles for human single-nucleotide polymorphisms using high-density oligonucleotide assays. *Nat. Genet.* 22:164–67

125. Goodman M. 1999. Molecular evolution '99: the genomic record of humankind's evolutionary roots. *Am. J. Hum. Genet.* 64:31–39

126. Czelusniak J, Goodman M, Hewett-Emmett D, Weiss ML, Venta PJ, Tashian RE. 1982. Phylogenetic origins and adaptive evolution of avian and mammalian haemoglobin genes. *Nature* 298(5871):297–300

127. Chiu C-H, Schneider H, Slightom JL, Gumucio DL, Goodman M. 1997. Dynamics of regulatory evolution in primate β-globin gene clusters: cis-medi-

ated acquisition of simian γ fetal expression patterns. *Gene* 205:47–57

128. Chiu C-H, Gregoire L, Gumucio DL, Muniz JAPC, Lancaster WD, Goodman M. 1999. Model for the fetal recruitment of simian γ-globin genes based on findings from two new world monkeys *Cebus apella* and *Callithrix jacchus* (Platyrrhini, primates). *J. Exp. Zool.* 285:27–40

129. Hayasaka K, Fitch DHA, Slightom JL, Goodman M. 1992. Fetal recruitment of anthropoid γ-globin genes. *J. Mol. Biol.* 224:875–81

130. McConkey EH, Goodman M. 1997. A human genome evolution project is needed. *Trends Genet.* 13:350–51

131. Dutrillaux B. 1979. Chromosomal evolution in primates: tentative phylogeny from *Microcebus murinus* (Prosimian) to man. *Hum. Genet.* 48:251–314

132. Yunis JJ, Prakash O. 1982. The origin of man: a chromosomal pictorial legacy. *Science* 215:1525–30

Annu. Rev. Pharmacol. Toxicol. 2000. 40:133–57

HIGH-THROUGHPUT SCREENING IN DRUG METABOLISM AND PHARMACOKINETIC SUPPORT OF DRUG DISCOVERY

Ronald E. White

Department of Drug Metabolism and Pharmacokinetics, Schering-Plough Research Institute, 2015 Galloping Hill Road, Kenilworth, New Jersey 07033–1300; e-mail: ronald.white@spcorp.com

Key Words   in vitro, in vivo, cytochrome P450, Caco-2, hepatocytes

■ **Abstract**   The application of rapid methods currently used for screening discovery drug candidates for metabolism and pharmacokinetic characteristics is discussed. General considerations are given for screening in this context, including the criteria for good screens, the use of counterscreens, the proper sequencing of screens, ambiguity in the interpretation of results, strategies for false positives and negatives, and the special difficulties encountered in drug metabolism and pharmacokinetic screening. Detailed descriptions of the present status of screening are provided for absorption potential, blood-brain barrier penetration, inhibition and induction of cytochrome P450, pharmacokinetics, biotransformation, and computer modeling. Although none of the systems currently employed for drug metabolism and pharmacokinetic screening can be considered truly high-throughput, several of them are rapid enough to be a practical part of the screening paradigm for modern, fast-moving discovery programs.

INTRODUCTION

Since the early 1990s, several new forces in drug discovery have changed the pursuit of this endeavor. We may group these forces into three main areas: chemistry, molecular biology, and robotics. Chemists have invented many new methodologies for production of large, diverse sets of novel organic compounds. We refer to these methodologies under the umbrella term combinatorial chemistry (1). The result has been a many-fold increase in the number of compounds available to sample so-called chemistry-space, that is, the multidimensional relation between molecular structure and biological activity (2). In addition, structural chemists have developed powerful new tools such as molecular docking algorithms (3), mapping of protein binding sites by nuclear magnetic resonance (SAR-by-NMR) (4), and homology modeling of proteins (5) that allow an unprecedented level of rational design to guide the synthesis of prospective drugs.

0362–1642/00/0415–0133$14.00   **133**

From another direction, molecular biology and genomics have allowed identification of many important new biological targets (6) and have provided the means to express these target proteins in in vitro systems that enable them to be used in high-throughput screening (7, 8). For both combinatorial chemistry and high-throughput screening, the enabling development has been the commercial availability of reliable, highly programmable, adaptable robots (9–11) that can carry out complex microscale laboratory operations to synthesize and test hundreds of thousands of new organic compounds. Recent advances in miniaturization and assay speed and sensitivity have allowed the use of 1536-well microtiter plates instead of the conventional 96-well plates and have prompted the use of the term ultrahigh-throughput screening. These forces have synergistically increased our ability to create pharmacologically interesting compounds, at least at the in vitro level.

As a practical matter, this increase has produced an enormous pressure to determine which of these thousands of biochemically active compounds have drug-like properties (i.e. which are biologically active). We can define a compound to be drug-like when it has the following properties.

1. Efficacy: the intrinsic ability of the compound to produce a desired pharmacological effect. Efficacy comprises the absolute amount of the compound necessary to achieve the effect (potency) and the magnitude of the maximum effect that can be achieved.
2. Availability: the ability of the compound to pass through multiple biological barriers to reach the target receptor. Normally we consider availability to comprise both oral bioavailability and adequate distribution to the target organ.
3. Persistence: sufficient residence time at the target receptor so that pharmacological effects have a clinically meaningful duration. Persistence is usually expressed as the plasma elimination half-life.
4. Safety: sufficient selectivity for the target receptor so that an adequate dose range exists in which the intended pharmacological action is essentially the only physiological effect of the compound.
5. Practicality: generally thought of as the pharmaceutical properties of the compound, including solubility and rate of dissolution, chemical stability, crystallinity, and so on, which allow the drug substance to be synthesized and the drug product to be formulated, distributed, handled, and dosed in a practical manner. For this discussion, we can ignore consideration of commercial success criteria such as size of patient population, marketing, production economics, and so on.

Each of the drug-like properties must be present in a successful clinical drug, although there is considerable latitude in each property. A major deficit in any of these properties will preclude an active compound from being used as a drug. All five properties must be in the acceptable range, even if it is not possible to fully optimize each property. Of these drug properties, only efficacy and safety can be considered to be optimized in any sense during the combinatorial synthesis/in vitro screening phase, inasmuch as the compound's intrinsic affinity for the receptor, the potential magnitude of the response (if the compound has an agonist action), and the selectivity of the compound for the particular receptor subtype are standard components of the screening phase.

Optimizing the other properties is much less straightforward for two reasons. First, to derive the full benefit from the great advances made in high-throughput screening, subsequent optimization steps must occur at a substantial fraction of the rate of production of compounds with acceptable biochemical activity, meaning that in vitro or accelerated in vivo methods must be used. Second, an in vitro method must have physiological relevance. That is, the method must be validated, or shown to have a good concordance with the desired in vivo parameter. Validation is surprisingly difficult with metabolic pathways and parameters such as intestinal absorption, half-life, or brain penetration. Often only in vivo measurements of these parameters are reliable enough to allow strategic decisions about the viability of a candidate compound. Unfortunately, in vivo measurements are generally so slow that they represent a considerable bottleneck for compound selection, largely negating the speed of creation and identification of potent compounds.

In this review we consider the problems of optimizing drug-like properties, with a focus on drug metabolism and pharmacokinetics (DMPK). We discuss the advances that have been made in recent years to increase the speed of assessment methods enough to achieve the rapidity of advancement through a drug discovery campaign that is theoretically possible. Truly high-throughput screening methods, such as those used to screen for early leads in compound libraries, may achieve rates of 50,000–100,000 compounds per week. In contrast, the fastest methods presently used in DMPK screening typically do not exceed 100 compounds per week. For in vivo methods, a throughput of 10 compounds per week might be considered high if the conventional methodology could handle only one compound in a week. Thus we use the term higher-throughput to denote the acceleration of the rate even though the absolute rate is very slow.

GENERAL CONSIDERATIONS FOR SCREENING

Criteria for Good Screens

The following five criteria should be met when designing and implementing a discovery screen.

1. Relevance: The result of the screen should have good concordance with the corresponding in vivo property of the drug (e.g. clearance, absorption, or brain penetration). This requires validation of the screen with standard compounds of known animal or human performance.

2. Effectiveness: The cutoff criterion should eliminate a substantial fraction of compounds. If almost all compounds survive the screen, it merely adds a useless extra step that delays the discovery process (but see "Counterscreens" below).
3. Speed: The experimental procedure must be fast enough to keep pace with the input rate of new compounds from chemistry. Rapidity is often achieved at the expense of absolute accuracy, but for screening purposes we can afford to relax our usual criteria for accuracy. An effective means to achieve speed is to use exactly the same assay, regardless of the compound being tested, but this is seldom possible with DMPK screens.
4. Robustness: The experimental procedure must be applicable to a wide variety of chemical structures. Ideally it should also work with different biological components (e.g. animal or human microsomes, S9 fractions, hepatocytes).
5. Accuracy and reproducibility: Obviously we want the screen to give the right result the first time (see "False Positives and False Negatives" below), and extensive retesting degrades the method's productivity. Because of relaxed accuracy to achieve speed, it may also make sense to widen the acceptance criterion window to account for greater-than-normal uncertainty in the measured value.

Counterscreens

In many cases, we are not trying to find the compounds that have a certain property; rather, we are trying to find the ones that lack a certain property. For instance, counterscreens are used for confirming high selectivity for the receptor of interest by showing that the compound does not bind well to other receptors. Likewise, we often use a counterscreen to assure that potent inhibitors of CYP 3A4 are eliminated from further consideration. Counterscreens have the same criteria as screens, except that for counterscreens the effectiveness criterion is reversed, because we want as many compounds as possible to survive the counterscreen.

Sequencing of Screens

Often the lead optimization phase of drug discovery has a battery of successive screens that must be passed. The general rule is that the screen with the best overall combination of speed and "veto power" should be highest in the succession of screens. All work done on a compound that has no potential to be a clinical drug is wasted effort, except when the compound is to be used only as an investigational agent in pharmacological proof-of-principle studies. Most frequently, then, the first screen is a high-throughput in vitro assay for antagonism or inhibition of the receptor or enzyme that is the biochemical target. This is usually readily adaptable from the high-throughput lead discovery phase, and the data from this screen are clearly interpretable in an absolute sense (i.e. a compound with a K_i of 1000 nM is clearly not active enough). Thus having this screen in the first position eliminates many more compounds than other screens would.

The next screen after the in vitro activity screen might be a counterscreen against related receptor types, or a cell-culture model. However, industry is increasingly using a screen for a desirable biopharmaceutical property (e.g. Caco-2 permeability as an indicator of intestinal absorption) or a counterscreen against an undesirable biopharmaceutical property (e.g. CYP 3A4 inhibition). This second-level screen can even be an in vivo pharmacokinetic screen based on cassette dosing or pooling of plasma samples, methods that can offer enough speed to be practical even at a relatively high position in the screening sequence.

Interpretation of Screens

The biopharmaceutical properties of drugs fall into two groups: those determined entirely by the molecular structure of the compound and those that depend on interaction with a biological component. Examples of the first type are pK_a, solubility, dissolution rate, crystallinity, and chemical instability. These properties are intrinsic to the compound and are, therefore, measurable by completely abiotic methods. The interpretation of values for intrinsic properties is straightforward, because the significance of slow dissolution rate or chemical instability is clear when considering the suitability of a compound to be a drug. Even for some of the properties of compounds that depend on a biological component, for example in vitro binding affinity to the target receptor, interpretation of in vitro data is straightforward (i.e. tighter binding is better). In stark contrast, most of the DMPK properties of a compound are the result of a complex interaction of the compound with membranes, binding proteins, transporters, and metabolizing enzymes as well as higher-level phenomena such as organ blood flows, glomerular filtration rate, and tissue uptake. These biological interactions make it difficult to assess the meaning and importance of a value for a particular property that is measured in vitro, especially when a cross-species comparison is required. Consequently, it is particularly important to establish the relevancy of the in vitro–measured property to the corresponding physiological property prior to application of the screen to a new series of compounds, and to check the continuing relevance as that property is improved in successive analogs.

False Positives and False Negatives

Any screening procedure has a characteristic error rate. This is almost inevitable, because it is usually necessary to sacrifice some accuracy or precision to achieve the requisite speed. Thus when a large number of compounds is carried through a particular screen, some of the compounds will be classified incorrectly. A screen may be used in an absolute sense, so that compounds that pass a certain criterion (e.g. Caco-2 permeability greater than that of a benchmark compound) are termed positives, whereas those that fail to meet the criterion are termed negatives. Compounds that pass but should have failed are false positives. In general, false positives are tolerable, if they are not too numerous, because they will be rectified later. Compounds that fail but should have passed are false negatives. False negatives may be lost forever if the failure eliminates them from further testing. However, as long as a reasonable number of true positives are being found, false negatives are also tolerable. Because the pass-fail criterion for a screen is arbitrary to a degree, the relative fractions of false positives to false negatives are adjustable by moving the acceptance criterion up or down, and the researcher may opt for more false positives and fewer false negatives for a direct screen and the converse for a counterscreen. A screen may also be used in a relative sense, to rank-order compounds for priority for subsequent testing. However, even for rank-ordering, false positives and false negatives can still cause the compound to be ranked incorrectly.

DRUG METABOLISM AND PHARMACOKINETICS SCREENING

General Considerations

The main subject of this review is the extensive effort presently occurring in industrial drug discovery organizations to increase the probability of ultimate success for a compound entering clinical trials (12). Obviously when a compound fails in clinical trials, failure was not expected. In fact, the three main reasons for clinical failure (lack of efficacy, toxicity, and unfavorable DMPK properties) are poorly understood and inherently difficult to predict. To illustrate, let us look at these reasons for failure. In contemporary drug discovery and development, most companies are investigating new pharmacology—that is, a novel approach, a novel molecular target, or a previously untreatable disease. Of course, the reason for this is that to be "first-in-market" with a new therapy is the sine qua non of the pharmaceutical business. The difficulty with being first is that clinical trials carry the additional burden of "proof-of-principle" with the new therapeutic concept, and sometimes the new pharmacology simply does not work in humans. This is something that can be determined only by clinical experience; thus, it is unpredictable preclinically. Similarly, a particular clinical toxicity is not normally expected, except in the special case of exaggerated pharmacology. For example, if the compound had shown hepatotoxicity in the preclinical animal toxicology studies, it would not have been taken to Phase I clinical trials, except for poorly treated, life-threatening indications. So, in most cases, an observed human toxicity was not predicted by animal toxicity.

The prediction of DMPK properties is similarly difficult, partly because of the vast number of possible metabolic pathways (13) and partly because of interspecies differences (14). At the same time, good DMPK properties are fundamental to the success of a drug candidate, and it is important to have some sort of procedure to assure their presence in the clinical candidate. For instance, although efforts continue to quantitatively predict pharmacokinetics, the current industry trend is to settle for categorization of candidates as clearly bad, marginal, or probably good (15). Candidates that are clearly bad are eliminated, and the good candidates are rank-order prioritized for more in-depth study. If enough good candidates are found, it may be unnecessary to make hard decisions about the marginal ones. As we discuss the screening for various DMPK properties in the next sections, we will see how the categorization concept is applied in each case.

Absorption Potential

Although in vivo studies are clearly the most reliable way to determine intestinal absorption, current in vivo methodology is far too slow to allow its application in discovery screening. Although a high-throughput in situ rat intraduodenal dosing model was used to guide synthesis of absorbable renin inhibitors (16), this method has not been applied widely, and researchers have mainly sought in vitro methods. The two chief determinants of in vivo intestinal absorption are solubility and intestinal permeability. Solubility is readily estimated on small quantities of a compound following synthesis, but permeability is much more difficult to assess. The most popular approach is to measure rates of compound diffusion down a concentration gradient across cultured Caco-2 cell monolayers (17).

Caco-2 permeability screening is used widely to screen drugs (18), prodrugs (19), and combinatorial libraries (20, 21). It is generally accepted that good permeability through Caco-2 monolayers is a reliable indicator of good absorption in vivo (22, 23), unless dissolution is a problem. The interpretation of low and intermediate Caco-2 permeabilities is not clear. Low molecular weight hydrophilic compounds, sugars, nucleosides, or small peptides may show very low permeabilities in vitro yet be well absorbed in vivo because alternative mechanisms of absorption are not well modeled by the Caco-2 monolayer, including paracellular passage or active transport (24). Even for drugs that have good Caco-2 permeability, in vivo absorption can occasionally be limited by the P-glycoprotein (PGP) efflux pump (see below). This ambiguity in interpretation makes it difficult to predict with confidence the net in vivo absorption of a candidate. Most groups eschew quantitative predictions entirely, preferring either to categorize compounds as having low, medium, or high permeability or to compare them to a structurally related benchmark compound with known in vivo absorption. A genetically engineered Caco-2 variant has been developed that stably expresses high levels of CYP 3A4, the intestinal P450 enzyme responsible for some first-pass metabolism, to allow a concurrent assessment of permeability and gut wall metabolism (25). It is difficult to quantitatively relate the degree of metabolism in such a system to the in vivo first-pass effect.

Reports of increasing throughput of the Caco-2 permeability assessment via automation are just beginning to appear in the peer-reviewed literature (26), but this technology is already becoming widely applied, with several automation companies offering specialized robots for the purpose. The usual approach is to separate the overall process into two regimens: (*a*) culture of the cells until confluency and tight junctions are achieved, and (*b*) the actual permeation experiment. Although neither of these steps can be considered truly high-throughput, the cell culture process is by far the slower of the two. This stage is accelerated by the simple expedient of maintaining many cultures in parallel. After an initial 3-week delay, monolayers can be staggered to be ready for a permeability experiment each day. If the automation is set up properly, every step from initial seeding of cells, through daily maintenance and medium changes, through running the permeability experiment, to the LC/MS/MS (liquid chromatography/tandem mass spectrometry) assay can be carried out with only a little human intervention, such as occasionally replenishing media reservoirs or manually moving microtiter plates from the robotic liquid handler to the LC sample-injector robot. Special 24-well plates are now available for Caco-2 cultures, allowing rates of a few hundred compounds per month to be realized. Although such a rate is far below that of true high-throughput screening, it is far better than the rate typically achievable with purely manual cell-culture methods, and it is usually sufficient to keep pace with the delivery of potent compounds through the primary in vitro activity screen. Another advantage is that automation allows cells to be maintained during holiday and vacation periods, which otherwise create blackout periods for Caco-2 determinations.

Two other methods for rapid assessment of absorption potential should be mentioned, both of which are based on completely artificial membrane-mimic systems. Immobilized artificial membrane (IAM) chromatography offers the advantages of experimental simplicity and familiarity to most chemists, compared with Caco-2 permeabilities. Good correlations have been shown between IAM chromatographic k' values and both Caco-2 permeabilities and in vivo intestinal absorption (27). Because retention times increase with increasing absorption potential, the chromatography sets limits on throughput that would have to be addressed in a high-throughput screening application. Recently, the parallel artificial membrane permeation assay (PAMPA) was introduced for in vitro assessment of passive absorption (28). The method utilizes permeation through an artificial phospholipid bilayer formed on a filter within the wells of a 96-well microtiter plate. The assay, based on simple ultraviolet absorbance of the effluent, allows high rates of compound assessment, in the range of hundreds per day. Like the Caco-2 permeability method, IAM and PAMPA may underestimate the absorption of compounds subject to active or paracellular transport in vivo. However, both methods, especially PAMPA, seem well suited to early drug discovery absorption counterscreening, in which the goal is to eliminate poorly absorbable compounds.

As mentioned above, a potential limitation of net absorption of compounds with good transport properties is the PGP efflux pump (29). For instance, PGP has been shown to limit the absorption of several HIV protease inhibitors by as much as fivefold (30). Thus there is interest in screening compounds as PGP substrates during discovery. A higher-throughput assay based on competition against ^{3}H-verapamil binding in PGP-overexpressing Caco-2 cells has been described (31). Two other methods are based on inhibition of efflux of a fluorescent PGP substrate (32–34), and these methods have been applied in an industrial setting. A limitation of all three methods is that they do not distinguish between PGP substrates and inhibitors.

The case of PGP screening illustrates the difficulty of screening for DMPK properties. Because PGP both limits intestinal absorption and excludes xenobiotics from the brain (30), a compound in which PGP recognition has been eliminated may be better absorbed but also show greater net brain penetration. Although brain penetration will be desirable for central nervous system (CNS) drugs, it is generally undesirable for other indications because of the potential for CNS side effects or toxicity. Also, a PGP substrate may competitively inhibit the brain efflux of a second co-dosed drug, increasing its potential for CNS toxicity (35). Therefore, one must carefully consider the therapeutic indication and likely co-dosed drugs before applying a PGP screen in a drug discovery program.

Blood-Brain Barrier

The ability of compounds to penetrate the blood-brain barrier is almost always of interest, either as a property to screen for in a CNS indication or to counterscreen against in non-CNS indications. Although this property is not usually considered an object of primary screening, requiring higher-throughput methodology, it is often set as the object of secondary or tertiary screening in CNS discovery programs, because many pharmacological models of CNS diseases are long and tedious. It is prudent to determine whether a compound can get past the blood-brain barrier before investing time in the in vivo assay. A good in vitro model is available for this purpose, bovine brain microvessel endothelial cell (BMEC) monolayers, which are used in a manner analogous to that of Caco-2 permeability screening (36, 37). BMEC monolayers have been applied to higher-throughput drug discovery screening for good brain penetration (38). Although BMEC permeability is determined quantitatively, it is usually sufficient to express the results qualitatively (i.e. good or poor brain penetration). A major disadvantage is that BMECs are not an immortal cell line; therefore, they must be primary-cultured from cow brain. Although the cells may be frozen after harvesting, they are an exhaustible resource that must be replenished regularly. Recent studies show that BMECs express a functional PGP system (39, 40) that may allow them to be used as an in vitro model of PGP-limited brain penetration in a screening mode. The BMEC system has not yet been reported to have been automated.

Enzyme Inhibition

Inhibition of a shared metabolic enzyme is a common source of adverse clinical interaction between co-dosed drugs (41–43). At the same time, enzyme inhibition is one of the easiest phenomena to measure in a higher-throughput mode, because of experimental simplicity and because the same assay can be used regardless of the test compound. As a result, most companies conduct enzyme inhibition counterscreening, and the main difference among companies is in the stage in the discovery process at which screening occurs. The only enzymes that have been subjected to higher-throughput inhibition screening are the cytochrome P450 enzymes, although others are certainly amenable if there were interest. Because the majority of drugs metabolized by P450 are substrates of either CYP 3A4 or CYP 2D6, these two enzymes have been subject to the most screening efforts, but CYP 2C9 has recently become recognized as an important enzyme for inhibition screening (44). It is also possible to determine which P450 enzyme is mainly responsible for the metabolism of a compound (45), but this is more difficult experimentally and is of less interest for counterscreening purposes. Flow diagrams to guide the application of hepatocytes in profiling of discovery compounds as both inhibitors and substrates of P450 have been published (46), and similar flow diagrams might be useful to those investigators contemplating higher-throughput screening.

The commercial availability of single P450 enzymes has made possible rapid inhibition assays in a 96-well format that are readily adaptable to automation (47, 48). Measurement of the enzymatic rate can be accomplished by a fluorimetric method (49, 50), but industrial laboratories are increasingly using LC/MS/MS because of advances in the speed of this technique and because of its ready availability in the industrial environment (51, 52).

Another aspect of P450 screening is whether the observed inhibition is direct or metabolism/mechanism-based, the distinction being that direct inhibition is the reversible, noncovalent binding of the test compound to a site on the enzyme that alters its Michaelis-Menten kinetic parameters, whereas metabolism/mechanism-based inhibition is the binding of a metabolic product of the test compound. To further elaborate this distinction, metabolism-based inhibition results from a metabolite that is a tighter binding reversible inhibitor, whereas mechanism-based inhibition results from covalent binding to the enzyme by a chemically reactive intermediate, which inactivates the enzyme (42). Metabolism/mechanism-based and direct inhibition are readily distinguished experimentally because the former increases with time whereas the latter is constant or may decrease with time.

If necessary, metabolism-based and mechanism-based inhibition may also be distinguished by removal of the metabolites through dilution or dialysis and rechallenge of the enzyme with fresh substrate. The enzyme would be affected reversibly by metabolism-based inhibition but irreversibly by the mechanism-based type. Because of the propensity of the P450 oxidative reaction mechanism to produce reactive intermediates, it is not unusual for a compound to be a weak direct inhibitor but a strong metabolism/mechanism-based inhibitor. Therefore, a complete assessment of the inhibition potential of a test compound should look for both types of inhibition. Commonly this is accomplished in the higher-throughput mode by determining the apparent IC_{50} of the test compound toward a standard substrate with and without a preincubation period of the enzyme with the test compound (53). Generally, compounds are classified as potent ($IC_{50} < 1$ μM), marginal ($1 \mu M < IC_{50} < 10 \mu M$), or weak inhibitors($IC_{50} > 10 \mu M$). Most companies are reluctant to advance a potent inhibitor. A large decrease (greater than 10-fold) in the apparent IC_{50} after preincubation with the test compound is evidence of metabolism/mechanism-based inhibition and usually terminates interest in the compound.

Enzyme Induction

Although a variety of drug-metabolizing enzymes are inducible by xenobiotic compounds, the main industrial interest is in the cytochromes P450 (54). There are two main, though disparate, reasons for this interest in P450 induction. The first reason is the obvious one, namely the involvement of P450 induction in some clinical drug interactions (42, 43). The second reason is that P450 induction appears to be related to the production of liver tumors in rodent oncogenicity studies during drug development (55), which provides a compelling reason to screen out this property in the discovery phase. Of course, rodent induction can be determined directly in discovery, but compound requirements and the necessity for days of dosing eliminate this approach for screening purposes, and it can be used only in the final testing phase of a potential clinical candidate just prior to selection for development. Therefore, as we discuss below, much faster methods requiring only milligram amounts of compound are required for practical screening. Unfortunately, rat enzyme induction does not predict human induction. For instance, phenobarbital induces mainly 2B enzymes in rats but 3A enzymes in humans (42). If human induction is also to be assessed preclinically, a separate, human-based in vitro system must be used.

Screening methods for P450 induction must necessarily use in vitro systems, of which two basic types exist: hepatocytes and cell-based gene-reporter constructs. Hepatocytes are used widely and can be applied to both rodent and human induction problems, now that human hepatocytes are commercially available (56, 57). Hepatocytes cannot be considered to be high-throughput or even higher-throughput methods. Even if we ignore the preincubation culture period of several days, the basic experiment requires at least 2 days of incubation of the cells with the test compound. As with Caco-2 culture, the throughput can be increased by parallel incubation of many cultures and test compounds, but the subsequent analysis of enzyme activities and Western blotting also offers a considerable barrier to rapid operation.

The utility of hepatocytes lies not in their speed but in their comparison to alternative methods for assessment of P450 induction. First, the amount of compound required is small in comparison to in vivo rodent studies. For instance, to conduct a 5-day induction study in three rats at doses of 30 and 100 mg/kg, a total of 600 mg of test compound is needed, compared to the ~2 mg needed for hepatocytes. Although this difference may seem unimportant when investigating the induction patterns of established drugs, for discovery purposes the total compound supply may be a paramount consideration, because the combinatorial synthesis may have produced only 10 mg of each of 500 compounds. In general, a compound must pass many in vitro and in vivo tests before it is of sufficient interest to warrant the synthesis of gram quantities, meaning that in vivo rat induction testing is limited to late-stage discovery compounds and is not suitable for early-stage screening. Second, there is no in vivo alternative to hepatocyte testing for human induction. Thus it is not surprising that discovery research has embraced the use of both rat and human hepatocytes for induction screening (58).

To achieve a higher-throughput induction assay, companies are now turning to promoter-gene-reporter constructs. Such cell-based systems may incorporate a fluorescent or luminescent reporter product (59, 60) to allow an automated spectrophotometric endpoint, and the entire induction experiment may require only a few hours. Each specific enzyme to be investigated would have a separate gene-construct-transfected cell line. We currently understand enough of the induction mechanisms for the 1A (61) and 3A families (62) for these systems to be practical realities. A method to investigate the 4A family has been reported, because CYP 4A is closely related to peroxisome proliferation (63). Although the induction of the 2B family has been poorly understood (64), recent advances in our understanding of the phenobarbital-response mechanism may also allow a construct that is useful for the assessment of the CYP 2B induction potential (65, 66). Based on the results of the induction screen, whether from hepatocytes or a reporter-gene system, the test compound would be categorized as a strong, weak, or non-inducer of P450 and as phenobarbital-like or methylcholanthrene-like.

Pharmacokinetics

In Vitro Screening

Metabolic Stability   The kinetic susceptibility of a compound to biotransformation is one determinant of oral bioavailability and systemic clearance. Although rates of in vitro biotransformation can be used in a more rigorous fashion to extrapolate in vivo clearances (see below), it is often adequate and useful merely to set up an appropriate in vitro metabolism model system and rank-order compounds in terms of their relative metabolic stability. The in vitro model system may be microsomes, cDNA-expressed enzymes, liver slices, or hepatocytes, and the availability of these biological components from common animal species and humans makes this a powerful technique for assessing metabolic stability through a long series of compounds as well as across species. When adapted to a 96-well plate format and to LC-MS assay of disappearance of parent compound, it is possible to implement a metabolic stability screen with throughput appropriate to apply in a fast-moving drug discovery program (67). In fact, throughput can be high enough that informatics software may be needed to capture, manipulate, and distribute the data. A helpful variation is to index the rate of metabolism of the test compounds to that of a benchmark compound whose in vivo persistence is to be matched or exceeded. The system can be adjusted to provide an intermediate rate of metabolism of the benchmark compound (e.g. 30% loss of parent). Compounds that are substantially more or less stable than the benchmark are discerned readily.

Two caveats are important when interpreting data of this type. First, it is easily possible to have no correlation between the in vitro stability data and the in vivo clearance of the drug. Thus it is important to carry out in vivo checking of the in vitro stability order before incorporating this method into the screening process. Second, the measured rate of disappearance of parent drug should ideally be the initial rate but likely is not because of substrate and cofactor depletion, accumulation of inhibitory products, and decay of enzyme activity. Therefore, the observed relative rates of decline of two compounds may be quite different from their true relative intrinsic clearances. Consequently, relative stability data through a compound series should not be interpreted too quantitatively. Nonetheless, microsomal stability screening is experimentally simple, and the data lend themselves to intuitive interpretation, making this method widely utilized.

In Vitro/In Vivo Scaling   A great deal of effort has been expended on the theory and practice of quantitative prediction of human hepatic clearance of drugs from rates of metabolic conversion observed in various in vitro systems such as microsomes, hepatocytes, and liver slices (15, 68–70). From the point of view of discovery screening, we can make two comments. First, scientific understanding of the in vitro and in vivo components of the predictions is presently insufficient for them to be more accurate than within a factor of two of the true value, on average. However, this situation may change as our understanding improves, and, indeed, hepatocytes may be used to rank compounds by their predicted hepatic extraction ratios (71). The problem of quantitative uncertainty is alleviated by lowering the expectation of the results and merely classifying a compound as low, medium, or high extraction. Second, although these methods may be useful for selecting among a few final clinical candidates at the end of a discovery program (72), they are not fast enough to serve as a practical means of screening compounds in the early phase. Thus these methods are not more useful in discovery of a suitable clinical candidate than is simple metabolic stability ranking, and they are considerably slower.

In Vivo Screening

Multicompound Dosing   This term refers to simultaneous administration of several compounds to a single animal and is also called cassette or *N*-in-one dosing. Multicompound dosing has become widely applied in DMPK screening because it offers enhanced rates of examination of compounds in vivo, avoiding the problem of in vitro/in vivo correlation (73–76). The enabling technology is LC/MS/MS, which allows the investigator to cleanly assay a particular analyte in the presence of many structurally similar compounds (77, 78). The rate acceleration comes from two efficiencies: (*a*) far fewer animals must be prepared and dosed, and (*b*) far fewer samples are generated for assay. The degree of acceleration depends on how many compounds are co-dosed (*N*), but there are practical limitations on *N* so that most applications use *N* of 10 or less. Both rats and dogs have been used. Because medicinal chemists have been very receptive to the introduction of multicompound dosing into discovery DMPK screening, it is worthwhile to discuss several caveats that accompany its use.

1. Care must be taken in selecting the mixture of compounds to be dosed because of the homogeneity of the typical compound set and the possible presence of metabolites in the plasma samples. Isomers may be co-dosed as long as they exhibit distinct daughter ions because the MS/MS technique is normally used. However, it is easily possible for a metabolite to have a structure identical to one of the original test compounds. For instance, if the test mixture contains both a tertiary methyl amine and the corresponding secondary amine, the *N*-desmethyl metabolite of the first compound is identical to the second compound. Similarly, if the test mixture contains both a phenyl compound and the corresponding phenol, the phenolic metabolite of the former will confound the assay of the latter.
2. Drug interactions can cause a distortion of the pharmacokinetics of one or more components of the co-dosed test mixture. Although this phenomenon is generally recognized, the following misconceptions exist: (*a*) One may guard against competitive inhibition of a shared metabolic enzyme (the main reason for drug interactions) by keeping doses small; (*b*) even if the absolute values are wrong, the correct rank order will be observed; (*c*) one can detect drug interactions by always including a control compound; and (*d*) drug interactions can lead only to false positives, which will be discovered later in the process. Consideration of pharmacokinetics shows that none of these assumptions is true.
3. The total pharmacological and toxicological load delivered to the animal must be considered. Most investigators take the position that it is better to keep the total amount of all compounds low so that pharmacological and toxicological effects do not become large enough to physiologically compromise the animal's ability to clear the drugs. The consequence is a limit to the total number of compounds that can be co-dosed, because the sensitivity of the assay will become limiting when the dose of each compound is very low.

Rapid Pharmacokinetic Screening   To avoid the problems of in vitro/in vivo scaling and drug interactions, several laboratories have developed methods to accelerate the acquisition of focused data from singly dosed animals. The approach in each case is to reduce the overall time for assessment of each drug candidate by minimizing both the in vivo and bioanalytical phases of the experiments. To minimize the in vivo phase, the collection period is reduced to 6–8 h, which is much shorter than that in conventional pharmacokinetic studies. The bioanalytical phase is minimized by the reduced number of samples accruing from the shorter collection period, by pooling at time points or across all time points, and by the use of an abbreviated standard curve. All higher-throughput in vivo pharmacokinetics methods depend on an accelerated assay technology to achieve meaningful rate increases (79). Interestingly, one group has reversed the trend to use LC/MS as the assay tool and has revived the use of bioassay of plasma concentrations for screening purposes because of the ease of automation of enzyme-based methodologies (80). Shortened, "one-in-one" in vivo pharmacokinetics procedures can result in a throughput that is still adequate to support many drug discovery programs, as long as the in vivo pharmacokinetic screening is somewhat downstream in the screening sequence so that no more than about 20–30 compounds are to be tested each week.

The first such procedure to be reported used pooling of plasma from several animals at each time point up to 8 h, LC/MS for sample assay, and normal pharmacokinetic analysis of the concentration-time data (81). This process was followed quickly by a variation in which samples were collected for 24 h and then pooled across all time points, yielding a single sample per animal per compound dosed (82). LC/MS/MS compound assay provided a single concentration that was multiplied by the collection period to yield an approximation of the AUC_{0-t} (t = time of last sample) for the test compound. A final variation, theoretically capable of the highest speed, was introduced later, in which the in vivo phase is reduced to 6 h, yielding a truncated area under the curve (AUC) value (83). Because of the truncated AUC value, a 6-h time point is also assayed to provide an indication of whether most of the area has been captured. The rapid AUC method is particularly useful for screening for plasma levels after oral dosing of a series of drug candidates because oral bioavailability is frequently an issue in discovery support. A simple method has been described for deriving the true AUC from these pooling methods and for approximating the fraction of the AUC_{∞} captured within the collection period (84). Another advantage of using LC/MS/MS for sample assay is that it is easy to concurrently examine the plasma for simple metabolites such as hydroxylated derivatives, which are monitored at $M+16$ (i.e. 16 mass units greater than the parent molecular weight) (85). A related but experimentally more difficult method is the continuous withdrawal technique, in which blood is drawn from the animal slowly but continuously for the entire collection period. The concentration of this sample, multiplied by the collection period, is the true AUC_{0-t} for the test compound (86).

Metabolic Transformation

Although there has been no pressure to add metabolite structure elucidation to the screening process, this does not mean that metabolite identification is without value in early-phase discovery. On the contrary, it can often be a critical component of the discovery of DMPK-competent drug candidates because every discovery program has periods in which high-speed screening is not producing compounds with adequate pharmacokinetics, and synthesis must be directed toward solving the pharmacokinetics problem. Usually the problem is poor absorption or a metabolic hot spot; in the latter case, rapid identification of the major metabolites is required, normally without the benefit of radiolabeled parent compound (87). The methods described in the next two sections are intended for this situation.

Methods for Metabolite Generation   The simplest system to use involves liver microsomes, which are easily obtainable from laboratory species and from humans. Because many metabolites are the result of P450-catalyzed oxidation, microsomes often give good results in generating the correct metabolites. However, in some cases liver microsomes fail to metabolize the test compound or they give a different pattern of metabolites than would be observed in vivo. Consequently it is a good idea to use hepatocytes (88, 89) or liver slices (90, 91) in conjunction with or in place of microsomes. Hepatocytes and liver slices have the additional advantage of being more integrated than microsomes, meaning that the full complement of metabolic enzymes and cofactors are present. Thus the metabolism is not biased toward oxidation, as occurs with microsomes. Incubation of the test compound with the microsomes, hepatocytes, or liver slices provides a relatively clean matrix to bring to the next step, metabolite isolation and identification. The highest level of integration is in vivo, and the use of whole animals has the advantage that all physiological processes that may affect metabolic pathways are present, including membrane transporters, nonhepatic clearance, blood flows, protein binding, and tissue distribution. Bile, urine, and plasma can be collected from animals, but these matrices are complex and make subsequent instrumental analysis of metabolites difficult. Modern methods such as LC/MS and LC/NMR (nuclear magnetic resonance) can accomplish metabolite analysis even in these fluids.

New Rapid Technology   Several ingenious new techniques have been described recently that accelerate or facilitate metabolite identification. These techniques involve innovative coupling of existing technologies, one of which is always a variant of mass spectrometry. For instance, a method has been devised in which liver microsomal incubations are conducted inside an ultrafiltration apparatus that is infused continuously with buffer (92). The effusate is free of protein, avoiding the slow extraction step, and can be introduced directly into an electrospray mass spectrometer for real-time analysis of metabolites. The authors suggested that very high rates of sample throughput are theoretically possible, up to 60 incubations per hour, limited by the number of ultrafiltration chambers that can be operated in parallel. Of course, until human operators are able to interpret the results of 60 mass spectrometer runs in an hour, such rates cannot be fully realized in the overall throughput.

In a related development, a means to find and identify active metabolites has been described in which chromatographic peaks from a biological sample are exposed to a receptor in an ultrafiltration device (93). After filtering the unbound (i.e. inactive) materials through the ultrafiltration membrane, the bound materials (i.e. parent and active metabolites) are released and introduced into the mass spectrometer for structural characterization. Although the method is easily applied in a 96-well format, the identification of active metabolites has not been a screening priority. Also, recently introduced innovations in instrument design, such as ion-trap and quadrupole-time-of-flight mass spectrometers, have facilitated metabolite identification, allowing it to be accomplished at speeds suitable for rapid discovery work, even from complex ex vivo samples (94).

As anyone conducting LC/MS can attest, it is difficult to determine, in the absence of radiolabel, that a particular chromatographic peak is a metabolite and not a background component. To determine the chemical structure is harder yet. Toward that end, industrial mass spectrometrists have begun introducing artificial intelligence into the process, taking advantage of the ability of modern mass spectrometric systems to monitor numerous ions and fragmentation processes during a chromatographic run. The computer is programmed to watch for various relationships among masses of the parent ions of the peaks and the resulting fragment ions. For a human, this kind of numerology is tedious and prone to error, whereas computers excel at such tasks. For example, automated simultaneous monitoring of the incremental differences from the molecular weight of the test compound due to common biotransformations such as hydroxylation ($M + 16$), oxidation of a methyl group to a carboxyl ($M + 30$), and demethylation ($M - 14$) considerably reduced the time required by the human operator to deconvolute the metabolic profile of in vitro incubations (95). A more sophisticated elaboration of this idea was described (96) in which the mathematical technique of correlation analysis was brought to bear, allowing the metabolites from mixtures of drugs to be recognized and characterized.

Just beginning to be developed widely in industry is the technique of LC/NMR, which generates a completely different kind of information to apply to the problem of metabolite recognition and identification (97). NMR has not previously been considered as useful as mass spectrometry for metabolite identification because of the need to present purified, concentrated samples to the instrument due to the relative insensitivity of the NMR technique. However, the intrinsic power of NMR to elucidate molecular structure has kept interest in the technique alive and has spurred development of new microflow cell designs that have improved dramatically the sensitivity. An advantage of NMR is that for molecules containing fluorine, phosphorus, or deuterium atoms, or functional groups uncommon in biology, the NMR signal is as definitive of drug-relatedness and as easy to find as a radiolabel. There is no reason to discuss whether LC/MS or LC/NMR is the better technique, because LC/MS/NMR has already been demonstrated (98), and one may expect its widespread implementation in the coming years.

Virtual Screening

A trend in higher-throughput discovery DMPK screening is the increasing applicability of computer models. The earliest such approach was a completely empirical and statistical method known as the Rule of Five, or Lipinski's Rules (99). The Rule of Five is summarized as follows: A molecule is more likely to be poorly absorbed when the molecular weight is greater than 500, the sum of OH and/or NH groups is more than 5, the sum of N and O atoms is more than 10, and the log P is greater than 5. Because these criteria are easily calculable from the molecular structure without experimental measurements, the Rule of Five is easy to incorporate into the compound registration process to provide an alert that the compound may exhibit poor absorption, and it may even be used prospectively when planning a combinatorial chemistry campaign. More theoretically derived estimates of absorption can be made with the use of physiologically based absorption models (100, 101), but these models presently require experimental input such as Caco-2 permeability and rate of dissolution.

Molecular modeling is now starting to be used to predict substrate recognition by P450 enzymes. Homology models are available for most liver microsomal forms, including 2B (102), 2C9 and 2C19 (103), 2D6 (104), and 3A4 (105). This approach has been most successful with CYP 2D6 (106, 107), but so far it has been applied only to the drug design process and not to screening. Pattern recognition has been applied to the identification of substrates for PGP (108). Two structural motifs were proposed, and simple small-molecule modeling can identify whether those structural features are present in a real or hypothesized molecule, allowing rapid prospective screening against PGP substrates and inhibitors. Two industrial groups have introduced computational methods for scoring molecules (109, 110). In this automated neural network process, numerous molecular descriptors are compared to the values for molecules in databases defined as drug-like (e.g. the World Drug Index) and non-drug-like (e.g. the Available Chemicals Directory) to create an individual score for each molecule that allows ranking of molecules in terms of drug-like properties. As with the Rule of Five, the utility of this approach is that no experimental measurements are needed, so that scoring may be done during the planning process for combinatorial synthesis to avoid wasting effort in making molecules that lack favorable DMPK properties. However, the scoring approach has not been applied widely, and it is probably too early to assess its ultimate value.

CONCLUSION

Although the fastest DMPK screening methods do not come within two orders of magnitude of the rates routinely achieved by truly high-throughput discovery screening, they are nonetheless absolutely essential in the screening paradigm. The technology for higher-throughput screening in most cases is already mature, and additional large rate enhancements will probably be achieved only at the cost of increasing the scientific gap between the measured quantity and its human in vivo correlate. The greatest need in DMPK screening for discovery support is a much better understanding of the integrated operation of in vivo absorption, first-pass metabolism, organ uptake and efflux mediated by transporters, plasma protein binding, competition among metabolic enzymes, and cellular determinants of intrinsic clearance. In the short term, we would be able to use current in vitro systems more reliably to anticipate the in vivo disposition of drug candidates. Discovery DMPK screening would then be accelerated as we would be able to reduce our reliance on slower in vivo work. Ultimately it might be possible to create physiologically based DMPK models that would use animal in vitro/in vivo data for training and validation and then be able to support rapid screening of drug candidates with only human in vitro data for input.

ACKNOWLEDGMENTS

The author wishes to thank Drs. CC Lin, WA Korfmacher, and AA Nomeir of the Schering-Plough Research Institute for a critical review of this manuscript, and Dr. AYH Lu for helpful discussions.

Visit the Annual Reviews home page at www.AnnualReviews.org.

LITERATURE CITED

1. Fecik RA, Frank KE, Gentry EJ, Menon SR, Mitscher LA, Telikepalli H. 1998. The search for orally active medications through combinatorial chemistry. *Med. Res. Rev.* 18:149–85

2. Gorse D, Rees A, Kaczorek M, Lahana R. 1999. Molecular diversity and its analysis. *Drug Discov. Today* 4:257–64

3. Burkhard P, Hommel U, Sanner M, Walkinshaw MD. 1999. The discovery of steroids and other novel FKBP inhibitors using a molecular docking program. *J. Mol. Biol.* 287:853–58

4. Shuker SB, Hajduk PJ, Meadows RP, Fesik SW. 1996. Discovering high-affinity ligands for proteins: SAR by NMR. *Science* 274:1531–34

5. Kiyama R, Tamura Y, Watanabe F, Tsuzuki H, Ohtani M, Yodo M. 1999. Homology modeling of gelatinase catalytic domains and docking simulations of novel sulfonamide inhibitors. *J. Med. Chem.* 42:1723–38

6. Fernandes PB. 1998. Technological advances in high-throughput screening. *Curr. Opin. Chem. Biol.* 2:597–603

7. Broach JR, Thorner J. 1996. High-throughput screening for drug discovery. *Nature* 384(Suppl.):14–16

8. Silverman L, Campbell R, Broach JR. 1998. New assay technologies for high-throughput screening. *Curr. Opin. Chem. Biol.* 2:397–403

9. Houston JG. 1997. The impact of automation on high-throughput screening. *Methods Find. Exp. Clin. Pharmacol.* 19(Suppl. A):43–45

10. Houston JG, Banks M. 1997. The chemical-biological interface: developments in automated and miniaturised screening technology. *Curr. Opin. Biotechnol.* 8:734–40

11. Persidis A. 1998. High-throughput screening. Advances in robotics and miniaturization continue to accelerate drug lead identification. *Nat. Biotechnol.* 16:488–89

12. Rodrigues AD. 1998. Rational high-throughput screening in preclinical drug metabolism. *Med. Chem. Res.* 8:422–33

13. Tarbit MH, Berman J. 1998. High-throughput approaches for evaluating absorption, distribution, metabolism and excretion properties of lead compounds. *Curr. Opin. Chem. Biol.* 2:411–16

14. Lin JH. 1995. Species similarities and differences in pharmacokinetics. *Drug Metab. Dispos.* 23:1008–21

15. Obach RS, Baxter JG, Liston TE, Silber BM, Jones BC, et al. 1997. The prediction of human pharmacokinetic parameters from preclinical and in vitro

metabolism data. *J. Pharmacol. Exp. Ther.* 283:46–58

16. Rosenberg SH, Spina KP, Woods KW, Polakowski J, Martin DL, et al. 1993. Studies directed toward the design of orally active renin inhibitors. 1. Some factors influencing the absorption of small peptides. *J. Med. Chem.* 36:449–59

17. Artursson P, Borchardt RT. 1997. Intestinal drug absorption and metabolism in cell cultures: Caco-2 and beyond. *Pharm. Res.* 14:1655–58

18. Caldwell GW, Easlick SM, Gunnet J, Masucci JA, Demarest K. 1998. In vitro permeability of eight beta-blockers through Caco-2 monolayers utilizing liquid chromatography/electrospray ionization mass spectrometry. *J. Mass Spectrom.* 33:607–14

19. Obermeier MT, Chong S, Dando SA, Marino AM, Ryono DE, et al. 1996. Prodrugs of BMS-183920: metabolism and permeability considerations. *J. Pharm. Sci.* 85:828–33

20. Taylor EW, Gibbons JA, Braeckman RA. 1997. Intestinal absorption screening of mixtures from combinatorial libraries in the Caco-2 model. *Pharm. Res.* 14:572–77

21. Stevenson CL, Augustijns PF, Hendren RW. 1999. Use of Caco-2 cells and LC/MS/MS to screen a peptide combinatorial library for permeable structures. *Int. J. Pharm.* 177:103–15

22. Yamashita S, Tanaka Y, Endoh Y, Taki Y, Sakane T, et al. 1997. Analysis of drug permeation across Caco-2 monolayer: implication for predicting in vivo drug absorption. *Pharm. Res.* 14:486–91

23. Yee S. 1997. In vitro permeability across Caco-2 cells (colonic) can predict in vivo (small intestinal) absorption in man—fact or myth. *Pharm. Res.* 14:763–66

24. Delie F, Rubas W. 1997. A human colonic cell line sharing similarities with enterocytes as a model to examine oral absorption: advantages and limitations of the Caco-2 model. *Crit. Rev. Ther. Drug Carrier Syst.* 14:221–86

25. Crespi CL, Penman BW, Hu M. 1996. Development of Caco-2 cells expressing high levels of cDNA-derived cytochrome P4503A4. *Pharm. Res.* 13:1635–41

26. Garberg P, Eriksson P, Schipper N, Sjostrom B. 1999. Automated absorption assessment using Caco-2 cells cultured on both sides of polycarbonate membranes. *Pharm. Res.* 16:441–45

27. Pidgeon C, Ong S, Liu H, Qiu X, Pidgeon M, et al. 1995. IAM chromatography: an in vitro screen for predicting drug membrane permeability. *J. Med. Chem.* 38:590–94

28. Kansy M, Senner F, Gubernator K. 1998. Physicochemical high throughput screening: parallel artificial membrane permeation assay in the description of passive absorption processes. *J. Med. Chem.* 41:1007–10

29. Wacher VJ, Silverman JA, Zhang Y, Benet LZ. 1998. Role of P-glycoprotein and cytochrome P450 3A in limiting oral absorption of peptides and peptidomimetics. *J. Pharm. Sci.* 87:1322–30

30. Kim RB, Fromm MF, Wandel C, Leake B, Wood AJ, et al. 1998. The drug transporter P-glycoprotein limits oral absorption and brain entry of HIV-1 protease inhibitors. *J. Clin. Invest.* 101:289–94

31. Doppenschmitt S, Langguth P, Regardh CG, Andersson TB, Hilgendorf C, Spahn-Langguth H. 1999. Characterization of binding properties to human P-glycoprotein: development of a [3H]verapamil radioligand-binding assay. *J. Pharmacol. Exp. Ther.* 288:348–57

32. Tiberghien F, Loor F. 1996. Ranking of P-glycoprotein substrates and inhibitors by a calcein-AM fluorometry screening assay. *Anticancer Drugs* 7:568–78

33. Krishna G, Tang X, Norton L, Kirschmeier P, Lin CC, Nomeir AA. 1999. Higher-throughput P-glycoprotein assay for screening compounds in drug discov-

ery. *Annu. Meet. Am. Assoc. Pharm. Sci.* (Abstr.)

34. Wang EJ, Casciano CN, Clement RP, Johnson WW. 1999. Flow cytometry method for assessing the ability of a candidate drug to inhibit P-glycoprotein-mediated drug efflux from multidrug resistant cells. *2nd AAPS Front. Symp.: Membrane Transporters and Drug Ther.,* Bethesda, MD (Abstr.)

35. Letrent SP, Pollack GM, Brouwer KR, Brouwer KL. 1999. Effects of a potent and specific P-glycoprotein inhibitor on the blood-brain barrier distribution and antinociceptive effect of morphine in the rat. *Drug Metab. Dispos.* 27:827–34

36. Shah MV, Audus KL, Borchardt RT. 1989. The application of bovine brain microvessel endothelial-cell monolayers grown onto polycarbonate membranes in vitro to estimate the potential permeability of solutes through the blood-brain barrier. *Pharm. Res.* 6:624–27

37. Takakura Y, Audus KL, Borchardt RT. 1992. Cultured brain microvessel endothelial cells as in vitro models of the blood-brain barrier. *NIDA Res. Monogr.* 120:138–52

38. Liu F, Kumari P, Chu I, Soares A, Lin CC, Nomeir AA. 1999. Use of an in vitro bovine brain endothelial cell culture to evaluate potential blood-brain penetration of drug discovery candidates. *Annu. Meet. Am. Assoc. Pharm. Sci.* (Abstr.)

39. Huai-Yun H, Secrest DT, Mark KS, Carney D, Brandquist C, et al. 1998. Expression of multidrug resistance-associated protein (MRP) in brain microvessel endothelial cells. *Biochem. Biophys. Res. Commun.* 243:816–20

40. Rose JM, Peckham SL, Scism JL, Audus KL. 1998. Evaluation of the role of P-glycoprotein in ivermectin uptake by primary cultures of bovine brain microvessel endothelial cells. *Neurochem. Res.* 23:203–9

41. Guengerich FP. 1997. Role of cytochrome

P450 enzymes in drug-drug interactions. *Adv. Pharmacol.* 43:7–35

42. Lin JH, Lu AY. 1998. Inhibition and induction of cytochrome P450 and the clinical implications. *Clin. Pharmacokinet.* 35:361–90

43. Pelkonen O, Maenpaa J, Taavitsainen P, Rautio A, Raunio H. 1998. Inhibition and induction of human cytochrome P450 (CYP) enzymes. *Xenobiotica* 28:1203–53

44. Miners JO, Birkett DJ. 1998. Cytochrome P4502C9: an enzyme of major importance in human drug metabolism. *Br. J. Clin. Pharmacol.* 45:525–38

45. Clarke SE. 1998. In vitro assessment of human cytochrome P450. *Xenobiotica* 28:1167–202

46. Rodrigues AD, Wong SL. 1997. Application of human liver microsomes in metabolism-based drug-drug interactions: in vitro-in vivo correlations and the Abbott Laboratories experience. *Adv. Pharmacol.* 43:65–101

47. Crespi CL, Miller VP, Penman BW. 1997. Microtiter plate assays for inhibition of human, drug-metabolizing cytochromes P450. *Anal. Biochem.* 248:188–90

48. Crespi CL, Miller VP, Penman BW. 1998. High throughput screening for inhibition of cytochrome P450 metabolism. *Med. Chem. Res.* 8:457–71

49. Palamanda JR, Favreau L, Lin CC, Nomeir AA. 1998. Validation of a rapid microtiter plate assay to conduct cytochrome P450 2D6 enzyme inhibition studies. *Drug Discov. Today* 3:466–70

50. Crespi CL. 1999. Assessing the potential for drug-drug interactions in an accelerated throughput mode. *Pharm. Sci. Technol. Today* 2:119–20

51. Ayrton J, Plumb R, Leavens WJ, Mallett D, Dickins M, Dear GJ. 1998. Application of a generic fast gradient liquid chromatography tandem mass spectrometry method for the analysis of cytochrome P450 probe substrates. *Rapid Commun. Mass Spectrom.* 12:217–24

52. Chu I, Favreau L, Soares T, Lin CC, Nomeir AA. 1999. Higher-throughput cytochrome P450 enzyme inhibition analysis by APCI-HPLC/MS/MS. *Proc. 47th ASMS Conf. Mass Spectrom. Allied Topics,* Dallas, pp. 1474–75

53. Favreau LV, Palamanda JR, Lin CC, Nomeir AA. 1999. Improved reliability of the rapid microtiter plate assay using recombinant enzyme in predicting CYP2D6 inhibition in human liver microsomes. *Drug Metab. Dispos.* 27: 436–39

54. Thompson TN. 1997. Experimental models for evaluating enzyme induction potential of new drug candidates in animals and humans and a strategy for their use. *Adv. Pharmacol.* 43:205–29

55. Whysner J, Ross PM, Williams GM. 1996. Phenobarbital mechanistic data and risk assessment: enzyme induction, enhanced cell proliferation, and tumor promotion. *Pharmacol. Ther.* 71:153–91

56. Li AP, Maurel P, Gomez-Lechon MJ, Cheng LC, Jurima-Romet M. 1997. Preclinical evaluation of drug-drug interaction potential: present status of the application of primary human hepatocytes in the evaluation of cytochrome P450 induction. *Chem. Biol. Interact.* 107:5–16

57. Madan A, DeHaan R, Mudra D, Carroll K, LeCluyse E, Parkinson A. 1999. Effect of cryopreservation on cytochrome P-450 enzyme induction in cultured rat hepatocytes. *Drug Metab. Dispos.* 27:327–35

58. Silva JM, Morin PE, Day SH, Kennedy BP, Payette P, et al. 1998. Refinement of an in vitro cell model for cytochrome P450 induction. *Drug Metab. Dispos.* 26: 490–96

59. Li H, Liu S, Kemper B. 1996. Sex- and tissue-specific expression of a cytochrome P450 2C2-luciferase transgene. *Mol. Cell. Endocrinol.* 120:77–83

60. Ogg MS, Williams JM, Tarbit M, Goldfarb PS, Gray TJ, Gibson GG. 1999. A reporter gene assay to assess the molec-ular mechanisms of xenobiotic-dependent induction of the human CYP 3A4 gene in vitro. *Xenobiotica* 29:269–79

61. Whitlock JP Jr. 1999. Induction of cytochrome P4501A1. *Annu. Rev. Pharmacol. Toxicol.* 39:103–25

62. Guengerich FP. 1999. Cytochrome P-450 3A4: regulation and role in drug metabolism. *Annu. Rev. Pharmacol. Toxicol.* 39:1–17

63. Giddings SJ, Clarke SE, Gibson GG. 1997. CYP4A1 gene transfection studies and the peroxisome proliferator-activated receptor: development of a high-throughput assay to detect peroxisome proliferators. *Eur. J. Drug Metab. Pharmacokinet.* 22: 315–19

64. Kemper B. 1998. Regulation of cytochrome P450 gene transcription by phenobarbital. *Prog. Nucleic Acid Res. Mol. Biol.* 61:23–64

65. Honkakoski P, Zelko I, Sueyoshi T, Negishi M. 1998. The nuclear orphan receptor CAR-retinoid X receptor heterodimer activates the phenobarbital-responsive enhancer module of the CYP2B gene. *Mol. Cell. Biol.* 18:5652–58

66. Sueyoshi T, Kawamoto T, Zelko I, Honkakoski P, Negishi M. 1999. The repressed nuclear receptor CAR responds to phenobarbital in activating the human CYP2B6 gene. *J. Biol. Chem.* 274: 6043–46

67. Korfmacher WA, Palmer CA, Nardo C, Dunn-Meynell K, Grotz D, et al. 1999. Development of an automated mass spectrometry system for the quantitative analysis of liver microsomal incubation samples: a tool for rapid screening of new compounds for metabolic stability. *Rapid Commun. Mass Spectrom.* 13: 901–7

68. Houston JB, Carlile DJ. 1997. Prediction of hepatic clearance from microsomes, hepatocytes, and liver slices. *Drug Metab. Rev.* 29:891–922

69. Ito K, Iwatsubo T, Kanamitsu S, Nakajima Y, Sugiyama Y. 1998. Quantitative

prediction of in vivo drug clearance and drug interactions from in vitro data on metabolism, together with binding and transport. *Annu. Rev. Pharmacol. Toxicol.* 38:461–99

70. Lin JH. 1998. Applications and limitations of interspecies scaling and in vitro extrapolation in pharmacokinetics. *Drug Metab. Dispos.* 26:1202–12

71. Lave T, Dupin S, Schmitt C, Valles B, Ubeaud G, et al. 1997. The use of human hepatocytes to select compounds based on their expected hepatic extraction ratios in humans. *Pharm. Res.* 14:152–55

72. Prueksaritanont T, Gorham LM, Breslin MJ, Hutchinson JH, Hartman GD, et al. 1997. In vitro and in vivo evaluations of the metabolism, pharmacokinetics, and bioavailability of ester prodrugs of L-767,679, a potent fibrinogen receptor antagonist: an approach for the selection of a prodrug candidate. *Drug Metab. Dispos.* 25:978–84

73. Olah TV, McLoughlin DA, Gilbert JD. 1997. The simultaneous determination of mixtures of drug candidates by liquid chromatography/atmospheric pressure chemical ionization mass spectrometry as an in vivo drug screening procedure. *Rapid Commun. Mass Spectrom.* 11:17–23

74. Allen MC, Shah TS, Day WW. 1998. Rapid determination of oral pharmacokinetics and plasma free fraction using cocktail approaches: methods and application. *Pharm. Res.* 15:93–97

75. Shaffer JE, Adkison KK, Halm K, Hedeen K, Berman J. 1999. Use of "N-in-one" dosing to create an in vivo pharmacokinetics database for use in developing structure-pharmacokinetic relationships. *J. Pharmaceut. Sci.* 88:313–18

76. Bayliss MK, Frick LW. 1999. High-throughput pharmacokinetics: cassette dosing. *Curr. Opin. Drug Discov. Dev.* 2:20–25

77. McLoughlin DA, Olah TV, Gilbert JD.

1997. A direct technique for the simultaneous determination of 10 drug candidates in plasma by liquid chromatography-atmospheric pressure chemical ionization mass spectrometry interfaced to a Prospekt solid-phase extraction system. *J. Pharm. Biomed. Anal.* 15:1893–901

78. Beaudry F, Le Blanc JC, Coutu M, Brown NK. 1998. In vivo pharmacokinetic screening in cassette dosing experiments; the use of on-line Prospekt liquid chromatography/atmospheric pressure chemical ionization tandem mass spectrometry technology in drug discovery. *Rapid Commun. Mass Spectrom.* 12:1216–22

79. Bryant MS, Korfmacher WA, Wang S, Nardo C, Nomeir AA, Lin CC. 1997. Pharmacokinetic screening for the selection of new drug discovery candidates is greatly enhanced through the use of liquid chromatography-atmospheric pressure ionization tandem mass spectrometry. *J. Chromatogr. A* 777:61–66

80. Singh J, Soloweij J, Allen M, Killar L, Ator M. 1996. Lead development: validation and application of high throughput screening for determination of pharmacokinetic parameters for enzyme inhibitors. *Bioorg. Med. Chem.* 4:639–43

81. Kuo BS, Van Noord T, Feng MR, Wright DS. 1998. Sample pooling to expedite bioanalysis and pharmacokinetic research. *J. Pharm. Biomed. Anal.* 16:837–46

82. Hop CE, Wang Z, Chen Q, Kwei G. 1998. Plasma-pooling methods to increase throughput for in vivo pharmacokinetic screening. *J. Pharm. Sci.* 87:901–3

83. Cox KA, Dunn-Meynell K, Korfmacher WA, Broske L, Nomeir AA, et al. 1999. Novel in vivo procedure for rapid pharmacokinetic screening of discovery compounds in rats. *Drug Discov. Today* 4:232–37

84. Krishna G, White RE, Nomeir AA, Broske L, Lin CC. 1999. Pharmacokinetics approaches to rapidly assess systemic availability of compounds in

discovery. *Annu. Meet. Am. Assoc. Pharm. Sci.* (Abstr.)

85. Bryant MS, Hsieh Y, Liu M, Korfmacher W, Gruela G, et al. 1999. Rapid pharmacokinetic screening in the mouse using sample pooling and HPLC-API/MS/MS. *Proc. 47th ASMS Conf. Mass Spectrom. Allied Topics,* Dallas, pp. 1137–38

86. Humphreys WG, Obermeier MT, Morrison RA. 1998. Continuous blood withdrawal as a rapid screening method for determining clearance or oral bioavailability in rats. *Pharm. Res.* 15:1257–61

87. Korfmacher WA, Cox KA, Bryant MS, Veals J, Ng K, et al. 1997. HPLC-API/MS/MS: a powerful tool for integrating drug metabolism into the drug discovery process. *Drug Discov. Today* 2:532–37

88. Guillouzo A, Morel F, Fardel O, Meunier B. 1993. Use of human hepatocyte cultures for drug metabolism studies. *Toxicology* 82:209–19

89. Ekins S, Williams JA, Murray GI, Burke MD, Marchant NC, et al. 1996. Xenobiotic metabolism in rat, dog, and human precision-cut liver slices, freshly isolated hepatocytes, and vitrified precision-cut liver slices. *Drug Metab. Dispos.* 24:990–95

90. Hashemi E, Dobrota M, Till C, Ioannides C. 1999. Structural and functional integrity of precision-cut liver slices in xenobiotic metabolism: a comparison of the dynamic organ and multiwell plate culture procedures. *Xenobiotica* 29:11–25

91. Ferrero JL, Brendel K. 1997. Liver slices as a model in drug metabolism. *Adv. Pharmacol.* 43:131–69

92. van Breemen RB, Nikolic D, Bolton JL. 1998. Metabolic screening using on-line ultrafiltration mass spectrometry. *Drug Metab. Dispos.* 26:85–90

93. Lim HK, Stellingweif S, Sisenwine S, Chan KW. 1999. Rapid drug metabolite profiling using fast liquid chromatography, automated multiple-stage mass spectrometry and receptor-binding. *J. Chromatogr. A* 831:227–41

94. Cox KA, Clarke N, Dunn-Meynell K, Korfmacher W, Lin C-C. 1999. Use of the Q-TOF, LCQ and triple quadrupole mass spectrometers for metabolite ID in support of drug discovery. *Proc. 47th ASMS Conf. Mass Spectrom. Allied Topics,* Dallas, pp. 1316–17

95. Lopez LL, Yu X, Cui D, Davis MR. 1998. Identification of drug metabolites in biological matrices by intelligent automated liquid chromatography/tandem mass spectrometry. *Rapid Commun. Mass Spectrom.* 12:1756–60

96. Fernandez-Metzler CL, Owens KG, Baillie TA, King RC. 1999. Rapid liquid chromatography with tandem mass spectrometry-based screening procedures for studies on the biotransformation of drug candidates. *Drug Metab. Dispos.* 27:32–40

97. Lindon JC, Nicholson JK, Sidelmann UG, Wilson ID. 1997. Directly coupled HPLC-NMR and its application to drug metabolism. *Drug Metab. Rev.* 29:705–46

98. Holt RM, Newman MJ, Pullen FS, Richards DS, Swanson AG. 1997. High-performance liquid chromatography/NMR spectrometry/mass spectrometry: further advances in hyphenated technology. *J. Mass Spectrom.* 32:64–70

99. Lipinski CA, Lombardo F, Dominy BW, Feeney PJ. 1997. Experimental and computational approaches to estimate solubility and permeability in drug discovery and development settings. *Adv. Drug Deliv. Rev.* 23:3–25

100. Grass GM, Bozarth CA, Vallner JJ. 1994. Evaluation of the performance of controlled release dosage forms of ticlopidine using in vitro intestinal permeability and computer simulations. *J. Drug Target.* 2:23–33

101. Sinko PJ, Leesman GD, Waclawski AP, Yu H, Kou JH. 1996. Analysis of intestinal perfusion data for highly permeable drugs

using a numerical aqueous resistance-nonlinear regression method. *Pharm. Res.* 13:570–76

102. Lewis DF, Lake BG. 1997. Molecular modelling of mammalian CYP2B isoforms and their interaction with substrates, inhibitors and redox partners. *Xenobiotica* 27:443–78

103. Lewis DF, Dickins M, Weaver RJ, Eddershaw PJ, Goldfarb PS, Tarbit MH. 1998. Molecular modelling of human CYP2C subfamily enzymes CYP2C9 and CYP2C19: rationalization of substrate specificity and site-directed mutagenesis experiments in the CYP2C subfamily. *Xenobiotica* 28:235–68

104. Lewis DF, Eddershaw PJ, Goldfarb PS, Tarbit MH. 1997. Molecular modelling of cytochrome P4502D6 (CYP2D6) based on an alignment with CYP102: structural studies on specific CYP2D6 substrate metabolism. *Xenobiotica* 27:319–39

105. Szklarz GD, Halpert JR. 1997. Molecular modeling of cytochrome P450 3A4. *J. Comput. Aided Mol. Des.* 11:265–72

106. Halliday RC, Jones BC, Park BK, Smith DA. 1997. Synthetic strategies to lower affinity for CYP2D6. *Eur. J. Drug Metab. Pharmacokinet.* 22:291–94

107. de Groot MJ, Ackland MJ, Horne VA, Alex AA, Jones BC. 1999. Novel approach to predicting P450-mediated drug metabolism: development of a combined protein and pharmacophore model for CYP2D6. *J. Med. Chem.* 42:1515–24

108. Seelig A. 1998. A general pattern for substrate recognition by P-glycoprotein. *Eur. J. Biochem.* 251:252–61

109. Sadowski J, Kubinyi H. 1998. A scoring scheme for discriminating between drugs and nondrugs. *J. Med. Chem.* 41:3325–29

110. Ajay, Walters WP, Murcko MA. 1998. Can we learn to distinguish between "drug-like" and "nondrug-like" molecules? *J. Med. Chem.* 41:3314–24

Annu. Rev. Pharmacol. Toxicol. 2000. 40:159–76

PHARMACOGENETICS OF SULFOTRANSFERASE

K. Nagata and Y. Yamazoe

Division of Drug Metabolism and Molecular Toxicology, Graduate School of Pharmaceutical Sciences, Tohoku University, Sendai 980–8578, Japan; e-mail: nagataki@mail.pharm.tohoku.ac.jp

Key Words SULT, classification, nomenclature system, allelic variant, gene correspondence

■ **Abstract** Cytosolic sulfotransferase catalyzes sulfoconjugation of relatively small lipophilic endobiotics and xenobiotics. At least 44 cytosolic sulfotransferases have been identified from mammals, and based on their amino acid sequences, these forms are shown to constitute five different families. In humans, 10 sulfotransferase genes have been identified and shown to localize on at least five different chromosomes. The enzymatic properties characterized in the recombinant forms indicate the association of their substrate specificity with metabolisms of such nonpeptide hormones as estrogen, corticoid, and thyroxine, although most forms are also active on the sulfation of various xenobiotics. Genetic polymorphisms are observed on such human sulfotransferases as ST1A2, ST1A3, and ST2A3.

INTRODUCTION

Cytosolic sulfotransferase (SULT) plays an important role in the detoxication and activation of endogenous and exogenous compounds (1–4). The reaction catalyzed by this enzyme involves transfer of a sulfonate group from 3'-phosphoadenosine-5'-phosphosulfate (PAPS) to the acceptor substrate to form either a sulfate or sulfamate conjugate (1, 2). Considerable numbers of cytosolic SULTs have been characterized at the mRNA level and divided into several gene families based on the similarity of their amino acid sequences and catalytic properties in mammals (5, 6). An international sulfotransferase nomenclature workshop suggested using "SULT" as the abbreviation for these enzymes and their genes. The names of individual forms, however, have not been universally agreed upon. In this context, a nomenclature system for SULTs is suggested here as a result of a comparison of currently characterized forms of mammalian SULTs.

The pharmacogenetics of drug sulfation by human platelets are known (7–9). Human platelet phenol SULT activity differs widely among individuals (8, 10) and now has been characterized by genotype using recent advanced molecular techniques (11–14). Current understanding of pharmacogenetics of human SULT is also summarized here.

SULT GENE

A nomenclature for the SULT gene family is not yet in common use, although "SULT" has been agreed upon to be used as the acronym. In fact, some groups use SULT1A1 for one of human phenol SULTs (12) and others for rat phenol sulfotransferase (PST) (15). A similar phenomenon is observed for other SULTs (15–17). As a result, the name SULT has become very confusing. Recent pharmacogenetic studies have revealed several alleles of SULT genes through discovery of mutations (11–14), and there is a need to use a universal nomenclature. Here, a nomenclature system that is based on the cytochrome P450 nomenclature system is shown (18, 19). Known mammalian SULT cDNA sequences are compared and listed in Table 1. Basically, SULTs in one gene family have less than 40% similarity to SULTs in other gene families. Within a gene family, any SULTs in one subfamily have 40–65% similarity to SULTs in any of the other subfamilies. Numbers in parentheses indicate the accession number obtained from the Entrez Protein database, which links with the accession number of the nucleotide database. Using an unweighted-pair-group method of analysis, we have made a dendrogram (Figure 1). The family and subfamily are classified based on homology. Individual numbers of families and forms are termed as sequential chronological numbers.

The first enzyme characterized at the cDNA level among all SULTs is bovine estrogen SULT (20), which was named ST1E1 for the first family and estrogen SULT. Rat phenol SULT was called ST1A1 because it was the first cDNA isolated in the SULT1A subfamily (21). We believe that this method, based on cDNA information, is better than the method based on the currently known human gene. The reasons are as follows: (a) We still don't know how many SULT genes exist in humans as well as in experimental animals. Partial sequences likely to correspond to unknown SULTs are found in the expression tag sequence (EST) database. (b) A gene referred to as orthologous in two species is driven from the ancestral gene that existed before the evolutionary divergence of the two species. For example, only one form of SULT1B was identified from rat, human, and mouse as ST1B1, ST1B2, and St1b3, respectively (17, 22–24). The three forms show 72–88% homology and preferentially catalyze the sulfation of thyroid hormone. These results suggest that these three genes may be orthologous. However, a number of species-specific gene duplications and gene-conversion events have been shown in several subfamilies of cytochrome P450 (18). In fact, highly similar SULT genes have also been found in human SULT1A and rat SULT2A subfamilies (6, 25). Therefore, a new gene of human SULT including the SULT1B subfamily could possibly be found in the future. The current information is still too primitive to verify this possibility at the gene level at the present time (18).

TABLE 1 Correspondences of cytosolic SULTs and GenBank accession numbers

ST1A1 rat (X52883) (21)	PST-1 (X52883) (21), Mx-STb (L19998) (68), ASTIV (X68640) (69), Tyrosine-ester (U323721)
ST1A2 human (X78282) (70)	SULT1A2 (NM_001054) (46), HAST4V (U28169) (71), HAST4 (U28170) (71), STP2 (U33886) (53)
ST1A3 human (X78283) (70)	SULT1A1 (NM_001055, AJ007418) (46), (72), HAST1, Hpsta (L10819) (73), TS PST1 (U52852) (72), HAST2 (U09031, L19955) (74), P-PST (L19999) (75), STP (X84654, U54701) (76), (44), H-PST (U26309) (77)
St1a4 mouse	mST_{p1} (L02331) (78)
ST1A5 human	SULT1A3, hTLPST (U20499) (79), HAST3 (L19956) (74), TL PST (U08032) (79), hEST (L25275) (80), STM (X84653, U37686) (76), (55), HAST5 (U34199)
ST1A6 bovine	PST (L33828, U35253) (81)
ST1A7 dog	dPST-1 (D29807)
ST1A8 rabbit (AB029494)	
ST1A9 monkey	monPST-1 (D85514)
ST1B1 rat (D89375) (23)	dopa/tyrosine SULT (U38419) (22)
ST1B2 human (D89479) (23)	hST1B2 (U95726) (24)
St1b3 mouse	mouse SULT1B1 (AF022894) (17)
ST1C1 rat (L22339) (29)	HAST-1 (L22339) (29)
ST1C2 human (AB008164) (30)	human SULT1C SULT 1 (AF026303) (31) human SULT1C1 (NM_001056) (32)
ST1C3 human	human SULT1C SULT 2 (AF055584) (31)
St1c4 mouse	P-ST (AF033653) (33)
ST1C5 rabbit	Stomach SULT (AF026304)
ST1C6 rat	sultK1 (AJ238391)
ST1C7 rat	sultK2 (AJ238392)
St1d1 mouse	SULT-N (AF026073) (34)
ST1D2 rat	tyrosine-ester SULT (U32372)
ST1E1 bovine	OST (X56395) (20)
ST1E2 rat	EST-1, Ste 1 (U50204), EST-3 (M86758, S76489) (36), (37)
ST1E3 guinea pig	EST (U09552) (82)
ST1E4 human	hEST (L25275, U08098, Y11195) (80), (83), hEST-1 (S77383) (61)
St1e5 mouse	testis-specific estrogen SULT (S78182) (84)

(continued)

TABLE 1 *Continued*

ST1E6 rat	EST-2, Ste2 (U50205) (85), EST-6 (S76490) (37)
ST2A1 rat (M31363) (39)	ST-20 (M31363) (39), ST-21a (D14987) (25), ST-21b (D14988) (25)
ST2A2 rat (M33329) (86)	ST-40 (M33329) (86), ST-41 (X63410) (40)
ST2A3 human	DHEA-SULT (U08025) (87), HST-hfa (U08024) (88), hSTa (S43859) (89), DHEA-ST8 (L20000) (90)
St2a4 mouse	mST$_{a1}$ (L02335) (91)
ST2A5 rat	ST-60 (D14989) (25)
ST2A6 guinea pig	gpHST1 (U06871) (63)
ST2A7 guinea pig	gp HST2 (U&35115) (92), Preg-ST (U55944) (93)
ST2A8 rabbit (AB006053) (64)	AST-RB2 (AB006053) (64),
St2a9 mouse	mST$_{a2}$ (L27121) (94)
ST2A10 monkey	monHST-1 (D85521)
ST2B1 human	SULT2B1a (U92314) (16), SULT2B1b (U92315) (16)
St2b2 mouse	mouse SULT2B1 (AF026072) (34)
ST3A1 rabbit (D86219) (27)	AST-RB1 (D86219) (27)
St3a2 mouse	SULT-X2 (AF026075)

CLASSIFICATION

Mammalian SULTs have been classified into two groups (SULT1 and SULT2 families) based on their similarity of amino acid sequences and enzymatic properties. Enzymes included in SULT1 and SULT2 families transfer sulfonate to hydroxy groups of phenols and alcohols, respectively (5, 6, 26). A SULT catalyzing the formation of a sulfamate has recently been isolated from rabbits (27). This form constitutes a third gene family of SULT (SULT3). In addition, unique SULT cDNAs consisting of two new families (SULT4 and SULT5) are found in the DNA database, although properties of enzymes encoded by these SULT cDNAs have not yet been characterized. As shown in Figure 1, mammalian SULTs are classified into five families that share less than 40% similarity with

Figure 1 The classification of cytosolic SULTs previously reported based on their primary amino acid sequences. This dendrogram was made with the GeneWorks program (Intelli Genetics). The nomenclature was modified from that proposed by Y Yamazoe et al (5). The classification was performed according to the nomenclature system for the cytochrome gene superfamily. Any SULT in one gene family has < 40% similarity to a SULT including other gene families. Within a gene family, any SULT in one subfamily is 40–65% similar to a SULT in any of the other subfamilies. Figures in parentheses represent the accession number in the protein database, which links to the nucleotide database.

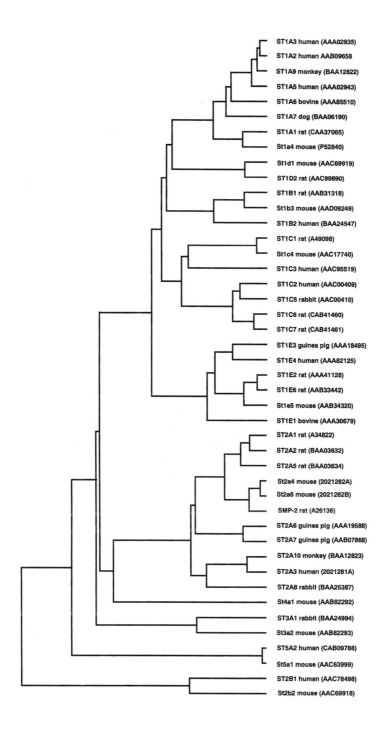

each other. SULT1 has the largest number of enzymes and is further divided into five subfamilies (SULT1A, SULT1B, SULT1C, SULT1D, and SULT1E). The SULT2 family is separated into two subfamilies (SULT2A and SULT2B).

At least nine SULT1A forms, from experimental animals and humans, are members of the SULT1A subfamily (Figure 1), but the properties of monkey, mouse, and rabbit SULT1A forms have not yet been determined. The ST1A forms, except for human ST1A5, commonly catalyze sulfations of p-nitrophenol and α-naphthol. ST1A5 catalyzes the sulfation of dopamine, although a limited activity for p-nitrophenol is observed (28).

ST1B1 and ST1B2 were isolated as a thyroid hormone SULT from rats and humans, respectively (22–24). Mouse St1b3 is also shown to have an activity for thyroid hormone (17). Therefore, this SULT family seems to have a thyroid hormone-sulfating activity as a common catalytic property.

ST1C1, which mediated the activation of N-hydroxy-2-acetylaminofluorene (N-OH-AAF) through sulfate formation, was first isolated from rats (29). Other members of this subfamily include ST1C2 and ST1C3 from human (30–32), St1c4 from mouse, ST1C5 from rabbit, and ST1C6 and ST1C7 from rat. Mouse St1c4, which is reported as an olfactory-specific form (33), shares a high extent of homology (94%) with ST1C1, but human ST1C2 and ST1C3, and rabbit CT1C5, show lower extents of homology with ST1C1. ST1C2, ST1C3, and St1c4 have been reported to catalyze the sulfation of N-OH-AAF, although ST1C2 did not mediate DNA binding of N-OH-AAF in our experiment (30).

SULT1D was recently identified as St1d1 from the mouse (34). This form catalyzes the sulfation of serotonin and ecosanoids as well as p-nitrophenol and dopamine (35). Isolation of rat ST1D2 is also reported.

Six forms of SULT1E have been identified from bovine, rat, mouse, guinea pig, and human. These forms show a high affinity for sulfation of estrogen. Bovine ST1E1 is the first form whose primary structure has been characterized at a molecular level (20). A single form is found in each experimental animal species except for rats. Two SULT1E forms, ST1E2 and ST1E6, have been isolated from rats (36, 37). The three-dimensional structure of mouse St1e4 has been determined from X-ray data analysis of the crystallized PAPS-bound form (38).

The sulfation of alcohols is mainly catalyzed by forms of the SULT2 family (SULT2A and SULT2B subfamilies). At least four different cDNAs of SULT2A forms (ST2A1, ST2A2, ST2A5, and SMP-2) have been reported in rats (25, 39–41). SMP-2 was at first reported as a senescence marker protein and later found to have a high homology to the SULT2A form (41). The mRNA and gene corresponding to SMP-2 have not been confirmed, and thus the existence of the gene exactly related to SMP-2 in rat is doubtful. SULT2B forms were isolated from human (ST2B1) and mouse (St2b2) through the EST database (16). SULT2B forms as well as SULT2A forms prefer dehydroepiandrostene as the substrate. Judging from the dendrogram shown in Figure 1, ST2B forms seemed to diverge early from an ancestral SULT to constitute an independent family. Human SULT2B1a and ST2B1b are composed of 350 and 365 amino acids, which are

53 and 68 amino acids longer than SULT2A3, respectively. Alignment of ST2A3 and ST2B1 forms showed 48% homology at the protein level, indicating that ST2A and ST2B forms are members of the same family.

A novel SULT (ST3A1) has been isolated from rabbit livers in the authors' laboratory (27). ST3A1 represents the third gene family, SULT3, and shows a selectivity for the conversion of amino compounds to sulfamates (42). An enzyme related to ST3A1 is not detected in human and rat livers by Western and Northern blotting procedures. A nucleotide sequence similar to that of ST3A1 was found in the mouse GenBank database, although the properties of the protein encoded by the cDNA have not been reported. Three nucleotide sequences related to SULT, which are not classified into the three known families described above, are found in the nucleotide database. Based on their deduced amino acid sequences, these genes are judged to consist of new families of SULT, SULT4 and SULT5. We arbitrarily termed them St4a1, St5a1, and ST5A2, respectively. Mouse St4a1 and St5a1 cDNAs are identified from mouse kidney and brain, respectively. ST5A2 is identified in human chromosome 22.

REGULATION OF SULT GENE EXPRESSION IN HUMAN

Plural types of cDNA for each human SULT are registered in the DNA database except for ST1E4 and ST2A3. These differences are confined to the 5'-untranslated region (UTR) and are thus attributed to the existence of alternative sites for transcription initiation (6). Until now, three different ST1A2 cDNAs, four ST1A3 cDNAs, and five ST1A5 cDNAs have been isolated from different human tissues, as shown in Figure 2. Human SULT genes, except for ST1B2, ST1C2, and ST1C3, have been isolated and the structures determined (43–47). The open reading flames of SULT1 and SULT2 families consist of 7 and 6 exons, respectively. A single exon 1 for ST1E4, two exon 1s (exon 1a and exon 1b) for ST1A2 and ST1A3, and three exon 1s (exon 1a, exon 1b, and exon 1c) for ST1A5 are identified by their genes and mRNAs, but these exons do not contain coding regions of their proteins (6). On the other hand, exon 1 for ST2A3 and ST2B1 encodes the N terminus (16, 43). Therefore, the variety of the 5'-UTR sequences for these SULTs is generated by alternative transcription initiation, alternative splicing, or both mechanisms. The expression of some SULTs is known to be regulated by hormones (48–50). However, the molecular mechanism of SULT gene expression has not been well characterized.

SULT1A

Three SULT1A forms have been identified in humans, as shown in Table 1. Classical pharmacogenetic studies of the human sulfation have been done to determine the substrate specificity, inhibitor sensitivity, or thermal stability (7–9).

Gene name	Gene structure	cDNA	Accession number	Tissue
ST1A2 (U34804, U71086, U76619)			(U34804)	Liver
			R09752*	Fetal liver/spleen
			U28169	Liver
			U28170	Liver
ST1A3 (AH003659, U37025, U52852)			L19955	Brain
			U26309	Hipppocampus
			U09031	Brain
			(U52852)	Liver
			(U52852)	Liver
			L19999	Liver
			L10819	Liver
			X84654	Platelet
			X78283	Liver
			H67938*	Fetal liver/spleen
ST1A5 (U20499, U37686)			AA325280*	Cerebellum
			W76361*	Fetal heart
			W81033*	Fetal heart
			L25275	Placenta
			L19956	Brain
			U20499	Liver Brain
ST1E4 (AH006624)			U08098	Liver
			AR003684	Unknown
			Y11195	Embryo
			AA460624*	Total fetus
			AA448993*	Total fetus
			N83541*	Fetal heart
			AA334071*	Embryo
ST2A3 (AH003200, AH006684)			L02337	Liver
			X84816	Fetus
			U08025	Liver
			T74488*	Liver
			L20000	Liver
			U08024	Liver
			T68221*	Liver
			Z21023*	Liver
			AA328456*	Embryo
ST2B1 (AH007006)		2B1a	U92314	Placenta
		2B1b	U92315	Placenta

SULTs catalyzing phenol sulfations are referred to as thermostable (TS)/phenol-preferring (P) PST and the thermolabile (TL)/monoamine-preferring (M) PST (8, 51). Two genes (ST1A2 and ST1A3) of TS PST have been identified and localized to chromosome 16p12.1–11.2 (46, 52, 53). ST1A2 is located in the approximately 45-kb distant region of ST1A3. ST1A2 and ST1A3 catalyze the sulfation of p-nitrophenol and the activation of heterocyclic amines. These forms are sensitive to 2,6-dichloro-4-nitrophenol, a typical inhibitor of SULT (28). ST1A3 shows higher catalytic activity and lower Km value for p-nitrophenol than does ST1A2 (28). A gene (ST1A5) corresponding to TL PST has been isolated and localized to chromosome 16p11.2 (54, 55). ST1A5 is mapped at about 100 kb from ST1A2 and ST1A3 (56).

Studies on individual variations of TS PST indicate that phenotypic variations in both platelet TS PST activity and thermal stability are associated with ST1A3 polymorphism (57). Four allelic variants accompanying amino acid exchange in ST1A3 have been identified (11, 12, 14). One of them, ST1A3*2, is associated with both low TS PST activity and low thermal stability. The ST1A3*2 allele has a G→T mutation at ST1A3 cDNA nucleotide 638 located in exon 7, resulting in an Arg 213→His change in amino acid (Table 2). The allele frequency of ST1A3*2 is reported to be 0.31 to 0.37 in Caucasians and Nigerians, as shown in Table 2. The frequencies of two other alleles are quite lower than that of ST1A3*2 and reported to be 0.01 and 0.003 for ST1A3*3 and ST1A3*4, respectively. A genetic polymorphism accompanying amino acid exchange in ST1A2 is also found with the frequency of 0.38 (ST1A2*2). The frequencies of the haplotypes ST1A2*1/ ST1A3*1 and ST1A2*2/ST1A3*2 are highly similar to allele frequencies of ST1A2*1 and ST1A2*2 or ST1A3*1 and ST1A3*2. These data suggest that ST1A2*2 and ST1A3*2 alleles are associated (58).

SULT1B

Human SULT1B (ST1B2) has been identified (23, 24). This form catalyzes sulfation of 3, 3', 5'-triiodothyronine and p-nitrophenol (28), although both sulfations are also catalyzed by other SULTs, including the SULT1 family (28). A recent study on their enzyme kinetics and expressions showed that 3, 3', 5'-triiodothyronine and p-nitrophenol are preferentially sulfated by ST1B2 and ST1A3, respectively, in human livers (28). Similar results were also obtained with rat ST1B1 (59). Kinetic parameters for PAPS and 3, 3', 5'-triiodothyronine are quite similar between ST1B2 and ST1B1. Chromosome localization and genetic

◄————————————————————————————

Figure 2   Structure of human SULT cDNA 5'-untranslated region. Gene structures are shown in only the first and second exons of individual genes. The figures in parentheses represent the accession numbers for SULT genes, and the asterisks represent the accession numbers for EST.

TABLE 2   Chromosomal localization and allele frequency of human SULTs

Chromosomal localization	Genotype	Substitution		Allele frequency
		Nucleotide	Amino acid	
16p12.1-p11.2	*ST1A2*1*			
	ST1A2*2	T20C, A706C	Ile7Thr, Asn235Thr	0.38
16p12.1-p11.2	*ST1A3*1*			
	ST1A3*2	G638A	Arg213His	0.31-0.37
	ST1A3*3	A667G	Met223Val	0.01
	ST1A3*4	G110A	Arg37Gln	0.003
16p11.2	*ST1A5*	–	–	–
–	*ST1B2*	–	–	–
2q11.1-q11.2	*ST1C2*	–	–	–
–	*ST1C3*	–	–	–
4q13.1	*ST1E4*	–	–	–
19q13.3	*ST2A3*1*			
	ST2A3*2	T170C	Met57Thr	0.027
	ST2A3*3	A557T	Glu186Val	0.038
19q13.3	*ST2B1*	–	–	–
22	*ST5A2*	–	–	–

polymorphism are still unknown, although a wide individual variation in the hepatic level of ST1B2 in human livers is observed (28).

SULT1C

SULT1C was first isolated from rat as an N-hydroxy-2-acetylaminofluorene (N-OH-AAF) SULT (ST1C1) (29). Two human SULT1C cDNAs (ST1C2 and ST1C3) have been identified through the EST database (30–32). Both amino acid sequences deduced from the nucleotide sequences shared about 63% identity with that of ST1C1. These human ST1C2 and ST1C3 shared 62.9% identity in their amino acid sequences with each other, which suggests that these three genes may have diverged from the same ancestor at an earlier era than when primates and rodents diverged. ST1C2 mRNA is expressed in adult human stomach, kidney, and thyroid, as well as in fetal kidney and liver (32). ST1C3 mRNA is expressed at higher levels in fetal lung and kidney and at lower levels in fetal heart, adult kidney, ovary, and spinal cord (31). An ST1C gene sharing a higher homology with ST1C1 was identified from humans (60). The amino acid sequence deduced from exon 7 and exon 8 showed 85.6% identity with that of ST1C1, although the expression has not been identified in human. The chromosome localization is reported to be on chromosome 2q11.1-q11.2 for ST1C2 (32).

SULT1E

A gene of human SULT1E (ST1E4) has been identified and located on chromosome 4q13.1 (45). ST1E4 is a typical estrogen sulfotransferase (28, 61). The Km value for β-estradiol is lowest (0.25 µM) among human SULTs (28). The hepatic level of ST1E4 in human is correlated with the sulfation activity of β-estradiol (r = 0.88). The level of ST1A3 is, however, also correlated with the sulfation activity of β-estradiol (r = 0.90) (28), when the activity is determined at 0.5 µM of the substrate concentration. These phenomena might be explained by differences in expressed levels of both forms in the tissue: In human livers, the ST1A3 level is nine times higher than that of ST1E4 (28). The plasma level of β-estradiol is known to be around 0.5 nM. These data thus suggest that estrogen sulfation is the main physiological role of ST1E4 in humans, although the pharmacological or physiological role of ST1A3 is not excluded. Although the expression level of ST1E4 varies among individuals, the genetic polymorphism has not been reported (28).

SULT2A

Plural SULT2A forms have been isolated from a rodent species and display different substrate specificity on the sulfation of hydroxysteroids (62–64). However, the single form, ST2A3, is contained in humans and catalyzes the sulfation of hydroxysteroids, including bile acids (43). ST2A3 is highly expressed in human adrenals and livers (47). Liver ST2A3 activity has been shown to vary more than fivefold and has shown bimodal distribution when approximately 25% of subjects were included in a high-activity subgroup (65). ST2A3 consists of 6 exons and is located on chromosome band 19q13 (66, 67). By analyses of numbers of ST2A3 genes, three allele variants with amino acid changes were identified (13). ST2A3*2 allele contains a T → C mutation at ST2A3 cDNA nucleotide 170, located within exon 2, resulting in a Met 57 → Thr change in the amino acid sequence. Another allele (ST2A3*3) contained an A → T mutation at nucleotide 557 within exon 4 resulting in a Glu 186 → Val change, as shown in Table 2. Recombinant ST2A3*2 (Met57Thr) and recombinant ST2A3*3 (Glu186Val) were shown to have decreased the thermal stability and activity for dehydroepiandrosterone as compared to the wild type (ST2A3*1). The allele frequencies for ST2A3*2 and ST2A3*3 are reported to be 0.024 and 0.038, respectively (13).

SULT2B

SULT2B1 was originally identified through the EST database from a human placenta cDNA library (16). The rapid amplification of cDNA end studies provided evidence that two ST2B1s (ST2B1a and ST2B1b) are transcribed from the same gene. ST2B1a and ST2B1b have different N-terminal amino acid sequences, which are transcribed from different exons as shown in Figure 2. ST2B1a is derived only from exon 2, whereas ST2B1b is from exon 1 and a part of exon 2. ST2B1a and ST2B1b thus consist of 350 and 365 amino acids, respectively, whose C-terminal sequences (342 amino acids) transcribed from a part of exon 2 to exon 6 are identical. Both forms are reported to catalyze sulfation of dehydroepiandrosterone, but not of other typical substrates for other SULTs (16). ST2B1 is expressed in human placenta, prostate, and trachea, and also slightly in the small intestine and lung. ST2B1 is on the long arm of chromosome 19 within band 19q13.3, which is the location similar to that of ST2A3 with an approximately 500-kb distance (16). Data on the genetic polymorphism are not yet available.

SULT5A

This SULT gene was identified by the Human Chromosome 22 Project Group. Information on the expression and enzymatic properties is not yet available. A part of the sequence is, however, observed in the EST database from human infant brain. The similar SULT sequence (St5a2) is also identified in the mouse brain cDNA library, although characterization of the St5a2 property has not been performed. It is worthwhile to note that amino acid sequences of both forms share 98% identity. These high sequence identities may suggest an important role of SULT5A in brain function.

SUMMARY AND FUTURE DIRECTIONS

A large number of cytosolic sulfotransferases has been identified from mammals and classified into five families based on their amino acid sequences. Recent studies on genetic polymorphism of SULT provide considerable amounts of information on allelic variants. These types of genetic information will likely increase in the near future.

The nomenclature system for SULTs is not yet universal, and confusion has already appeared. For this reason, we have proposed a comprehensive SULT nomenclature system. Cytosolic sulfotransferase (CST) other than those in mammals can be included based on structural similarity. Information on membrane-bound types of sulfotransferase (MST) is also increasing, but a relationship between CST and MST remains unclear. Family numbers of SULT for vertebrates start from 1 for vertebrates, as shown above. Nonvertebrate forms may be started from 50, plant forms from 100, and bacteria forms from 200. We hope that this nomenclature system will be discussed and adapted and will be useful in the sulfotransferase research field.

Visit the Annual Reviews home page at www.AnnualReviews.org.

LITERATURE CITED

1. Sekura RD, Duffel MW, Jakoby WB. 1981. Aryl sulfotransferases. In *Detoxication and Drug Metabolism: Conjugation and Related Systems,* ed. WB Jakoby, pp. 197–206. New York: Academic
2. Mulder GJ. 1984. Sulfation-metabolic aspects. In *Progress in Drug Metabolism,* ed. JW Bridges, LF Chasseaud, pp. 35–100. London: Taylor & Francis
3. Yamazoe Y, Kato R. 1995. Structure and function of sulfotransferase. In *Advances in Drug Metabolism in Man,* ed. GM Pacifici, GN Fracchia, pp. 659–78. Luxembourg: Eur. Comm.
4. Falany CN. 1997. Sulfation and sulfotransferases. Introduction: changing view of sulfation and the cytosolic sulfotransferases. *FASEB J.* 11:1–2
5. Yamazoe Y, Nagata K, Ozawa S, Kato R. 1994. Structural similarity and diversity of sulfotransferases. *Chem.-Biol. Interact.* 92:107–17
6. Weinshilboum RM, Otterness DM, Aksoy IA, Wood TC, Her C, et al. 1997. Sulfation and sulfotransferases 1: Sulfotransferase molecular biology: cDNAs and genes. *FASEB J.* 11:3–14
7. Sundaram RS, Van Loon JA, Tucker R, Weinshilboum RM. 1989. Sulfation pharmacogenetics: correlation of human platelet and small intestinal phenol sulfotransferase. *Clin. Pharmacol. Ther.* 46:501–9
8. Weinshilboum R. 1990. Sulfotransferase pharmacogenetics. *Pharmacol. Ther.* 45:93–107

9. Weinshilboum R, Aksoy I. 1994. Sulfation pharmacogenetics in humans. *Chem.-Biol. Interact.* 92:233–46
10. Pacifici GM, De'Santi C. 1995. Human sulphotransferase. Classification and metabolic profile of major isoforms. The point of view of the clinical pharmacologist. In *Advances in Drug Metabolism in Man,* ed. GM Pacifici, GN Fracchia, pp. 311–49. Luxembourg: Eur. Comm.
11. Ozawa S, Tang YM, Yamazoe Y, Kato R, Lang NP, et al. 1998. Genetic polymorphisms in human liver phenol sulfotransferases involved in the bioactivation of N-hydroxy derivatives of carcinogenic arylamines and heterocyclic amines. *Chem.-Biol. Interact.* 109:237–48
12. Raftogianis RB, Wood TC, Otterness DM, Van Loon JA, Weinshilboum RM. 1997. Phenol sulfotransferase pharmacogenetics in humans: association of common SULT1A1 alleles with TS PST phenotype. *Biochem. Biophys. Res. Commun.* 239:298–304
13. Wood TC, Her C, Aksoy I, Otterness DM, Weinshilboum RM. 1996. Human dehydroepiandrosterone sulfotransferase pharmacogenetics: quantitative Western analysis and gene sequence polymorphisms. *J. Steroid Biochem. Mol. Biol.* 59:467–78
14. Coughtrie MW, Gilissen RA, Shek B, Strange RC, Fryer AA, et al. 1999. Phenol sulphotransferase SULT1A1 polymorphism: molecular diagnosis and allele frequencies in Caucasian and African populations. *Biochem. J.* 337:45–49
15. Dunn RT 2nd, Klaassen CD. 1998. Tis-

sue-specific expression of rat sulfotransferase messenger RNAs. *Drug Metab.
Dispos.* 26:598–604

16. Her C, Wood TC, Eichler EE, Mohrenweiser HW, Ramagli LS, et al. 1998.
Human hydroxysteroid sulfotransferase
SULT2B1: two enzymes encoded by a
single chromosome 19 gene. *Genomics*
53:284–85

17. Saeki Y, Sakakibara Y, Araki Y, Yanagisawa K, Suiko M, et al. 1998. Molecular
cloning, expression, and characterization
of a novel mouse liver SULT1B1 sulfotransferase. *J. Biochem.* 124:55–64

18. Nelson DR, Kamataki T, Waxman DJ,
Guengerich FP, Estabrook RW, et al.
1993. The P450 superfamily: update on
new sequences, gene mapping, accession
numbers, early trivial names of enzymes,
and nomenclature. *DNA Cell Biol.* 12:1–
51

19. Nelson DR, Koymans L, Kamataki T,
Stegeman JJ, Feyereisen R, et al. 1996.
P450 superfamily: update on new
sequences, gene mapping, accession
numbers and nomenclature. *Pharmacogenetics* 6:1–42

20. Nash AR, Glenn WK, Moore SS, Kerr J,
Thompson AR, et al. 1988. Oestrogen
sulfotransferase: molecular cloning and
sequencing of cDNA for the bovine placental enzyme. *Aust. J. Biol. Sci.* 41:507–
16

21. Ozawa S, Nagata K, Gong DW, Yamazoe
Y, Kato R. 1990. Nucleotide sequence of
a full-length cDNA (PST-1) for aryl sulfotransferase from rat liver. *Nucleic
Acids Res.* 18:4001

22. Sakakibara Y, Takami Y, Zwieb C,
Nakayama T, Suiko M, et al. 1995. Purification, characterization, and molecular
cloning of a novel rat liver Dopa/tyrosine
sulfotransferase. *J. Biol. Chem.* 270:
30470–78

23. Fujita K, Nagata K, Ozawa S, Sasano H,
Yamazoe Y. 1997. Molecular cloning and
characterization of rat ST1B1 and human
ST1B2 cDNAs, encoding thyroid hor-

mone sulfotransferases. *J. Biochem.*
122:1052–61

24. Wang J, Falany JL, Falany CN. 1998.
Expression and characterization of a
novel thyroid hormone-sulfating form of
cytosolic sulfotransferase from human
liver. *Mol. Pharmacol.* 53:274–82

25. Watabe T, Ogura K, Satsukawa M,
Okuda H, Hiratsuka A. 1994. Molecular
cloning and functions of rat liver hydroxysteroid sulfotransferases catalysing covalent binding of carcinogenic polycyclic
arylmethanols to DNA. *Chem.-Biol. Interact.* 92:87–105

26. Strott CA. 1996. Steroid sulfotransferases. *Endocr. Rev.* 17:670–97

27. Yoshinari K, Nagata K, Ogino M, Fujita
K, Shiraga T, et al. 1998. Molecular cloning and expression of an amine sulfotransferase cDNA: a new gene family of
cytosolic sulfotransferases in mammals.
J. Biochem. 123:479–86

28. Fujita K, Nagata K, Yamazaki T, Watanabe
E, Shimada M, et al. 1999. Enzymatic
characterization of human cytosolic sulfotransferases: identification of ST1B2 as
a thyroid hormone sulfotransferase. *Biol.
Pharm. Bull.* 22:446–52

29. Nagata K, Ozawa S, Miyata M, Shimada
M, Gong DW, et al. 1993. Isolation and
expression of a cDNA encoding a male-
specific rat sulfotransferase that catalyzes
activation of N-hydroxy-2-acetylamino-
fluorene. *J. Biol. Chem.* 268:24720–25

30. Yoshinari K, Nagata K, Shimada M,
Yamazoe Y. 1998. Molecular characterization of ST1C1-related human sulfotransferase. *Carcinogenesis* 19:951–53

31. Sakakibara Y, Yanagisawa K, Katafuchi
J, Ringer DP, Takami Y, et al. 1998.
Molecular cloning, expression, and characterization of novel human SULT1C sulfotransferases that catalyze the sulfonation
of N-hydroxy-2-acetylaminofluorene. *J.
Biol. Chem.* 273:33929–35

32. Her C, Kaur GP, Athwal RS, Weinshilboum RM. 1997. Human sulfotransferase

SULT1C1: cDNA cloning, tissue-specific expression, and chromosomal localization. *Genomics* 41:467–70

33. Tamura HO, Harada Y, Miyawaki A, Mikoshiba K, Matsui M. 1998. Molecular cloning and expression of a cDNA encoding an olfactory-specific mouse phenol sulphotransferase. *Biochem. J.* 331:953–58

34. Sakakibara Y, Yanagisawa K, Takami Y, Nakayama T, Suiko M, et al. 1998. Molecular cloning, expression, and functional characterization of novel mouse sulfotransferases. *Biochem. Biophys. Res. Commun.* 247:681–86

35. Liu MC, Sakakibara Y, Liu CC. 1999. Bacterial expression, purification, and characterization of a novel mouse sulfotransferase that catalyzes the sulfation of eicosanoids. *Biochem. Biophys. Res. Commun.* 254:65–69

36. Demyan WF, Song CS, Kim DS, Her S, Gallwitz W, et al. 1992. Estrogen sulfotransferase of the rat liver: complementary DNA cloning and age- and sex-specific regulation of messenger RNA. *Mol. Endocrinol.* 6:589–97

37. Falany JL, Krasnykh V, Mikheeva G, Falany CN. 1995. Isolation and expression of an isoform of rat estrogen sulfotransferase. *J. Steroid Biochem. Mol. Biol.* 52:35–44

38. Kakuta Y, Pedersen LG, Carter CW, Negishi M, Pedersen LC. 1997. Crystal structure of estrogen sulphotransferase. *Nat. Struct. Biol.* 4:904–8

39. Ogura K, Kajita J, Narihata H, Watabe T, Ozawa S, et al. 1989. Cloning and sequence analysis of a rat liver cDNA encoding hydroxysteroid sulfotransferase. *Biochem. Biophys. Res. Commun.* 165:168–74

40. Ogura K, Satsukawa M, Okuda H, Hiratsuka A, Watabe T. 1994. Major hydroxysteroid sulfotransferase STa in rat liver cytosol may consist of two microheterogeneous subunits. *Chem.-Biol. Interact.* 92:129–44

41. Chatterjee B, Majumdar D, Ozbilen O, Murty CV, Roy AK. 1987. Molecular cloning and characterization of cDNA for androgen-repressible rat liver protein, SMP-2. *J. Biol. Chem.* 262:822–25

42. Shiraga T, Iwasaki K, Hata T, Yoshinari K, Nagata K, et al. 1999. Purification and characterization of two amine N-sulfotransferases, AST-RB1 (ST3A1) and AST-RB2 (ST2A8), from liver cytosols of male rabbits. *Arch. Biochem. Biophys.* 362:265–74

43. Otterness DM, Her C, Aksoy S, Kimura S, Wieben ED, et al. 1995. Human dehydroepiandrosterone sulfotransferase gene: molecular cloning and structural characterization. *DNA Cell Biol.* 14:331–41

44. Bernier F, Soucy P, Luu-The V. 1996. Human phenol sulfotransferase gene contains two alternative promoters: structure and expression of the gene. *DNA Cell Biol.* 15:367–75

45. Her C, Aksoy IA, Kimura S, Brandriff BF, Wasmuth JJ, et al. 1995. Human estrogen sulfotransferase gene (STE): cloning, structure, and chromosomal localization. *Genomics* 29:16–23

46. Her C, Raftogianis R, Weinshilboum RM. 1996. Human phenol sulfotransferase STP2 gene: molecular cloning, structural characterization, and chromosomal localization. *Genomics* 33:409–20

47. Luu-The V, Dufort I, Paquet N, Reimnitz G, Labrie F. 1995. Structural characterization and expression of the human dehydroepiandrosterone sulfotransferase gene. *DNA Cell Biol.* 14:511–18

48. Gong DW, Murayama N, Yamazoe Y, Kato R. 1992. Hepatic triiodothyronine sulfation and its regulation by growth hormone and triiodothyronine in rats. *J. Biochem.* 112:112–16

49. Ueda R, Shimada M, Hashimoto H, Ishikawa H, Yamazoe Y. 1997. Distinct regulation of two hydroxysteroid sulfotransferases, ST2A1 and ST2A2, by growth hormone: a unique type of

growth hormone regulation in rats. *J. Pharmacol. Exp. Ther.* 282:1117–21

50. Klaassen CD, Liu L, Dunn RT 2nd. 1998. Regulation of sulfotransferase mRNA expression in male and female rats of various ages. *Chem.-Biol. Interact.* 109: 299–313

51. Falany CN. 1991. Molecular enzymology of human liver cytosolic sulfotransferases. *Trends Pharmacol. Sci.* 12:255–59

52. Dooley TP, Obermoeller RD, Leiter EH, Chapman HD, Falany CN, et al. 1993. Mapping of the phenol sulfotransferase gene (STP) to human chromosome 16p12.1-p11.2 and to mouse chromosome 7. *Genomics* 18:440–43

53. Gaedigk A, Beatty BG, Grant DM. 1997. Cloning, structural organization, and chromosomal mapping of the human phenol sulfotransferase STP2 gene. *Genomics* 40:242–46

54. Aksoy IA, Callen DF, Apostolou S, Her C, Weinshilboum RM. 1994. Thermolabile phenol sulfotransferase gene (STM): localization to human chromosome 16p11.2. *Genomics* 23:275–77

55. Dooley TP, Probst P, Munroe PB, Mole SE, Liu Z, et al. 1994. Genomic organization and DNA sequence of the human catecholamine-sulfating phenol sulfotransferase gene (STM). *Biochem. Biophys. Res. Commun.* 205:1325–32

56. Dooley TP. 1998. Cloning of the human phenol sulfotransferase gene family: three genes implicated in the metabolism of catecholamines, thyroid hormones and drugs. *Chem.-Biol. Interact.* 109:29–41

57. Price RA, Spielman RS, Lucena AL, Van Loon JA, Maidak BL, et al. 1989. Genetic polymorphism for human platelet thermostable phenol sulfotransferase (TS PST) activity. *Genetics* 122:905–14

58. Engelke CEH, Meinl W, Boeing H, Glatt H. 1999. Association between functional genetic polymorphism of human sulfotransferases 1A1 and 1A2. *Pharmacogenetics.* In press

59. Fujita K, Nagata K, Watanabe E, Shimada M, Yamazoe Y. 1999. Bacterial expression and functional characterization of a rat thyroid hormone sulfotransferase, ST1B1. *Jpn. J. Pharmacol.* 79: 467–75

60. Nagata K, Yoshinari K, Ozawa S, Yamazoe Y. 1997. Arylamine activating sulfotransferase in liver. *Mutat. Res.* 376: 267–72

61. Falany CN, Krasnykh V, Falany JL. 1995. Bacterial expression and characterization of a cDNA for human liver estrogen sulfotransferase. *J. Steroid Biochem. Mol. Biol.* 52:529–39

62. Homma H, Ogawa K, Hirono K, Morioka Y, Hirota M, et al. 1996. Site-directed mutagenesis of rat hepatic hydroxysteroid sulfotransferases. *Biochim. Biophys. Acta* 1296:159–66

63. Lee YC, Park CS, Strott CA. 1994. Molecular cloning of a chiral-specific 3α-hydroxysteroid sulfotransferase. *J. Biol. Chem.* 269:15838–45

64. Yoshinari K, Nagata K, Shiraga T, Iwasaki K, Hata T, et al. 1998. Molecular cloning, expression, and enzymatic characterization of rabbit hydroxysteroid sulfotransferase AST-RB2. *J. Biochem.* 123: 740–46

65. Aksoy IA, Sochorova V, Weinshilboum RM. 1993. Human liver dehydroepiandrosterone sulfotransferase: nature and extent of individual variation. *Clin. Pharmacol. Ther.* 54:498–506

66. Durocher F, Morissette J, Dufort I, Simard J, Luu-The V. 1995. Genetic linkage mapping of the dehydroepiandrosterone sulfotransferase (STD) gene on the chromosome 19q13.3 region. *Genomics* 29:781–83

67. Otterness DM, Mohrenweiser HW, Brandriff BF, Weinshilboum RM. 1995. Dehydroepiandrosterone sulfotransferase gene (STD): localization to human chromosome band 19q13.3. *Cytogenet. Cell Genet.* 70:45–47

68. Hirshey SJ, Dooley TP, Reardon IM,

Heinrikson RL, Falany CN. 1992. Sequence analysis, in vitro translation, and expression of the cDNA for rat liver minoxidil sulfotransferase. *Mol. Pharmacol.* 42:257–64

69. Yerokun T, Etheredge JL, Norton TR, Carter HA, Chung KH, et al. 1992. Characterization of a complementary DNA for rat liver aryl sulfotransferase IV and use in evaluating the hepatic gene transcript levels of rats at various stages of 2-acetylaminofluorene-induced hepatocarcinogenesis. *Cancer Res.* 52:4779–86

70. Ozawa S, Nagata K, Shimada M, Ueda M, Tsuzuki T, et al. 1995. Primary structures and properties of two related forms of aryl sulfotransferases in human liver. *Pharmacogenetics* 5:S135–40

71. Zhu X, Veronese ME, Iocco P, McManus ME. 1996. cDNA cloning and expression of a new form of human aryl sulfotransferase. *Int. J. Biochem. Cell Biol.* 28: 565–71

72. Raftogianis RB, Her C, Weinshilboum RM. 1996. Human phenol sulfotransferase pharmacogenetics: STP1 gene cloning and structural characterization. *Pharmacogenetics* 6:473–87

73. Zhu X, Veronese ME, Sansom LN, McManus ME. 1993. Molecular characterization of a human aryl sulfotransferase cDNA. *Biochem. Biophys. Res. Commun.* 192:671–76

74. Zhu X, Veronese ME, Bernard CC, Sansom LN, McManus ME. 1993. Identification of two human brain aryl sulfotransferase cDNAs. *Biochem. Biophys. Res. Commun.* 195:120–27

75. Wilborn TW, Comer KA, Dooley TP, Reardon IM, Heinrikson RL, et al. 1993. Sequence analysis and expression of the cDNA for the phenol-sulfating form of human liver phenol sulfotransferase. *Mol. Pharmacol.* 43:70–77

76. Jones AL, Hagen M, Coughtrie MW, Roberts RC, Glatt H. 1995. Human platelet phenolsulfotransferases: cDNA cloning, stable expression in V79 cells and identification of a novel allelic variant of the phenol-sulfating form. *Biochem. Biophys. Res. Commun.* 208:855–62

77. Hwang SR, Kohn AB, Hook VY. 1995. Molecular cloning of an isoform of phenol sulfotransferase from human brain hippocampus. *Biochem. Biophys. Res. Commun.* 207:701–7

78. Kong ANT, Ma MH, Tao DL, Yang LD. 1993. Molecular cloning of cDNA encoding the phenol/aryl form of sulfotransferase (mSTp1) from mouse liver. *Biochim. Biophys. Acta* 1171:315–18

79. Aksoy IA, Weinshilboum RM. 1995. Human thermolabile phenol sulfotransferase gene (STM): molecular cloning and structural characterization. *Biochem. Biophys. Res. Commun.* 208:786–95

80. Bernier F, Lopez Solache I, Labrie F, Luu-The V. 1994. Cloning and expression of cDNA encoding human placental estrogen sulfotransferase. *Mol. Cell Endocrinol.* 99:R11–R15

81. Henry T, Kliewer B, Palmatier R, Ulphani JS, Beckmann JD. 1996. Isolation and characterization of a bovine gene encoding phenol sulfotransferase. *Gene* 174:221–24

82. Oeda T, Lee YC, Driscoll WJ, Chen HC, Strott CA. 1992. Molecular cloning and expression of a full-length complementary DNA encoding the guinea pig adrenocortical estrogen sulfotransferase. *Mol. Endocrinol.* 6:1216–26

83. Aksoy IA, Wood TC, Weinshilboum R. 1994. Human liver estrogen sulfotransferase: identification by cDNA cloning and expression. *Biochem. Biophys. Res. Commun.* 200:1621–29

84. Song WC, Moore R, McLachlan JA, Negishi M. 1995. Molecular characterization of a testis-specific estrogen sulfotransferase and aberrant liver expression in obese and diabetogenic C57BL/KsJ-db/db mice. *Endocrinology* 136:2477–84

85. Rikke BA, Roy AK. 1996. Structural relationships among members of the

mammalian sulfotransferase gene family. *Biochim. Biophys. Acta* 1307:331–38

86. Ogura K, Kajita J, Narihata H, Watabe T, Ozawa S, et al. 1990. cDNA cloning of the hydroxysteroid sulfotransferase STa sharing a strong homology in amino acid sequence with the senescence marker protein SMP-2 in rat livers. *Biochem. Biophys. Res. Commun.* 166:1494–500

87. Otterness DM, Weinshilboum R. 1994. Human dehydroepiandrosterone sulfotransferase: molecular cloning of cDNA and genomic DNA. *Chem.-Biol. Interact.* 92:145–59

88. Forbes KJ, Hagen M, Glatt H, Hume R, Coughtrie MW. 1995. Human fetal adrenal hydroxysteroid sulphotransferase: cDNA cloning, stable expression in V79 cells and functional characterisation of the expressed enzyme. *Mol. Cell Endocrinol.* 112:53–60

89. Kong ANT, Yang LD, Ma MH, Tao D, Bjornsson TD. 1992. Molecular cloning of the alcohol/hydroxysteroid form (hSTa) of sulfotransferase from human liver. *Biochem. Biophys. Res. Commun.* 187: 448–54

90. Comer KA, Falany JL, Falany CN. 1993. Cloning and expression of human liver dehydroepiandrosterone sulphotransferase. *Biochem. J.* 289:233–40

91. Kong ANT, Tao DL, Ma MH, Yang LD. 1993. Molecular cloning of the alcohol/ hydroxysteroid form (mSTa1) of sulfotransferase from mouse liver. *Pharm. Res.* 10:627–30

92. Luu NX, Driscoll WJ, Martin BM, Strott CA. 1995. Molecular cloning and expression of a guinea pig 3-hydroxysteroid sulfotransferase distinct from chiral-specific 3α-hydroxysteroid sulfotransferase. *Biochem. Biophys. Res. Commun.* 217: 1078–86

93. Dufort I, Tremblay Y, Belanger A, Labrie F, Luu-The V. 1996. Isolation and characterization of a stereospecific 3β-hydroxysteroid sulfotransferase (pregnenolone sulfotransferase) cDNA. *DNA Cell Biol.* 15:481–87

94. Kong ANT, Fei PW. 1994. Molecular cloning of three sulfotransferase cDNAs from mouse liver. *Chem.-Biol. Interact.* 92:161–68

Annu. Rev. Pharmacol. Toxicol. 2000. 40:177–91

DRUG DISCOVERY IN THE NEXT MILLENNIUM

Eliot H. Ohlstein, Robert R. Ruffolo Jr., and John D. Elliott

Departments of Cardiovascular Pharmacology and Medicinal Chemistry, Research & Development, SmithKline Beecham Pharmaceuticals, King of Prussia, Pennsylvania 19406–0939; e-mail: ohlstein@sbphrd.com, robert_r_ruffolo@sbphrd.com, john_d_elliott@sbphrd.com

Key Words   target validation, functional genomics, proteomics, high-throughput screening, combinatorial chemistry, cheminformatics, gene therapy

■ **Abstract**   Selection and validation of novel molecular targets have become of paramount importance in light of the plethora of new potential therapeutic drug targets that have emerged from human gene sequencing. In response to this revolution within the pharmaceutical industry, the development of high-throughput methods in both biology and chemistry has been necessitated. This review addresses these technological advances as well as several new areas that have been created by necessity to deal with this new paradigm, such as bioinformatics, cheminformatics, and functional genomics. With many of these key components of future drug discovery now in place, it is possible to map out a critical path for this process that will be used into the new millennium.

INTRODUCTION

The Human Genome Project was initiated on October 1, 1990, and according to the original plan, the complete DNA sequence of the human genome would be achieved by the year 2005 (1). However, improvements in technology and an increase in interest in human DNA sequence have placed the project 2 years ahead of schedule; it is now anticipated that the Human Genome Project will be completed in the year 2003. Furthermore, a partial blueprint of the human genome is scheduled to be available as early as March 2000. Gene identification provides a new paradigm for understanding human disease at its most fundamental level; a knowledge of the genetic control of cellular functions will constitute the conceptual underpinnings of future strategies for the prevention and treatment of disease. It is of interest that the identification in the 1980s of the gene believed to be responsible for cystic fibrosis took researchers approximately 9 years to discover, whereas the gene responsible for Parkinson's disease was recently identified within a period of several weeks (2). This quantum leap in the ability to associate a specific gene with a disease can be attributed primarily to the extraordinary

0362–1642/00/0415–0177$14.00

progress that has been made in the areas of gene sequencing and information technologies.

TARGET VALIDATION

Several thousand molecular targets have been cloned and are available as potential novel drug discovery targets. These targets include more than 750 G-protein–coupled receptors (GPCRs), over 100 ligand-gated ion channels, more than 60 nuclear receptors and 50 cytokines, and approximately 20 reuptake/transport proteins (3). A new potential therapeutic approach for the treatment of a known disease is published nearly every week, as a result of the exponential proliferation of novel molecular and biochemical targets. The sheer volume of genetic information being produced has shifted the emphasis from the generation of novel DNA sequences to the determination of which of these many new targets offer the greatest opportunity for drug discovery. Thus, with several thousand potential targets available, target selection and validation has become the most critical component of the drug discovery process and will continue to be so in the future.

An example of the new paradigm of target selection comes as a result of the pairing of the orphan GPCR, GPR-14, with its cognate neuropeptide ligand, urotensin II. Urotensin II is the most potent vasoconstrictor identified to date, being approximately one order of magnitude more potent than endothelin-1 (4). Thus, GPR-14/urotensin II represents an attractive therapeutic target for the treatment of disorders related to or associated with enhanced vasoconstriction, such as hypertension, congestive heart failure, and coronary artery disease, to name but a few.

The human genome contains approximately 100,000 genes, and any individual tissue expresses between 15,000 and 50,000 of these genes in differing amounts. In diseased tissue, gene expression levels often differ from those observed in normal tissues, with certain genes being over- or underexpressed, or new genes being expressed or completely absent. The localization of this differential gene expression is one of the first crucial steps in identifying an important potential molecular target for drug discovery. In addition to the traditional techniques of Northern blotting analysis, there are a number of newer methods used to localize gene expression. The techniques that typically yield the highest-quality data are in situ hybridization and immunocytochemistry, both of which are labor intensive. For example, in situ hybridization or immunohistochemical localization of a prospective molecular target to a particular tissue or subcellular region is likely to yield valuable information concerning gene function. Recent examples of the success of this approach include the case of the orexin peptides and receptors whose hypothalamic regional localization suggested an involvement in feeding (5). Furthermore, positional cloning of the gene encoding the leptin peptide from ob/ob mice and its subsequent localization to adipocytes has identified this peptide as an important lipostatic factor (6).

Each of these localization techniques has its advantages and disadvantages. In situ hybridization can be initiated immediately following gene sequencing and cloning; however, gene detection is only at the transcriptional mRNA level. Immunocytochemistry, on the other hand, offers the ability to measure protein expression but requires the availability of antibodies having the requisite affinity and selectivity, which may often take several months to generate. With either of these techniques, target localization within the cell is possible at the microscopic level, but it is dependent on the availability of high-quality normal and diseased human tissues, which often represents yet another problem.

The localization of a gene in a particular tissue does not necessarily shed light on all the functions of that gene. As an example, the previously mentioned discovery of orexin as a putative regulator of energy balance and feeding was initially concluded as a result of localization in the dorsal and lateral hypothalamic regions of the brain (5). However, more recently, this gene product was discovered through a positional cloning approach to be a major sleep-modulating neurotransmitter that may represent the gene responsible for narcolepsy (7).

In recent years, new technologies such as microarray gridding (gene-chip) and TaqMan polymerase chain reaction have emerged that would appear destined to play a more prominent role in the high-throughput localization of genes, and the identification of their regulation in disease (8). Gene-chip technology has evolved into two platforms: oligonucleotide (9, 10) and cDNA fragment arrays (11). The inherent problem with oligonucleotide arrays stems from the use of a short hybridization sequence, which can lead to artifacts. cDNA arrays, as a result of their extended sequence, provide higher-quality information due to the specificity and stringency of hybridization. The latter approach does, however, require the generation of long (300–750 bp) cDNAs.

Microarray gridding is already evolving into a procedure that will allow for the comprehensive evaluation of differences in gene expression patterns in normal, diseased, or pharmacologically manipulated systems (8). For genes expressed in low abundance, more sensitive techniques may be required, and reverse transcriptase polymerase chain reaction–based TaqMan technology offers the ability to detect changes in gene expression with as little as two copies per cell. TaqMan technology also has the potential to be developed into a robust methodology for high-throughput tissue localization.

PROTEOMICS

Proteomics offers an alternative, and complimentary, approach to genomic-based technologies for the identification and validation of protein targets, and for the description of changes in protein expression under the influence of disease or drug treatment. Much interest has been expressed by the pharmaceutical industry in proteomics in anticipation of the value of this technology to both discovery and development of new drugs (12).

Proteomics involves the identification and quantitation of gene expression at the protein level. Additionally, proteomics may help to identify protein interaction partners and members of multiprotein complexes. Furthermore, this technique may assist in following time-dependent changes in protein expression levels resulting from selective excitation of a biological pathway, and thereby delineating a cellular protein network, a methodology that has been referred to as functional proteomics.

A recent example of the successful application of a proteomics approach was demonstrated by the identification of a protein (HMG-1) that is a potential late mediator of endotoxin lethality in mice (13). This particular study is noteworthy because it detected changes in HMG-1 release from macrophages induced by endotoxin treatment, whereas the mRNA expression of HMG-1 was not affected by endotoxin treatment, indicating that protein release is not necessarily regulated by gene transcription. These authors further demonstrated that HMG-1 itself is toxic and that anti–HMG-1 antibodies prevent lethality, implicating HMG-1 as a potential target for therapeutic intervention (13). This example clearly demonstrates the complementary nature of proteomic- and genomics-based methods.

In contrast to genomic-based approaches, proteomics is not nearly as well developed as a high-throughput methodology, for a number of reasons. First, proteins have more variable physicochemical properties than does DNA, affecting their behavior, separation, and identification. Second, the abundance of proteins often varies widely. For example, transcription factors are present only at the level of a few copies per cell, whereas very abundant proteins, such as actin, may be present at 10^8 copies/cell. Recently, however, considerable progress has been made in improving detection of low copy proteins through enhancement of gel-loading techniques and enrichment strategies such as affinity-based purification two-dimensional gel separation. Finally, enhanced protein staining/detection methods are now becoming available, and mass spectrometry is pushing the bounds of detection to even more sensitive limits (14). Notwithstanding the technical difficulties that remain, sufficient evidence exists, even at this early stage of the technology, to warrant that proteomics will provide crucial information for the discovery and development of novel therapeutic targets.

HIGH-THROUGHPUT SCREENING

Throughout the 1990s, the pharmaceutical industry has sought to expand its collections of compounds for the purpose of high-throughput screening (HTS) against novel molecular targets (15). A notable early success using this paradigm was the discovery of CP-96,345 (16) (Figure 1), a potent, nonpeptide, neurokinin-1 receptor antagonist. During the past decade, many lead structures have subsequently been unearthed through HTS, particularly for GPCR targets (17, 18). Although the example cited above was a spectacular success (i.e. CP-96,345 has a 50% inhibitory concentration of 3 nM for the NK1 receptor), it has been more

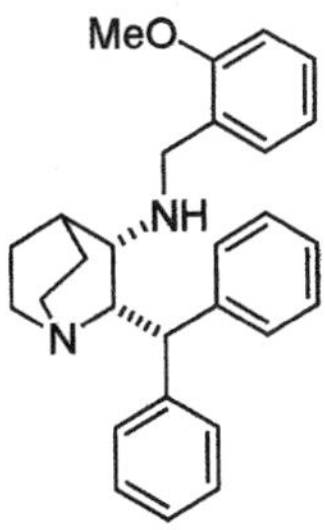

Figure 1 The structure of CP-96,345, a potent neurokinin-1 receptor antagonist obtained by high-throughput screening and compounds 1 and 2, rationally designed cathepsin K inhibitors.

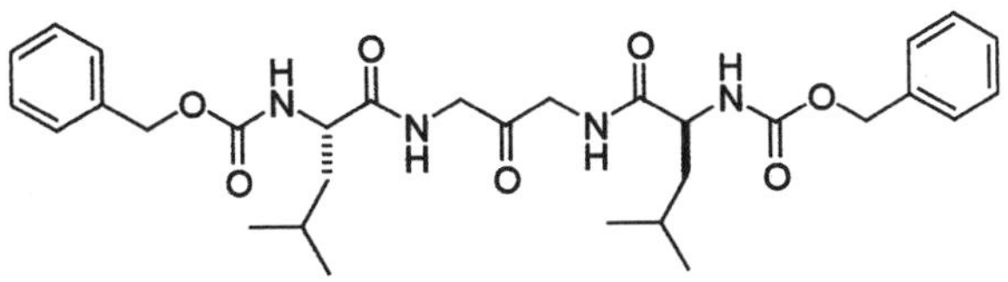

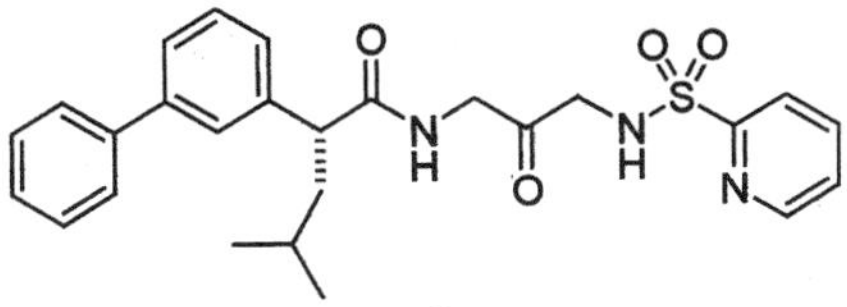

commonly the case that "hits" emerging from HTS require more substantial chemical optimization to provide therapeutic agents with the desired level of potency, selectivity, and suitable pharmacokinetic properties (19). Furthermore, the data available from HTS efforts have been of limited utility from the point of view of generating structure-activity relationships capable of directing medicinal chemistry efforts. The combinatorial chemical revolution has led to a situation in which chemotypes previously represented by a few examples in compound collections are now available as arrays of analogs. Thus, at the outset of research programs in the future, more valuable data will be available to guide a medicinal chemistry effort. To fulfill the potential that is promised by this technology, several challenges are currently being addressed. First, industrial compound collections have grown from tens of thousands of compounds in the mid-1990s to hundreds of thousands of compounds today. Fueled by combinatorial chemistry, most major pharmaceutical companies will be screening a million or so discrete compounds against each novel molecular target early into the next millennium.

In rising to the challenge of providing this quantity of data in a timely fashion, the scientist involved in high-throughput screening has sought increasing use of automation, as well as miniaturization, to reduce the demands on precious protein reagents and chemical supplies. Traditional radioligand binding assays are giving way to more rapid and easily miniaturizable homogeneous fluorescence-based methods, a trend almost certain to continue in the future. The increased efficiency of ultra-HTS offers the potential, which will be realized in the not-too-distant future, to screen discrete collections of a million or more single compounds, at multiple concentrations. This vast body of useful structure-activity relationship information will be made available at the nascence of a medicinal chemical effort.

Traditional medicinal chemical endeavors have involved the analysis of detailed biological data from hundreds or perhaps thousands of compounds. It is not surprising that the prospect of such an explosive growth of information both from screening and from program-directed combinatorial chemistry has driven the evolution of cheminformatics (20), in much the same way that genomic sequencing gave rise to the science of bioinformatics.

So what should the medicinal chemist expect from HTS when beginning a new research program early into the third millennium? In many cases, the molecule(s) of requisite potency needed for biological proof-of-concept studies will come directly from the HTS. As the HTS of compound collections becomes more dependent on combinatorial chemistry, the properties of lead structures may be enhanced rapidly using previously established high-throughput synthetic methods. The latter effort may be significantly aided by the incorporation of desirable developability characteristics (i.e. bioavailability, drug metabolism, and pharmacokinetics) into the design of libraries for lead generation, an area of further impact for the cheminformatics practitioners of the future (21).

MEDICINAL CHEMISTRY

During the past 50 years, the total synthesis of many exceedingly complex natural products has been achieved, representing a major accomplishment for organic chemistry (22). Although these efforts have been greatly facilitated by advances in the use of spectroscopic techniques, the underlying scientific principles are the same as those that guided synthetic organic chemical pioneers at the turn of this century. Organic synthesis is, and is likely to be for some time, the cornerstone upon which medicinal chemistry is built. However, as part of an exciting development still taking place as the millennium closes, these disciplines have witnessed a paradigm shift as great as any in their history, namely the introduction of parallel or combinatorial synthesis. For some time now, the synthesis of peptides and oligonucleotides has been conducted by automated methods, a paradigm rendered more accessible by the modular nature of these macromolecules. The revolution that has gripped medicinal chemistry over the past 5 years has brought a similar philosophy to the construction of more "drug-like" small-molecules, using both solid- and solution-phase methods. Although early attempts to automate solid-phase small-molecule synthesis used modified peptide synthesizers, such machines were less than optimal. However, custom designed devices are now available that handle both solution and solid-phase protocols. Further refinement of these devices will continue into the new millennium, and the use of parallel synthesis will likely become part of the armamentarium of every medicinal chemist. In addition to the introduction of combinatorial methods, the 1990s have witnessed further refinement of rational drug design based upon molecular modeling and the use of protein X-ray crystallography. In the future, the availability of structural information early in a research program will no doubt enhance its impact, especially with the further development of de novo–design molecular modeling protocols.

The positive impact that structural information has on a medicinal chemistry program is evident from many efforts in recent years, notably those directed toward inhibitors of HIV protease (23) and cathepsin K (24). Thus, an initial design hypothesis for cathepsin K inhibitors, based upon the X-ray cocrystallography of aldehyde-type structures bound to papain, led to the synthesis of potent and selective 1,3-bis(acylamino-2-propanone, compound 1 ($K_{i,app}$ = 22 nM) (Figure 1) (24). Subsequent elaboration of compound 1 based upon further cocrystallization experiments with cathepsin K itself, and molecular modeling, led to the synthesis of even more potent analogs, such as compound 2 ($K_{i,app}$ = 1.4 nM) (Figure 1) (25).

Given the importance of GPCRs as targets in the pharmaceutical industry, the recently disclosed X-ray crystal structure of the archetypal protein of this class, bacteriorhodopsin (26), assumes special significance. In the first decade of the next century, it is likely that the three-dimensional structure of therapeutically relevant GPCRs will become available, enhancing our understanding of these targets at a molecular level and opening the way for rational drug design.

The impact of nuclear magnetic resonance (NMR) spectroscopy on rational drug design has recently come to the fore with the description of the so-called structure-activity relationships by NMR technique (27). This and other NMR techniques (28) that probe molecular interactions will no doubt receive attention in the coming decade, providing a new technique for HTS. Furthermore, NMR structural studies may become applicable to larger proteins than heretofore examined through the development of recently described segmental labeling protocols (29).

The successful medicinal chemical drug discovery effort for the new millennium will rely on a hybrid approach of parallel and iterative (single-molecule) synthesis. As HTS collections are built up through parallel synthesis, lead structures will be amenable to high-throughput follow-up. Iterative analog preparation directed at specific questions, which will influence the design of the parallel analog syntheses, will, however, continue to play a key role in the medicinal chemical effort of the future. As a research program begins to define more clearly the chemical structure of a compound that is appropriate for drug development, a greater level of iterative synthesis will likely become necessary to fine-tune the molecule to enhance specific properties of the drug in order to make the compound more suitable for drug development (e.g. potency, selectivity, pharmacokinetic profile). Structure-based design will continue to positively impact medicinal chemical efforts. In this area, the ability of parallel synthesis to explore hypotheses with a greater number of analogs should offer a distinct advantage in overcoming inevitable uncertainties with even the best X-ray or NMR-derived models.

CHEMINFORMATICS

The ability of combinatorial synthetic methods to provide large numbers of compounds rapidly does not ensure that screening collections built up by this means make the most effective use of HTS resources. To maximize the opportunity for lead generation from a given compound collection, the constituents of the collection should be as diverse as possible. However, such comparisons are complicated by the fact that any measure of chemical diversity is dependent on the parameter being considered. Certain molecular features have been considered desirable in drug candidate molecules, such as molecular weights of <500, a limited number of H-bond acceptors (<10) and donors (<5), and a cLogP of <5, and these characteristics have been recognized in what have become known as the Lipinski "rule of five" (21). Notwithstanding a desire to populate screening databases with molecules embodying these favorable characteristics, attempts are being made to maximize diversity within these limits. The development of such diversity tools by cheminformatic scientists is still in its infancy, and their value will only really become apparent when chemical libraries thus designed have been screened against a battery of structurally diverse targets. Database mining of these screening data may then provide an understanding of which molecular characteristics are most important for a given target. In this manner, commonalties of molecular properties of compounds known to interact with a given protein family can be used to enrich databases with small molecules bearing these features, so-called biased libraries. Thus, the likelihood of finding a lead structure for a novel member of such a class of proteins may be enhanced. In essence, this approach, although more rigorous, is a development of the empirical observation that certain structural similarities exist among small-molecule ligands of GPCRs, the so-called permissive or promiscuous structures (8). Thus, at least two classes of endothelin receptor antagonists arose from the discovery of a lead structure that had been previously prepared as an antagonist of another GPCR, the angiotensin AT-1 receptor (30) (Figure 2).

Although many classes of receptors and enzymes have had small-molecule agonists/substrates and antagonists/inhibitors discovered for them, protein-protein interactions have proven to be more difficult to influence, an exception being certain integrins. This has been found to be the case despite a large number of such targets having been subjected to HTS (15). It is also true, however, in the case of the integrins, that structures synthesized for one target, such as GP $II_b/$ III_a, have provided lead molecules for another member of the integrin family, $\alpha_v\beta_3$ (31). In the mid-1990s, a study of the complex between human growth hormone and the extracellular domain of the human growth hormone receptor highlighted, through site-directed mutagenesis, a relatively small area of interaction, or a "hot spot," responsible for the more than three quarters of the binding free energy (32). Although this observation bodes well for the possible ability to identify an inhibitor of the protein-protein interaction with a small molecule, the

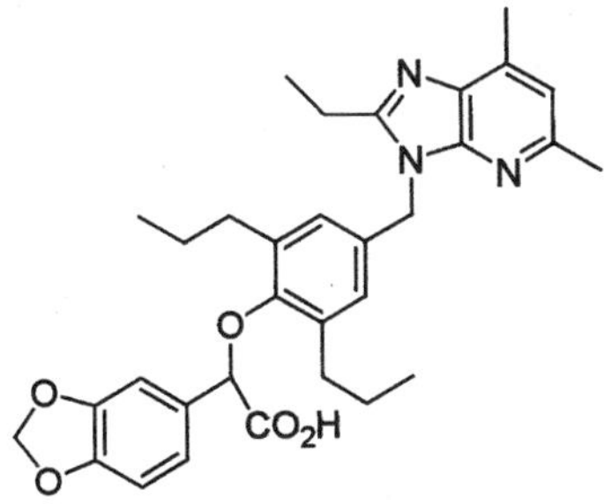

L-162,659
IC$_{50}$'s:
ET$_A$ = 38nM
ET$_B$ = 230nM
AT-1 = 2.5nM

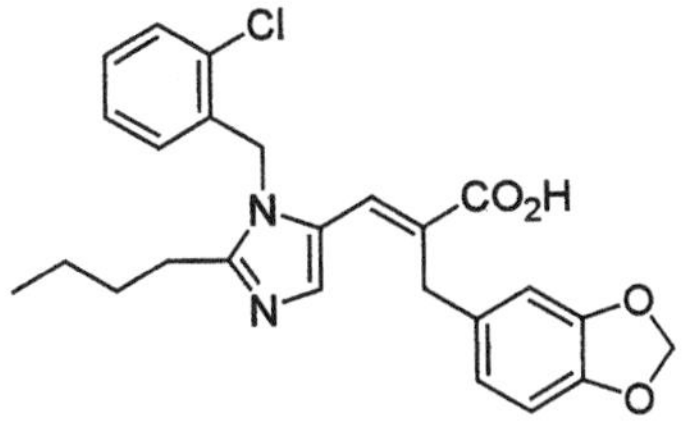

SK&F 107328
IC$_{50}$'s:
ET$_A$ = 400nM
ET$_B$ = 3,400nM
AT-1 = 180nM

Figure 2 Two classes of endothelin receptor antagonists obtained by screening collections of compounds made for another G-protein–coupled seven-transmembrane receptor, angiotensin II AT-1. IC$_{50}$, 50% inhibitory concentration; ET$_A$, endothelin-A receptor subtype; ET$_B$, endothelin-B receptor subtype; SK&F, SmithKline and French.

generality of this paradigm remains uncertain. As structural information for protein-protein interactive targets becomes more plentiful, combined with site-directed mutagenesis data, the medicinal chemist of the future may be able to predict which of these targets are more likely to be susceptible to small-molecule therapeutic intervention. A further breakthrough in this area has been achieved recently with the discovery of a small-molecule agonist of the GCSF receptor, which acts by oligomerization of receptor proteins (33). As examples of small molecules influencing protein-protein interactions accumulate, cheminformatic analysis of the data, as described above, could expand the influence of medicinal chemistry within this important area.

FUNCTIONAL GENOMICS

The term functional genomics is now being used to describe the post–genome project era, which will begin early in the new millennium and will encompass the many efforts needed to elucidate gene function. Indeed, the phenotyping of genetically manipulated animals will be critical in the determination of biological function of a particular gene. But, in reality, the discipline of functional genomics has its foundation in the physiological and pharmacological sciences. This is gratifying to the "traditional" pharmacologist, whose expertise will be drawn on even more in the future to unravel the mysteries of genetics. Although the evaluation of genetically manipulated animals will require a thorough understanding of physiology and pharmacology, the experimental approach will involve many new technologies. These methods will include in vivo imaging (i.e. magnetic resonance imaging, micro–positron emissions tomography, ultrafast computed tomography, infrared spectroscopy), mass spectrometry, and microarray hybridization, all of which should enhance the speed and accuracy at which functional genomics is achieved.

There are two general systematic approaches to the generation of mutations in the mammalian genome, one genotype driven and the other phenotype driven. Genotype-driven mutagenesis involves classic transgenic approaches whereby constructs introduced into the genome by pronuclear injection lead to insertional mutagenesis. Alternatively, homologous recombination in embryonic stem cells can be used to introduce new mutations into known genes. This approach is not easily scalable to the recovery of a large number of mutations on a genome-wide basis.

Because the phenotyping of mutant animals is usually driven by preconceived notions concerning the biological function of the manipulated gene, critical data can be overlooked. Thus, in the case of the endothelin-B receptor knockout mouse, anticipated to be hypertensive, more rigorous phenotyping implicated this receptor as an important sensory pain mediator (34).

Phenotype-driven approaches have focused on random mutagenesis systems to identify novel genes and pathways. One type of phenotype-driven mutagenesis employs the chemical mutagen, N-ethyl-N-nitrosourea. This potent mutagen can deliver mutation frequencies of approximately 1 in 1000 gametes and is therefore effective in accomplishing saturation mutagenesis of the entire mouse genome. Obviously, this approach draws heavily on the appropriate biological screens used to identify phenotypes of interest.

GENE THERAPY

Gene therapy as a therapeutic technique offers the possibility of introducing a functioning gene into somatic cells of a patient to correct a defective gene and thereby restore biological function. The major interest of the pharmaceutical industry in gene therapy will undoubtedly be centered around in vivo treatment protocols, although more invasive ex vivo methods (whereby cells are removed from the patient, transfected with the gene of interest, and then placed back into the patient) may be acceptable for certain serious diseases (e.g. cancer). Currently, genetic information can be transferred into cells by a number of protocols, including the use of DNA plasmids, DNA liposomes, or a variety of viruses. The most effective transforming agents are viral vectors, such as adenovirus, adeno-associated viruses, and retroviruses. Although retroviruses require cell division to incorporate the new information into the genome, adenovirus and adeno-associated viruses will transfer their information into nonreplicating cells. Despite considerable efforts that have gone into vector design during the past decade, delivery of genes still represents one of the major problems associated with the gene therapeutic approach. Encouragingly, recent work has demonstrated the ability of certain viral vectors to stably incorporate genetic material in vivo, resulting in expression of the resultant proteins, which can be maintained for periods of several months (35).

The Food and Drug Administration has approved approximately 90 clinical studies involving gene therapy, which represents one of the fastest growing areas in biomedical research. Safety is, and will continue for some time to be, an issue with this approach, and many of the clinical trials involving gene therapy are directed toward patients with life-threatening diseases (e.g. cancer patients already receiving conventional therapy). Most reports to date have been phase I clinical studies confirming gene transfection and demonstrating safety, but evidence of efficacy has been anecdotal. Properly controlled phase II and phase III clinical trials involving gene therapy are yet to be done and will tax the current development capacity within the pharmaceutical industry.

Some published examples of clinical studies of gene therapy in the cardiovascular arena have appeared. For example, the intra-arterial gene transfer of a plasmid that encodes for vascular endothelial growth factor has been tested for its ability to increase coronary and peripheral angiogenesis (36, 37). The initial results from these early clinical trials suggest that vascular endothelial growth factor gene transfer produces angiogenesis and reduces ischemic symptoms. However, as mentioned above, these studies are inadequately controlled and the results can only be considered anecdotal.

Gene therapy has received much attention for the treatment of inherited metabolic diseases. One such disease in which preclinical data suggest promise targets familial hypercholesterolemia. Replacement of the low-density-lipoprotein receptor gene by adenovirus transfection into mice in which the gene for this receptor had been knocked out resulted in correction of the dyslipidemia (38).

PROTEIN THERAPEUTICS

The development of proteins as drugs has been the principal focus of the biotechnology industry as well as a component of the drug pipeline of several larger pharmaceutical companies for some time. With the anticipated disclosure of the blueprint of the human genome scheduled for the spring of 2000, further interest is likely to emerge in the area of novel proteins as drugs. Although the focus of the pharmaceutical industry is likely to remain principally on small-molecule agents, there have been some notable successes with protein agents (e.g. erythropoietin). Human genome sciences have already converted genomic information obtained from high-throughput sequencing into potential therapeutic proteins in clinical trials. Thus, myeloid progenitor inhibitory factor-1 is currently in phase II clinical trials as a stem cell protector in cancer therapy. In addition, keratinocyte growth factor-1 is in phase II clinical trials for wound healing.

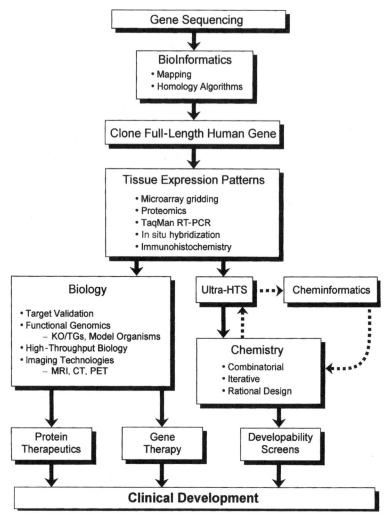

Figure 3   Progression of molecular targets to novel therapeutics under a new paradigm for drug discovery. HTS, High-throughput screening; RT-PCR, reverse transcriptase polymerase chain reaction; MRI, magnetic resonance imaging; CT, computed tomography; PET, positron emissions tomography.

CONCLUSIONS

The tremendous impact of genomic sequencing is currently being felt across all areas of drug discovery, and major challenges for the pharmaceutical industry into the next millennium will be in the areas of drug target selection and validation. The progression of new molecular targets into novel drugs under this new paradigm for drug discovery is shown in Figure 3. One can already anticipate the future availability of genetic structure and susceptibility to disease at the individual level. With such information available early in a research program, the drug discovery scientist is faced with the unprecedented opportunity to address the individual variability to drug therapy and safety prior to advancing a compound into clinical trials. The exponential growth of attractive novel molecular targets for potential drug therapy has heavily taxed the core disciples of drug discovery, and automated methods of compound synthesis and biological evaluation will play an even more dominant role in the pharmaceutical industry of the twenty-first century.

Visit the Annual Reviews home page at www.AnnualReviews.org.

LITERATURE CITED

1. Natl. Inst. Health. *The National Human Genome Research Institute.* http://www.nhgri.nih.gov.

2. Venkatesh TV, Bowen B, Lim HA. 1999. Bioinformatics, pharma and farmers. *Trends Biotechnol.* 17:85–88

3. Stadel JM, Wilson S, Bergsma D. 1997. Orphan G protein-coupled receptors: a neglected opportunity for pioneer drug discovery. *Trends Pharmacol. Sci.* 18: 430–37

4. Ames RS, Sarau HM, Chambers J, Willette RN, Aiyar N, et al. 1999. Human urotensin-II, the most potent vasoconstrictor identified, is a ligand at the novel receptor GPR-14. *Nature* 401:282–86

5. Sakurai T, Amemiya A, Ishii M, Matsuzaki I, Chemelli RM, et al. 1998. Orexins and orexin receptors: a family of hypothalamic neuropeptides and G protein-coupled receptors that regulate feeding behavior. *Cell* 92:573–85

6. Zhang Y, Proenca R, Maffei M, Barone M, Leopold L, Friedman JM. 1994. Positional cloning of the mouse obese gene and its human homologue. *Nature* 372: 425–32

7. Lin L, Faraco J, Li R, Kadotani H, Rogers W, et al. 1999. The sleep disorder canine narcolepsy is caused by a muta-tion in the hypocretin (orexin) receptor 2 gene. *Cell* 98:365–76

8. Debouck C, Metcalf B. 2000. The impact of genomics on drug discovery. *Annu. Rev. Pharmacol. Toxicol.* 40:193–208

9. Pease AC, Solas D, Sullivan EJ, Cronin MT, Holmes CP, Fodor SA. 1994. Light-generated oligonucleotide arrays for rapid DNA sequence analysis. *Proc. Natl. Acad. Sci. USA* 91:5022–26

10. Lipshutz RJ, Fodor SPA, Gingeras TR, Lockhard DJ. 1999. High density synthetic oligonucleotide arrays. *Nat. Genet. Suppl.* 21:20–24

11. Schena M, Shalon D, Heller R, Chai A, Brown PO, Davis RW. 1996 Parallel human genome analysis: microarray-based expression monitoring of 1000 genes. *Proc. Natl. Acad. Sci. USA* 93: 10614–19

12. Blackstock WP, Weir MP. 1999. Proteomics: quantitative and physical mapping of cellular proteins. *Trends Biotechnol.* 17(3): 121–27

13. Wang H, Bloom O, Zhang M, Vishnubhakat JM, Ombrellino M, et al. 1999. HMG-1 as a late mediator of endotoxin lethality in mice. *Science* 9:248–51

14. Carr SA, Huddleston MJ, Annan RS. 1996. Selective detection and sequencing

of phosphopeptides at the femtomole level by mass spectrometry. *Anal. Biochem.* 1:239(2):180–92

15. Spencer RW. 1998. High-throughput screening of historic collections: observations on file size, biological targets, and file diversity. *Biotechnol. Bioeng.* 61(1):61–67

16. Snider RM, Constantine JW, Lowe JA III, Longo KP, Lebel WS, et al. 1991. A potent nonpeptide antagonist of the substance P (NK₁) receptor. *Science* 251: 435–37

17. Doherty AM, Patt WC, Edmunds JJ, Berryman KA, Reisdorph BR, et al. 1995. Discovery of a novel series of orally active non-peptide endothelin-A (ETA) receptor-selective antagonists. *J. Med. Chem.* 38:1259–63

18. White JR, Lee JM, Young PR, Hertzberg RP, Jurewicz AJ, et al. 1999. Identification of a potent, selective non-peptide CXCR2 antagonist that inhibits interleukin-8-induced neutrophil migration. *J. Biol. Chem.* 273:10095–98

19. Ohlstein EH, Nambi P, Douglas SA, Edwards RM, Gellai M, et al. 1994. SB 209670, a rationally designed potent nonpeptide endothelin receptor antagonist. *Proc. Natl. Acad. Sci. USA* 91:8052–56

20. Polinsky A. 1999. Combichem and cheminformatics. *Curr. Opin. Drug Discov. Dev.* 2(3):197–203

21. Lipinski CA, Lombardo F, Dominy BW, Feeney PJ. 1997. Experimental and computational approaches to estimate solubility and permeability in drug discovery and development settings. *Adv. Drug Deliv. Rev.* 23:3–25

22. Service RF. 1999. Race for molecular summits. *Science* 285:184–85

23. Eyermann CJ, Jadhav PK, Hodge CN, Chang C-H, Rodgers JD, Lam PYS. 1997. The role of computer-aided and structure-based design techniques in the discovery and optimization of cyclic urea inhibitors of HIV protease. *Adv. Amino Acid Mimetics Pept.* 1:1–40

24. Yamashita DS, Smith WW, Zhao B, Janson CA, Tomaszek TA, et al. 1997. Structure and design of potent and selective cathepsin K inhibitors. *J. Am. Chem. Soc.* 119:11351–52

25. DesJarlais RL, Yamashita DS, Oh H-J, Uzinskas IN, Erhard KF, et al. 1998. Use of X-ray co-crystal structures and molecular modeling to design potent and selective non-peptide inhibitors of cathepsin K. *J. Am. Chem Soc.* 120:9114–18

26. Leucke H, Schobert B, Richter H-T, Cartailler J-P, Lanyi JK. 1999. Structure of bacteriorhodopsin at 1.55 Å resolution. *J. Mol. Biol.* 291(4):899–911

27. Shuker SB, Hajduk PJ, Meadows RP, Fesik SW. 1996. Discovering high-affinity ligands for proteins—SAR by NMR. *Science* 274:1531–34

28. Lin M, Shapiro MJ, Wareing JR. 1997. Diffusion-edited NMR—affinity NMR for direct observation of molecular interactions. *J. Am. Chem. Soc.* 119:5249–50

29. Yamazaki T, Otomo T, Oda N, Kyogoku Y, Uegaki K, et al. 1998. Segmental isotope labeling for protein NMR using peptide splicing. *J. Am. Chem. Soc.* 120: 5591–91

30. Peishoff CE, Lago MA, Ohlstein EH, Elliott JD. 1995. Endothelin receptor antagonists. *Curr. Pharm. Design* 1:425–40

31. Keenan RM, Miller WH, Kwon C, Ali FE, Callahan JF, et al. 1997. Discovery of potent nonpeptide vitronectin receptor (αᵥβ₃) antagonists. *J. Med. Chem.* 40: 2289–92

32. Clackson R, Wells JA. 1995. A hot spot of binding energy in a hormone-receptor interface. *Science* 267:383–86

33. Tian S-S, Lamb P, King AC, Miller SG, Kessler L, et al. 1998. A small, nonpeptidyl mimic of granulocyte-colony-stimulating factor. *Science* 281:257–59

34. Griswold DE, Douglas SA, Martin LD, Davis L, Schultz LB, Ohlstein EH. 1999. Modulatory role of the endothelin B receptor in inflammatory pain and

cutaneous inflammation in gene target-disrupted knockout mice. *Mol. Pharmacol.* In press

35. Ye R, Rivera VM, Zoltick P, Cerasoli F Jr, Schnell MA, et al. 1999. Regulated delivery of therapeutic proteins after in vivo somatic cell gene transfer. *Science* 283:88–91

36. Losordo DW, Vale PR, Symes JF, Dunnington CH, Esakof DD, et al. 1998. Gene therapy for myocardial angiogenesis: initial clinical results with direct myocardial injunction of phVEGF165 as sole therapy for myocardial ischemia. *Circulation* 98:2800–4

37. Isner JM, Pieczek A, Schainfeld R, Clair R, Haley L, et al. 1996. Clinical evidence of angiogenesis after arterial gene transfer of phVEGF165 in patient with ischaemic limb. *Lancet* 348:370–74

38. Kozarsky KF, Jooss K, Donahee M, Strauff JF III, Wilson JM. 1996. Effective treatment of familial hypercholesterolaemia in the mouse model using adenovirus-mediated transfer of the VLDL receptor gene. *Nat. Genet.* 13:54–62

Annu. Rev. Pharmacol. Toxicol. 2000. 40:193–208

THE IMPACT OF GENOMICS ON DRUG DISCOVERY

C. Debouck and B. Metcalf

Discovery Chemistry & Platform Technologies, SmithKline Beecham Pharmaceuticals, Research & Development, King of Prussia, Pennsylvania 19406; e-mail: Christine_M_Debouck@sbphrd.com, Brian_Metcalf@sbphrd.com

Key Words EST, cathepsin K, G-protein coupled receptors, microarrays, proteomics

■ **Abstract** High-throughput gene sequencing has revolutionized the process used to identify novel molecular targets for drug discovery. Thousands of new gene sequences have been generated but only a limited number of these can be converted into validated targets likely to be involved in disease. We describe here some of the approaches used at SmithKline Beecham to select and validate novel targets. These include the identification of selective tissue gene product expression, such as for cathepsin K, a novel osteoclast-specific cysteine protease. We also describe the discovery and functional characterization of novel members of the G-protein coupled receptor superfamily and their pairing with natural ligands. Lastly, we discuss the promises of gene microarrays and proteomics, developing technologies that allow the parallel analyses of tissue expression patterns of thousands of genes or proteins, respectively.

THE PARADIGM SHIFT—FROM GENE TO SCREEN

Traditionally, the identification of molecular targets in drug discovery has been biologically driven. An interesting enzyme or receptor activity implicated in normal physiology or disease was characterized and isolated, usually from animal tissues. Micropurification, monitored by functional assays such as radioligand binding or other techniques, led to the cloning of the gene encoding the target of interest. Following the expression of the gene in a recombinant host, the desirable activity was confirmed and used to run a high-throughput compound screen or to support rational drug design. This "from-function-to-gene" process was time consuming, but it delivered defined targets whose function was understood. The advent of high-throughput gene sequencing resulted in the rapid identification of thousands of novel genes, most without known function. As a result, the drug discovery scientists have had the challenging task of leveraging genes of unknown function into attractive therapeutic targets, a paradigm shift often referred to as the "from-gene-to-screen" process. We describe here a number of approaches

0362–1642/00/0415–0193$14.00

applied in SmithKline Beecham (SB) laboratories to identify and validate novel therapeutic targets from the wealth of gene sequence information currently available.

EST Sequencing

High-throughput sequencing was first applied to complementary DNA (cDNA) libraries by Adams et al (1) and has since rapidly led to a buildup of expressed sequence tags (ESTs) in corporate and public (2) databases. By definition, this approach gives partial sequences of expressed genes from the various cells and tissues used for the cDNA library preparation, but it does not include the sequence of the intervening noncoding DNA. This "junk" DNA constitutes about 97% of the human genome. Although these ESTs are only partial sequences of 200–600 nucleotides, bioinformatic approaches are able to assemble ESTs derived from the same gene through the identification of overlapping fragments. Assemblies of EST (contigs) are then created, giving an estimate of the number of expressed genes (as distinct from gene fragments) in the library under consideration. Taken to their logical conclusion, such approaches could eventually identify the complete repertoire of expressed human genes and, thereby, an extremely large number of potential human drug targets. The full complement of the human genome is estimated to be 80,000–100,000 genes. Analogously, application of high-throughput sequencing techniques to microbial genomes has made possible the sequence determination of several entire bacterial genomes. This wealth of sequence information will allow researchers to characterize shared pathways and metabolic networks, and to identify all possible targets for intervention in infection control (3).

"Smart" Libraries

The approach initially taken by scientists at SB is illustrated in Figure 1. Here, "smart" cDNA libraries are prepared from various sources likely to either play a role in disease etiology or be enriched in cell surface or secreted proteins. For example, libraries were prepared from tissues of particular therapeutic interest, such as prostate, kidney, left heart ventricle, bone marrow, or subsections of the brain, or from cell lines where an activated form can be compared with a resting form. In collaboration with Human Genome Sciences, we constructed more than 500 cDNA libraries, subjected them to random sequencing from the 5′ end, searched for sequence homology, and assembled contigs. After first-pass sequencing of 500 ESTs, the libraries that were deemed high quality were further sequenced, to a depth of 2,000–10,000 ESTs. Because many genes are expressed at low level, this type of "shallow" sequencing is expected to identify genes that are moderately to abundantly expressed in the tissue under study. The relative abundance of ESTs for a given gene in a given library can be a selection criterion for choosing a novel gene as a molecular target, as illustrated below for cathepsin K. On the other hand, random EST sequencing, much like the lottery, can draw

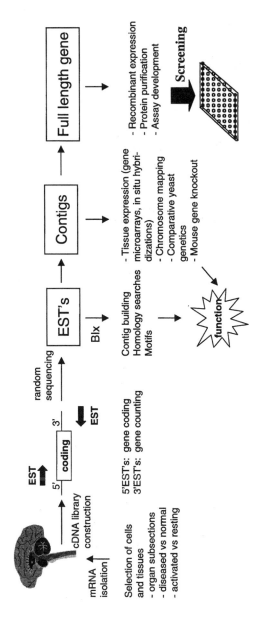

Figure 1 Outline of the gene-to-screen process. The main experimental steps for the identification and validation of novel drug targets are depicted and discussed further in the text. EST, Expressed sequence tags.

some low-abundance, important novel genes, such as the orphan G-protein coupled receptors also discussed in this chapter. In order to reduce the continuing identification of abundantly expressed clones and thereby increase the probability of identifying distinct novel genes, including those expressed at low levels, our group and others made serious attempts to construct normalized cDNA libraries. However, sequence analysis of such libraries revealed that normalization only resulted in limited removal of redundant genes and did not justify the investment of additional time and effort (4).

Identifying Novel Protein Sequences

ESTs are obtained by single-pass sequencing of the ends of cDNA inserts using library vector-specific primers, thereby affording sequence information at higher speed and lower cost compared with gene-specific primers. Thus, sequencing can be conducted from the 5′ or the 3′ end of the inserts or from both ends, and this choice impacts the potential for novel gene discovery. Because reverse transcriptase synthesizes cDNA starting from the 3′ end of the mRNA, all cDNA inserts derived from the same gene have the same 3′ EST sequence. This feature is useful when the primary interest is gene counting to determine the gene expression profiles in a given tissue. However, because 3′ untranslated regions can be long, 3′-derived EST sequences often lack protein coding information. On the other hand, reverse transcriptase tends to stall and fall off the mRNA during cDNA synthesis and will often not reach the 5′ end of the mRNA, producing incomplete and ragged 5′ ends from a given gene. As a result, 5′-derived EST sequences typically contain protein coding information, and those derived from the same gene tend to overlap with one another, leading to the generation of in silico full-length gene sequences. For this reason, we focused our efforts on 5′ EST sequencing to favor the novel gene discovery process. We also felt that electronic gene counting would not be accurate because of the libraries not being sequenced in depth and that it would be supplanted by high-throughput "wet" gene expression profiling technologies (see below).

The protein sequences translated from the EST contigs often represent enough coding sequence for the molecular function of the gene to be recognized by homology to known human, animal, or other available sequences, for example a cysteine protease, a zinc finger, a G-protein coupled receptor, etc. In addition, appropriate probes can be derived from these partial sequences to carry out tissue distribution studies, e.g. by in situ hybridization. When coupled with the source of the cDNA library and the putative function of the gene product, enough information may be obtained to suggest further interest. The full-length gene is then cloned and expressed in an appropriate recombinant host. It should be noted that although the molecular function of the gene may be surmised at this stage, the physiological function is by no means certain. Drug discovery programs that are commenced based on this information have some degree of risk, owing to lack of knowledge of the physiological role of the selected target. Further work, such as construction of transgenic animals, can be undertaken to further underpin the importance of the target.

Millions of ESTs have been generated (e.g. 1,048,756 at http://www.tigr.org/ and 1,505,046 at http://www.ncbi.nlm.nih.gov/dbEST/) and subjected to extensive bioinformatic analyses, including assembly into contigs, and nucleic acid and protein homology searches. The challenge for drug discovery scientists is to identify those genes that play critical roles in normal physiology or in the etiology of diseases, and to elucidate their function both biochemically and biologically. This is then followed by the development of assays for high-throughput screening and the establishment of the relevant animal models for preclinical testing of compounds. Sequence homology and tissue distribution of a novel gene are two critical pieces of the large jigsaw puzzle of its function. Other high-throughput as well as more specialized, low-throughput techniques need to be deployed to add more pieces to the puzzle and to start discerning the picture of their role in normal physiology or disease. We describe below examples of how scientists at SB have selected novel therapeutic targets starting from hundreds of thousands of ESTs: the protease cathepsin K and the orphan G-protein coupled receptor superfamily.

CATHEPSIN K—A PROTOTYPIC GENOMICS-DERIVED DRUG DISCOVERY TARGET

If one were interested in discovering a treatment for osteoporosis, for example, a logical starting point in the context of genomics would be the osteoclast, a highly specialized cell that is responsible for bone resorption during the bone remodeling process. An imbalance between bone resorption and formation results in pathological states such as osteoporosis. Clearly one would make a cDNA library from the human osteoclast (see Figure 1). Because there is no cell line representative of the osteoclast, the SB approach was to use surgical specimens of osteoclastoma tumor, from which osteoclasts could be extracted using osteoclast-specific antibodies attached to magnetic beads (5). Upon sequencing a cDNA library prepared from human osteoclasts, it was found that approximately 4% of the ESTs generated encoded a novel cysteine protease, which was named cathepsin K (6). ESTs encoding other cysteine proteases were rare in the osteoclast library. Subsequent studies at both the message and the protein level demonstrated that cathepsin K was expressed exclusively in osteoclasts. Indeed, in situ hybridizations showed high levels of expression in osteoclasts but not other bone cells, whereas immunocytochemistry revealed a polar distribution of the enzyme right at the site of contact between the osteoclasts and the bone resorption pit, which suggests proteolytic digestion of the bone "in the making."

A research program was started involving the cloning and recombinant expression of full-length cathepsin K and the detailed characterization of its proteolytic properties (7). At the time, the conceptual underpinnings of the decision to commit to a program that eventually could cost as much as $400 million (the cost of development of a new drug) and to initiate a drug discovery program were limited to the following: The target is highly expressed in a human cell of interest, the osteoclast; the target is selectively expressed in the osteoclast; and the target is a new cysteine protease. It was assumed that inhibition of cathepsin K would lead to treatments for osteoporosis. Starting extensive drug discovery efforts with such a paucity of information seemed a high-risk strategy. Hence, firmer demonstration of the involvement of cathepsin K in bone resorption was important.

Pycnodysostosis—The Human Cathepsin K Knockout

When efforts on cathepsin K were under way, the mutations causative for the rare inherited osteochrondrodysplasia, pycnodysostosis, were localized to the cathepsin K gene. Affected individuals present with osteopretrosis and bone fragility. In humans, three separate mutations that could lead to loss of function of cathepsin K have been identified. Osteoclasts from such individuals demineralize normally but do not degrade the bone protein matrix. Cathepsin K was thereby confirmed to be the major protease responsible for degradation of the bone matrix (8). It should be noted that cathepsin K–deficient mice have since been constructed. These also exhibit an osteopetrotic phenotype and produce osteoclasts impaired in bone resorptive activity (9, 10).

The results of this human genetic study (and the mouse knockout) put the drug discovery program aimed at inhibiting cathepsin K on a firmer conceptual footing. Cathepsin K was confirmed as the major protease in human osteoclasts, and loss of function was shown to lead to an impairment in bone resorption. Our laboratories determined the crystal structure of cathepsin K (11) and undertook inhibitor design and synthesis (12). We further demonstrated that inhibitors of cathepsin K inhibit bone resorption both in vitro and in vivo (13). The gene-to-function-to-potential-drug paradigm was thus demonstrated.

Are Genes that Are Expressed in High Abundance Ideal Drug Targets?

The traditionalist might well question the EST paradigm with the choice of cathepsin K as a drug target. If high message abundance were to translate to high protein abundance, then the efficacy of a drug directed at that target might be limited by the sheer amount of protein it must bind to. A compelling example is the development of resistance to the antitumor drug, PALA, and hence perhaps its clinical failure as a result of induced expression of its target enzyme, aspartic acid transcarbamylase (14). Conversely, the success of the statins as cholesterol-lowering agents reflects the status of their molecular target, HMGCo-A reductase, as the rate-limiting enzyme in cholesterol biosynthesis (15). Cathepsin K was chosen as a drug target in part because of the high abundance of its expression in the target cell. Although the abundance of cathepsin K has not resulted in lack of efficacy of its inhibitors in animal models of osteoporosis (M Lark & G Stroup, unpublished data), high levels of expression could prove to be a fatal flaw in the EST strategy for other abundantly expressed targets.

AN ALTERNATIVE APPROACH—YOUR FAVORITE GENE SUPERFAMILY

The choice of cathepsin K as a molecular target for osteoporosis resulted primarily from identification of its high and selective expression in human osteoclasts. As it was a cysteine protease, its enzymatic mechanism of action could be extrapolated from studies on prototypic cysteine proteases. Therefore, approaches to its inhibition could be envisaged by experienced medicinal chemists. The drug discovery program thus appeared from the outset to be chemically tractable. Alternatively, the most abundantly expressed gene product could have been a partner in a spurious protein-protein interaction with no enzymatic activity and involved in unknown functions. Such a scenario would not have presented an attractive target for drug discovery.

To bias toward chemical tractability, one could select all members of gene superfamilies that have proven records in drug discovery and then attempt to assign biological function to them. Such superfamilies, when translated into protein families, could be the G-protein coupled receptors [also known as 7 transmembrane receptors (7TMRs)], ion channels, nuclear hormone receptors, and proteases, or more tenuously kinases. We chose to focus initially on the identification and functional characterization of novel 7TMRs.

The G-Protein Coupled Receptor Superfamily

Recent internal analysis pointed out that 37 marketed drugs are targeted at 21 distinct 7TMRs, representing $21 billion dollars in annual worldwide sales in 1997 (M Birkeland & P Agarwal, personal communication). There are currently over 250 known human 7TMRs, not including sensory olfactory receptors. It is estimated that the human genome will be shown to contain over 5000 members of this family, with 500–1000 being unrelated to odor-detecting receptors and, hence, of likely interest for drug discovery. Given the proven chemical tractability of agonism and antagonism within this superfamily, this represents a formidable opportunity.

At SB, we have identified 170 novel 7TMRs. Full-length cDNA clones have already been isolated for 117 of these, and 35 have been linked with ligands either in-house or by other groups. Our approach to functionally characterize these orphan receptors has been to first identify native or surrogate ligands for these receptors (16). To this end, we use stably or transiently transfected mammalian cell lines to guide biofractionation from various tissues following cytosolic calcium mobilization to detect agonist activity. In parallel, we test a bank of known bioactive substances. Once the agonist is detected, the receptor/agonist pair is configured into a high-throughput screening assay. Biological function is then sought using a combination of technologies to identify tissue distribution and responses in pharmacological assays chosen to reflect the tissue distribution. This approach also offers the tangible possibility that low-molecular-weight antagonists might be discovered early in the program by high-throughput screening and hence could serve as tool compounds to allow the function of the molecular target to be more readily assigned.

The discovery of the orexins 1 and 2 and their receptors and the pairing of melanin-concentrating hormone (MCH) to its receptor serve to illustrate these approaches.

Orexins and Orexin Receptors

Fifty stable transfectant HEK293 cell lines, each harboring a novel orphan 7TMR, were challenged with high-performance liquid chromatography fractions derived from various tissue extracts, with monitoring of cytoplasmic Ca^{2+} mobilization as a measure of agonism of the transfected receptor (17). In order to identify responses from endogenous receptors, three different transfectants, each expressing a distinct orphan 7TMR, were monitored and only those signals that were unique to a single cell line were pursued.

With this approach, several fractions from rat brain extracts elicited responses in a transfectant that expressed HFGAN72, a receptor originally identified as an EST from human brain. Purification of the active fractions exposed two peptides, which were called orexin-A and orexin-B. Orexin-A is a 33–amino acid peptide with an N-terminal pyroglutamate, a C-terminal amidation, and four cysteine residues that form two intramolecular disulfide bonds. Orexin-B, a 28–amino acid peptide, was 46% identical to orexin-A and was C-terminally amidated. Subsequent cloning of the cDNA for orexin-A revealed that the open reading frame encoded both orexin-A and orexin-B. Orexin-A and orexin-B are therefore expressed as a prepropeptide and processed proteolytically at dibasic amino acid residues like many known bioactive peptides. As orexin-B was considerably less active on HGFAN72 than was orexin-A, the presence of an orexin-B receptor was postulated. Such a receptor was subsequently identified in a BLAST search of the GenBank database using the sequence of HFGAN72 to identify paralogs. Subsequently OX_1R (HFGAN72) was found to be 64% identical to OX_2R at the protein sequence level.

Tissue Distribution of Orexin and Orexin Receptors and Potential Therapeutic Indication of Orexin Receptor Antagonists

In situ hybridization and immunohistochemical analyses in rat brains showed that orexin-containing neurons were present in the lateral and posterior hypothalamic areas. Because the lateral hypothalamic area has been implicated in the regulation of feeding behavior, orexins-A and -B may be involved in feeding behavior. To investigate this hypothesis, orexin-A was administered acutely into the lateral ventricle of male rats. A dramatic stimulation of feeding behavior was observed. Intuitively, an antagonist of orexin-A would appear to offer approaches to the treatment of obesity, diabesity, and diabetes mellitus.

The Receptor for Melanin-Concentrating Hormone

As part of the battery of orphan 7TMRs under study, a 353–amino acid human orphan known as SLC-1 was cloned from a human fetal brain cDNA library and expressed in HEK 293 cells (18). These cells were then challenged with a collection of known bioactive subtances, including >500 neuropeptides. Of these, only the cyclic neuropeptide MCH elicited a robust, dose-dependent elevation of intracellular calcium. MCH has long been implicated in the regulation of food intake and energy balance, but its receptor has been unknown. SLC-1 was shown for the first time by in situ hybridization and immunohistochemical techniques to be expressed in two nuclei of the hypothalamus, the ventromedial and dorsomedial nuclei, areas known to be involved in feeding. The pairing of MCH with SLC-1 allows configuration of a high-throughput screen and opens the route for the discovery of antagonists, which are likely to be useful in the treatment of obesity.

The Promiscuous Paradigm

The success in drug discovery engendered by members of the 7TMR superfamily as drug targets is not unrelated to a degree of promiscuity of ligand structures that cross-react among family members. The interplay of dopamine, epinephrine, norepinephrine, and serotonin (5-HT) is illustrative. This cross-reactivity of ligands probably reflects the derivation of discrete family member receptors from common ancestors. The promiscuity of ligands transfers to promiscuous structural templates found in antagonists of disparate receptors. An example of a promiscuous template is the biphenyl moiety found in the structure of the angiotensin antagonist losartan (Figure 2A) (19) and in various 5-HT1B receptor antagonists (Figure 2B) (20). Angiotensin II is an acidic ligand whereas 5-HT is a basic one, yet antagonists for their respective receptors can be presented on the same biphenyl scaffold.

Another example comes from SB programs with the commonality of the imidazoleacrylate scaffold of the angiotensin antagonist (Figure 3A) and the endothelin antagonist (Figure 3B) (21). In this case, cross-screening of angiotensin antagonists in an enthothelin receptor screen led to leads that could be converted into selective endothelin antagonists.

Combinatorial Libraries Based on Promiscuous Templates

Linking the two concepts of pairing novel orphan receptors within the 7TMR family with their ligands and antagonist structural promiscuity suggests the interfacing of combinatorial libraries based on promiscuous templates with the stable

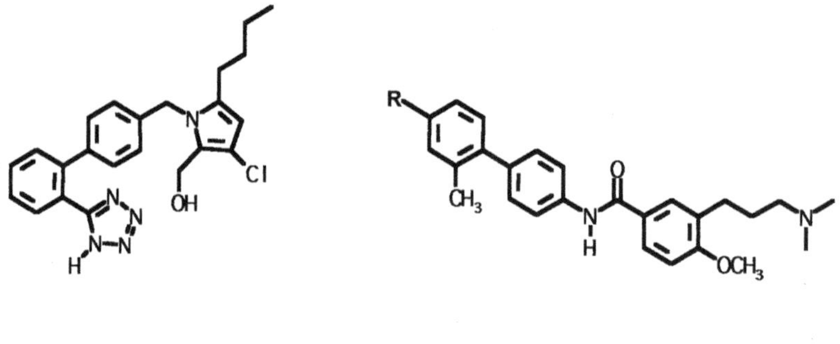

Figure 2   The structure of the angiotensin antagonist losartan (*A*) and the 5-HT1B receptor antagonist (*B*).

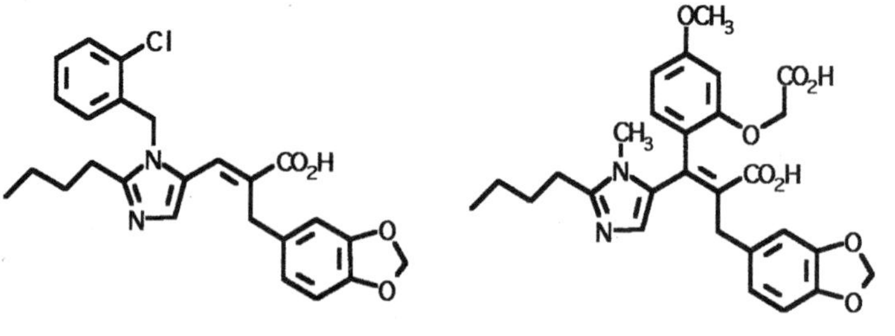

Figure 3   The imidazoleacrylate scaffold of the angiotensin antagonist (*A*) and the endothelin antagonist (*B*).

transfectants of orphan receptors in a high-throughput screening mode. For example, a combinatorial library was prepared based on the biphenyl scaffold and is proving to be a useful resource in the search for antagonists for novel 7TMRs (22). Similarly, the imidazole acrylate substructure common in Figure 3*A* and *B* would also offer a likely template for combinatorial expansion.

THE MOLECULAR TECHNOLOGIES REQUIRED

The prototypical examples cited above of the discovery of cathepsin K and its tantalizing validation as a drug discovery target, and the generic approach to the discovery and characterization of novel 7TMRs, their cognate ligands, and their antagonists, rely on a number of platform technologies. These include rapid full-length cDNA cloning, tissue localization, combinatorial chemistry, high-throughput screening, and the underlying automation and data management. Given the multiplicity of the target opportunities presented by genomics, a major investment in these downstream platform technologies is required. These different technologies each have their own evolution, although striking convergence is seen between genomics, combinatorial chemistry, and high-throughput screening with respect to handling thousands of objects, dependence on miniaturization and laboratory automation, creation of information and data tidal waves, and need for effective data management and mining.

Many approaches are needed to appropriately validate novel drug discovery targets. These include tissue distribution in normal and diseased tissues, chromosome localization, and analysis of orthologous genes in model systems such as yeast, the worm *Caenorhabditis elegans,* fruit flies, or mice. Yeast and *C. elegans* are particularly powerful systems because their entire genome sequence has been determined (23, 24), and ingenious genetic techniques are available allowing facile gene disruption, gene complementation, etc. Because the estimated number of human genes is high (80,000–100,000), scientists are striving to develop high-throughput technologies in which all or many genes are analyzed in parallel. For example, a critical technology in target validation is the use of high-density gene microarrays to monitor spatial and temporal gene expression. In addition, the correlation or lack of correlation of mRNA levels with translated protein and subsequent posttranslational processing and modifications can be accessed by proteomics.

The Gene Microarrays

Gene microarrays allow the rapid parallel analysis of the expression of thousands of genes against hundreds of tissues, cell types, and conditions whether using oligonucleotide arrays (25) or arrays of gene fragments (26). Because of the compatibility of glass with fluorescently labeled probes, the most effective gene microarrays are those constructed on glass surfaces, as opposed to arrays on nylon membranes (27). Because fluorescent probes exhibit little-to-no signal dispersion, very dense array spacing is possible, and deposition of DNA samples at densities of thousands of discrete DNA spots per 1.0 cm^2 have been attained. Another advantage of dense arrays on small glass surfaces is that the volumes required for hybridization are very small, thereby allowing the use of probes from small amounts of tissues.

The number and variety of microarray applications is virtually unlimited (28). Gene microarrays are being used extensively to generate broad and in-depth data on gene expression patterns in normal and diseased tissues, both in human and in animal systems. Although many effective drugs have been developed against targets that are widely expressed in the body (e.g. the angiotensin converting enzyme), highly selective tissue expression of a drug target, such as that seen for cathepsin K, is attractive, as the potential for unwanted side effects may be more restricted. Perhaps the most promising application of microarrays is the study of differential expression in disease. The up- or down-regulation of a gene can be the cause of the disease or its result. In addition, microarrays are a powerful tool to help dissect the mechanism of action of drugs and drug candidates. They will also increasingly contribute to the analysis of metabolic pathways for drugs, the understanding and prediction of toxic or adverse events in vitro and in vivo, as well as the potential identification of surrogate markers to follow the dose and even efficacy of a drug in the clinical setting.

Microarray-based assays yield several hundred data points for thousands of genes, and this in turn demands the development of fully automated and standardized software systems for the collection, quality scoring, and tracking of all data points. The rush to apply this new technology should not ignore quality assurance because low-quality data will only generate poor biological conclusions. It will therefore be critical that strict and broadly accepted quality standards be developed, so that data from different laboratories can be compared and even combined.

Microarrays are not the panacea for gene expression analysis. They have a number of limitations that must be addressed by complementary technologies. First, the sensitivity of detection is about 1 in 100,000. More sensitive but lower throughput methods such as quantitative polymerase chain reaction, e.g. the recently automated Taqman technology (29), must be utilized for the analysis of genes that are expressed in low abundance. Second, the labor-intensive in situ hybridization and immunocytochemistry methods will continue to make important contributions because they provide a critical link to histology and cytology that the best microdissection of cells from tissues is unlikely to provide. Third, mRNA levels may not be paralleled at the protein level. To address this, high-throughput methods for the analysis of differential expression at the protein level are being developed to characterize translational and posttranslation regulation. This emerging technology is referred to as proteomics (30).

Proteomics

Recent technological advances in protein analysis have paved the way for proteomics, which characterizes the protein complement, proteome, of a cell or tissue as opposed to the mRNA transcripts, transcriptome, studied by microarrays. These advances were made possible by significant progress in two-dimensional gel electrophoresis and ultrasensitive mass spectrometry. The improvements to two-dimensional gel electrophoresis included larger format to allow separation of thousands of protein spots and reproducibility and image scanning to position spots and to quantitate their intensity between gels. Mass spectrometry has provided a quantum leap in sensitivity, as even the most sensitive Edman sequencers could not sequence the majority of the spots. Currently, the extensive deployment of proteomic approaches to support target validation is limited by the inherent low throughput of the method. Early applications are likely to be restricted to selected subsets of the proteome, such as phosphorylated proteins where the proteins under study are defined by those revealed by anti-phosphotyrosine or phos-phoserine antibodies (31), or to the bacterial proteome. Other defined subsets of the proteome that are yielding to these approaches include the ribosomal protein complexes where interacting partners can be defined (32).

FUTURE OPPORTUNITIES

By the spring of 2000, 90% of the human genome will be sequenced, inaugurating the twenty-first century with a historical achievement for mankind. Bioinforma-ticians and molecular biologists will be challenged to select the protein coding information out of 2.9 billion noncoding nucleotides. Gene-calling algorithms are being developed to allow the rapid identification of open reading frames, which will need to be confirmed as truly expressed genes as opposed to pseudogenes. This exercise will be greatly facilitated by the availability of the millions of ESTs generated to date (33, 34). Regulatory sequences, including promoters and enhancers, will become available for study and will facilitate therapeutic inter-vention at the level of transcription. The study of regulatory elements will benefit tremendously from being interfaced with tissue expression data generated by microarray analysis, prompting identification of common regulatory features in genes with coregulated expression profiles (35).

The accuracy of genome sequence data will be very high (99.99%), and hence, nucleotide sequence differences, known as single-nucleotide polymorphisms, in the same gene derived from different individuals will be reliable. These single-nucleotide polymorphisms will constitute the basis for pharmacogenetic studies of differences between individuals with respect to drug efficacy and to manifes-tation of adverse events (36). The completion of animal genome sequences will be expected not too long after that of the human genome, allowing for unprece-dented comparisons of biochemical pathways and physiological phenomena between humans, mice, and other animal models used in research for decades.

High-throughput screening will migrate from the current 384 format to a high-density 1536 format, aided by fluorescent detection methodologies (37). Com-binatorial chemistry will evolve in high-speed medicinal chemistry where thousands of compounds can be prepared as singles, rather than as mixtures. These advances are discussed elsewhere in this edition (38).

Visit the Annual Reviews home page at www.AnnualReviews.org.

LITERATURE CITED

1. Adams MD, Kelley JM, Gocayne JD, Dubnick M, Polymeropoulos MH, et al. 1991. Complementary DNA sequencing: expressed sequence tags and human genome project. *Science* 252:1651–56
2. Pandey A, Lewitter F. 1999. Nucleotide

sequence databases: a gold mine for biologists. *Trends Biochem. Sci.* 24:276–80

3. Karp PD, Krummenacker M, Paley S, Wagg J. 1999. Integrated pathway-genome databases and their role in drug discovery. *Trends Biotechnol.* 17:275–81

4. Hillier LD, Lennon G, Becker M, Bonaldo MF, Chiapelli B, et al. 1996. Generation and analysis of 280,000 human expressed sequence tags. *Genome Res.* 6:807–28

5. James IE, Walsh S, Dodds RA, Gowen M. 1991. Production and characterization of osteoclast-selective monoclonal antibodies that distinguish between multinucleated cells derived from different human tissues. *J Histochem. Cytochem.* 39:905–14

6. Drake FH, Dodds R, James I, Connor J, Debouck C, et al. 1996. Cathepsin K but not cathepsins B, L or S is abundantly expressed in human osteoclasts. *J. Biol. Chem.* 271:12511–16

7. Bossard MJ, Tomaszek TA, Thompson SK, Amegadzie BY, Hanning CR, et al. 1996. Proteolytic activity of human osteoclast cathepsin K: expression, purification, activation and substrate identification. *J. Biol. Chem.* 271:12517–24

8. Gelb BD, Shi G-P, Chapman HA, Desnick RJ. 1996. Pycnodysostosis, a lysosomal disease caused by cathepsin K deficiency. *Science* 273:1236–38

9. Saftig P, Hunziker E, Wehmeyer O, Jones S, Boyde A, et al. 1998. Impaired osteoclastic bone resorption leads to osteopetrosis in cathepsin-K-deficient mice. *Proc. Natl. Acad. Sci. USA* 95:13453–58

10. Gowen M, Lazner F, Dodds R, Field J, Tavaria M, et al. 1999. Cathepsin K knockout mice develop osteopetrosis due to a deficit in matrix degradation but not demineralization. *J. Bone Miner. Res.* In press

11. Zhao B, Janson C, Amegadzie B, D'Alessio K, Griffin C, et al. 1997. Crystal structure of human osteoclast cathep-

sin K complex with E64. *Nat. Struct. Biol.* 4:109–11

12. Yamashita DS, Smith WW, Zhao B, Janson CA, Tomaszek TA, et al. 1997. Structure and design of potent and selective cathepsin K inhibitors. *J. Am. Chem. Soc.* 119:11351–52

13. Votta BJ, Levy MA, Badger A, Bradbeer J, Dodds RA, et al. 1997. Peptide aldehyde inhibitors of cathepsin K inhibit bone resorption both in vitro and in vivo. *J. Bone Miner. Res.* 12:1396–406

14. Kensler TW, Mutter G, Hankerson JG, Reck LJ, Harley C, et al. 1981. Mechanism of resistance of variants of the Lewis lung carcinoma to N-(phosphonacetyl)-L-aspartic acid. *Cancer Res.* 41:894–904

15. Shapiro DJ, Rodwell VW. 1971. Regulation of hepatic 3-hydroxy-3-methylglutaryl coenzyme A reductase and cholesterol synthesis. *J. Biol. Chem.* 246: 3210–16

16. Stadel JM, Wilson S, Bergsma DJ. 1997. Orphan G protein-coupled receptors: a neglected opportunity for pioneer drug discovery. *Trends Pharmacol. Sci.* 18: 430–37

17. Sakurai T, Amemiya A, Ishii M, Matsuzaki I, Chemelli RM, et al. 1998. Orexins and orexin receptors: a family of hypothalamic neuropeptides and G protein-coupled receptors that regulate feeding behavior. *Cell* 92:573–85

18. Chambers J, Ames RS, Bergsma DJ, Muir A, Fitzgerald LR, et al. 1999. Melanin-concentrating hormone is the cognate ligand for the orphan G-protein-coupled receptor SLC-1. *Nature* 400: 261–65

19. Chiu AT, McCall DE, Price WA, Wong PC, Carini DJ, et al. 1990. Nonpeptide angiotensin II receptor antagonists. VII. Cellular and biochemical pharmacology of DuP 753, an orally active antihypertensive agent. *J. Pharm. Exp. Ther.* 252:711–18

20. Clitherow JW, Scopes DIC, Skingle M, Jordan CC, Feniuk W, et al. 1994. Evolution of a novel series of [(N,N-dimethylamino)propyl]- and piperazinylbenzanilides as the first selective 5-HT$_{1D}$ antagonists. *J. Med. Chem.* 37:2253–57

21. Elliott JD, Bryan DL, Nambi P, Ohlstein EH. 1996. A novel series of non-peptide endothelin receptor antagonists. In *Peptides: Chemistry, Structure and Biology,* ed. PTP Kaumaya, RS Hodges, pp. 673–75. Kingswinford, UK: Mayflower Sci.

22. Chenera B, Finkelstein JA, Veber DF. 1995. Photodetachable arylsilane polymer linkages for use in solid phase organic synthesis. *J. Am. Chem. Soc.* 117:11999–2000

23. Mewes HW, Albermann K, Bahr M, Frishman D, Gleissner A, et al. 1997. Overview of the yeast genome. *Nature* 387(Suppl):7–65

24. *C. elegans* Sequencing Consort. 1998. Genome sequence of the nematode *Caenorhabditis elegans.* A platform for investigating biology. *Science* 282:2012–18

25. Lockhart DJ, Dong H, Byrne MC, Follettie MT, Gallo MV, et al. 1996. Expression monitoring by hybridization to high-density oligonucleotide arrays. *Nat. Biotechnol.* 14:1675–80

26. Schena M, Shalon D, Davis RW, Brown PO. 1995. Quantitative monitoring of gene expression patterns with a complementary DNA microarray. *Science* 270:467–70

27. Mooney J, Kayne P, O'Brien S, Debouck C. 2000. Construction and applications of gene microarrays on nylon membranes. In *PCR5: Differential Display: A Practical Approach,* ed. R Leslie, H Robertson. New York: Oxford Univ. Press. In press

28. Debouck C, Goodfellow P. 1999. DNA microarrays in drug discovery and development. *Nat. Genet.* 21:48–50

29. Wang T, Brown MJ. 1999. mRNA quantification by real time TaqMan polymerase chain reaction: validation and comparison with RNase protection. *Anal. Biochem.* 269:198–201

30. Blackstock WP, Weir MP. 1999. Proteomics: quantitative and physical mapping of cellular proteins. *Trends Biotechnol.* 17:121–27

31. Soskic V, Görlach M, Poznanovic S, Boehmer FD, Godovac-Zimmermann J. 1999. Functional proteomics analysis of signal transduction pathways of the platelet-derived growth factor β receptor. *Biochemistry* 38:1757–64

32. Link AJ, Eng J, Schieltz DM, Carmack E, Mize GJ, et al. 1999. Direct analysis of protein complexes using mass spectrometry. *Nat. Biotechnol.* 17:676–82

33. Marra MA, Hillier L, Waterston RH. 1998. Expressed sequence tags—establishing bridges between genomes. *Trends Genet.* 14:4–7

34. Bailey LC Jr, Searls DB, Overton GC. 1998. Analysis of EST-driven gene annotation in human genomic sequence. *Genome Res.* 8:362–76

35. Bucher P. 1999. Regulatory elements and expression profiles. *Curr. Opin. Struct. Biol.* 9:400–7

36. Kleyn PW, Vesell ES. 1998. Genetic variation as a guide to drug development. *Science* 281:1820–21

37. Pope AJ, Haupts UM, Moore KJ. 1998. Homogeneous fluorescence readouts for miniaturized high-throughput screening: theory and practice. *Drug Disc. Today* 4:350–62

38. Ohlstein EH, Ruffolo RR Jr, Elliott JD. 2000. Drug discovery in the next millennium. *Annu. Rev. Pharmacol. Toxicol.* 40:177–90

Annu. Rev. Pharmacol. Toxicol. 2000. 40:209–34

SIMULATION OF CLINICAL TRIALS

N. H. G. Holford,[1,2] H. C. Kimko,[2] J. P. R. Monteleone,[1] and C. C. Peck[2]

[1]Department of Pharmacology & Clinical Pharmacology, University of Auckland, Private Bag 92019, Auckland, New Zealand; [2]Center for Drug Development Sciences, Department of Pharmacology, Georgetown University Medical Center, Washington, DC 20007; e-mail: n.holford@auckland.ac.nz, koh@compuserve.com, j.monteleone@auckland.ac.nz, carl_peck@compuserve.com

Key Words design optimization, pharmacokinetics, pharmacodynamics

■ **Abstract** Computer simulation of clinical trials has evolved over the past two decades from a simple instructive game to "full" simulation models yielding pharmacologically sound, realistic trial outcomes. The need to make drug development more efficient and informative and the awareness that many industries make extensive use of simulation in product development have advanced considerably the use of simulation of clinical trials in pharmaceutical product development over the past decade. The structural and stochastic components of trial simulation models are explained as a prelude to a listing of representative simulation projects, reflecting investigative applications of statistical methods, trial design comparisons, and full simulation of new drugs being developed. Lessons learned from these projects are reviewed in the context of their current impact and potential for influencing the future of drug development.

INTRODUCTION

Computer simulation is the process of building a mathematical model that mimics a real-world situation and then using the model to conduct experiments in order to describe, explain, investigate, and predict the behavior of that situation (1). Simulation furnishes scientists with a conceptual tool for translating often-complex, real-world subject matter into a simplified form (a mathematical model), generalizing detail and exposing important assumptions. The model should capture all crucial aspects of the physical situation being described. By employing the model, simulation experiments can explore assumptions made about the model's structure and parameters. Additionally, model-based simulations may enable the investigation of actual experiment designs, which, in turn, might shed light on the model's assumptions.

The clinical trial is the preferred modern strategy for empirical evaluation of medical therapy (2). As such, it serves as a key component of the drug development process, when adequately designed and conducted, by providing information with which to weigh the risks and benefits of a compound. This information is used in risk management at various levels: at a regulatory level when a government agency determines, based on this information, whether or not a candidate compound may be marketed; and in a clinical setting when a physician decides whether, and if so, how a drug should be administered to a patient (2).

Clinical trial simulation is the abstraction of the clinical trial process. It is used to investigate assumptions and to influence trial design in order to maximize the amount of pertinent information gained throughout this process about the drug. Simulation is applicable to many areas of the clinical trial process. The focus here centers on the use of simulation with models based upon the dose-concentration-effect relationship (3) that reflect the disposition and effect of drugs as observed in clinical trials. In this chapter, we describe (*a*) motivations and history, (*b*) the general methodology of clinical trial simulation, including a brief description of current software available for performing such simulations, (*c*) some examples and lessons learned from using simulation in clinical trial design, and finally (*d*) our view of the current and future impact and directions for this powerful technology in drug development.

Motivations

Computer simulation has been used in the automotive and aerospace industry for over 20 years, improving the safety and durability of new products at a reduced development cost (4, 5). Similarly, the fundamental motivation for clinical trial simulation in pharmaceutical product development is to increase the efficiency of development, e.g. minimizing cost and time, while maximizing the informativeness of data generated from the trial. Clinical trial simulation aims to integrate relevant information and enable critical assessment of assumptions before resources are invested in conducting the actual clinical trial.

Before the 1990s, the drug development process, from initiation of preclinical studies through drug approval, took up to 12 years: 3.5 years for the preclinical phase; 1, 2, and 3 years, respectively, for clinical phases I, II, and III; and approximately 2.5 years for the Food and Drug Administration (FDA) review phase (6). Despite significant reductions in preclinical and regulatory review times, the clinical phase of development continues to consume up to 50% of overall drug development time. In 1997, research and development costs were estimated to be greater than $359 million US dollars (7), the majority of which was associated with the conducting of clinical trials. Nearly one third of the cost and over one half of the time (7.2 years) necessary to bring one new drug through FDA approval is spent on clinical development (8).

Why has drug development been so time-consuming and expensive? Often trials have had to be repeated because of flaws in trial design and performance that resulted in inadequate information about the safety or effectiveness of the new drug being tested (9). Identifying why a trial failed and how to prevent the failure in future trials is an additional use of clinical trial simulation. Often a deeper understanding of drug disposition and action may be achieved during the simulation model building process, and this understanding can influence the design of subsequent trials to increase the potential for successfully achieving the scientific goals of the program.

History

The term clinical trial simulation may have been first used to describe a game entitled "Instant Experience" (10) during a teaching course for doctors and scientists interested in learning about practical difficulties and sources of error in clinical trial design and performance. Patient information was "simulated" by the game organizers, and participants were split into groups charged with designing a clinical trial to detect whether a therapeutic difference existed between two drugs, with gender as the sole prognostic factor. While developing the game rules, the organizers created a computer program to generate simulated patients for future games.

The computer program was used at other workshops (11–13), as more simulation programs began appearing to explore complex statistical aspects of clinical trial design. For example, prognostic factors influence a patient's ability to respond to treatment and often in clinical trials the number of combinations of these factors approaches the sample size. Traditional methods are inadequate for analyzing these situations, so when a new sequential treatment assignment method was developed, it was subsequently tested using simulation (14). Other aspects of trials that were explored using clinical trial simulation included sample size, influence of dropouts (15), and problems with early termination of a clinical trial (16). It was recognized that as designs were becoming more complex, traditional statistical theory was no longer valid. Simulation, however, offered the means for generating complex data sets, which included prognostic factors, for testing new analysis methods (17).

Despite new developments in statistical analysis, the underlying goal remained the same: to design a clinical trial to detect a statistically significant difference between treatments. The question being asked in the trial was simply does the drug work rather than how much does the drug work (18).

In the 1980s, clinical trial simulation entered a more informative phase, with several advances, making simulation more than only a tool for statisticians. The desktop computer was becoming more powerful and prevalent, giving researchers easy access to a tool for creating complex mathematical models reflecting fundamental pharmacological principles, e.g. pharmacokinetics and the dose-response relationship. In 1986, Tiefenbrunn et al (19) used a physiologically-based computer simulation of biochemical reactions in response to concentrations of circulating tissue-type plasminogen activator (t-PA) to prospectively characterize its pharmacodynamics, using six patients given t-PA for coronary thrombosis. The findings from this model development and simulation process permitted the prospective evaluation of dosing regimens for t-PA in clinical trials. Using this model and computer simulation studies, it was shown that the degree of fibrinogenolysis induced by t-PA administration was almost independent of the dosing schedule (19, 20). This was an early example of applying simulation to clinical trials that yielded more than just a binary result.

In clinical pharmacology, models are created to describe data and provide a logical, biological explanation for observed drug disposition and pharmacologic effect. The early 1980s witnessed an explosion in the development of compartmental modeling analysis in clinical pharmacology (21, 22). Software (23) became available for modeling the population nature of clinical data, and literature on modeling concentration-effect (24) relationships and simultaneous pharmacokinetic and pharmacodynamic modeling (25) described how clinical pharmacology could benefit from a modeling approach. A series of papers by Sheiner & Beal (26–28) compared the population approach to traditional methods of clinical data analysis, demonstrating the limitations of traditional methods (see Table 2).

Simulation was a natural progression from the increased use of mathematical models in clinical pharmacology and has been used as an informative tool for evaluating complex clinical trial designs. One such design is the randomized concentration-controlled trial (RCCT) (29, 30). Simulation was used to investigate trial designs that efficiently provide accurate and precise estimates of pharmacokinetic parameters characterizing the dose-concentration-effect relationship in the face of high between-subject pharmacokinetic variability (see Table 4).

Prior to the early 1990s, there were no known attempts to simulate realistically an entire clinical trial based on the simultaneous integration of (a) a pharmacokinetic-pharmacodynamic (PKPD) drug action model, (b) a disease progress or placebo effect model, and (c) trial subject demographic covariates, between-subject variability and unexplained variability, and typical protocol deviations (e.g. dropouts, partial compliance). Simultaneously, this new and complex ("full") level of clinical trial simulation was initiated by two groups. For purposes of teaching, the educationally sponsored (31) RIDO (RIght DOse first time) software (32) was developed. The RIDO program, which incorporated the full clinical trial simulation capability, was developed to educate pharmaceutical scientists about the basic principles of clinical pharmacology and the role of variability in understanding why clinical trials are difficult to design. A pharmaceutical developer, motivated by the FDA to evaluate the feasibility of a proposed concentration controlled trial, employed full clinical trial simulation to determine not only feasibility but also trial design features such as individualized dose adjustment procedure and sample size (56, 57) (see Table 4). The evolution of applications and software for full clinical trial simulation technology has accelerated during the past 5 years, as evinced by several key conferences and workshops (33–35) sponsored by two centers that have championed methodological advances in drug development science (31, 36).

Any software that allows for the modeling of data may be used to perform a simulation [e.g. SAS (SAS Institute, Cary, NC), NONMEM (UCSF, San Francisco, CA), Mathcad (MathSoft, Inc. Seattle, WA)], but since 1996, two innovative commercial simulation software products have provided special capabilities dedicated to simulation of clinical trials: Pharsight Trial Designer (37) and MGA-ACSL Biomed (38). The ACSL Biomed clinical trial simulation program incorporated new routines based on a mature simulation language, advanced continuous simulation language (CACSL) (38), into existing biomedical modeling and simulation software. Use of these software packages (now both owned by Pharsight Corp.) is reflected in several recent clinical trial simulations (see Table 4). A more detailed account of the history and evolution of clinical trial simulation software in recent years is available (39).

So rapidly has this field evolved in the past few years that a draft guideline describing good practices for modeling and simulation of clinical trials in drug development has recently been published and public comment has been invited (40). Figure 1 lists the main sections and topics described in these guidelines. A key concept in these guidelines is the recommendation that clinical trial simulation be approached as an "experiment." The simulation experiment should have a well-defined plan developed by those who will be directly involved in performing the simulation and applying the results of the experiment. Execution of the planned simulations will usually lead to modification of the plan as new results are made available. The simulation plan is therefore a dynamic document. To reap the full benefits of the simulation, it is essential for the plan to include a formal strategy for assessment. For consistency, the remainder of this review follows the terminology and conceptual framework recommended in the draft guideline. Readers are encouraged to study the draft guideline in conjunction with this chapter for a fuller understanding of the current state of the art of clinical trial simulation.

ANATOMY OF A CLINICAL TRIAL SIMULATION

The steps in performing any type of computer simulation are similar, with each step expected to lead to the next. Often work on a step may reveal problems with a previous step, which will then have to be revisited. This iterative process ultimately aids the trial design team in understanding underlying assumptions impacting the quality of information obtained from the trial.

Clinical Trial Simulation Questions

Clinical trial simulation has developed in the context of increased understanding of clinical pharmacology and deals with questions that are raised about how to incorporate this knowledge into the design of clinical trials. Sheiner (18) has pointed out a useful conceptual framework for the epistemology of drug development. Phase III clinical trials are usually undertaken to answer a yes/no question ("Does the drug work?") that is approached statistically by a test of the null hypothesis. This is a confirming type of trial. Earlier in drug development, trials aim to investigate properties of the drug that may be elucidated using statistical estimation—e.g. the treatment effect size and dose-response relationship, etc. This is a learning type of trial.

1 PLANNING A SIMULATION PROJECT

1.1 Simulation Team
1.2 Simulation Plan
1.3 Overall Objectives and Specific Aims
1.4 Assumptions
1.5 Design of the Simulation Project
1.6 Simulation Project Design
1.6.1 Experimental Design
1.6.2 Replications
1.6.3 Trial Design Properties
1.7 Models for Simulation
1.7.1 Input-Output Models
1.7.2 Covariate Distribution Models
1.7.3 Execution Models
1.7.4 Source of Models
1.8 Computational Methods
1.8.1 Random Number Generation
1.8.2 Simulation of Probability Densities
1.8.3 Differential Equation Solvers
1.8.4 Computer Requirements
1.9 Analyses
1.10 Critical Assessment of Simulation Results
1.11 Reporting

2 EXECUTION OF THE SIMULATION PROJECT

2.1 Model Building
2.2 Model Checking and Validation
2.3 Analyses
2.3.1 Replication Analysis
2.3.2 Simulation Study Analysis
2.4 Report Contents

3 CRITICAL ASSESSMENT OF SIMULATION

3.1 Prospective Evaluation
3.2 Retrospective Evaluation
3.3 Cumulative Evaluation

Figure 1 From the Table of Contents of Simulation in Drug Development: Good Practices (40).

Confirming: Power

Confirming-type trials are designed to give an answer to such simple binary or categorical questions as whether or not the drug works. If the null hypothesis is rejected, then a clear answer is obtained. If the null hypothesis is not rejected, it could be because the drug does not actually work or because the design or analysis of the trial was not sufficiently powerful. A priori power analysis seeks to protect against this kind of "Still don't know" answer to the "Does the drug work?" question. There is extensive theory and experience of evaluating the power of a design to answer a yes/no question for many common design and analysis method combinations.

Learning: Power, Bias, and Precision

In addition to an affirmative answer to the yes/no question of whether a drug works, questions of direct interest to the patient and prescriber, such as the size of the effect or when the peak effect occurs, must also be answered. From a statistical perspective, these are estimation problems, and analyses that address these main questions of learning trials are rare. In this instance, clinical trial simulation can be a powerful tool. Responses are predicted using reasonable models of drug action and disease progress, along with stochastic elements such as patient variability and measurement error.

Modeling assumptions, trial design properties, and analysis methods can all be evaluated to understand the power of a design to answer more informative yes/no questions based on complex underlying concepts, e.g. whether an offset drug effect model can be distinguished from a slope effect model (54). Simulation can also be used to evaluate the bias and precision of the estimates of quantitative descriptors reflecting treatment effect size, time to peak effect, etc.

Simulation Model

Computer simulation requires a mathematical model that adequately reflects the actual situation being simulated. The model employed in a clinical trial simulation must, at a minimum, approximate a description of the clinical effect of a drug and, optimally, should be based upon the dose-concentration-effect relationships for the drug. The rapidly developing interest in clinical trial simulation has led to a variety of overlapping terms. The terminology used for defining a simulation model is listed in Table 1 and is further elaborated in the following sections. A simulation model is made up of three components (40): input-output model, covariate distribution model, and trial execution model.

Input-Output Model   The input-output (IO) model incorporates all scientific knowledge about the disease and drug. It may include (but is not limited to) the following components:

Structural Model   The structural model incorporates pharmacokinetics, pharmacodynamics, disease status and progress, and placebo responses.

Covariate Model   The covariate model serves to integrate patient-specific features (covariates such as age, weight, etc) that are associated with systematic differences between individuals. Covariate models are used to predict model parameters typical of an individual with a particular combination of covariates.

TABLE 1   Terminology for models involved in clinical trial simulations

Model	Components	Partially descriptive synonyms
Input-output model	Pharmacokinetics Pharmacodynamics[a] Disease progress Placebo response Covariate model relating covariates to typical parameter values Population parameter variability that includes between- and within-subject variability Residual unexplained variability that includes measurement error and model misspecification error Pharmacoeconomics	Structural model Variance model Pharmacostatistical model Outcome model PKPD model[b] Drug intervention model
Covariate distribution model	Demographic covariates (e.g. age, weight, gender, disease severity, concurrent treatment) Distribution and covariance of demographic covariates	Population Model demographics Trial subject inclusion/exclusion criteria
Trial execution model	Nominal design (protocol) Deviations from nominal protocol	Trial design Deviation from protocol model Compliance model Subject withdrawal Missing observations Adaptive design model

[a]Pharmacodynamics includes drug effects on biomarkers, surrogate endpoints, and clinical endpoints and outcomes.
[b]PKPD, pharmacokinetics pharmacodynamics.

Pharmacoeconomic Model   Project resource models, when employed, are considered part of the IO model because they predict responses (e.g. costs) as a function of the trial design and execution.

Stochastic Models   The IO model includes stochastic components that include the following. (*a*) Population parameter variability comprises between-subject and within-subject variability in model parameters. In practical terms, within-subject variability is largely defined by between-occasion variability (42) but includes stochastic variation in parameters, such as clearance, that may occur within an occasion (within-occasion variability). A term often used for population parameter variability is inter-individual variability. (b) Residual unexplained variability accounts for model misspecification and measurement error. A term often used for residual unknown variability is intra-individual variability.

Covariate Distribution Model   The distribution of demographic covariates in the trial subject sample is obtained from a model for the distribution of covariates in the target trial population. Such a model reflects the expected frequency distribution of the various covariates and, more importantly, the relationships among the covariates, e.g. age and renal function are related, such that renal function typically decreases with age in an adult population. The covariate distribution model should not be confused with the covariate model used to relate covariates to IO model parameters (see above).

Trial Execution Model   Although in real clinical trial practice, good faith attempts are made to perform or execute the trial according to the (nominal) trial protocol, human behavior and real-world events always intervene, and deviations or violations of the protocol are common. Thus, clinical trial simulations must recognize that the nominal trial protocol will never be executed with absolute perfection. There will be protocol deviations, e.g. subjects may withdraw, doses may not be taken as prescribed, or observations may be missing. Computer instructions that reflect both the nominal protocol and models for protocol deviations define the trial execution model.

Analysis of Simulated Data

Analysis of a Single Trial Replication   Simulation may be used to define responses across subjects within a single trial. For the single clinical trial, the unit for replication is each individual in the trial. The outcome of the trial can be defined qualitatively, in terms of whether or not it supported the rejection of a statistical null hypothesis (in the case of a confirming trial), or quantitatively, when it provided estimates of the trial outcome measure effect size(s) (in a learning trial). An individual subject outcome measure might be a statistic such as the time of peak drug effect or slope of a dose-response curve.

Analysis of the Simulation Experiment   Simulation may be used to define responses across trials. For the simulation experiment, the unit for replication is each clinical trial. The outcome of a simulation experiment will be based on the analysis of the outcome measures obtained from each clinical trial replication. The power of a specific clinical trial design is determined from the number of trials that reject the null hypothesis. Bias and precision of statistics such as the estimated treatment effect size, or parameters such as the maximum drug effect, are typically computed. When simulation is employed to investigate influence of various trial design features, a sensitivity analysis may be employed in a meta-analysis framework to compare power or estimation properties of the varying design factors.

CLINICAL TRIAL SIMULATION SOFTWARE

Numerous techniques are available for clinical trial simulation and most of the work reported to date has used general-purpose modeling and statistical software such as SAS. Clinical trial simulation involves several steps, each of which may be performed using different software tools.

Development of a Simulation Model

Input-Output Model   PKPD model building and parameter estimation, typically using data from previous clinical trials, may be done using either individual non-linear regression programs [e.g. WinNonlin (Pharsight, Mountain View, CA), ADAPT II (Biomedical Simulations Resource, Los Angeles, CA)] or population mixed effect modeling programs [e.g. NONMEM (23), NPML (44)].

Covariate Distribution Model   We are not aware of specific software for developing a model of the distribution of covariates in a target population for a clinical trial, thus general-purpose software is employed. Large databases exist that could be used to create such a model, e.g. NHANES (45).

Trial Execution Model   Models accounting for the nominal trial protocol and deviations such as subject withdrawal, variable compliance with medication, and missing observations have typically been based on ad hoc procedures within the simulation software program employed for the simulation. Software for collecting and reviewing medication compliance is available from suppliers of electronic monitoring systems (46). Attempts have been made to use such data to develop a model suitable for simulation (47).

Simulation

The same software program used for development of the IO model may be used to simulate clinical trial response data. The key element is the ability to add random (stochastic) variability to the model as residual error (measurement and model misspecification error) and IO model parameter variability. More realistic simulations will also include stochastic variation in sampling subject specific values from the covariate distribution model, and in the deviations from the nominal protocol defined by the trial execution model. Standard statistical software—e.g. SAS and S-Plus (MathSoft, Seattle, WA), or more specialized programs such as NONMEM and Pharsight Trial Designer—can accomodate all of these features. General statistical software is least convenient because all components of the simulation model must be created by the user. NONMEM has a comprehensive library of pharmacokinetic models but requires the user to create a data file to specify doses, covariates, and observation times for each subject. Dedicated commercial simulation software such as Pharsight Trial Simulator can be expected to provide more convenient trial simulations with predefined model and trial design libraries, and for integration of all routines and procedures necessary for accomplishing the simulation.

Analysis of Simulated Data

For statistical analysis of a single simulated clinical trial, standard statistical software will most commonly be used for confirmatory-type trials but more complex model-based procedures (e.g. mixed effects nonlinear modeling with NONMEM) will be preferred for more informative learning trials (18). Commercial simulation software should allow the user to conveniently select from a variety of typical trial outcome measures (e.g. response at a specified time, peak response, area under the curve of a response) and perform standard analyses (e.g. analysis of variance). Most of the user-written software is employed to perform a set of replication level analyses and to summarize the simulation experiment results, e.g. clinical trial simulator, developed by one of us (NHG Holford).

For analysis of either a single trial replication or a simulation experiment, the distribution of individual or trial responses may be informatively displayed in graphical form, e.g. showing the scatter of responses as a function of time after the start of treatment or the distribution of outcomes from many trials. Meta-analysis of comparative power or estimation properties across varying trial design factors may be accomplished using standard analysis of variance or regression procedures.

REVIEW OF CLINICAL TRIAL SIMULATION PROJECTS

Below, we present representative examples of research projects or practical applications known to us that have used simulation in relation to clinical trial questions. Much recent work in this area has only been reported in abstract form or has been communicated primarily at conferences. Therefore, we have drawn extensively from our own experiences and describe them using the format of Holford et al (40). We acknowledge that the tables are incomplete in many places and apologize to authors whose work we may have incorrectly interpreted or of which we are unaware. We intend the tables to provide a view of what questions have been investigated and what techniques have been used. The "Lessons Learned" columns (Tables 2, 3, and 4) indicate what we think are key new knowledge and insights that have been derived with respect to the overall application of clinical trial simulation. Each project may have had other objectives but we have chosen not to elaborate on them.

We have identified three levels of simulation projects. The first deals with evaluations of statistical properties and analytical methods used as the basic tools of clinical trial simulation. The second entails the application of simulation to investigate the general properties of certain classes of clinical trial designs. The third deals with full clinical trial simulations applied to specific drugs and specific designs.

Investigations of Statistical Properties and Analytical Methods

Simulation has long been used by mathematical statisticians and others to investigate properties and performance of statistical and data analysis methods. Illustrative examples of such investigations applied to two widely employed PKPD model building and parameter estimation techniques can be seen in Table 2. These methodological investigations bear primarily on the properties of estimation methods that are widely used in the specific projects detailed below.

Simulations of a typical pharmacokinetic experiment, analyzed by two nonlinear regression estimation methods, enabled Peck et al (48) to describe the less biased and more precise parameter estimates derived from maximum likelihood estimation using a general parametric residual variance model (extended least squares) versus weighted least squares regression analysis. Likewise, Sheiner & Beal (28) demonstrated via simulation that estimation of population PK parameters using mixed-effects modeling enabled efficient use of sparse data compared with the two-stage weighted least squares method.

Investigations of Trial Designs

Simulation has also been used to investigate power and estimation properties of various clinical trial designs. Six illustrative examples that have utilized PKPD-type IO models in simulation models of common clinical trial designs are listed in Table 3. Simulations of competing clinical trial designs have been useful in evaluating their comparative advantages and limitations. Optimal sampling design methods, aimed at the timing of a minimum number of pharmacokinetic observations for estimation of model parameters with minimum bias and variance, were investigated by D'Argenio (49) comparing optimal designs with standard intensive sampling schemes. The investigation of randomized concentration controlled trial (RCCT) designs reported by Sanathanan & Peck (50) investigated the extent of improvement in sample size efficiency that can be gained from the RCCT design in comparison to the traditional randomized dose controlled trial design when between-subject PK variability is high. Following the theoretical investigation by simulation of escalation designs in learning type trials (51) pointed to a reevaluation of the merits of cross-over and dose-titration trials. The investigation by Holford (53) of the enrichment design used in confirmatory trials of tacrine (for Alzheimer's disease) showed that the criterion used to identify responders during a titration phase was little different from simple randomization, because of the unrecognized contribution of between-occasion variation in observing the cognitive response to treatment. The difficulties in distinguishing different drug effects on disease progression was highlighted by simulating trials of a pseudo-drug, pstat (54). This study also pointed out the value of considering monetary costs of alternative study designs. Finally, El-Tahtawy et al (55) used Monte-Carlo simulation to investigate bioequivalence trial designs applied to

TABLE 2 Simulation projects evaluating statistical and data analysis methods used in simulation of clinical trials

Statistical Property or Analytical Method	Reference	I/O Model				Covariate Distribution Model		Trial Execution Model				Simulation Experiment				Replication Analysis			Simulation Experiment Analysis			Lessons Learned
		Structural Model	Stochastic Component	Software	Data Source	Covariate	Data Source	Nominal Trial Design	Protocol Deviation Model	Source	Software	Model Factors	Design or Analysis Factors	Software	Replications	Null hypothesis	Descriptive Aims	Software	Confirmatory Hypothesis	Learning Hypothesis	Software	
Extended Least Squares Estimation	48	PK	RUV	LSNLR (61)	Authors	None		Individual PK experiment	None	NA	NA	PPV, RUV, randomization seed	ELS vs WLS (various weights), initial PK parameter estimates	LSNLR	100 subjects	Estimation methods equally accurate and precise	Bias and precision of estimates	LSNLR	Power (capacity to estimate true model parameters)	Comparative bias and precision of ELS vs WLS estimates	Simple Statistics	Simulation is a valuable procedure for evaluating novel nonlinear parameter estimation methods
Nonlinear mixed effects modeling (NONMEM)	28	PK	PPV, RUV	NONMEM	Authors	None		Individual PK experiment	None	NA	NA	RUV	NONMEM vs 2-stage WLS	NONMEM	50 trials	Estimation methods equally accurate and precise	Precision	NONMEM	Capacity to estimate true model parameters	Bias and precision of NONMEM vs 2-stage WLS estimates	Simple Statistics	Simulation is a valuable procedure for evaluating novel population PK estimation methods

NA: Not Applicable

TABLE 3 Simulation projects evaluating trial designs

Experimental Design Aspect	Reference	I/O Model			Covariate Model		Trial Execution Model		Simulation Experiment			Replication Analysis			Simulation Experiment Analysis			Lessons Learned
		Structural Model	Stochastic Component	Software Data Source	Covariate	Data Source	Nominal Trial Design	Software Source	Model Factors	Design or Analysis Factors	Software Replications	Null hypothesis	Descriptive Aims	Software	Confirmatory Hypothesis	Learning Hypothesis	Software	(in all cases: simulation was a valuable procedure for evaluating competing clinical trial designs)
Optimal Sampling Times	49	PK	PPV, RUV	ADAPT / Author	None		Sequential population PK trial	None / NA / NA	PPV, RUV	Sampling times	ADAPT / 30 trials	Optimal vs. conventional sampling trials	PK estimates	ADAPT	Capacity to estimate true population parameters	Bias, precision	Simple statistics	"Optimal sampling and preexperiment simulation may be useful tools for designing informative pharmacokinetic experiments"
Randomized Concentration-Controlled Trial (RCCT) and Dose-Controlled Trial (RDCT) Designs	50	PK, PD	PPV, RUV	SAS / Authors	None		Parallel dose- & concentration response trial	none / NA / SAS	PPV, RUV	Concentration and dose control methods	SAS / 5000 trials	Dose vs concentration control	Concentration – Effect slope estimate	SAS	Power	Bias and precision	SAS	RCCT is more powerful & efficient than RDCT when PK PPV is high
Escalation Design	51, 52	PD	PPV, RUV	Author / NA	None		Parallel, Crossover, Escalation	None / NA / NA	None	Parallel, Crossover, Escalation	NONMEM / 50 trials	Treatments not different	Treatment effect size	NONMEM	Power	Bias	Simple statistics	Escalation designs are valuable for learning type trials.

Study (No.)	PK, PD, DP, PL	Smoker effect on drug sensitivity	Parallel, titration, enrichment	Fixed	Treatments not different	Power	
Enrichment Design (Tacrine) — 53	PPV, RUV NONMEM Sponsor data	Sponsor data	None None N/A	Number and timing of observations, Enrichment design Trial Designer 100trials	PK, PD, DP, PL model Parameter estimates NONMEM	Power Bias and Precision CTS	Enrichment design for certain tacrine trials were flawed. Titration design is powerful. Automated procedures were required for complex simulation experiment and numerically intensive analysis
Designs for Evaluating Disease Progress (Pstat) — 54	PK, PD, DP,PL, PEC PPV, RUV NONMEM Sponsor data	None	Parallel	Offset, slope, both drug effects with linear DP model. Number and timing of observations, dose size, number of subjects Trial Designer 100 trials	Drug has no effect PK, PD, DP, PL model parameter estimates NONMEM	Power Bias and Precision Cost CTS	Spread out sampling is essential to distinguish drug effects on disease progress. Cost is a major factor in evaluating designs.
Bioequivalence trials of highly variable drugs — 55	PK PPV, RUV NA Authors	None	Crossover None NA	Formulation release rate, RUV, parameter correlation Single vs multiple dose regimens SAS 1000 trials	Power independent of RUV Bioequivalence SAS	Power SAS	Served as basis for regulatory policy for bioequivalence designs

NA: Not Applicable

highly variable drugs. These simulations were used to justify regulatory guidance documents (55; AA El-Tahtawy, personal communication).

Drug-Specific Clinical Trials

Tables 4 and 5 list characteristics of 19 recent clinical trial simulation projects involving specific drugs (some drug products are not identified to respect confidential information), nine of which were undertaken by the authors. These nine simulations, as well as the pioneer simulation of mycophenolate mofetil, are reported in greatest detail, whereas all others (Table 5) are less completely reported because of the lack of publicly available information. The entries in Tables 4 and 5 are similar, with the exception of the final right hand column, which reflects lessons learned from the author's simulation projects (Table 4) or stated goal of the other reported simulations (Table 5).

The simulation by Hale et al (56, 57) of a proposed concentration controlled trial was the first reported demonstration of the practical utility of a full clinical trial simulation that determined trial feasibility and influenced trial design features for an actual drug in development. It is important to note that this project was motivated by a specific request for the simulation by the FDA, signaling official regulatory interest and receptivity to this novel technology. Regulatory interest has persisted, as evinced not only by the FDA's acceptance of trial simulation in other regulatory submissions (see Table 4) but also Agency cosponsorship of several recent conferences and guidelines encompassing population modeling and trial simulation.

Evaluation of a new and evolving technology is essential as a guide to future directions for research, application, and evaluation. Table 4 lists several impediments for simulation, including difficulties encountered with retrospective data retrieval, nonavailability of adequate modeling databases (especially placebo and disease progress data), time pressures interfering with completeness of simulations, and useful prerequisites such as the need for input from disease experts, value of IO model features reflecting drug discontinuation and rebound effects, and value of standards for model diagnostics and model evaluation techniques. Although some of these matters have been considered in the good simulation practices guideline (40), others are philosophical and require cultural and attitudinal changes. For example, prospective integration of modeling and clinical trial simulation in a drug development program should optimally commence in the preclinical phase, leading to use of simulation in planning the first human clinical trial (58).

IMPACT AND FUTURE DIRECTIONS

Application of clinical trial simulation in contemporary drug development programs is variable and often absent or incomplete—hence, measurable impact is modest at best. Simulation of PK properties of a new drug, derived primarily from phase I normal volunteer studies, is sometimes utilized to define dosage regimens

TABLE 4 Simulation projects evaluating drug specific clinical trials

Drug / Reference		Mycophenolate Mofetil 56,57	Seroquel (62) and unpublished results (CDDS, 1998)
I/O Model	Structural Model	PK, PD	PK, PD, PL, DP
	Stochastic Component	PPV, RUV	PPV, RUV
	Software	SAS	NONMEM
	Data Source	1 Phase 1 trial	1 Phase 1 and 1 Phase 2 trials
Covariate Distribution Model	Covariate	None supported by data	None supported by data
	Data Source	1 phase 2 trial	1 Phase 1 and 1 Phase 2 trials
Trial Execution Model	Nominal Trial Design / Protocol Deviation Model	RCCT / None	Parallel / Random subject dropout
	Software	NA	ACSL Biomed
	Source	NA	Sponsor experience
Simulation Experiment	Model Factors / Design or Analysis Factors	Fixed / Number of subjects, maximum daily dose	Fixed
	Software	SAS	ACSL Biomed
	Replications	5000 trials	100 trials
Replication Analysis	Null hypothesis	Treatments not different / Treatment effect siz	Treatments not different / Dose-response slope zero
	Descriptive Aims		Drug and placebo effect sizes
	Software	SAS	SAS
Simulation Experiment Analysis	Confirmatory Hypothesis / Learning hypothesis	Power / Comparison with actual trial	Power / Comparison with actual trial
	Software	SAS	SAS
Lessons Learned		Modeling enabled prediction of graft-rejection probability with respect to AUC, while simulation affirmed study feasibility and led to design of a successful trial	Retrospective data retrieval was difficult. Placebo prediction based on inadequate database

225

TABLE 4 (continued) Simulation projects evaluating drug specific clinical trials

	PK	Fed/fasted	Cross-over	Fixed	formulations not different formulations equivalent	Power	Value of diagnostics of IO model for model selection Unexplained poor prediction of effect size
NSAID Formulations (63) and unpublished results) CDDS, 1999)	PK PPV, RUV	Dog and human PK	None	number of subjects, duration of sampling	Covariate and treatment effect size	Comparison with actual trial	Value of diagnostics of IO model for model selection Unexplained poor prediction of effect size
	NONMEM Literature, in vitro study, dog and human PK		NA	NONMEM 100 trials	SAS	SAS	
Anticoagulant Unpublished results (CDDS, 1999)	PK, PD, PL, DP PPV, RUV	Disease severity	Parallel None considered	Fixed and escalation scheme Dose, infusion duration	None Treatment effect size	NA Dose-response relationship	Time pressure interfered with completeness of M&S. Rapid and simple simulation provided decision support by sponsor and regulatory agency.
	NONMEM 4 Phase 1 trials	4 Phase 1 and 1 Phase 2 trials	NA NA	ACSL-Biomed 10 subjects	Simple statistics	Simple statistics	
Antihypertensive Unpublished results (CDDS, 1999)	PK, PD, PL, DP PPV, RUV	Clearance–creatinine	Parallel Random subject dropout Noncompliance	Fixed Fixed	Treatments not different Drug and placebo effect size	Power Comparison with actual trial	Placebo prediction based on inadequate database IO model may have been suboptimal for lack of model for drug

Therapeutic area	Reference	Model	Variability	Estimation method / Data	Covariates / Data	Trial design	Design elements	Fixed / varied factors; Tool; Size	Assumption; Quantity; Method	Metric; Parameter; Method	Conclusions
CNS drug	Unpublished results (CDDS, 1999)	PK, PD	PPV, RUV	NONMEM 4 preclinical studies	None 4 preclinical studies	None considered	NA NA	Fixed; Dose, administration route; Trial Designer; 20 subjects	Feasibility of sufficient exposure; None; Simple statistics	Power; PK; Simple statistics	Simulation facilitated No Go decision of first trial in human from preclinical information.
CNS drug	Unpublished results (CDDS, 1999)	PK, PD	PPV, RUV	NONMEM 2 Phase 2 and 1 Phase 3 trials	Baseline severity Normal 2 Phase 2 and 1 Phase 3 trials	Cross over	None NA NA	Fixed; Fixed; SAS; 18 subjects	Formulations therapeutically equivalent; None; SAS	Therapeutic equivalence; NA; SAS	Therapeutic equivalence between two formulations may be investigated via simulation with a firm understanding of PK/PD relationship
Anti-arthritic drug	Unpublished results (CDDS, 1999)	PK, PD, DP	PPV, RUV	NONMEM Literature, sponsor experience	Age, gender, weight, renal function Multivariate Normal Disease expert	Parallel	Random subject dropout Random missing observations NA Sponsor experience	Subject dropouts, missing observation; Dosing schedule; Trial Designer; 100 trials	Treatments not different; PD and DP parameter estimates; NONMEM	Power; Bias, precision; CTS	Disease expert's opinion was helpful in developing and justifying complex simulation models.
Deep Brain Stimulation for Parkinson's Disease	Unpublished results (CDDS, 1999)	PD, DP	PPV, RUV	NA Investigator Experience	None NA	Incomplete crossover	None NA NA	None; Timing and number of observations; Trial Designer; 100 trials	Treatment has no effect on disease progress; NA; NONMEM	Power; NA; CTS	Longer trial duration required than originally planned
Anti-Parkinson's Disease Drug	Work in progress (CDDS, 1999)	PD, DP	PPV, RUV	NONMEM DATATOP(64)	None NA	Parallel	None NA NA	Drug effect on disease progress; Number and timing of observations; Trial Designer; 100 trials	Treatment has no effect on disease progress; Treatment effect size; Trial Designer	Power; Bias and precision (Actual trial results will be compared with simulation predictions); CTS	Work in progress

TABLE 5 Simulation projects evaluating drug specific clinical trials: published reports with incomplete information

Drug	Reference	I/O Model	Cov. Dist. Model	Trial Execution Model	Simulation Experiment	Replication Analysis	Simulation Experiment Analysis	Goal
		Structural Model Stochastic Component Software Data Source	Covariate Data Source	Nominal Trial Design Protocol Deviation Model Software Source	Model Factors Design or Analysis Factors Software Replications	Null Hypothesis Descriptive Aims Software	Confirmatory Hypothesis Learning Hypothesis Software	
Treatment of Migraine	65 (abstract)	PK, PD UA NONMEM UA	UA UA	Parallel UA UA UA	Absorption rate, potency Study duration, number of subjects, dose, Trial Designer 100 trials	Treatments not different Treatment effect size S-Plus	Power Dose-response relationship S-Plus	To evaluate design strategies and model assumptions
Ketorolac	66	PK, PD Mixture of PPV & RUV NONMEM "several clinical trials"	None	Parallel None NA NA	Fixed Fixed NONMEM 1000 subjects	None Treatment effect size S-PLUS	NA Dose-response relationship S-PLUS	To evaluate design strategies and model assumptions
GW262570 Anti-diabetic Drug	67 (abstract)	PK UA UA UA	UA UA	Parallel UA UA UA	ED50, Emax Dose, duration UA UA	Treatments not different none UA	Power NA UA	To find a study design to detect a drug effect.
Docetaxel	68 (abstract)	PK, PD Median SAS 180 patients	Body surface area, protein binding, hepatic function 180 patients	Parallel None NA NA	Fixed Protein level ACSL Biomed 100 trials	None Treatment effect size Simple statistics	NA Dose-response relationship Simple statistics	To predict safety profiles.

TABLE 5 (continued) Simulation projects evaluating drug specific clinical trials: published reports with incomplete information

Agent	Ref									Objective
Anticholinergic agent	69 (abstract)	PK, PD	UA	UA	None	Study size, dose	Treatment effect size	Dose-response relationship		To examine the impact of trial design on the ability to characterize the dose-response relationship and demonstrate efficacy over placebo
		UA	"data and publications available at the time"		NA	UA	UA	UA		
					NA	UA				
GI198745 5-a-reductase	70 (abstract)	PK, PD	Dose	Parallel	Fixed	None	NA			To predict dose vs DHT reduction
		UA	48 subjects	None	Fixed	SCI Clinical Trials Forecaster	Treatment effect size	Dose-response relationship		
		48 subjects					Simple statistics	Simple plot		
Capecitabine Anti-cancer	43	PK, PD	UA	Parallel	Fixed	None	NA			To Predict tumor size and adverse reaction to decide dosing schedule
		UA	NA	None	Dosing time	ACSL BioMed	Treatment effect size	Dose-response relationship		
			NA			50 subjects	Simple statistics	Simple statistics		
GPIIB/IIIA antagonist	71 (abstract)	PK, PD	UA	Parallel	Fixed	Treatments not different	Power			To decide if a Phase II trial could improve the success rate of a Phase III trial.
		UA	NA	None	Dose	Treatment effect size	Dose-response relationship			
		UA	"Phase I data" and published data	NA	UA	UA	UA			
				NA	500 subjects					
GM-0911	72 (abstract)	PK, PD	Baseline severity	Parallel	Formulation, tolerance	Treatments not different	Power			To predict the impact of tolerance on a new formulation in a trial
		UA		UA	UA	UA	UA			
		UA		UA	UA	UA	UA			
		UA		UA	UA					

UA: Unavailable or unclear

229

for evaluation in phase II trials. As this procedure is often performed without taking into account between-subject variability or pharmacodynamic linkages, an opportunity is lost to influence trial design features such as dosages and dosage intervals, or "go/no go" decisions for direction of product development. Two important exceptions provide instructive illustrations of the power of clinical trial simulation in a drug development program.

As highlighted above, PKPD-based clinical trial simulation of the organ anti-rejection agent, mycophenolate mofetil, was employed to evaluate study feasibility and to influence multiple trial design features of a proposed RCCT in renal transplant patients (56). The simulation model, derived from 41 patients, employed a binary-outcome clinical response (transplant rejection, yes or no) and guided the design of a RCCT that, when completed, was adjudged to have successfully met its scientific objectives (57). In the case of the antiretroviral agent, alovudine (R Desjardins, personal communication), PKPD-based simulations of alovudine activity and toxicity, derived from two concentration controlled trials (RCCT) in HIV patients (59), provided a strong rationale to halt the further development of the drug. The 12-h area under the alovudine concentration-time curve value above which unacceptable hematologic toxicity occurred (>300 ng ml^{-1} h^{-1}), was less than threefold that of the area under the alovudine concentration-time curve above which a 50% or greater reduction in viral serum HIV antigen concentration (p24) was observed. When between-subject PK variability was taken into consideration, simulations predicted unacceptable toxicity in a high proportion of patients at dosages necessary to achieve antiretroviral effectiveness.

Despite the modest impact of current applications of clinical trial simulation in drug development, there is reason to expect increasing incorporation of this technology in all phases, from discovery to phase IV. Several major pharmaceutical firms are committing major resources to the establishment of intellectual and computational capabilities for prospective incorporation of modeling (41) and for clinical trial simulation in selected drug development programs.

In the near term, lessons learned from experience in recent years with clinical trial simulation (e.g. Table 4) provide direction for the next steps in the realm of research and development management and education. Thus, drug developers that plan to benefit from this technology should provide for trained personnel and resources to enable prospective integration of modeling and clinical trial simulation in drug development programs (to mitigate problems cited above with retrospective data retrieval, company cultural resistance or lack of cooperativeness, unrealistic time pressures, etc), commencing in the preclinical phase, and fully integrating the modeling and simulation approach in all subsequent clinical phases. This step alone has major implications for education and training of personnel needed for this bold evolution in drug development. Because the trained personnel needed for this approach are already scarce, consideration should be given to expansion of existing, and establishment of new, educational programs to develop the large number (hundreds) of experts in clinical trial simulation that will be needed.

Comprehensive databases and models for adequately modeling the disease progress and placebo response patterns in various diseases and treatments are sorely needed. Equally needed is an understanding of the consequences to subjects of the interruptions and resumptions of drug regimens (60) that often occur during clinical trials, leading to loss or exaggeration of drug effects, rebound effects, tolerance, and other nonlinear deviations from simple models of drug effect. Evaluating, improving, and implementing the draft simulation good practices guidance (40) is another valuable next step in advancing the quality, utility, and confidence in this novel technology.

In the far future, we foresee a central role for clinical trial simulation in a revolutionary paradigm shift in drug development practices. Today, drug development continues its inefficient tradition of many tens to hundreds of clinical trials per new drug application, supporting a mostly empirically derived safety-and-effectiveness database—with modest or no role of trial simulations. In our vision of a very different future, clinical trial simulations will be the principle scientific activity, and actual clinical trials will be few, aimed at informing simulation models and confirming simulation predictions. The impact of clinical trial simulations in this vision of the future will go well beyond the success and efficiency of actual development activities. It will impact the selection and training of scientific personnel involved in drug development, as well as the demography of clinical trial subjects, and possibly even the economics of development— virtual clinical trials may reduce overall cost of drug development by reducing the total number of trials, especially ones that are prone to failure or that are unnecessary.

ACKNOWLEDGMENT

We appreciate the efforts of Ms. Jeanine Sawler of the Center for Drug Development Science in editorial assistance of the manuscript.

Visit the Annual Reviews home page at www.AnnualReviews.org.

LITERATURE CITED

1. Hoover SV, Perry RF. 1989. *Simulation: A Problem Solving Approach.* New York: Addison-Wesley
2. Sheiner LB, Rubin DB. 1995. Intention-to-treat analysis and the goals of clinical trials. *Clin. Pharmacol. Ther.* 57:6–15
3. Holford NHG. 1995. The target concentration approach to clinical drug development. *Clin. Pharmacokinet.* 29(5): 287–91
4. Kaufmann WJ, Smarr LL. 1993. *Supercomputing and the Transformation of Science.* New York: Sci. Am.
5. Johnson SCD. 1998. The role of simulation in the management of research: What can the pharmaceutical industry learn from the aerospace industry? *Drug Inf. J.* 32(4):961–70
6. Heilman R. 1995. Drug development: history, "overview," and what are GCPs? *Qual. Assur.* 4(1):75–79
7. Watling KJ, Milius RA, Williams M. 1997. Recent advances in drug discovery. *RBI Neurotrans.,* Nov., pp. 1–5
8. DiMasi JA. 1996. A new look at United States drug development and approval times. *Am. J. Ther.* 3:1–11
9. Peck CC. 1997. Drug development:

improving the process. *Food Drug Law J.* 52(2):163–67

10. Maxwell C, Domenet JG, Joyce CRR. 1971. Instant experience in clinical trials: a novel aid to teaching by simulation. *J. Clin. Pharmacol.* 11(5):323–31

11. Marsh BT. 1975. The planning of a clinical trials workshop. *Br. J. Clin. Pharmacol.* 2(5):455–61

12. Madsen BW, Woodings TL, Ilett KF, Shenfield GM, Potter JM, et al. 1978. Clinical trial experience by simulation: a workshop report. *Br. Med. J.* 2(6148): 1333–35

13. Bland JM. 1986. Computer simulation of clinical trial as an aid to teaching the concept of statistical significance. *Stat. Med.* 5:193–97

14. Pocock SJ, Simon R. 1975. Sequential treatment assignment with balancing for prognostic factors in the controlled clinical trial. *Biometrics* 31(1):103–15

15. Jones DR. 1979. Computer simulation as a tool for clinical trial design. *Int. J. Bio-Med. Comp.* 10:145–50

16. DeMets DL. 1981. Practical aspects of decision making in clinical trials: the coronary drug project as a case study. *Control Clin. Trials* 1(4):363–76

17. Lee KL, Frederick M, Starmer CF, Harris PJ, Rosati RA. 1980. Clinical judgement and statistics: lessons from a simulated randomized trial in coronary artery disease. *Circulation* 61(3):508–15

18. Sheiner LB. 1997. Learning versus confirming in clinical drug development. *Clin. Pharmacol. Ther.* 61(3):275–91

19. Tiefenbrunn AJ, Graor RA, Robison AK, Lucas FV, Hotchkiss A, et al. 1986. Pharmacodynamics of tissue-type plasminogen activator characterized by computer-assisted simulation. *Circulation* 73(6): 1291–99

20. Noe DA, Bell WR. 1987. A kinetic analysis of fibrinogenolysis during plasminogen activator therapy. *Clin. Pharmacol. Ther.* 41(3):297–303

21. Sheiner LB, Grasela TH. 1984. Experience with NONMEM: analysis of routine

phenytoin clinical pharmacokinetic data. *Drug Metab. Rev.* 15(1–2):293–303

22. Grasela TH, Sheiner LB. 1984. Population pharmacokinetics of procainamide from routine clinical data. *Clin. Pharmacokinet.* 9(6):545–54

23. Boeckmann AJ, Sheiner LB, Beal SL. 1990. *NONMEM Users Guides.* San Francisco: Univ. Calif. NONMEM Proj. Group. 5th ed.

24. Holford NHG, Sheiner LB. 1981. Understanding the dose-effect relationship: clinical application of pharmacokinetic-pharmacodynamic models. *Clin. Pharmacokinet.* 6:429–53

25. Colburn WA. 1981. Simultaneous pharmacokinetic and pharmacodynamic modeling. *J. Pharmacokinet. Biopharm.* 9(3): 367–87

26. Sheiner LB, Beal SL. 1980. Evaluation of methods for estimating population pharmacokinetics parameters. I. Michaelis-Menten model: routine clinical pharmacokinetic data. *J. Pharmacokinet. Biopharm.* 8(6):553–71

27. Sheiner BL, Beal SL. 1981. Evaluation of methods for estimating population pharmacokinetic parameters. II. Biexponential model and experimental pharmacokinetic data. *J. Pharmacokinet. Biopharm.* 9(5):635–51

28. Sheiner LB, Beal SL. 1983. Evaluation of methods for estimating population pharmacokinetic parameters. III. Monoexponential model: routine clinical pharmacokinetic data. *J. Pharmacokinet. Biopharm.* 11(3):303–19

29. Sanathanan LP, Peck C, Temple R, Lieberman R, Pledger G. 1991. Randomization, PK-controlled dosing, and titration: an integrated approach for designing clinical trials. *Drug Inf. J.* 25:425–31

30. Endrenyi L, Zha J. 1994. Comparative efficiencies of randomized concentration- and dose-controlled clinical trials. *Clin. Pharmacol. Ther.* 56:331–38

31. Eur. Cent. Pharm. Med. http://www.ecpm.ch/html/pg_home.html

32. Amstein R, Steimer J, Holford N, Guentert T, Racine A, et al. 1996. RIDO: Multimedia CD-Rom software for training in drug development via PK/PD principles and simulation of clinical trials. *Pharm. Res.* 13:S452 (Abstr.)
33. Cent. Drug Dev. Sci. 1996. *Frontiers in Drug Development—Computer Simulation and Modeling.* Basel, Switzerland: Eur. Cent. Pharm. Med.
34. Cent. Drug Dev. Sci. 1997. *Modeling and Simulation of Clinical Trials in Drug Development and Regulation.* Reston, VA: Cent. Drug Dev. Sci.
35. Cent. Drug Dev. Sci. 1999. *Modeling and Simulation: Best Practices Workshop.* 1999. Arlington, VA: Cent. Drug Dev. Sci.
36. Cent. Drug Dev. Sci. http://www.dml. georgetown.edu/cdds
37. Pharsight Corp. 1997. *Pharsight Trial Designer User's Guide.* Mountain View, CA: Pharsight Corp.
38. Mitchell EEL. 1978. Advanced continuous simulation language (ACSL). In *Numerical Methods for Differential Equations and Simulation,* ed. AW Bennet, R Vichnevetsky. Amsterdam: North-Holland Publ.
39. Regalado A. 1998. Re-engineering drug development. I: Simulating clinical trials. *Start Up,* Jan. pp. 13–18
40. Holford NHG, Hale M, Ko HC, Steimer J-L, Sheiner LB, et al. 1999. *Simulation in Drug Development: Good Practices.* http://www.dml.georgetown.edu/cdds/ SDDGP.html
41. Sheiner LB, Steimer J-L. 2000. Pharmacokinetic/pharmacodynamic modeling in drug development. *Annu. Rev. Pharmacol. Toxicol.* 40:67–95
42. Karlsson MO, Sheiner LB. 1993. The importance of modeling interoccasion variability in population pharmacokinetic analyses. *J. Pharmacokinet. Biopharm.* 21(6):735–50
43. Gieschke R, Reigner BG, Steimer J-L. 1997. Exploring clinical study design by computer simulation based on pharmacokinetic/pharmacodynamic modelling. *Int.*

44. Mallet A, Mentré F, Steimer JL, Lokiec F. 1988. Nonparametric maximum likelihood estimation for population pharmacokinetics, with application to cyclosporine. *J. Pharmacokinet. Biopharm.* 16(3):311–27
45. National Center for Health Statistics. 1994. *The Third National Health and Nutrition Examination Survey, 1988–94 (NHANES III).* http://www.cehn.org/ cehn/resource guide/nhanes.html
46. Kastrissios H, Blaschke TF. 1997. Medication compliance as a feature in drug development. *Annu. Rev. Pharmacol. Toxicol.* 37:451–75
47. Girard P, Blaschke T, Kastrissios H, Sheiner L. 1998. A Markov mixed effect regression model for drug compliance. *Stat. Med.* 17:2313–33
48. Peck CC, Beal SL, Sheiner LB, Nichols AI. 1984. Extended least squares nonlinear regression: a possible solution to the "choice of weights" problem in analysis of individual pharmacokinetic parameters. *J. Pharmacokinet. Biopharm.* 12(5): 545–57
49. D'Argenio DZ. 1981. Optimal sampling times for pharmacokinetic experiments. *J. Pharmacokinet. Biopharm.* 9(6):739–56
50. Sanathanan LP, Peck CC. 1991. The randomized concentration-controlled trial: an evaluation of its sample size efficiency. *Control Clin. Trials* 12:781–94
51. Sheiner LB, Beal SL. 1989. Study designs for dose-ranging. *Clin. Pharmacol. Ther.* 46:63–77
52. Sheiner LB, Hashimoto Y, Beal SL. 1991. A simulation study comparing designs for dose ranging. *Stat. Med.* 10:303–21
53. Holford NHG. 1998. Simulation based evaluation of an enrichment trial design for Alzheimer's disease. *Clin. Pharmacol. Ther.* 63(2):200
54. Holford NHG. 1997. Modelling therapeutic effects and disease progress. In *Modeling and Simulation of Clinical Tri-*

J. Clin. Pharmacol. Ther. 35(10):469–74

als in *Drug Development and Regulation*, pp. 61–62. Washington, DC: Cent. Drug Dev. Sci., Georgetown Univ. Med. Cent.

55. El-Tahtawy AA, Jackson AJ, Ludden TM. 1995. Evaluation of bioequivalence of highly variable drugs using Monte Carlo simulations. I. Estimation of rate of absorption for single and multiple dose trials using Cmax. *Pharm. Res.* 12(11):1634–41

56. Hale MD. 1997. Using population pharmacokinetics for planning a randomized concentration-controlled trial with a binary response. In *European Cooperation in the Field of Scientific and Technical Research*, ed. L Aarons, LP Balant, M Danhof, pp. 227–35. Geneva, Switzerland: Eur. Comm.

57. Hale MD, Nicholls AJ, Bullingham RES, Hene RH, Hoitsman A, Squifflet JP, et al. 1998. The pharmacokinetic-pharmacodynamic relationship for mycophenolate mofetil in renal transplantation. *Clin. Pharmacol. Ther.* 64:672–83

58. Bies R, Ko HC, Gobburu J, Burak E, Slusher B, et al. 1999. The relationship of pharmacokinetic metrics to efficacy in pre-clinical rat middle cerebral artery occlusion (MCAO) studies for NAAL-1, a novel NAALADASE inhibitor. *Pharm. Res.* In press

59. Flexner C, van der Horst C, Jacobson MA, Powderly W, Duncanson F, et al. 1994. Relationship between plasma concentrations of 3'-deoxy-3'-fluorothymidine (alovudine) and antiretroviral activity in two concentration-controlled trials. *J. Infect. Dis.* 170:1394–403

60. Metry JM, Meyer UA, eds. 1998. *Drug Regimen Compliance: Issues in Clinical Trials and Patient Management.* West Sussex, UK: Wiley

61. Peck CC, Barrett BB. 1979. Nonlinear least-squares regression: programs for microcomputers. *J. Pharmacokinet. Biopharm.* 7:537–41

62. Krall RL, Engleman KH, Ko HC, Peck CC. 1998. Clinical trial modeling and simulation—work in progress. *Drug Inf. J.* 32(4):971–76

63. Gobburu JVS, Holford NHG, Ko HC, Peck CC. 1999. Model optimization, via "lateral validation" for purposes of clinical trial simulation. *Clin. Pharm. Ther.* 65(2):164

64. The Parkinson Study Group. 1996. Impact of deprenyl and tocopherol treatment on Parkinson's disease in DATATOP subjects not requiring levodopa. *Ann. Neurol.* 39:29–36

65. Mandema JW. 1997. Design and analysis of dose-ranging studies for analgesics. See Ref. 73, pp. 65–66

66. Mandema JW, Stanski DR. 1996. Population pharmacodynamic model for ketorolac analgesia. *Clin. Pharmacol. Ther.* 60:619–35

67. Muir KT. 1997. Simulation of phase I and II studies for a new oral antidiabetic agent. See Ref. 73, pp. 45–46

68. Veyrat-Follet C, Bruno R, Montay G, Rhodes GR. 1999. Application of clinical trial simulation in exploring the safety profile of docetaxel in cancer patients. *Clin. Pharm. Ther.* 65(2):198

69. Schoenhoff MBM, Mandema J. 1999. Clinical trial simulation: retrospective analysis of dose ranging trials in detrusor instability with tolterodine. *Clin. Pharm. Ther.* 65(2):203

70. Herman D, Weiner D. 1997. A Phase II PK/PD simulation: study of a 5-alpha reductase inhibitor. See Ref. 73, pp. 49–51

71. Wada DR, Engleman K, Ellis S, Warwick M, Marshall P, et al. 1999. Design of a phase II efficacy trial for a GPIIB/IIIA antagonist using computer simulation. *Clin. Pharmacol. Ther.* 65(2):182

72. Gastonguay MR, Pentikis HS, Alexander MT, Lee L. 1999. Applying modeling and simulation to improve the design of a clinical efficacy trial. *Clin. Pharmacol. Ther.* 65(2):181

73. Cent. Drug Dev. Sci. 1997. *Modeling and Simulation of Clinical Trials in Drug Development and Regulation.* Herndon, VA: Cent. Drug Dev. Sci.

Annu. Rev. Pharmacol. Toxicol. 2000. 40:235–71

THE REGULATOR OF G PROTEIN SIGNALING FAMILY

Luc De Vries, Bin Zheng, Thierry Fischer, Eric Elenko, and Marilyn G. Farquhar

Department of Cellular and Molecular Medicine, University of California, San Diego, La Jolla, California 92093; e-mail: ldevries@ucsd.edu, bzheng@ucsd.edu, tfischer@ucsd.edu, eelenko@ucsd.edu, mfarquhar@ucsd.edu

Key Words   RGS, GAP, G protein, signal transduction

■ **Abstract**   Regulator of G protein signaling (RGS) proteins are responsible for the rapid turnoff of G protein–coupled receptor signaling pathways. The major mechanism whereby RGS proteins negatively regulate G proteins is via the GTPase activating protein activity of their RGS domain. Structural and mutational analyses have characterized the RGS/Gα interaction in detail, explaining the molecular mechanisms of the GTPase activating protein activity of RGS proteins. More than 20 RGS proteins have been isolated, and there are indications that specific RGS proteins regulate specific G protein–coupled receptor pathways. This specificity is probably created by a combination of cell type–specific expression, tissue distribution, intracellular localization, posttranslational modifications, and domains other than the RGS domain that link them to other signaling pathways. In this review we discuss what has been learned so far about the role of RGS proteins in regulating G protein–coupled receptor signaling and point out areas that may be fruitful for future research.

RGS PROTEINS: INTRODUCTION TO A FAMILY OF GAPS FOR Gα SUBUNITS

Regulation of G Protein–Coupled Receptor Signaling

G protein–coupled receptor (GPCR) signaling pathways are involved in cellular responses to extracellular stimuli and need to be tightly regulated, both short-term and long-term. Most of the short-term regulation takes place at the level of the receptor and the heterotrimeric G protein. The best-described receptor regulatory mechanism is the agonist-dependent "disconnection" of the β-adrenergic receptor from the transducing G protein via phosphorylation of the receptor by G protein–coupled receptor kinases (GRKs), arrestin binding, followed by receptor dephosphorylation in endosomes and recycling to the plasma membrane (PM) (1). At the G protein level, phosphorylation of G_z and acetylation of G_s have been

0362–1642/00/0415–0235$14.00

shown to play a short-term regulatory role (2, 3), and myristoylation and reversible palmitoylation changes the affinity of G proteins for membranes (4, 5). Long-term modulation of certain G protein mRNA levels by transcriptional regulation has been documented, but at the protein level G proteins are generally very stable molecules with long half-lives (6). None of the above-described regulatory mechanisms can explain the rapid turnoff of G protein signaling with satisfaction. Rapid turnoff of G proteins can be accomplished by accelerating their return to the inactivated state, and this is exactly one of the mechanisms of regulator of G protein signaling (RGS) protein function.

The ability of cells to negatively regulate signaling on both the receptor and G protein level might appear redundant, but RGS proteins and GRKs play distinct roles in turning off signaling. GRKs prevent additional ligands from acting on receptors, whereas RGS proteins shorten signals that have already been generated by inactivating G proteins.

The activation-inactivation cycle of G proteins and the factors that influence the kinetics of this cycle are represented in Figure 1. Factors that regulate the speed of the different steps in the G protein cycle clearly have a major impact on the kinetics of the GPCR signaling system. These factors are GTPase activating proteins (GAPs) and guanine exchange factors (GEFs) isolated more than 10 years ago for the small G proteins (7). In the classical G protein paradigm at the PM, the receptor activates the G protein, but a fast turnoff mechanism generally appli-

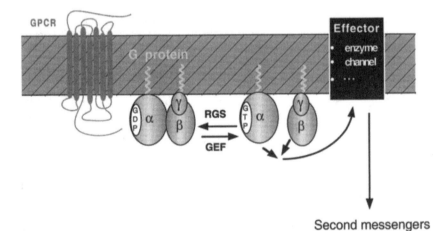

Second messengers

Figure 1 Effect of regulator of G protein signaling (RGS) proteins on the classical G protein cycle at the plasma membrane. A G protein–coupled receptor (GPCR) serves as a guanine nucleotide exchange factor (GEF) that activates the G protein by enhancing GDP dissociation from the Gα subunit. Gα and Gβγ dissociate and stimulate their respective effectors. RGS proteins serve as GTPase activating proteins that accelerate GTP hydrolysis and thereby return the Gα subunit to its inactivated GDP-bound form, followed by reassembly of the heterotrimer.

cable to (almost) all G proteins emerged only 4 years ago with the discovery of the mammalian RGS protein family. Soon thereafter the GAP activity of RGS proteins was shown to be the major mechanism of negative regulation (8). Since then, a number of reviews on RGS proteins have been published (9–17).

Although all of the above-described regulatory events take place at the PM, it should be noted that G proteins have also been found on intracellular membranes such as Golgi membranes, and the regulation of G proteins on intracellular membranes might be different from the classical G protein paradigm at the PM (18).

Discovery of the RGS Family

RGS proteins evolutionarily stem from the Sst2 gene in *Saccharomyces cereviseae,* involved in desensitization of the yeast pheromone response (19, 20).

The recognition of a distinct mammalian family took place when a 130-residue homologous domain—defined as the RGS domain—was described in several proteins at approximately the same time (21–23), and the RGS domain was demonstrated to be responsible for binding of the RGS protein to the Gα subunit (21). Genetic studies in yeast also suggested a direct interaction between Sst2, the yeast RGS, and Gpa1, the pheromone receptor–linked Gα subunit (24–26). That RGS proteins can regulate G protein–mediated signaling events in vivo was demonstrated by the findings that RGS1, RGS2, RGS3, and RGS4 could attenuate mitogen-activated protein kinase (MAPK) activation by interleukin 8 (IL-8) and RGS2 and RGS4 can complement the defective pheromone response in yeast *sst2* mutants, which suggests that they play a role in the negative regulation of G protein signaling (23, 27). In the 4-year period since the family was originally recognized, many more mammalian RGS homologs have been isolated (17). To date, approximately 25 different RGS proteins have been identified in mammals (Figure 2). They all contain the diagnostic RGS domain, and many contain additional domains with different functions that link RGS proteins to other signaling pathways (17).

In this review we summarize our present knowledge of the function of RGS proteins in GPCR signaling and what has been learned so far about their regulation, expression, localization, and molecular structure, including the importance of non-RGS domains in certain RGS proteins. It is also our goal to point out what we do not know and by doing so to stimulate research in these directions.

THE FUNCTION OF RGS PROTEINS IN GPCR SIGNALING PATHWAYS

Molecular Mechanisms of RGS Protein Function

There are three known mechanisms by which most RGS proteins act in vivo to turn off signaling pathways. First and foremost, RGS proteins are GAPs, initially demonstrated by in vitro assays using recombinant proteins (8, 28–32) or receptor/

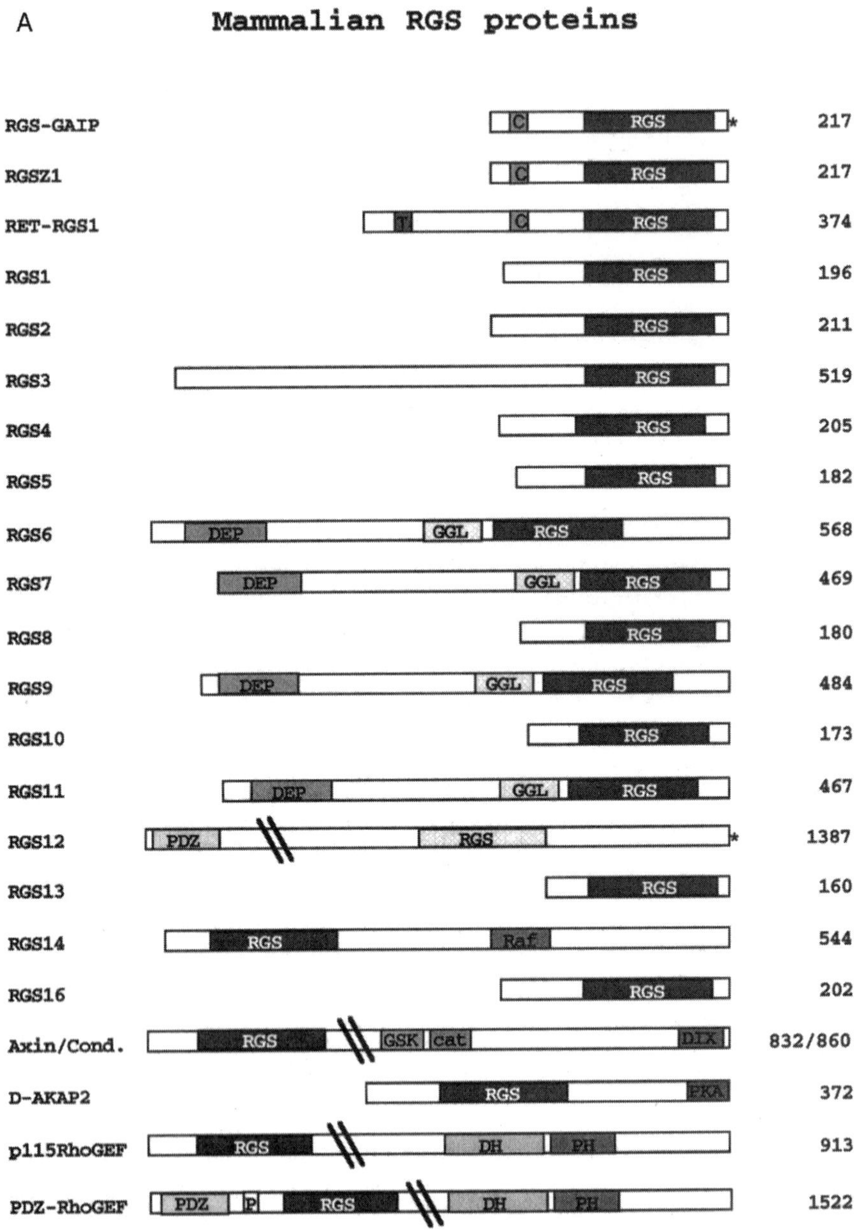

A   **Mammalian RGS proteins**

RGS-GAIP	217
RGSZ1	217
RET-RGS1	374
RGS1	196
RGS2	211
RGS3	519
RGS4	205
RGS5	182
RGS6	568
RGS7	469
RGS8	180
RGS9	484
RGS10	173
RGS11	467
RGS12	1387
RGS13	160
RGS14	544
RGS16	202
Axin/Cond.	832/860
D-AKAP2	372
p115RhoGEF	913
PDZ-RhoGEF	1522

Figure 2   For legend and Figure 2b see next page.

B   **Non-mammalian RGS proteins**

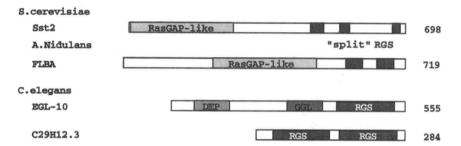

Figure 2   Schematic representation of mammalian (A) and nonmammalian (B) regulator of G protein signaling (RGS) proteins. The total number of amino acids for each family member are indicated to the right. RGS, RGS domain. Because of space limitations, most *Caenorhabditis elegans* and none of the *Drosophila* RGS proteins are included. RasGAP, RasGAP-like domain; C, cysteine string domain; Cat, β-catenin binding domain; DEP, DEP domain (Dishevelled/EGL-10/pleckstrin homology); DH, double homology domain; DIX, dishevelled homology domain; GGL, GGL (G protein gamma-like) domain (homology to Gγ); GSK, glycogen synthase kinase 3b binding domain; *, PDZ-binding motif; PDZ, PDZ domain (PSD95/Dlg/ZO1 homology); PH, pleckstrin homology domain; PID, PID domain (phosphotyrosine interacting domain); PKA, PKA-anchoring domain; Raf, B-raf homology domain; T, transmembrane domain.

G protein/effector complexes reconstituted in phospholipid vesicles (33). Their GAP function was later confirmed in vivo in a number of systems. For example, RGS4 and G alpha interacting protein (GAIP) attenuated bradykinin (G_q-mediated) and somatostatin (G_i-mediated) signaling when overexpressed in HEK293 cells, and this effect was shown to be due to their GAP activity (34).

Second, RGS proteins can act as effector antagonists that prevent G proteins from binding to their effectors by physically blocking this interaction. For example, recombinant PLC-β1 can displace RGS4 bound to G_q-GDP-AlF$_4^-$ (which mimics the GTP → GDP transition state). Furthermore, RGS4 is able to inhibit PLC-β1–catalyzed phosphoinositol hydrolysis induced by GTPγS-activated G_q (33).

Third, RGS proteins can alter the number of free βγ subunits available to interact with their effectors by enhancing the affinity of Gα subunits for βγ subunits after GTP hydrolysis, thus accelerating reformation of the heterotrimer. Evidence for this mechanism came from the findings that (a) overexpression of RGS4 attenuated MAPK activation by IL-8 (G_i) and bombesin (G_q), a process that involves the βγ subunit of the G protein (23, 35), and (b) overexpression of RGS1,

RGS2, RGS4, and RGS8 accelerated the turning off of G protein–coupled inwardly rectifying K^+ channels (GIRKs) (30, 36), known to be activated (opened) by direct binding of $\beta\gamma$ subunits to the channel (37, 38). Unexpectedly, overexpression of the same RGS proteins also results in increased activation of GIRKs (30, 36, 39–41). Transfection of a chimeric protein that can act as a $\beta\gamma$ "sink" reduced the ability of RGS4 to accelerate the kinetics of GIRK activation (39), and the results conflict with the idea that RGS proteins deactivate channels by reducing the number of available $\beta\gamma$ subunits. The mechanism whereby RGS protein increases both the activation and the turnoff of GIRK channels remains a mystery.

The Role of RGS Proteins on GPCR Signaling in Various Cell Types

Considerable work has been focused on demonstrating the importance of RGS proteins in the function of various cell types (Table 1). Every cell type seems to express several RGS proteins (17), but their functions have only begun to unfold. Studies involving in situ hybridization (32, 42–47) or reverse transcriptase–polymerase chain reaction (48) demonstrated that numerous RGS proteins are expressed in the brain, where they display a cell type–specific distribution pattern, but there is little or no information available on which RGSs are found in specific cell types and which GPCR pathways are regulated by each. The presence of many different types of serpentine receptors and G protein–regulated channels in the nervous system suggests that RGS proteins could play a role in the selective regulation of signaling pathways activated by neurotransmitters and psychogenic agents. Indeed there are already indications that this is the case (see below). To decipher the complexity of the regulation of GCPR signaling pathways, including the role of RGS proteins in different parts of the brain, represents a challenging task for the future.

Ten different RGS proteins have been found in cardiac myocytes (49), but the only RGS protein whose functions have been investigated in detail in this system is RGS4. Overexpression of RGS4 attenuated hypertrophy induced by phenylephrine (G_i- or G_q-coupled) or endothelin-1 (G_q-coupled) in neonatal rat cardiomyocytes (50). Also, in both a cell culture model and in living animals, RGS4 mRNA levels increased during cardiac hypertrophy (51). This implies that RGS4 is induced in the heart to keep the process of hypertrophy in check following cardiac overload and suggests the existence of a negative feedback loop for long-term regulation of cardiac hypertrophy.

Secretion of many hormones is mediated by GPCR signaling, but so far little is known about their regulation by RGS proteins in any system. The best examples to date are as follows: (a) In Cos cells, overexpression of RGS3 inhibited the ability of gonadotropin-releasing hormone to raise inositol trisphosphate levels (52), and (b) in the pancreatic beta TC3 cell line overexpression of RGS2 abolished the ability of glucose-dependent insulinotropic polypeptide (GIP), via its

TABLE 1 Effects of overexpression of RGS proteins on second messengers and other cellular functions[a]

RGE	Transfected cell lines	Responses	References
GAIP	HT-29, Caco-2 (colon)	Stimulates $G\alpha_{i3}$-inhibited autophagy	82
	LLC-PK$_1$ (kidney)	Retards trafficking of secretory protein	103
	Dorsal (microinjected) root ganglia	Accelerates GABA- and NE-induced desensitization of N-type Ca^{2+} channel currents	61
GAIP, RGS4	NG108 neuronal cells	Reduces leu-enkephalin inhibition of adenylyl cyclase	33
	HEK293T cells	Reduces SST-induced inhibition of adenylyl cyclase	162
		Inhibits IP3 formation by bradykinin	
RGS1	HS-Sultan (B cells)	Reduces PAF-induced MAPK activation	23
RGS1, −2, −4	Myocytes, CHO	Accelerates ACh-induced deactivation of GIRK	36
RGS1, −2, −3, −4, −16	HEK293	Reduces IL-8–and carbachol-induced MAPK activation	92, 36
RGS2, −9	βTC3 (pancreatic), L293	Inhibits GIP-induced cAMP response	53
	Melanophores (electroporation)	Decreases pigment aggregation induced by morphine	46
RGS3	HIT-15 (pancreatic)	Reverses inhibition of insulin secretion induced by epinephrine	163
	COS-1	Suppresses IP3 release induced by GnRH	52
	HMC (mesangial)	Decreases ET-1–induced Ca^{2+} response and MAPK activation	164
	L1/2 cells (lymphoi)	Inhibits chemoattractant (IL-8, MCP-1)-induced migration and integrin-dependent adhesion	55
RGS3, −8	HEK293	Releases carbachol-induced N-type calcium channels inhibition	165

(*continued*)

G_s-coupled GPCR, to cause secretion of insulin (53). It is interesting that GIP induced an agonist-dependent interaction between RGS2 and G_s, shown by immunoprecipitation in RGS2-transfected L293 cells (53). The mRNAs of at least nine

TABLE 1 (*continued*) Effects of overexpression of RGS proteins on second messengers and other cellular functions[a]

RGE	Transfected cell lines	Responses	References
RGS4	*Xenopus* oocytes (microinjected) CA1 hippocampal neurons	Blocks glutamate-induced activation of $I_{C1(Ca)}$ and I_{Girk} as well as glutamate-induced activation of I_{AHP}	166
	Cardiomyocytes	Blocks ANF and MLC-2 gene transcription induced by ET-1 and epinephrine as well as myofilament organization and cell growth	50
	COS-7	Inhibits bombesin- and dopamine-induced activation of MAPK and IP3 formation	35
	Pancreatic acini (microinjected)	Inhibits Ca^{2+} mobilization and $C1^-$ current induced by carbachol, bombesin and CCK	62
	Xenopus oocytes (microinjected)	Potentiates μ-opioid agonist-induced GIRK desensitization	41
	HEK293, CHO-K1	Induces basal $I_{K(ACh)}$ currents; induces basal N-type Ca^{2+} channels currents	39
RGS4, −10	Superior cortical ganglions (intranuclear injections)	Accelerate deactivation of NE-induced N-type calcium channels currents	167
RGS7	CHO transfected	Reduces 5-HT–induced Ca^{2+} mobilization	43
RGS7, −8	*Xenopus* oocytes	Accelerates dopamine- and ACh-induced GIRK deactivation	30, 40
RGS9	CHO	Accelerates decay of quinpirole (dopaminergic agonist)-induced activation of GIRK	47
RGS12	NIH3	Blocks basal and agonist-mediated (thrombin and LPA) SRF activation	85
RGS16	EcR-CHO	Suppresses PAF-activated p38 MAPK activation	168
	COS-7	Suppresses carbachol-induced MAPK activation	64

[a]ACh, acetylcholine; ANF, atrial natriuretic factor; BK, bradykinin; CCK, cholecystokinin; ET-1, endothelin 1; GABA, γ-amino-n-butyric acid; GIP, glucose-dependent insulinotropic polypeptide; GIRK, G protein–coupled inward rectifying K^+ channels; GnRH, gonadotropin-releasing hormone; 5-HT, serotonin; IL-8, interleukin-8; LPA, lysophosphatidic acid; MLC-2, myosin light chain-2; MCP-1, monocyte chemoattractant protein; NE, norepinephrine; PAF, platelet activating factor; RGS, regulator of G protein signaling; SEF, serum response factor.

RGS proteins are expressed in pituitary, but no cell type–specific expression has been documented in this gland (54).

Another system where GPCR signaling pathways are diverse is the immune system. RGS proteins have been shown to play a role in regulating the actions of cytokines/chemokines secreted by immune cells (15). Overexpression of RGS3 in L1/2 pre-B lymphoma cells stably expressing the chemokine IL-8/CXCR1 receptor (coupled to G_i) abolished IL-8–triggered chemotaxis (55). The ability of the same cells to bind to vascular cell adhesion molecule 1 when stimulated with formyl-methionyl-leucyl-phenylalanine, which has its own G_i-coupled receptor, was also attenuated by overexpression of RGS3 (55). This clearly suggests the involvement of RGS3 in regulating signaling during chemotaxis and cell adhesion signaling. The role of G protein in general and of RGS protein function in the immune system in particular is still in its infancy.

Nearly all the studies to date involve overexpression of RGS proteins. Overexpression studies might give misleading information about the actual role that RGS proteins play within a system. The finding that overexpressed RGS1, RGS2, RGS3, and RGS4 can all complement a yeast strain that is deficient in Sst2 (23) indicates not only that RGS proteins can function in settings that are not physiologically relevant, but also that their RGS domains can act promiscuously. The use of an antisense strategy or RGS knockouts in mice (56–58) will be helpful in determining the specific roles of different RGS proteins.

How Do RGS Proteins Selectively Act on a GPCR Signaling Pathway?

The mechanisms identified so far are the localization of RGS proteins (cell type–specific and intracellular localization), the timing of their expression (transcription), and the presence of other domains outside of the RGS domain that connect to other signaling pathways (17).

For instance, the distinct regional and cell type–specific localization patterns of RGS mRNAs within the brain suggest that spatial segregation allows RGS proteins to specifically associate with neurotransmitter pathways found within particular brain areas (42). Spatial segregation might also be coupled to developmental regulation, as is the case for RGS9. The small transcript of RGS9 is expressed in total brain in embryonic and early postnatal stages (44) but is specifically expressed only in the retina of adult rats (59, 60).

Domains outside the RGS domain are also important for specificity. This was demonstrated in presynaptic N-type Ca^{2+} channels of dorsal root ganglion neurons, which are inhibited by norepinephrine through G_i and G_o pathways. RGS4 and GAIP can selectively accelerate the turnoff rate of these G_i and G_o pathways, respectively (61). When the N terminus of GAIP was deleted, leaving only the RGS domain and the C terminus, selectivity toward the $G\alpha_o$-mediated pathway was lost. Similarly, the N-terminal domain of RGS4 is capable of discriminating between specific G_q-coupled receptors (62). These results collectively imply that

GAIP and RGS4 confer selectivity via two different domains: the RGS domain for Gα specificity and the N-terminal domain for receptor specificity as well as targeting to the PM (see below).

Elucidating the factors that control specificity in the interaction between specific RGS proteins and particular signal transduction pathways clearly requires more research.

GENE STRUCTURE, TISSUE-SPECIFIC EXPRESSION, AND REGULATION

Gene Structure and Chromosomal Localization

Although the RGS domain is present in the yeast Sst2 protein, it is not clear how RGS proteins diverged and/or duplicated from this ancestor to give rise to more than 20 mammalian RGS proteins. Analysis of the gene structure of RGS proteins should help clarify the situation.

The genomic structure of only five mammalian RGS proteins has been described to date—RGS2, RGS3, RGS9, RGS16 [also called RGS-r (63) and a28-RGS14p (64)], and Axin (46, 65–68). Gene sizes vary greatly, from 4 kb (RGS16) to 56 kb (Axin), generally reflecting protein size and number of exons. The open reading frames of the small RGS proteins—RGS2, RGS3, and RGS16—are encoded by five exons. The RGS domain itself in RGS2, RGS3, RGS9, and RGS16 is encoded by three exons, and the sites of the two introns in the RGS domain are conserved in RGS2, RGS3, and RGS16, which suggests a common ancestor gene (66, 67). RGSZ1 also possesses two introns in its RGS domain, but the site of the first intron is not conserved, which suggests it diverged separately from the other RGS genes (69). In contrast to the gene structure of other RGS proteins, the Axin gene has its entire RGS domain, located N terminally, encoded in exon 2 (68). The intron/exon boundaries of the RGS domain of the *Caenorhabditis elegans* gene, EGL-10, do not coincide with those of the small mammalian RGS proteins (22, 66).

Recently, based on protein sequence homologies of RGS domains, the existence of six subfamilies of RGS proteins has been proposed (70). So far, data coming from gene structure analysis fit well with these subfamily designations. Exploring the gene structure should facilitate the classification of RGS proteins into subfamilies and will determine sites of alternative splicing.

Chromosomal localization (see Table 2) should be helpful in determining the potential involvement of RGS proteins in genetic diseases. At least seven RGS genes have been mapped to chromosome 1 by radiation hybrid and fluorescent in situ hybridization analyses (65, 67, 71, 72) (L De Vries, unpublished data). The RGS9 gene has been mapped to the same site on chromosome 17 (q23–24) as the retinitis pigmentosa gene, which suggests a potential involvement of RGS9 in this degenerative retinal disease (47). RGS6 has been mapped to chromosome 14q24.3, a region known to contain an early onset Alzheimer disease gene (72).

TABLE 2 Multiple RGS mRNAs found in tissues and cell types analyzed for their presence by in situ hybridization and Northern blotting[a]

RGS	Chromosomal localization	Tissue expression	Alternative splicing	References
GAIP	20	Ubiquitous, low in brain	NC	21
RET-RGS1	ND	Retina	Yes	32
RGSZ1	ND	Brain	No	69
RGS1	1q31	B-lymphocytes, lung	Yes	71, 75
RGS2	1q31	Ubiquitous	No	169
RGS3	9q31	Ubiquitous	Yes	23, 66
RGS4	1q21	Brain, heart	No	23
RGS5	1q23	Ubiquitous	Yes	170
RGS6	14q24.3	Brain	Yes	72, 141
RGS7	1q42	Brain, B-cells	Yes	156
RGS8	ND	Brain	Yes	30
RGS9	17q23-24	Retina, neurons	Yes	47, 60
RGS10	10	Brain	No	28
RGS11	16p13.3	Brain	Yes	138
RGS12	4p16.3	Lung, brain, spleen, testis	Yes	151
RGS13	1	Lung	ND	unpublished data
RGS14	5qter	Brain, spleen, lung	Yes	151
RGS15	ND	ND	ND	unpublished data
RGS16	1q25-q31	Retina, pituitary, liver, ubiquitous?	NC	63, 67
Axin	16	Ubiquitous, greatest in thymus, testis	NC	68
Conductin (Axil)	17q23-q24	Lung, thymus	No	159, 171
D-AKAP2	ND	Ubiquitous, greatest in testis	Yes	34
p115RhoGEF	ND	Ubiquitus, leukocytes	Yes	145
PDZ-RhoGEF	ND	Ubiquitous, low in liver, lung, colon	Yes	133

[a]Information compiled from published data or data submitted to GenBank. For some regulator of G protein signaling (RGS) proteins, little information is available. ND, Not determined; NC, not clear.

RGS mRNAs Are Widely Expressed and Show Multiple Alternatively Spliced Forms

Multiple RGS mRNAs have been found in all tissues and cell types analyzed for their presence by in situ hybridization and Northern blotting (Table 2). At least nine different RGS mRNAs are expressed in pituitary (54) and in specific regions of the brain (42). Some RGS mRNAs, such as RGS3, RGS5, and GAIP, show a broad tissue distribution, which suggests a more general function (21, 23, 73). Other RGS mRNAs, such as RET-RGS1 (retina), RGSZ1 (caudate nucleus-brain), RGS8 (brain), and RGS1 (lymphocytes), show a narrow tissue expression (30, 32, 69, 74, 75), hinting that they have more specialized roles. The expression of RET-RGS1 has recently been shown to be restricted to the plexiform layers of the retina, implicating this molecule in retina-specific synaptic transduction rather than in phototransduction (76). The detection of mRNAs of RGS proteins by Northern blot analysis or in situ hybridization has provided useful information on cell type– or tissue-specific expression of these RGS proteins, but only in combination with data coming from tissue distribution, intracellular localization of the protein, and in vivo studies can we hope to establish the function of RGS proteins in specific locations.

The existence of alternatively spliced forms of RGS proteins was suggested when two major transcripts of different size were detected for RGS3 (23). Since then, alternative transcripts have been observed for many RGS proteins, but for the most part they have remained uncharacterized (Table 2). The most interesting examples of alternatively spliced RGS mRNAs are RGS12 and RGS9. RGS12 contains an N-terminal PDZ domain (PSD-95–Dishevelled–ZO1 homology, see below) and an extreme C-terminal PDZ-binding motif (ATFV). Four alternatively spliced forms of RGS12 allow a full combination of presence or absence of both its PDZ domain and its PDZ-binding motifs. Results obtained by surface plasmon resonance suggest that in the case of the alternatively spliced form of RGS12 that contains both motifs, the PDZ domain interacts with the PDZ-binding motif (77). This intramolecular interaction would create an additional regulatory mechanism for RGS12.

The RGS9 gene produces two major alternatively spliced mRNAs that give rise to substantially different C termini. RGS9–1—which is 191 amino acids shorter than RGS9–2—is specifically expressed in the retina, where it serves as a specific GAP for transducin (59, 60), and RGS9–2 is specifically expressed in the striatum, where it is involved in desensitization of $G_{i/o}$-coupled μ-opioid receptors (46, 47). The specific functions of the different C termini of RGS9–1 and RGS9–2 are currently unknown, but this region is likely to contain information that dictates specific interactions (17).

It is clear that alternative splicing of RGS proteins significantly expands the interaction possibilities of these proteins in GPCR signaling pathways and their possible functional consequences.

Transcriptional Regulation of RGS Proteins: Role in Desensitization

The majority of the data on desensitization or long-term (as opposed to short-term) regulation by RGS proteins fits into the paradigm of the negative feedback loop, summarized as follows: The continuous action of a ligand on a GPCR-linked signaling pathway increases the level of a particular RGS, which then turns off signaling through one of the three mechanisms mentioned earlier. The negative feedback paradigm was first shown for the yeast Sst2 gene: Prolonged pheromone treatment induces increased transcription of Sst2 mRNA (24, 26). The first mammalian negative feedback loop was described for RGS1, which is induced by platelet activating factor via a GPCR. Transiently induced RGS1 attenuates platelet activating factor–induced MAPK activity (23).

Generally, the levels of G protein expression do not vary significantly under various physiological conditions, but as already indicated, several RGS mRNAs have been shown to do so. This suggests that transcriptional regulation of RGS proteins is an important factor in turning down G protein signaling. But higher levels of a particular RGS mRNA do not necessarily mean more GAP activity on a specific G protein signaling pathway, as regulation at the protein level is also important (see posttranslational modifications). Enhanced expression of RGS proteins would be expected to lead to long-term regulation, resulting in diminished signaling through G protein linked pathways (i.e. desensitization).

RGS mRNAs can be induced by a variety of factors. RGS1 and RGS2 were originally isolated because their mRNA is transcriptionally up-regulated in B-lymphocytes and mononuclear cell mitogens (phorbol myristate acetate) and concanavalin A, respectively (65, 71, 75, 78). It is assumed that they negatively regulate GPCR signaling leading to cell proliferation in hematopoietic cells, where mediation via Gα subunits has been implicated (15). RGS2 mRNA levels increase in response to the calcium ionophore, ionomycin, in mononuclear cells (79) and to GIP, which raises cAMP levels in pancreatic β-cells (53), which suggests that agonist-stimulated Ca^{2+} and cAMP induce RGS2 mRNA. Again, these data fit the negative feedback loop scenario mentioned above.

In brain, RGS2 mRNA is rapidly induced in neurons of the hippocampus, cortex, and striatum by plasticity-evoking stimuli, and thus RGS2 may play an important role in the long-term regulation of neuro- and psycho-pharmacological signaling pathways (80). A "survey" study of RGS mRNA expression in the rat striatum after a single amphetamine injection showed that the level of RGS2 mRNA rapidly increases and subsequently decreases, whereas RGS3 and RGS8 mRNAs increase steadily and RGS9 mRNA decreases steadily (81). Prior exposure to amphetamine did not the reduce the induction of RGS2 and RGS3 mRNAs. This suggests that transcription of these genes is not turned off as a result of amphetamine-induced tolerance (81). These findings suggest that transcription of RGS mRNAs are differentially regulated by neuronal stimuli, which may give clues as to the function of RGS proteins.

The mRNA level for GAIP decreases during enterocyte differentiation. This decrease was mimicked in undifferentiated enterocytes by interrupting the G_{i3} GTPase cycle (pertussis toxin treatment or overexpression of a GTPase-deficient mutant). Thus, the expression of GAIP is dependent on G_{i3} activity and on the differentiation state of the enterocytes (82).

RGS16 mRNA is induced by serum and by the p53 tumor suppressor, and overexpression of the protein inhibits the activation of the MAPK pathway (64). These findings define RGS16 as a transcriptionally inducible component of a p53-controlled negative-feedback mechanism involved in cell proliferation and/or apoptosis.

To date, the promoters of relatively few RGS genes have been studied. In the case of RGS2, binding sites for several transcription factors (AP1, CRE, and others) have been described (65). Of particular interest is the fact that the RGS2 promoter also has putative binding sites for NFAT, a transcription factor activated by cyclosporin A. Because cyclosporins are involved in cell cycle progression, this suggests a role for RGS2 in regulating cell cycle progression of mononuclear cells (83). The RGS16 promoter probably contains serum response elements and p53 binding sites, because both serum and p53 induce RGS16 gene expression (64).

An important issue that has not been addressed is the role of RGS mRNA stability on the expression levels of RGS proteins. The exception is the study of the RGS4 mRNA, whose half-life of 3 h remained unchanged after forskolin treatment of PC12 cells (84).

There is evidence that RGS proteins can themselves indirectly regulate the transcription of other genes. A recent and very interesting example is the inhibitory role of RGS12 in the activation of the serum response factor, which is mediated by G_q and G_{12} (85, 86).

Promoter analysis and studies on transcriptional regulation of RGS genes should contribute significantly to our knowledge of incoming signaling pathways that induce or silence their expression.

INTRACELLULAR LOCALIZATION OF RGS PROTEINS

Posttranslational Modifications

Posttranslational modifications of signaling proteins generally play a role in their cellular localization and their stability and/or conformation. Palmitoylation (on cysteine residues in the N terminus) and myristoylation (on glycine residues in the N terminus) are two such modifications that have been reported to play a role in the affinity of G proteins for membranes and their translocation from the cytosol to the plasma membrane (87, 88). A parallelism can be drawn for certain RGS proteins whose posttranslational modifications may also affect their function.

GAIP, RGSZ1, and RET-RGS1 have a cysteine string motif in their N terminus (32, 69, 89). This motif is heavily palmitoylated in the cysteine string protein family and is responsible for their membrane attachment (90). Palmitoylated GAIP is detected only in membrane fractions (89), but the direct involvement of the cysteine string motif as well as of the palmitoylation itself in membrane association, although likely, remains to be demonstrated. It is intriguing that

RGS4, which lacks a cysteine string motif, can also be palmitoylated, but palmitoylation is not required for the translocation of RGS4 from the cytosol to the PM. Instead, the entire N terminus seems to be necessary for its PM localization (91). Similar results were obtained for RGS16, which contains the same conserved palmitoylation sites as RGS4 and RGS5. The level of its membrane association and its in vitro GAP activity was unchanged in palmitoyl-defective RGS16. However, its negative effect on G_i (cAMP levels) and G_q (MAPK activity) pathways was significantly attenuated in vivo (92). The authors suggest that palmitoylation might be important for localizing RGS and G proteins on the same membranes or membrane microdomains or it might play a role in the affinity of these proteins for one another.

Several RGS proteins contain putative myristoylation sites in their N termini, but the function of myristoylation, including its role in membrane attachment of RGS proteins has not yet been investigated.

Many of the components of the GPCR cascade undergo phosphorylation, including receptors (93), α and β subunits of G proteins [for review see Neer (94)] and effectors (95). Indications are that this may also be true for RGS proteins. Several RGS proteins, including GAIP (21), contain conserved potential phosphorylation sites for casein kinase II and for protein kinase C in their RGS domain as well as nonconserved sites outside their RGS domain. Recently it was shown that GAIP is phosphorylated and that only the membrane-associated pool is phosphorylated (95a). This suggests that the membrane association of GAIP may be regulated in part by phosphorylation. Putative phosphorylation sites are located in GAIP's RGS domain, which could regulate its GAP activity, and in its N terminus, which could modify its membrane association. Recombinant GAIP could be phosphorylated at its N terminus by purified casein kinase II, and Ser24 was identified as one of the phosphorylation sites (95a). The role of phosphorylation of RGS proteins has not yet been been linked to their function. Phosphorylation can be expected to represent an important regulatory event in controling the effect of RGS proteins on G protein signaling and localization.

Membrane Attachment and Intracellular Localization

The specificity of an RGS protein depends on its intracellular localization: It cannot assume its role as a GAP without making direct contact with its $G\alpha$ partner. G proteins are classically assumed to be localized on the cytoplasmic face of the PM in close contact with transmembrane receptors, but some $G\alpha$ subunits have also been localized on intracellular membranes (96, 97), where they have been assumed to play a role in vesicular trafficking (18). G proteins have also been detected on caveolae and reported to interact directly with caveolin (98). This suggests RGS proteins may also be found on several types of membranes, including membrane microdomains defined as lipid rafts, which are rich in cholesterol and sphingolipids (99).

Most RGS proteins are present in the cell in two pools, a cytosolic and a membrane-bound pool, and the available evidence suggests that many RGS proteins can be translocated from a cytoplasmic pool onto membranes (17, 25).

Few RGS proteins have been precisely localized inside the cell. Sst2, GAIP, RGSZ1, RGS3, RGS4, RGS7, and RGS9 are all membrane bound to a certain extent (25, 52, 59, 60, 69, 89, 91, 100, 101), but only RGS4, Sst2, RGS9, and GAIP have been localized at the subcellular level. Both membrane-bound and cytosolic pools of endogenous GAIP were found whose ratio seems to depend on the cell type (89, 102–104). By immunoelectron microscopy, endogenous GAIP was localized on clathrin-coated pits and vesicles (CCVs) close to the PM in liver and on budding CCVs in the *trans* Golgi region in pituitary (102), which suggested a role for GAIP in vesicular transport. In addition, GAIP on isolated liver CCVs was shown to be an active GAP in vitro for G_{i3} (105). GAIP was also reported on nonclathrin-coated vesicles close to Golgi stacks in LLC-PK1 epithelial cells (103). In this cell type, overexpression of GAIP retarded trafficking along the secretory pathway. Sst2 was found both at the PM and in the Golgi region by immunofluorescence in yeast (25). The membrane attachment of RET-RGS1 is likely because it has a putative transmembrane region and a cysteine string motif (32). RGS9, the specific GAP for transducin, is tightly associated with membranes and not detectable in a cytosolic form (59, 60). The presence of a DEP domain (from Dishevelled, EGL-10, and pleckstrin) in the N terminus of RGS9 might facilitate its tight membrane attachment (see below), but electrostatic interactions with membranes have also been proposed (59).

The membrane-bound pool of RGS4 localizes at the PM and overexpression of the activated form of G_{i2} (G_{i2}Q205L) results in translocation of RGS4 from the cytoplasm to the PM, as detected by immunofluorescence in 293T cells (100).

Each RGS protein may have its own mechanism for binding to membranes, but a common factor seems to be that attachment of RGS proteins to membranes in the proximity of $G\alpha$ subunits would enhance their performance, and translocation could be a supplementary regulatory component. One key question remains: If multiple RGS proteins are expressed and localized on membranes in the same cell, are they associated with the same or with different membranes?

In summary, the subcellular distribution of RGS proteins is still poorly documented, yet in order to elucidate the G-protein signaling pathways they regulate, their precise intracellular localization is essential.

MOLECULAR STRUCTURE OF RGS PROTEINS

Primary Structure of RGS Proteins

An alignment of RGS domains from different mammalian RGS proteins is depicted in Figure 3. From the alignment it can be seen that most of the RGS domains (RGS1–16, GAIP, RGSZ1, RET-RGS) are closely related, displaying

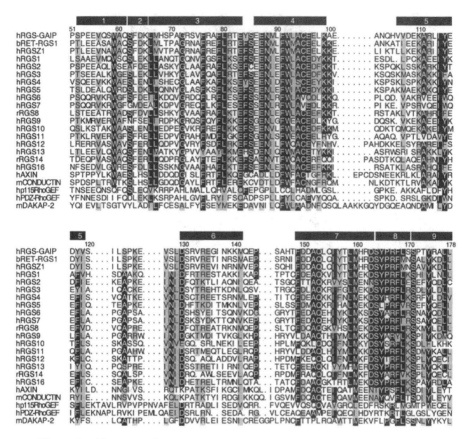

Figure 3 Alignment of RGS domains for mammalian regulator of G protein signaling (RGS) proteins. Amino acid sequences of RGS domains from 23 mammalian RGS proteins were aligned using Clustal W 1.7 and manual adjustments. (*Black, gray*) Conserved residues and similar residues, respectively, shaded by MacBoxshade2.15. The regions of RGS domains are defined based on work by Tesmer et al (106). Regions of the nine alpha helixes found in RGS4 are indicated (*black frames above the alignment*). h, *Homo Sapiens;* m, *Mus musculus;* r, *Rattus norvegicus;* b, *Bos taurus.* The accession numbers for the sequences used are as follows: hRGS-GAIP, P49795; bRET-RGS1, P79348; hRGSZ1, NP_003693; hRGS1, NP_002913; hRGS2, NP_002914; hRGS3, P49796; hRGS4, P49798; hRGS5, NP_003608; hRGS6, NP_004287; hRGS7, AAD34290; rRGS8, BAA23680; hRGS9, AAC64040; hRGS10, NP_002916; hRGS11, AAC69175; hRGS12, O14924; hRGS13, NP_002918; rRGS14, O08773; hRGS16, O15492; hAxin, AAC51624; mConductin, AAC26047; hp115-RhoGEF, NP_004697; hPDZ-RhoGEF, BAA20834; mD-AKAP2, AAC61898.

approximately 35–55% identity, whereas the RGS domains in Axin, D-AKAP2, conductin, p115 RhoGEF, and PDZ-Rho GEF are more distantly related to the others, sharing only ∼10–30% identity.

By contrast, the regions outside the RGS domain are diverse (Figure 2). Some RGS proteins are relatively small, approximately 20–25 kDa in size, and contain very short regions around the RGS domain. Others contain large N-terminal and/ or C-terminal regions. The regions outside the RGS domain usually have other structural and functional features, such as coiled-coil, DEP, DH, GGL, PDZ, PH, and PTB domains (discussed below).

RGS proteins have also been found in other eukaryotic organisms. In the *Saccharomyces* Sst2 protein and the *Aspergillus* FlbA protein, the RGS domains are interrupted and divided into segments (Figure 2*B*), which reportedly would not cause dramatic changes in their three-dimensional structure (106). Analysis of the nearly complete *C. elegans* genome revealed that it has 12 RGS domain–containing proteins (107). One contains two RGS domains (Figure 2*B*). In *Drosophila,* four RGS domain–containing proteins—dRGS7 (108), Loco (109), d-Axin (110), and dRhoGEF2 (111)—have been identified. The functional roles of most of the invertebrate RGS proteins remain to be investigated.

An intriguing finding is that the N-terminal region of most GRKs share significant sequence similarity (up to 30%) with the RGS domain (27). The function of this region in GRKs is currently under active investigation.

Three-Dimensional Structure of RGS Proteins

RGS4-Gi1 Complex   The crystal structure of the RGS domain of RGS4 in complex with G_{i1} in its transition state (RGS4-G_{i1}-Mg^{2+}-GDP-AlF_4^-) was determined by Tesmer and colleagues (106). In this complex, the RGS domain is made up of nine alpha helices that form two subdomains—a terminal subdomain ($\alpha1$–$\alpha3$, $\alpha8$–$\alpha9$) and a four-helix bundle subdomain ($\alpha4$–$\alpha7$) (Figure 4). The base of the four-helix bundle, including the $\alpha3$–$\alpha4$, $\alpha5$–$\alpha6$, and $\alpha7$–$\alpha8$ loops, constitutes the G_{i1}-contacting surface. In G_{i1}, the RGS4 binding sites are located in the three switch regions, where there are dramatic conformational changes during the GTP cycle and GTPase hydrolysis (112).

Mechanism of GAP Activity: Comparison with GAPs for Small GTPases
Besides G_{i1}-RGS4, the crystal structures of several small GTPases in complex with their corresponding GAPs were also resolved recently, including Ras-RasGAP (113), Rho-RhoGAP (114), Cdc42-Cdc42GAP (115), and ARF1-ARF-GAP (116). The structures of these complexes revealed two common features that characterize the molecular mechanism of GTPase activation: (*a*) A catalytic "arginine finger" is present at the active site of the GTPase in *trans* (from the GAP) or in *cis* (from the GTPase), and (*b*) switch regions of the GTPase, particularly a catalytic glutamine residue, are stabilized on the binding of the GAP to the GTPase (117–119).

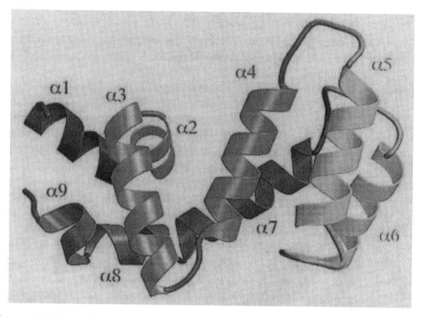

Figure 4   Ribbon diagram depicting the tertiary structure of RGS4. The RGS4 box consists of nine helices that form two subdomains. The terminal subdomain is formed by $\alpha1$, $\alpha2$, $\alpha3$, $\alpha8$, and $\alpha9$, and the bundle subdomain is formed by $\alpha4$, $\alpha5$, $\alpha6$, and $\alpha7$. The majority of residues that contact G_{i1} are found along the bottom of the bundle subdomain, as shown here. Insertions found in lower eukaryotes occur at the top of the bundle subdomain, opposite the G_{i1}-binding surface, and between $\alpha1$ and $\alpha2$ (106).

It was shown that both RasGAP (113) and RhoGAP (114) contribute a highly conserved arginine finger to the active site of Ras and Rho, respectively. At the same time, they can also stabilize the switch regions of the GTPase through protein-protein interaction. Unlike RasGAP and RhoGAP, it was deduced that RGS4 does not directly contribute an arginine residue or any other catalytic residue to the active site of G_{i1} for GTP hydrolysis (106). Subsequent mutational studies (discussed below) confirmed this assumption. In fact, the $G\alpha$ subunit has a "built-in" arginine residue in the extra helical domain that projects into the catalytic active site in the opposite direction compared with Ras and Rho (117). It is inferred that RGS4 exerts its GAP activity mainly through binding to the switch regions, reducing the flexibility and stabilizing the transition state of G_{i1} (106). In the case of ARF1-ARFGAP complex, the arginine finger is speculated to be supplied by the ARF effector coatomer instead of ARFGAP or ARF1 itself (116). Similar to RGS4, ARFGAP functions by stabilizing the switch regions.

Mutational Analysis of RGS Proteins

Mutagenesis has been used to study the mechanisms of GAP function and to search for dominant negative mutants of RGS proteins that would be useful for in vivo studies.

Early experiments demonstrated that the intact RGS domain itself is sufficient and necessary for the GAP activity in vitro but not for function in vivo (31, 32, 54). Before the crystal structure of the RGS4-G_{i1} complex was known, Chen et al (54) performed mutagenesis analysis on the RGS domain of RGS16 based on the conserved residues in several RGS proteins. For example, the RGS16 (G74R) mutant that retained binding ability to the transition state of G_i fails to attenuate pheromone signaling in yeast (54). This showed for the first time that the physical interaction between the RGS domain and the $G\alpha$ subunit could be separated from the GAP activity of the RGS protein on G protein signaling pathways. These results, however, need to be confirmed in a mammalian signaling system.

Implications for the Mechanism of GAP Activity   With the solving of the crystal structure of RGS4-G_{i1}, several mutagenesis studies have been conducted to further investigate the mechanisms of GAP activity. From the crystal structure of the RGS4-G_{i1} complex, the Asn128 residue of RGS4 appears to be important for GAP activity by making contact with the catalytic glutamine residue of G_{i1} (106). The RGS4 (N128A) mutant essentially lost all its GAP activity on G_i and its affinity for G_{i2} in vitro, which confirms that this residue is critical for RGS4 activity (120). When different Asn128 mutants of RGS4 (Ala, Gly, Phe, Ser, Val) were tested on four $G\alpha$ targets (G_o, G_{i1}, G_q, and G_z) by two distinct GAP assays (solution-based single-turnover assay and vesicle-based steady state assay), several mutations significantly decreased the apparent affinity for $G\alpha$ subunits but showed only modest effects on GTP hydrolysis (121). Based on these findings, it was suggested that Asn128 of RGS4 is predominantly involved in $G\alpha$ substrate binding. Similarly, when the equivalent Asn131 residue in RGS16 was mutated (into Ala, Asp, Gln, His, Leu, Ser) or deleted (122), the mutants showed substantial decreases in their ability to bind G_t to different degrees. The GAP activity of four of these mutants was essentially abolished, but two, N131S and N131Q, retained partial GAP activity (V_{max} ~80% and 60%, respectively).

It is intriguing to note that the critical N128 residue in RGS4 is not strictly conserved in all RGS proteins; it can be a Ser (GAIP, RET-RGS1, and RGSZ1), Gln (Axin), or Gly (D-AKAP2) (Figure 3). GAIP with a Ser in the equivalent position is a GAP, but no GAP activity has yet been demonstrated for Axin. A recent nuclear magnetic resonance study on the RGS domain of GAIP revealed it has a nine-alpha helical structure similar to that of RGS4 (123). The major differences between the RGS domains of RGS4 and GAIP are a displacement in the packing of some of the helices and the relative orientation of the loop connecting helices $\alpha 5$ and $\alpha 6$, where the critical residue for GAP activity is located (RGS4-Asn128, GAIP-Ser156). Biochemical data have shown that GAIP has comparable binding affinities for the transition state (GDP-AlF$_4^-$) and the GTP-bound state of G_{i3} (89), whereas RGS4 has a much higher affinity for the transition state than for the GDP- or GTP-bound states of G_i (124). The connection between the structural variations and the functional differences between these two proteins is still unknown. Further understanding is likely to come from structural studies of other RGS domains.

An extensive mutational analysis of the RGS domain of RGS4 using GAP activity and $G\alpha$ binding properties of these mutants supports the idea that RGS4 exerts its GAP activity primarily through stabilizing the transition state conformation of the switch regions of the $G\alpha$ subunit (120). All the GAP-defective RGS4 mutants tested were unable to bind $G\alpha$ in vitro. Besides residues directly involved in the RGS4-$G\alpha$ binding, other conserved residues distal to the interface are also critical for GAP activity, which suggests these residues may contribute to the overall conformational stability of RGS4.

Dominant Negative Mutants   Dominant negative mutants, i.e. those that uncouple the interaction between $G\alpha$ subunits and RGS proteins, represent valuable tools to determine the importance of a particular RGS protein in a specific signaling pathway. Mutational analysis and genetic screening have been employed to search for dominant negative mutants of RGS proteins and $G\alpha$ subunits, respectively.

Evidence was obtained that R167M/A and F168A mutants of RGS4 are incapable of binding to the transition state of G_{i1}. Instead, in contrast to the wild-type protein, they bind preferentially to the activated (GTPγS bound) form of G_{i1} (124a). More intriguing, it was shown that these mutants serve as RGS antagonists in a G_{i1} GAP assay and in an IL-8–induced G_i-mediated MAPK activation assay. However, the dominant negative effects of these mutants were not substantial. For example, the GAP activity of wild-type RGS4 was inhibited only 25% by a 10-fold excess of R167A mutant. It would be interesting to test similar mutants of other RGS proteins to examine their potential dominant negative roles.

Two recent reports demonstrated the usefulness of $G\alpha$ mutants for uncoupling RGS-$G\alpha$ interaction. A yeast $G\alpha$ mutant (Gpa1^{sst}) in which a conserved Gly residue in the switch I region was mutated into Ser was obtained that shows reduced binding to Sst2p (125). A similar mutation in G_o, G_{i1}, and G_q was shown to be insensitive to the GAP activity of RGS4 and RGS7, presumably because of the low affinity between the RGS proteins and the $G\alpha$ mutants (125, 126). The Gly-to-Ser mutations in $G\alpha$ did not significantly change effector coupling, intrinsic GTPase hydrolysis, or GDP release behavior. These $G\alpha$ mutants represent useful tools to study the relationship of an endogenous RGS protein and a particular $G\alpha$ subunit.

Relationship Between $G\alpha$ Effectors and RGS Proteins

Structural Basis for RGS as an Effector Antagonist   As indicated earlier, biochemical data have suggested that besides GAP function, some RGS proteins serve as effector antagonists. It was shown that RGS4 and GAIP are able to compete with phospholipase Cβ (PLCβ) for binding to GTPγS-G$_q$, and to inhibit the activation of PLCβ by GTPγS-G$_q$ (33). Similar partial attenuation effects were also observed for RGS16 (33), RGS4 (127), and GAIP (127) with G$_t$ and the cGMP phosphodiesterase γ subunits (PDEγ), the inhibitory subunit of PDE. These results are in agreement with the initial prediction based on the crystal structure of RGS4-G$_{i1}$ that Gα-effector binding sites may partially overlap with G$_i$-RGS binding sites at the switch regions (106). However, subsequent analysis of the crystal structure of G$_s$ associated with the catalytic domain of adenylate cyclase indicated that G$_i$ may be able to accommodate RGS4 and adenylate cyclase simultaneously (128). Mapping studies of PDEγ-binding sites on G$_t$ also suggested that there is no significant overlap between PDEγ and RGS16 binding surfaces on G$_t$ (129), but it should be noted that RGS16 is not the physiological partner for G$_t$.

Thus, the structural basis for the competition between RGS and effector is not yet well established. It is to be hoped that the structural analysis of other Gα-effector complexes will provide insight into the mechanisms underlying the effector-antagonist behavior of some RGS proteins.

Cooperative Action Between Effector and RGS   It has become clear that an effector-antagonist function does not apply to every RGS protein. Instead, unlike the RGS proteins mentioned above, the GAP activity of RGS9 on G$_t$ is enhanced by the PDEγ subunit (60). Similar to RGS9 and PDEγ, ARFGAP and the ARF effector, coatomer, were shown to have a synergistic effect on the GAP activity of the small GTPase ARF (116). The kinetic analysis of RGS9 binding to the G$_t$-PDEγ complex suggested that there was no steric hindrance to assembly of the ternary G$_t$-RGS9-PDEγ complex, which may provide the structural basis for this cooperative action (130). A more recent study (131) suggested that the α3-α5 region in the RGS domain of RGS9 is responsible for the effect of PDEγ on the GAP activity of RGS9 for G$_t$. It would be interesting to study whether this cooperative action is a unique feature for RGS9 or whether it is also found for other RGS proteins, at least for the closely related RGS6, RGS7, and RGS11 proteins.

RGS-Gα Partner: Specificity or Promiscuity?

One major question in the RGS field is whether there is specificity in the RGS-Gα interaction. Most of the RGS proteins tested so far are GAPs for G$_i$ and/or G$_q$, except that p115RhoGEF is a specific GAP for G$_{12}$ and G$_{13}$ (132) and probably also PDZ-RhoGEF (133). No RGS protein has yet been found to serve as a GAP for G$_s$. This has been explained by the finding that Asp229 in the switch 2 region of G$_s$ is a major structural barrier to its interaction with known RGS proteins (134, 135).

Regarding specificity toward different G$_i$ and G$_q$ subunits, in vitro data accumulated from GTPase assays show that some RGS proteins (e.g. RGS4) are relatively promiscuous, displaying little preference for different G$_i$ and G$_q$ subunits, whereas others (e.g. RGSZ1) have selectivity for certain $G\alpha$ subunits. RGS2 was shown to bind selectively to G_q and had no GAP activity on G_i in a solution-based single-turnover GTPase assay (136). However, in a reconstituted lipid vesicle–based GAP assay, RGS2 displayed GAP activities to both G_{i1} and G_q (80). These results are an indication of the limits of in vitro assays, and assessments of the specificity of RGS proteins for their $G\alpha$ partner(s) should include in vivo approaches whenever possible.

GAIP interacts more strongly with G_{i3}, G_{i1}, and G_o than with G_{i2} (89). A single residue at the far N terminus of switch 3 in G_i (Asp 229 of G_{i1} and the equivalent Ala 230 of G_{i2}) was shown to be the determinant for the selectivity for G_{i1} over G_{i2} (137). RGS9 was shown to have a high specificity for G_t over other G_i subunits in a GAP assay using urea-washed rod-outer-segment (ROS) membranes, and the molecular determinant for this specificity appears to be located in the helical domain of G_t (130). Finally, by an unknown mechanism, RGSZ1 displayed great selectivity of binding affinity and GAP activity for G_z over other $G\alpha$ subunits (69).

Although only a few examples of selective in vitro interaction between RGS and $G\alpha$ partners have been shown so far, greater specificity of RGS proteins for different $G\alpha$ subunits may arise in vivo because of different tissue expression patterns and different subcellular localizations of RGS proteins from their $G\alpha$ partner.

NON-RGS DOMAINS IMPLY LINKS TO OTHER SIGNALING PATHWAYS

GGL (Giggle) and DEP Domains

RGS6, RGS7, RGS9, RGS11, and EGL-10 (*C. elegans*) contain a domain with homology to $G\gamma$ subunits, termed G protein gamma-like (GGL or Giggle) (138) and a DEP domain (from Dishevelled, EGL-10, and Pleckstrin) (144). The fact that the 100–amino acid-long DEP domains are found exclusively in RGS proteins that have GGL domains suggests some functional link between the two. A first step toward understanding the role of the GGL domain was made when RGS7 was identified in a complex with the G protein $\beta 5$ subunit in the retina (139) and when RGS11 was shown to specifically interact with $G\beta 5$ (138). The photoreceptor-specific RGS9 protein also forms a complex with the long splice variant of $G\beta 5$ (140). In the case of RGS6, the specificity of interaction was narrowed to a specific tryptophan residue in the GGL domain (141). More detailed studies revealed that $G\beta 5$-RGS/GGL complexes may play a role in the affinity or selectivity for $G\alpha$ subunits (138, 142). The functional implication of $G\beta 5$ binding to the GGL domain in RGS proteins is still not clear and should be studied in its physiologically relevant context.

The presence of GGL domains in some RGS proteins significantly extends their interaction possibilities and suggests that these RGS proteins are part of a macromolecular complex that includes the receptor, G protein, and effector. This would certainly enhance the overall efficiency of the signaling pathway.

The DEP domain present in all RGS proteins that have a GGL domain may dictate membrane localization, as the DEP domain of the Dishevelled protein from *Drosophila* is responsible for localization of the protein to membranes (143). In keeping with this assumption is the finding that EGL-10 fused to GFP localizes to sarcoplasmic reticulum–like structures in *C. elegans* (22), and RGS9 is tightly attached to ROS membranes (59, 60), but this remains to be confirmed for other members of this RGS subfamily (70).

DH/PH Domains and Links to Small GTPases

An exciting direct link between heterotrimeric G proteins and small GTPases was recently unveiled, and the linking molecule p115 RhoGEF belongs to the RGS family. p115RhoGEF was discovered as a GEF of Rho GTPase, whose GEF activity is mediated through its DH (double homology) domain (145). Activated G_{12} and G_{13} were shown to induce cytoskeletal and mitogenic changes typically transmitted by the Rho family of small GTPases, but the nature of the connection to Rho remained obscure (146, 147). This link became obvious when it was demonstrated that activated G_{12} and G_{13} stimulate the GEF activity of p115RhoGEF, which has an N-terminal RGS domain that shows GAP activity on G_{12} and G_{13} (132, 148). This connection solved the longtime outstanding enigma of how GPCR ligands such as thrombin and lyso phosphatidic acid can induce cytoskeletal changes in the cell (149). Thus, p115RhoGEF serves as an effector molecule for G_{13}, which activates the GEF function of the DH domain by G_{13}/RGS domain interaction. The RGS protein p115RhoGEF occupies a crucial position in the signaling pathway that links an extracellular ligand via a heterotrimeric G protein to a small G protein that promotes downstream morphological changes in the cell. It is also the first example of an RGS protein that acts as an effector.

The Rho GEF family has recently been expanded to include p115RhoGEF, PDZ-RhoGEF, and the lsc oncogene. All have PH domains (pleckstrin homology) located immediately C-terminal of their DH domains and are required for the in vivo activity of these GEFs (150). PH domains may also facilitate translocation to membranes (150), but this remains to be verified.

Although p115RhoGEF is a GAP for both G_{13} and G_{12} in vitro, its GAP activity was 10-fold higher on G_{13} than on G_{12}. Furthermore, G_{12} does not stimulate the GEF activity of p115RhoGEF and does not activate the downstream serum response factor (85, 86, 132, 148). Clearly, the relationship between G_{12} and p115RhoGEF still needs to be worked out, but some of the possibilities include the following: (*a*) G_{12} activates the GEF of another family member of p115RhoGEF, or (*b*) G_{13} but not G_{12} interacts with an additional site in p115RhoGEF.

A new member of the RhoGEF family, PDZ-RhoGEF, that also interacts with $G_{12/13}$, was shown to have a PDZ domain N-terminal of its RGS domain (133). The role of the PDZ domain in this molecule remains unknown, but it was suggested that it may interact with the C terminus of the lyso phosphatidic acid receptor, which is coupled to $G_{12/13}$ and has a putative PDZ binding motif.

Another example of a link between heterotrimeric and small G proteins is provided by RGS14. It was also reported (151) to be a Rap1/Rap2 interacting protein (GenBank# U85055), which suggests that RGS14 might also link to small GTPases. Although the Rap1/Rap2 binding site in RGS14 has not been established, a 70–amino acid region with homology to B-raf kinase, an effector of Ras, is a potential candidate. In Raf kinase, this region homologous to B-raf kinase is part of the Ras-binding site, and the Raf-binding domain of Ras (amino acids 32–40, the effector domain) is very conserved in Rap1A (115). It is important to determine the in vivo $G\alpha$ specificity of RGS14 to establish which signal transduction pathways RGS14 might connect.

PDZ and PDZ Binding, PID/PTB and PKA Anchor Domains

Two RGS proteins contain PDZ domains, which bind to consensus C-terminal motifs in target proteins and play an important role in organizing protein networks on membranes (152). Generally, a PDZ domain in one protein binds to a PDZ-binding motif in another. RGS12, the largest RGS protein described so far, has an N-terminal PDZ domain that binds in vitro to the CXCR2 interleukin-8 receptor, but its in vivo target remains to be identified (77, 151). The C-terminal PDZ binding motif of RGS12 is also in search of a partner, but theoretically it could form an intramolecular link with its own PDZ domain. GAIP also has a PDZ binding motif in its short (extra-RGS) C terminus. A novel protein—GIPC (for GAIP interacting protein C terminus)—was recently isolated that binds, via a central PDZ domain, to the C terminus of GAIP (153). GIPC's function is unknown but, like GAIP, it is found on vesicles close to the cell membrane, which suggests a role in intracellular transport. Recently, GIPC was also isolated through interaction of its PDZ domain with the C terminus of several transmembrane proteins, including the glucose 1 transporter (154) and semaphorin F (154a). This suggests that GIPC, like other PDZ domain proteins, may serve to cluster signaling molecules and membrane proteins (152).

RGS12 contains a PID/PTB or phosphotyrosine interacting domain, that directly binds to a phosphotyrosine residue on the alpha subunit of the N-type Ca^{2+} channel (M Diversé, personal communication).

The protein kinase A (PKA) anchoring protein, D-AKAP2, has an N-terminal RGS-like domain and a C-terminal region that binds the regulatory subunits of PKA (PKA anchor), but no GAP activity or $G\alpha$ binding was yet shown for this protein (34). D-AKAP2 could form a novel link between G protein signaling and cAMP signaling, in addition to the established G_s/G_i–adenylate cyclase pathway, but the functional implications of this connection remain to be established.

PEST Domains

PEST (proline, glutamine, serine, threonine-rich) domains reportedly confer protein instability and are often found in signal transduction molecules with rapid turnover (155). RGS3 has four PEST domains in its N terminus (23), and GAIP also has one (L De Vries, unpublished results). RGS7 has two PEST sequences within its GGL domain and is rapidly degraded via the ubiquitin-proteosome pathway unless it interacts with the C-terminal tail of polycystin, an integral membrane protein (156). Rapid degradation and/or stabilization through interaction with membrane proteins could become a more general mechanism of regulation of RGS proteins.

Wnt Signaling

Axin and its homolog conductin (also named axil or axin-like) are important scaffold proteins in the Wnt signaling pathway, which involves the seven transmembrane Frizzled receptors (with no G protein connection demonstrated yet) and plays a role in cell-cell signaling and tissue development (157). Both axin and conductin negatively regulate Wnt signaling and have an N-terminal RGS domain for which an interacting Gα partner remains to be found (68, 158–160). However, the RGS domain of both proteins was shown to interact directly with the tumor suppressor, adenomatous polyposis coli (APC), a non–Gα-like molecule, which suggests that APC and a Gα might compete for the RGS domain. The region in APC that interacts with conductin is limited to three previously unidentified repeated motifs with the SAMP (Ser-Ala-Met-Pro) signature; mutation of the serine to alanine in the signature abolished binding to the RGS domain (158, 161). Deletion of the RGS domain down-regulates signaling through β-catenin or its *Drosophila* homolog armadillo (68, 110), which normally activates specific transcription factors inducing genes involved in cell adhesion, morphology, and motility. These results imply that Axin and conductin are involved in switching the cell from a proliferative to a more differentiated state. Future research should establish whether the Frizzled receptors are true GPCRs and which Gα subunit binds to the RGS domain of axin/conductin. This would also strengthen the association of heterotrimeric G proteins and RGS proteins with developmental processes.

SUMMARY

In this review we have summarized what is known to date on RGS proteins. The RGS protein family is only 4 years old, and already it has had a major impact on the way we think about the mechanisms of G protein signaling. The data available today reflect major progress in our understanding of the molecular mechanisms of the RGS-Gα interaction, but we have only begun to recognize the importance of factors that regulate RGS function, such as tissue-specific expression, transcriptional and posttranslational modifications, and intracellular localization. In order to establish the specificity of RGS proteins on the vast number of G protein signal transduction pathways implicated in processes such as cell proliferation, differentiation, motility, and vesicular trafficking, many more in vivo studies will be necessary.

PERSPECTIVES

The fact that levels of RGS proteins are tightly regulated suggests their importance in influencing G protein–coupled signaling pathways. Dysregulation might lead to a pathological state. For example, a defect in the transcriptional machinery that leads to overexpression of RGS proteins could affect the turnoff of GPCR signaling. Likewise, if there is a defect in the transcriptional machinery so that RGS proteins could not be expressed, or if RGS proteins are mistargeted and thus become nonfunctional, G protein signaling would be prolonged. The observation of pathological phenotypes in either transgenic or targeted knockout mice as well as chromosomal mapping will be helpful in determining the role of RGS proteins in normal cell processes as well as in disease. It should be noted, however, that several Gα knockout mice did not show evident phenotypes. The same may hold for RGS knockout mice.

Given that overexpression of RGS proteins alters signaling cascades, RGS proteins represent potential targets for therapeutic agents. Administering a compound that results in up-regulation of an RGS protein might be as effective as administering an antagonist to prevent initiation of the signaling pathway. Understanding the particular signaling pathways with which specific RGS proteins associate will be critical in designing such therapeutic agents. The use of RGS proteins in the context of therapeutics is one of the most difficult but arguably the most important challenges currently facing investigators studying RGS proteins.

ACKNOWLEDGMENTS

We wish to thank all colleagues who provided preprints of unpublished material. We thank Dr. Sprang for his permission to use Figure 4. This work was supported by National Institutes of Health grants DK 17780 and CA 58689 (to MGF). BZ is a member of the Molecular Pathology Graduate Program, University of California at San Diego, and is supported by the HUANG Memorial Scholarship. EE is a graduate student in the Biomedical Sciences Graduate Program, University of California at San Diego.

NOTE ADDED IN PROOF

After this paper was submitted, a new member of the RGS family, RGS17, was reported (171). It appears to be a member of the subfamily A and shares the characteristic cysteine string and subfamily-specific Ser residue (70).

Visit the Annual Reviews home page at www.AnnualReviews.org.

LITERATURE CITED

1. Krupnick JG, Benovic JL. 1998. The role of receptor kinases and arrestins in G protein-coupled receptor regulation. *Annu. Rev. Pharmacol. Toxicol.* 38:289–319

2. Fields TA, Casey PJ. 1995. Phosphorylation of $G_z\alpha$ by protein kinase C blocks interaction with the $\beta\gamma$ complex. *J. Biol. Chem.* 270:23119–25

3. Wedegaertner PB, Bourne HR. 1994. Activation and depalmitoylation of $G_s\alpha$. *Cell* 77:1063–70

4. Mumby SM. 1997. Reversible palmitoylation of signaling proteins. *Curr. Opin. Cell Biol.* 9:148–54

5. Wedegaertner PB. 1998. Lipid modifications and membrane targeting of $G\alpha$. *Biol. Signals Recept.* 7:125–35

6. Milligan G. 1993. Agonist regulation of cellular G protein levels and distribution: mechanisms and functional implications. *Trends Pharmacol. Sci.* 14:413–18

7. Boguski MS, McCormick F. 1993. Proteins regulating Ras and its relatives. *Nature* 366:643–53

8. Berman DM, Wilkie TM, Gilman AG. 1996. GAIP and RGS4 are GTPase-activating proteins for the G_i subfamily of G protein α subunits. *Cell* 86:445–52

9. Koelle MR. 1997. A new family of G-protein regulators—the RGS proteins. *Curr. Opin. Cell Biol.* 9:143–47

10. Neer EJ. 1997. Turning down G-protein signals. *Curr. Biol.* 7:31–33

11. Dohlman HG, Thorner J. 1997. RGS proteins and signaling by heterotrimeric G proteins. *J. Biol. Chem.* 272:3871–74

12. Zerangue N, Jan LY. 1998. G-protein signaling: fine-tuning signaling kinetics. *Curr. Biol.* 8:R313–16

13. Dohlman HG, Song J, Apanovitch DM, DiBello PR, Gillen KM. 1998. Regulation of G protein signalling in yeast. *Semin. Cell Dev. Biol.* 9:135–41

14. Berman DM, Gilman AG. 1998. Mammalian RGS proteins: barbarians at the gate. *J. Biol. Chem.* 273:1269–72

15. Kehrl JH. 1998. Heterotrimeric G protein signaling: roles in immune function and fine-tuning by RGS proteins. *Immunity* 8:1–10

16. Arshavsky VY, Pugh EN Jr. 1998. Lifetime regulation of G protein-effector complex: emerging importance of RGS proteins. *Neuron* 20:11–14

17. De Vries L, Farquhar MG. 1999. RGS proteins: more than just GAPs for heterotrimeric G proteins. *Trends Cell Biol.* 9:138–44

18. Helms JB. 1995. Role of heterotrimeric GTP binding proteins in vesicular protein transport: indications for both classical and alternative G protein cycles. *FEBS Lett.* 369:84–88

19. Chan RK, Otte CA. 1982. Isolation and genetic analysis of *Saccharomyces cerevisiae* mutants supersensitive to G1 arrest by a factor and alpha factor pheromones. *Mol. Cell Biol.* 2:11–20

20. Chan RK, Otte CA. 1982. Physiological characterization of Saccharomyces cerevisiae mutants supersensitive to G1 arrest by a factor and α factor pheromones. *Mol. Cell Biol.* 2:21–29

21. De Vries L, Mousli M, Wurmser A, Farquhar MG. 1995. GAIP, a protein that specifically interacts with the trimeric G protein $G\alpha_{i3}$, is a member of a protein family with a highly conserved core domain. *Proc. Natl. Acad. Sci. USA* 92:11916–20

22. Koelle MR, Horvitz HR. 1996. EGL-10 regulates G protein signaling in the *C. elegans* nervous system and shares a conserved domain with many mammalian proteins. *Cell* 84:115–25

23. Druey KM, Blumer KJ, Kang VH, Kehrl JH. 1996. Inhibition of G-protein-mediated MAP kinase activation by a new mammalian gene family. *Nature* 379:742–46

24. Dohlman HG, Apaniesk D, Chen Y, Song J, Nusskern D. 1995. Inhibition of G-protein signaling by dominant gain-of-function mutations in Sst2p, a pheromone desensitization factor in *Saccharomyces cerevisiae*. *Mol. Cell. Biol.* 15:3635–43

25. Dohlman HG, Song J, Ma D, Courchesne WE, Thorner J. 1996. Sst2, a negative regulator of pheromone signaling in the yeast *Saccharomyces cerevisiae:* expression, localization, and genetic interaction and physical association with Gpα1 (the G-protein α subunit). *Mol. Cell. Biol.* 16:5194–209

26. Dietzel C, Kurjan J. 1987. Pheromonal regulation and sequence of the *Saccharomyces cerevisiae* SST2 gene: a model for desensitization to pheromone. *Mol. Cell. Biol.* 7:4169–77

27. Siderovski DP, Hessel A, Chung S, Mak TW, Tyers M. 1996. A new family of regulators of G-protein-coupled receptors? *Curr. Biol.* 6:211–12

28. Hunt TW, Fields TA, Casey PJ, Peralta EG. 1996. RGS10 is a selective activator of $G\alpha_i$ GTPase activity. *Nature* 383:175–77

29. Watson N, Linder ME, Druey KM, Kehrl JH, Blumer KJ. 1996. RGS family members: GTPase-activating proteins for heterotrimeric G-protein α-subunits. *Nature* 383:172–75

30. Saitoh O, Kubo Y, Miyatani Y, Asano T, Nakata H. 1997. RGS8 accelerates G-protein-mediated modulation of K+ currents. *Nature* 390:525–29

31. Popov S, Yu K, Kozasa T, Wilkie TM. 1997. The regulators of G protein signaling (RGS) domains of RGS4, RGS10, and GAIP retain GTPase activating protein activity in vitro. *Proc. Natl. Acad. Sci. USA* 94:7216–20

32. Faurobert E, Hurley JB. 1997. The core domain of a new retina specific RGS protein stimulates the GTPase activity of transducin in vitro. *Proc. Natl. Acad. Sci. USA* 94:2945–50

33. Hepler JR, Berman DM, Gilman AG, Kozasa T. 1997. RGS4 and GAIP are GTPase-activating proteins for $G_q\alpha$ and block activation of phospholipase Cβ by γ-thio-GTP-$G_q\alpha$. *Proc. Natl. Acad. Sci. USA* 94:428–32

34. Huang LJ, Durick K, Weiner JA, Chun J, Taylor SS. 1997. D-AKAP2, a novel protein kinase A anchoring protein with a putative RGS domain. *Proc. Natl. Acad. Sci. USA* 94:11184–89

35. Yan Y, Chi PP, Bourne HR. 1997. RGS4 inhibits Gq-mediated activation of mitogen-activated protein kinase and phosphoinositide synthesis. *J. Biol. Chem.* 272:11924–27

36. Doupnik CA, Davidson N, Lester HA, Kofuji P. 1997. RGS proteins reconstitute the rapid gating kinetics of gbeta-gamma-activated inwardly rectifying K+ channels. *Proc. Natl. Acad. Sci. USA* 94:10461–66

37. Logothetis DE, Kurachi Y, Galper J, Neer EJ, Clapham DE. 1987. The βγ subunits of GTP-binding proteins activate the muscarinic K+ channel in heart. *Nature* 325:321–26

38. Huang CL, Slesinger PA, Casey PJ, Jan YN, Jan LY. 1995. Evidence that direct binding of G βγ to the GIRK1 G protein-gated inwardly rectifying K+ channel is

important for channel activation. *Neuron* 15:1133–43

39. Bunemann M, Hosey MM. 1998. Regulators of G protein signaling (RGS) proteins constitutively activate Gβγ-gated potassium channels. *J. Biol. Chem.* 273:31186–90

40. Saitoh O, Kubo Y, Odagiri M, Ichikawa M, Yamagata K, Sekine T. 1999. RGS7 and RGS8 differentially accelerate G protein-mediated modulation of K+ currents. *J. Biol. Chem.* 274:9899–904

41. Chuang H, Yu M, Jan YN, Jan LY. 1998. Evidence that the nucleotide exchange and hydrolysis cycle of G proteins causes acute desensitization of G-protein gated inward rectifier K+ channels. *Proc. Natl. Acad. Sci. USA* 95:11727–32

42. Gold SJ, Ni YG, Dohlman HG, Nestler EJ. 1997. Regulators of G-protein signaling (RGS) proteins: region-specific expression of nine subtypes in rat brain. *J. Neurosci.* 17:8024–37

43. Shuey DJ, Betty M, Jones PG, Khawaja XZ, Cockett MI. 1998. RGS7 attenuates signal transduction through the Gα_q family of heterotrimeric G proteins in mammalian cells. *J. Neurochem.* 70:1964–72

44. Thomas EA, Danielson PE, Sutcliffe JG. 1998. RGS9: a regulator of G-protein signalling with specific expression in rat and mouse striatum. *J. Neurosci. Res.* 52:118–24

45. Nomoto S, Adachi K, Yang LX, Hirata Y, Muraguchi S, Kiuchi K. 1997. Distribution of RGS4 mRNA in mouse brain shown by *in situ* hybridization. *Biochem. Biophys. Res. Commun.* 241:281–87

46. Rahman Z, Gold SJ, Potenza MN, Cowan CW, Ni YG, et al. 1999. Cloning and characterization of RGS9-2: a striatal-enriched alternatively spliced product of the RGS9 gene. *J. Neurosci.* 19:2016–26

47. Granneman JG, Zhai Y, Zhu Z, Bannon MJ, Burchett SA, et al. 1998. Molecular characterization of human and rat RGS 9L, a novel splice variant enriched in

dopamine target regions, and chromosomal localization of the RGS 9 gene. *Mol. Pharmacol.* 54:687–94

48. Bruch RC, Medler KF. 1996. A regulator of G-protein signaling in olfactory receptor neurons. *NeuroReport* 7:2941–44

49. Kardestuncer T, Wu H, Lim AL, Neer EJ. 1998. Cardiac myocytes express mRNA for ten RGS proteins: changes in RGS mRNA expression in ventricular myocytes and cultured atria. *FEBS Lett.* 438:285–88

50. Tamirisa P, Blumer KJ, Muslin AJ. 1999. RGS4 inhibits G-protein signaling in cardiomyocytes. *Circulation* 99:441–47

51. Zhang S, Watson N, Zahner J, Rottman JN, Blumer KJ, Muslin AJ. 1998. RGS3 and RGS4 are GTPase activating proteins in the heart. *J. Mol. Cell. Cardiol.* 30:269–76

52. Neill JD, Duck LW, Sellers JC, Musgrove LC, Scheschonka A, et al. 1997. Potential role for a regulator of G protein signaling (RGS3) in gonadotropin-releasing hormone (GnRH) stimulated desensitization. *Endocrinology* 138:843–46

53. Tseng CC, Zhang XY. 1998. Role of regulator of G protein signaling in desensitization of the glucose-dependent insulinotropic peptide receptor. *Endocrinology* 139:4470–75

54. Chen C, Zheng B, Han J, Lin SC. 1997. Characterization of a novel mammalian RGS protein that binds to Gα proteins and inhibits pheromone signaling in yeast. *J. Biol. Chem.* 272:8679–85

55. Bowman EP, Campbell JJ, Druey KM, Scheschonka A, Kehrl JH, Butcher EC. 1998. Regulation of chemotactic and proadhesive responses to chemoattractant receptors by RGS (regulator of G-protein signaling) family members. *J. Biol. Chem.* 273:28040–48

56. Kleuss C, Hescheler J, Ewel C, Rosenthal W, Schultz G, Wittig B. 1991. Assignment of G-protein subtypes to

specific receptors inducing inhibition of calcium currents. *Nature* 353:43–48

57. Kleuss C, Scherubl H, Hescheler J, Schultz G, Wittig B. 1993. Selectivity in signal transduction determined by gamma subunits of heterotrimeric G proteins. *Science* 259:832–34

58. Offermanns S, Toombs CF, Hu YH, Simon MI. 1997. Defective platelet activation in $G\alpha_q$-deficient mice. *Nature* 389:183–86

59. Cowan CW, Fariss RN, Sokal I, Palczewski K, Wensel TG. 1998. High expression levels in cones of RGS9, the predominant GTPase accelerating protein of rods. *Proc. Natl. Acad. Sci. USA* 95:5351–56

60. He W, Cowan CW, Wensel TG. 1998. RGS9, a GTPase accelerator for phototransduction. *Neuron* 20:95–102

61. Diverse-Pierluissi MA, Fischer T, Jordan JD, Schiff M, Ortiz DF, et al. 1999. Regulators of G protein signaling proteins as determinants of the rate of desensitization of presynaptic calcium channels. *J. Biol. Chem.* 274:14490–94

62. Xu X, Zeng W, Popov S, Berman DM, Davignon I, et al. 1999. RGS proteins determine signaling specificity of Gq-coupled receptors. *J. Biol. Chem.* 274:3549–56

63. Chen CK, Wieland T, Simon MI. 1996. RGS-r, a retinal specific RGS protein, binds an intermediate conformation of transducin and enhances recycling. *Proc. Natl. Acad. Sci. USA* 93:12885–89

64. Buckbinder L, Velasco-Miguel S, Chen Y, Xu N, Talbott R, et al. 1997. The p53 tumor suppressor targets a novel regulator of G protein signaling. *Proc. Natl. Acad. Sci. USA* 94:7868–72

65. Siderovski DP, Heximer SP, Forsdyke DR. 1994. A human gene encoding a putative basic helix-loop-helix phosphoprotein whose mRNA increases rapidly in cycloheximide-treated blood mononuclear cells. *DNA Cell Biol.* 13:125–47

66. Chatterjee TK, Eapen A, Kanis AB, Fisher RA. 1997. Genomic organization, 5'-flanking region, and chromosomal localization of the human RGS3 gene. *Genomics* 45:429–33

67. Snow BE, Antonio L, Suggs S, Siderovski DP. 1998. Cloning of a retinally abundant regulator of G-protein signaling (RGS-r/RGS16): genomic structure and chromosomal localization of the human gene. *Gene* 206:247–53; Erratum. 1998. *Gene* 213:223

68. Zeng L, Fagotto F, Zhang T, Hsu W, Vasicek TJ, et al. 1997. The mouse fused locus encodes axin, an inhibitor of the Wnt signaling pathway that regulates embryonic axis formation. *Cell* 90:181–92

69. Wang J, Ducret A, Tu Y, Kozasa T, Aebersold R, Ross EM. 1998. RGSZ1, a G_z-selective RGS protein in brain. Structure, membrane association, regulation by $G\alpha_z$ phosphorylation, and relationship to a G_z GTPase-activating protein subfamily. *J. Biol. Chem.* 273:26014–25

70. Zheng B, De Vries L, Farquhar MG. 1999. Divergence of RGS proteins: evidence for the existence of six mammalian RGS subfamilies. *Trends Biochem. Sci.* 24:411–14

71. Newton JS, Deed RW, Mitchell EL, Murphy JJ, Norton JD. 1993. A B cell specific immediate early human gene is located on chromosome band 1q31 and encodes an α helical basic phosphoprotein. *Biochim. Biophys. Acta* 1216:314–16

72. Seki N, Hattori A, Hayashi A, Kozuma S, Hori T, Saito T. 1999. The human regulator of G-protein signaling protein 6 gene (RGS6) maps between markers WI-5202 and D14S277 on chromosome 14q24.3. *J. Hum. Genet.* 44:138–40

73. Seki N, Sugano S, Suzuki Y, Nakagawara A, Ohira M, et al. 1998. Isolation, tissue expression, and chromosomal assignment of human RGS5, a novel G-protein signaling regulator gene. *J. Hum. Genet.* 43:202–5

74. Glick JL, Meigs TE, Miron A, Casey PJ. 1998. RGSZ1, a G_z-selective regulator of G protein signaling whose action is sensitive to the phosphorylation state of $G_z\alpha$. *J. Biol. Chem.* 273:26008–13

75. Hong JX, Wilson GL, Fox CH, Kehrl JH. 1993. Isolation and characterization of a novel B cell activation gene. *J. Immunol.* 150:3895–904

76. Faurobert E, Scotti A, Hurley JB, Chabre M. 1999. RET-RGS, a retina-specific regulator of G-protein signaling, is located in synaptic regions of the retina. *Neurosci. Lett.* 269:61–66

77. Snow BE, Hall RA, Krumins AM, Brothers GM, Bouchard D, et al. 1998. GTPase activating specificity of RGS12 and binding specificity of an alternatively spliced PDZ (PSD-95/Dlg/ZO-1) domain. *J. Biol. Chem.* 273:17749–55

78. Siderovski DP, Blum S, Forsdyke RE, Forsdyke DR. 1990. A set of human putative lymphocyte G0/G1 switch genes includes genes homologous to rodent cytokine and zinc finger protein-encoding genes. *DNA Cell Biol.* 9:579–87

79. Heximer SP, Cristillo AD, Forsdyke DR. 1997. Comparison of mRNA expression of two regulators of G-protein signaling, RGS1/BL34/1R20 and RGS2/G0S8, in cultured human blood mononuclear cells. *DNA Cell Biol.* 16:589–98

80. Ingi T, Krumins AM, Chidiac P, Brothers GM, Chung S, et al. 1998. Dynamic regulation of RGS2 suggests a novel mechanism in G-protein signaling and neuronal plasticity. *J. Neurosci.* 18: 7178–88

81. Burchett SA, Volk ML, Bannon MJ, Granneman JG. 1998. Regulators of G protein signaling: rapid changes in mRNA abundance in response to amphetamine. *J. Neurochem.* 70:2216–19

82. Ogier-Denis E, Petiot A, Bauvy C, Codogno P. 1997. Control of the expression and activity of the Gα-interacting protein (GAIP) in human intestinal cells. *J. Biol. Chem.* 272:24599–603

83. Cristillo AD, Heximer SP, Russell L, Forsdyke DR. 1997. Cyclosporin A inhibits early mRNA expression of G0/ G1 switch gene 2 (G0S2) in cultured human blood mononuclear cells. *DNA Cell Biol.* 16:1449–58

84. Pepperl DJ, Shah-Basu S, VanLeeuwen D, Granneman JG, MacKenzie RG. 1998. Regulation of RGS mRNAs by cAMP in PC12 cells. *Biochem. Biophys. Res. Commun.* 243:52–55

85. Mao J, Yuan H, Xie W, Simon MI, Wu D. 1998. Specific involvement of G proteins in regulation of serum response factor-mediated gene transcription by different receptors. *J. Biol. Chem.* 273:27118–23

86. Mao J, Yuan H, Xie W, Wu D. 1998. Guanine nucleotide exchange factor GEF115 specifically mediates activation of Rho and serum response factor by the G protein α subunit $G\alpha_{13}$. *Proc. Natl. Acad. Sci. USA* 95:12973–76

87. Degtyarev MY, Spiegel AM, Jones TL. 1994. Palmitoylation of a G protein α_i subunit requires membrane localization not myristoylation. *J. Biol. Chem.* 269:30898–903

88. Wedegaertner PB, Bourne HR, von Zastrow M. 1996. Activation-induced subcellular redistribution of $G_s\alpha$. *Mol. Biol. Cell* 7:1225–33

89. De Vries L, Elenko E, Hubler L, Jones TL, Farquhar MG. 1996. GAIP is membrane-anchored by palmitoylation and interacts with the activated (GTP-bound) form of $G\alpha_i$ subunits. *Proc. Natl. Acad. Sci. USA* 93:15203–8

90. Gundersen CB, Mastrogiacomo A, Faull K, Umbach JU. 1994. Extensive lipidation of a torpedo cysteine string protein. *J. Biol. Chem.* 269:19197–99

91. Srinivasa SP, Bernstein LS, Blumer KJ, Linder ME. 1998. Plasma membrane localization is required for RGS4 func-

tion in *Saccharomyces cerevisiae. Proc. Natl. Acad. Sci. USA* 95:5584–89

92. Beadling C, Druey KM, Richter G, Kehrl JH, Smith KA. 1999. Regulators of G protein signaling exhibit distinct patterns of gene expression and target G protein specificity in human lymphocytes. *J. Immunol.* 162:2677–82

93. Premont RT, Inglese J, Lefkowitz RJ. 1995. Protein kinases that phosphorylate activated G protein-coupled receptors. *Faseb J.* 9:175–82

94. Neer EJ. 1995. Heterotrimeric G proteins: organizers of transmembrane signals. *Cell* 80:249–57

95. Nishida E, Gotoh Y. 1993. The MAP kinase cascade is essential for diverse signal transduction pathways. *Trends Biochem. Sci.* 18:128–31

95a. Fischer T, Elenko E, Wan L, Thomas G, Farquhar MG. 2000. Membrane associated GAIP is a phosphoprotein and can be phosphorylated by clathrin coated vesicles. *Proc. Natl. Acad. Sci. USA* 97: In press

96. Stow FL, de Almeida JB, Narula N, Hotzman EF, Ausiello DA. 1991. A heterotrimeric G protein, Gαi3, on Golgi membranes regulates the secretion of heparan sulfate proteoglycan in LLC-PK1 epithelial cells. *J. Cell Biol.* 114:1113–24

97. Wilson BS, Komuro M, Farquhar MG. 1994. Cellular variations in heterotrimeric G protein localization and expression in rat pituitary. *Endocrinology* 134:233–44

98. Li S, Okamoto T, Chun M, Sargiacomo M, Casanova JE, et al. 1995. Evidence for a regulated interaction between heterotrimeric G proteins and caveolin. *J. Biol. Chem.* 270:15693–701

99. Harder T, Simons K. 1997. Caveolae, DIGs, and the dynamics of sphingolipid-cholesterol microdomains. *Curr. Opin. Cell Biol.* 9:534–42

100. Druey KM, Sullivan BM, Brown D, Fischer ER, Watson N, et al. 1998.

101. Khawaja XZ, Liang JJ, Saugstad JA, Jones PG, Harnish S, et al. 1999. Immunohistochemical distribution of RGS7 protein and cellular selectivity in colocalizing with Gα_q proteins in the adult rat brain. *J. Neurochem.* 72:174–84

102. De Vries L, Elenko E, McCaffery JM, Fischer T, Hubler L, et al. 1998. RGS-GAIP, a GTPase-activating protein for Gα_i heterotrimeric G proteins, is located on clathrin-coated vesicles. *Mol. Biol. Cell* 9:1123–34

103. Wylie F, Heimann K, Le TL, Brown D, Rabnott G, Stow JL. 1999. GAIP, a Gα_i-3-binding protein, is associated with Golgi-derived vesicles and protein trafficking. *Am. J. Physiol.* 276:C497–506

104. Petiot A, Ogier-Denis E, Bauvy C, Cluzeaud F, Vandewalle A, Codogno P. 1999. Subcellular localization of the Gα_{i3} protein and Gα interacting protein, two proteins involved in the control of macroautophagy in human colon cancer HT-29 cells. *Biochem. J.* 337:289–95

105. Fischer T, Elenko E, McCaffery JM, De Vries L, Farquhar MG. 1999. Clathrin-coated vesicles bearing GAIP possess GTPase-activating protein activity in vitro. *Proc. Natl. Acad. Sci. USA* 96:6722–27

106. Tesmer JJ, Berman DM, Gilman AG, Sprang SR. 1997. Structure of RGS4 bound to AlF4–activated G(i α1): stabilization of the transition state for GTP hydrolysis. *Cell* 89:251–61

107. Bargmann CI. 1998. Neurobiology of the *Caenorhabditis elegans* genome. *Science* 282:2028–33

108. Elmore T, Rodriguez A, Smith DP. 1998. dRGS7 encodes a *Drosophila* homolog of EGL-10 and vertebrate RGS7. *DNA Cell Biol.* 17:983–89

109. Granderath S, Stollewerk A, Greig S, Goodman CS, O'Kane CJ, Klumbt C.

1999. Loco encodes an RGS protein required for *Drosophila* glial differentiation. *Development* 126:1781–91

110. Hamada F, Tomoyasu Y, Takatsu Y, Nakamura M, Nagai S, et al. 1999. Negative regulation of wingless signaling by D-axin, a *Drosophila* homolog of axin. *Science* 283:1739–42

111. Barrett K, Leptin M, Settleman J. 1997. The Rho GTPase and a putative RhoGEF mediate a signaling pathway for the cell shape changes in *Drosophila* gastrulation. *Cell* 91:905–15

112. Sprang SR. 1997. G protein mechanisms: insights from structural analysis. *Annu. Rev. Biochem.* 66:639–78

113. Scheffzek K, Ahmadian MR, Kabsch W, Wiesmuller L, Lautwein A, et al. 1997. The Ras-RasGAP complex: structural basis for GTPase activation and its loss in oncogenic Ras mutants. *Science* 277:333–38

114. Rittinger K, Walker PA, Eccleston JF, Smerdon SJ, Gamblin SJ. 1997. Structure at 1.65 A of RhoA and its GTPase-activating protein in complex with a transition-state analogue. *Nature* 389: 758–62

115. Nassar N, Hoffman GR, Manor D, Clardy JC, Cerione RA. 1998. Structures of Cdc42 bound to the active and catalytically compromised forms of Cdc42GAP. *Nat. Struct. Biol.* 5:1047–52

116. Goldberg J. 1999. Structural and functional analysis of the ARF1-ARFGAP complex reveals a role for coatomer in GTP hydrolysis. *Cell* 96:893–902

117. Bourne HR. 1997. G proteins. The arginine finger strikes again. *Nature* 389:673–74

118. Scheffzek K, Ahmadian MR, Wittinghofer A. 1998. GTPase-activating proteins: helping hands to complement an active site. *Trends Biochem. Sci.* 23:257–62

119. Gamblin SJ, Smerdon SJ. 1998. GTPase-activating proteins and their complexes. *Curr. Opin. Struct. Biol.* 8:195–201

120. Srinivasa SP, Watson N, Overton MC, Blumer KJ. 1998. Mechanism of RGS4, a GTPase-activating protein for G protein α subunits. *J. Biol. Chem.* 273:1529–33

121. Natochin M, McEntaffer RL, Artemyev NO. 1998. Mutational analysis of the Asn residue essential for RGS protein binding to G-proteins. *J. Biol. Chem.* 273:6731–35

122. Posner BA, Mukhopadhyay S, Tesmer JJ, Gilman AG, Ross EM. 1999. Modulation of the affinity and selectivity of RGS protein interaction with Gα subunits by a conserved Asparagine/Serine residue. *Biochemistry* 38:7773–79

123. de Alba E, De Vries L, Farquhar MG, Tjandra N. 1999. Solution structure of human GAIP (Gα interacting protein). A regulator of G protein signaling. *J. Mol. Biol.* 29:927–39

124. Berman DM, Kozasa T, Gilman AG. 1996. The GTPase-activating protein RGS4 stabilizes the transition state for nucleotide hydrolysis. *J. Biol. Chem.* 271:27209–12

124a. Druey KM, Kehrl JH. 1997. Inhibition of regulator of G protein signaling function by two mutant RGS4 proteins. *Proc. Natl. Acad. Sci. USA* 94:12851–56

125. DiBello PR, Garrison TR, Apanovitch DM, Hoffman G, Shuey DJ, et al. 1998. Selective uncoupling of RGS action by a single point mutation in the G protein alpha-subunit. *J. Biol. Chem.* 273:5780–84

126. Lan KL, Sarvazyan NA, Taussig R, Mackenzie RG, DiBello PR, et al. 1998. A point mutation in Gα$_o$ and Gα$_i$1 blocks interaction with regulator of G protein signaling proteins. *J. Biol. Chem.* 273:12794–97

127. Nekrasova ER, Berman DM, Rustandi RR, Hamm HE, Gilman AG, Arshavsky VY. 1997. Activation of transducin guanosine triphosphatase by two proteins of the RGS family. *Biochemistry* 36:7638–43

128. Sunahara RK, Tesmer JJ, Gilman AG, Sprang SR. 1997. Crystal structure of the adenylyl cyclase activator G$_s\alpha$. *Science* 278:1943–47

129. Natochin M, Lipkin VM, Artemyev NO. 1997. Interaction of human retinal RGS with G-protein α-subunits. *FEBS Lett.* 411:179–82

130. Skiba NP, Yang CS, Huang T, Bae H, Hamm HE. 1999. The α-helical domain of galphat determines specific interaction with regulator of G protein signaling 9. *J. Biol. Chem.* 274:8770–78

131. McEntaffer RL, Natochin M, Artemyev NO. 1999. Modulation of transducin GTPase activity by chimeric RGS16 and RGS9 regulators of G protein signaling and the effector molecule. *Biochemistry* 38:4931–37

132. Kozasa T, Jiang X, Hart MJ, Sternweis PM, Singer WD, et al. 1998. p115 RhoGEF, a GTPase activating protein for Gα_{12} and Gα_{13}. *Science* 280:2109–11

133. Fukuhara S, Murga C, Zohar M, Igishi T, Gutkind JS. 1999. A novel PDZ domain containing guanine nucleotide exchange factor links heterotrimeric G proteins to Rho. *J. Biol. Chem.* 274:5868–79

134. Natochin M, Artemyev NO. 1998. A single mutation Asp229 → Ser confers upon Gs alpha the ability to interact with regulators of G protein signaling. *Biochemistry* 37:13776–80

135. Natochin M, Artemyev NO. 1998. Substitution of transducin ser202 by asp abolishes G-protein/RGS interaction. *J. Biol. Chem.* 273:4300–3

136. Heximer SP, Watson N, Linder ME, Blumer KJ, Hepler JR. 1997. RGS2/G0S8 is a selective inhibitor of G$_q\alpha$ function. *Proc. Natl. Acad. Sci. USA* 94:14389–93

137. Woulfe DS, Stadel JM. 1999. Structural basis for the selectivity of the RGS protein, GAIP, for Gα_i family members. Identification of a single amino acid determinant for selective interaction of Gα_i subunits with GAIP. *J. Biol. Chem.* 274:17718–24

138. Snow B, Krumins AM, Brothers GM, Lee S-F, Wall MA, et al. 1998. A G protein γ subunit-like domain shared between RGS11 and other RGS proteins specifies binding to Gβ5 subunits. *Proc. Natl. Acad. Sci. USA* 95:13307–12

139. Cabrera JL, de Freitas F, Satpaev DK, Slepak VZ. 1998. Identification of the Gβ5-RGS7 protein complex in the retina. *Biochem. Biophys. Res. Commun.* 249:898–902

140. Makino ER, Handy JW, Li T, Arshavsky VY. 1999. The GTPase activating factor for transducin in rod photoreceptors is the complex between RGS9 and type 5 G protein β subunit. *Proc. Natl. Acad. Sci. USA* 96:1947–52

141. Snow BE, Betts L, Mangion J, Sondek J, Siderovski DP. 1999. Fidelity of G protein β-subunit association by the G protein γ-subunit-like domains of RGS6, RGS7, and RGS11. *Proc. Natl. Acad. Sci. USA* 96:6489–94

142. Levay K, Cabrera JL, Satpaev DK, Slepak VZ. 1999. Gβ5 prevents the RGS7-Gα_o interaction through binding to a distinct Gγ-like domain found in RGS7 and other RGS proteins. *Proc. Natl. Acad. Sci. USA* 96:2503–7

143. Axelrod JD, Miller JR, Shulman JM, Moon RT, Perrimon N. 1998. Differential recruitment of Dishevelled provides signaling specificity in the planar cell polarity and Wingless signaling pathways. *Genes Dev.* 12:2610–22

144. Ponting CP, Bork P. 1996. Pleckstrin's repeat performance: a novel domain in G-protein signaling? *Trends Biochem. Sci.* 21:245–46

145. Hart MJ, Sharma S, el Masry N, Qiu RG, McCabe P, et al. 1996. Identification of a novel guanine nucleotide exchange factor for the Rho GTPase. *J. Biol. Chem.* 271:25452–58

146. Buhl AM, Johnson NL, Dhanasekaran N, Johnson GL. 1995. Gα12 and Gα13 stimulate Rho-dependent stress fiber for-

mation and focal adhesion assembly. *J. Biol. Chem.* 270:24631–34

147. Fromm C, Coso OA, Montaner S, Xu N, Gutkind JS. 1997. The small GTP-binding protein Rho links G protein-coupled receptors and Gα12 to the serum response element and to cellular transformation. *Proc. Natl. Acad. Sci. USA* 94:10098–103

148. Hart MJ, Jiang X, Kozasa T, Roscoe W, Singer WD, et al. 1998. Direct stimulation of the guanine nucleotide exchange activity of p115 RhoGEF by Gα13. *Science* 280:2112–14

149. Hall A. 1998. G proteins and small GTPases: distant relatives keep in touch. *Science* 280:2074–75

150. Whitehead IP, Khosravi-Far R, Kirk H, Trigo-Gonzalez G, Der CJ, Kay R. 1996. Expression cloning of lsc, a novel oncogene with structural similarities to the Dbl family of guanine nucleotide exchange factors. *J. Biol. Chem.* 271:18643–50

151. Snow BE, Antonio L, Suggs S, Gutstein HB, Siderovski DP. 1997. Molecular cloning and expression analysis of rat Rgs12 and Rgs14. *Biochem. Biophys. Res. Commun.* 233:770–77

152. Craven SE, Bredt DS. 1998. PDZ proteins organize synaptic signaling pathways. *Cell* 93:495–98

153. De Vries L, Lou X, Zhao G, Zheng B, Farquhar MG. 1998. GIPC, a PDZ domain containing protein, interacts specifically with the C terminus of RGS-GAIP. *Proc. Natl. Acad. Sci. USA* 95:12340–45

154. Bunn RC, Jensen MA, Reed BC. 1999. Protein interactions with the glucose transporter binding protein GLUT1CBP that provide a link between GLUT1 and the cytoskeleton. *Mol. Biol. Cell* 10:819–32

154a. Wang LH, Kalb RG, Strittmatter SM. 1999. A PDZ protein regulates the distribution of the transmembrane sema-phorin, M-SemF. *J. Biol. Chem.* 274:14137–46

155. Rechsteiner M, Rogers SW. 1996. PEST sequences and regulation by proteolysis. *Trends Biochem. Sci.* 21:267–71

156. Kim E, Arnould T, Sellin L, Benzing T, Comella N, et al. 1999. Interaction between RGS7 and polycystin. *Proc. Natl. Acad. Sci. USA* 96:6371–76

157. Ben-Ze'ev A, Geiger B. 1998. Differential molecular interactions of β-catenin and plakoglobin in adhesion, signaling and cancer. *Curr. Opin. Cell Biol.* 10:629–39

158. Behrens J, Jerchow BA, Wurtele M, Grimm J, Asbrand C, et al. 1998. Functional interaction of an axin homolog, conductin, with beta-catenin APC, and GSK3beta. *Science* 280:596–99

159. Yamamoto H, Kishida S, Uochi T, Ikeda S, Koyama S, et al. 1998. Axil, a member of the axin family, interacts with both glycogen synthase kinase 3beta and beta-catenin and inhibits axis formation of *Xenopus* embryos. *Mol. Cell. Biol.* 18:2867–75

160. Ikeda S, Kishida S, Yamamoto H, Murai H, Koyama S, Kikuchi A. 1998. Axin, a negative regulator of the Wnt signaling pathway, forms a complex with GSK-3β and β-catenin and promotes GSK-3β-dependent phosphorylation of β-catenin. *Embo J.* 17:1371–84

161. Kishida S, Yamamoto H, Ikeda S, Kishida M, Sakamoto I, et al. 1998. Axin, a negative regulator of the wnt signaling pathway, directly interacts with adeno-matous polyposis coli and regulates the stabilization of β-catenin. *J. Biol. Chem.* 273:10823–26

162. Huang C, Hepler JR, Gilman AG, Mumby SM. 1997. Attenuation of Gi- and Gq-mediated signaling by expression of RGS4 or GAIP in mammalian cells. *Proc. Natl. Acad. Sci. USA* 94:6159–63

163. Zhang H, Yasrebi-Nejad H, Lang J. 1998. G-protein betagamma-binding domains

regulate insulin exocytosis in clonal pancreatic beta-cells. *FEBS Lett.* 424:202–6

164. Dulin NO, Sorokin A, Reed E, Elliott S, Kehrl JH, Dunn MJ. 1999. RGS3 inhibits G protein-mediated signaling via translocation to the membrane and binding to Gα11. *Mol. Cell. Biol.* 19:714–23

165. Melliti K, Meza U, Fisher R, Adams B. 1999. Regulators of G protein signaling attenuate the G protein-mediated inhibition of N-type Ca channels. *J. Gen. Physiol.* 113:97–110

166. Saugstad JA, Marino MJ, Folk JA, Hepler JR, Conn PJ. 1998. RGS4 inhibits signaling by group I metabotropic glutamate receptors. *J. Neurosci.* 18:905–13

167. Jeong SW, Ikeda SR. 1998. G protein alpha subunit G alpha z couples neurotransmitter receptors to ion channels in sympathetic neurons. *Neuron* 21:1201–12

168. Zhang Y, Neo SY, Han J, Yaw LP, Lin SC. 1999. RGS16 attenuates Gα$_q$-dependent p38 mitogen-activated protein kinase activation by platelet-activating factor. *J. Biol. Chem.* 274:2851–57

169. Wu HK, Heng HH, Shi XM, Forsdyke DR, Tsui LC, et al. 1995. Differential expression of a basic helix-loop-helix phosphoprotein gene, G0S8, in acute leukemia and localization to human chromosome 1q31. *Leukemia* 9:1291–98

170. Mai M, Qian C, Yokomizo A, Smith DI, Liu W. 1999. Cloning of the human homolog of conductin (AXIN2), a gene mapping to chromosome 17q23-q24. *Genomics* 55:341–44

171. Jordan JD, Carey KD, Stork PJ, Iyengar RJ. 1999. *J. Biol. Chem.* 274:21507–10

Annu. Rev. Pharmacol. Toxicol. 2000. 40:273–82

Parallel Array and Mixture-Based Synthetic Combinatorial Chemistry: Tools for the Next Millennium

Richard A. Houghten

Torrey Pines Institute for Molecular Studies, San Diego, California 92121;
e-mail: rhoughten@tpims.org

Key Words deconvolution, iterative, libraries, positional scanning, screening

■ **Abstract** Technological advances continue to be a central driving force in the acceleration of the drug discovery process. Combinatorial chemistry methods, developed over the past 15 years, represent a paradigm shift in drug discovery. Initially viewed as a curiosity by the pharmaceutical industry, combinatorial chemistry is now recognized as an essential tool that decreases the time of discovery and increases the throughput of chemical screening by as much as 1000-fold. The use of parallel array synthesis approaches and mixture-based combinatorial libraries for drug discovery is reviewed.

INTRODUCTION

The philosophical and practical concepts encompassed by the varied approaches now termed combinatorial chemistry have fundamentally altered drug discovery. The first synthetic combinatorial chemistry methods were presented by Geysen et al (individual compounds chemically synthesized on plastic "pins") (1) and Houghten (simultaneous multiple compound synthesis on polystyrene resin "tea bags") (2) in 1984 and 1985, respectively. Both of these methods are based on Merrifield's pioneering work in solid-phase peptide synthesis (3). Even with the advent of automated means to carry out solid-phase peptide synthesis, the number of peptides available remained the limiting factor in virtually all studies. This was also true for the solution phase synthesis of classical heterocycles and other small molecule organic compounds. It is of note that Leznoff & Wong (4, 5) and Crowley & Rapoport (6) first carried out the solid-phase synthesis of heterocycles in 1973 and 1976, respectively, but this powerful approach remained unappreciated until work by Bunin & Ellman in 1992 (7). In the author's laboratory, the value of the parallel preparation of large numbers of peptides was shown in a 1988 study, in which more than 500 analogs of the 23-residue peptide

0362–1642/00/0415–0273$14.00

magainin were prepared (8). This increased synthetic capability (at the time, approximately 10-fold greater for peptides) has led to the successful clinical trial of the magainin analog Cytolex™ (MSI-78) and other therapeutic peptides (9). Furthermore, these approaches have made possible a range of basic research studies that were previously impractical due to economic or timeframe factors (reviewed in 10, 11).

As is true for all combinatorial chemistry approaches, the pin and tea-bag methods for solid-phase synthesis were first used to prepare peptides (1, 2, 11–14). They are now widely used to prepare large individual compound libraries of virtually all types, including peptidomimetics (15–19), oligonucleotides (20, 21), oligosaccharides (22–24), and heterocycles (25, 26). The widespread success of solid-phase synthesis is due to the ability to drive reactions to completion (often >99.8%) on polymer supports, the ability to readily remove excess reagents or starting materials, and automation (2, 7, 25). Despite the great increase in synthesis capability made possible by the pin and tea-bag techniques, it was soon clear that the barrier in virtually all studies still remained the number of compounds that could be synthesized. The successful preparation of mixture-based combinatorial libraries, in combination with earlier parallel-array synthesis approaches, has now pushed aside the synthesis limitations that were inherent in the drug-discovery process. Our laboratory's efforts have remained focused on the use of parallel-array synthesis for the preparation of very large, mixture-based combinatorial libraries.

MIXTURES VERSUS INDIVIDUAL COMPOUND ARRAYS

It is well accepted that the screening of natural product extracts is a productive source of therapeutic compounds. Such extracts are typically composed of hundreds to thousands of different compounds in varying concentrations. Additionally, highly active individual compounds have been found that were present in extracts at one part per 100,000 or less. In spite of the fact that natural products and, indeed, the very nature of biological interactions are inherently mixture-based, and the fact that these interactions do not occur in an environment made up of single compounds and single acceptors, an intense debate continues on the relative merits of the preparation and screening of individual compound arrays versus mixture-based combinatorial libraries of the same compounds. The central issue is the tradeoff between the time and cost necessary to acquire complete information about every compound making up an individual compound array, versus a somewhat less complete information set derived from the same compounds in a mixture-based library. Our experience over the past 15 years has found the generation and use of mixture-based combinatorial libraries to be an extremely effective and cost-efficient means to generate highly active, therapeutically relevant individual compounds.

SYNTHESIS OF MIXTURES

Divide-Couple-Recombine (Split-and-Mix) Synthesis

One important issue in library synthesis is to obtain as close to equimolar representation as possible of all individual compounds within a mixture-based library for ease of deconvolution. For peptides, therefore, the various amino acids have to be incorporated into each of the library positions in a ratio as close to equimolar as possible. When using resin beads as the solid support for library synthesis, this can be achieved using a process known as "divide-couple-recombine" (DCR) (27), "split-and-mix synthesis" (28), or "portioning-mixing" (29). This process involves the coupling of each protected amino acid to be used for the library to separate portions of resin, followed by combining and mixing all resin portions, before dividing the resin again for the next coupling step. By repeating this process for a total of five couplings, and using 20 amino acids as building blocks, a library of 3,200,000 (20^5) pentapeptides can be readily prepared. Due to the physical separation of the resins prior to incorporating the individual amino acids, the DCR process yields libraries containing an individual, unique compound on each resin bead.

Coupling of Mixtures of Incoming Reagents

An alternative means for the introduction of mixture positions is through the coupling of mixtures of incoming reagents, such as protected amino acids. Due to the differences in coupling rates of the various amino acids, coupling of an equimolar amino acid mixture to resin-bound amino groups, as typically used in solid-phase peptide synthesis, will lead to nonequimolar incorporation of amino acids into the mixture positions. This ultimately will result in a highly nonequimolar distribution of individual peptides within the library. To overcome this problem, the ratio of protected amino acids within the coupling mixture is adjusted according to their different coupling rates, i.e. the higher the coupling rate of a particular amino acid, the lower the concentration of that amino acid in the coupling mixture (30, 31). Such ratios are established by adjusting the relative concentration of each amino acid according to its incorporation ratio after coupling of an equimolar amino acid mixture, as determined by amino acid analysis or HPLC. Because these amino acid mixtures are coupled in a large (i.e. 5- to 10-fold) molar excess over resin-bound amino groups, the coupling can be considered a pseudo-first-order reaction. The ratio of coupling rates of the amino acids within the mixture is therefore independent of the amino acid it is being coupled to.

DECONVOLUTION—FINDING THE NEEDLE
IN THE HAYSTACK

Iterative Deconvolution

Geysen's early use of very large peptide mixtures immobilized on pins, while clearly of conceptual importance, has not been found to be generally useful. To deconvolute pin-immobilized peptide mixtures, Geysen et al used an iterative approach (30), as did the author's laboratory for soluble libraries (27). This approach steadily decreases the number of compounds per mixture while steadily defining successive positions. Iterative deconvolution of soluble (i.e. not immobilized on a solid support) mixture-based libraries has been found to be successful in a wide range of studies (reviewed in 32). The primary limitation of iterative deconvolution is the cost and time associated with the need for repetitive synthesis and screening steps, typically equal to the number of variable positions.

Positional Scanning Deconvolution

A rapid means to gather information about all possible variable positions in a library was presented by the author's laboratory in 1992 (33). An illustration of the positional scanning deconvolution approach for a simple tripeptide combinatorial library is shown in Figure 1. Four different amino acids are incorporated at each of the three diversity positions, resulting in 64 (4^3) individual peptides. When the same diversity is arranged as a positional scanning synthetic combinatorial library (PS-SCL), only 12 peptide mixtures (4 separate mixtures for each of the 3 positions) need to be synthesized. Each of the three positional sublibraries, namely OXX, XOX, and XXO, contain exactly the same diversity of peptides, differing only in the location of the position defined. Each of the O positions is singularly defined with one of the four amino acids, whereas the remaining two positions are mixtures (X) of the same four amino acids.

In this example, assume that the sequence RAT is the sole tripeptide having activity. Since each positional sublibrary contains the exact same diversity of peptides, the RAT tripeptide (outlined below each sublibrary in Figure 1) is present in all three positional sublibraries. Thus, the only mixtures with activity will be RXX, XAX, and XXT because the only active sequence, RAT, is present only in those mixtures. These three amino acids in their respective positions yield the tripeptide RAT, which can then be synthesized and tested for its individual activity. It should be noted that the activity observed for each of the three mixtures (RXX, XAX, and XXT) is due to the presence of the tripeptide RAT within each of these mixtures and is not due to the individual amino acids (R, A, and T) that occupy the defined positions. As expected, and found experimentally in more complex libraries, more than one mixture is usually found to have activity at each position. Selection of the building blocks for the synthesis of individual compounds is based first on the overall activity of the mixture and then on differences

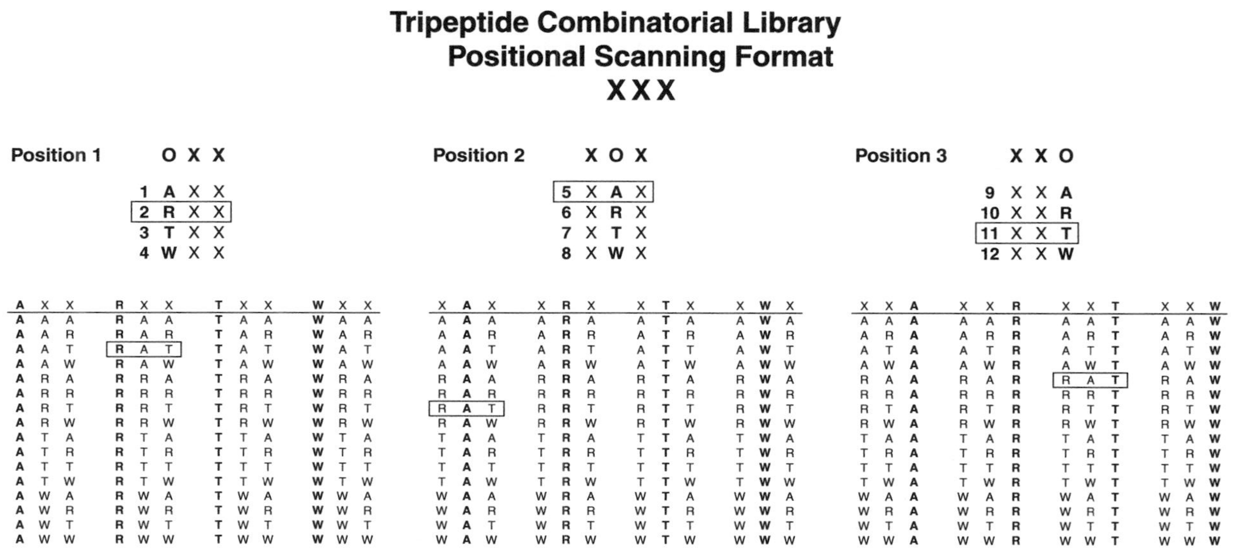

Tripeptide Combinatorial Library
Positional Scanning Format
X X X

Position 1   O X X

Position 2   X O X

Position 3   X X O

```
1 A X X        5 X A X        9  X X A
2 R X X        6 X R X        10 X X R
3 T X X        7 X T X        11 X X T
4 W X X        8 X W X        12 X X W
```

Figure 1 Tripeptide combinatorial library—positional scanning format.

in the chemical character of the building block (to reduce the number of individual compounds to be made). Freier and coworkers have presented an excellent discussion of the theoretical and experimental aspects of iterative and positional scanning deconvolution (34, 35).

The use of mixtures of compounds in a positional scanning combinatorial library format versus the use of individual compound arrays is clearly cost beneficial, thus allowing biotechnology companies, universities, and research institutes to carry out basic research and the initial stages of the drug-discovery process. Thus, previously unimagined numbers of compounds can be prepared and screened to yield highly active individual compounds.

The author's laboratory has successfully identified uniquely active and selective peptides from libraries made up of L-, D-, and unnatural amino acids totaling 6.25 million tetrapeptides (36), 52 million hexapeptides (27), and 6 trillion decapeptides (37). In practical terms, we believe that the cost and time savings make the use of mixtures in the positional scanning format a powerful alternative to the use of large individual compound arrays. A wide variety of classic heterocycles and other acyclic organic compounds can now be prepared using solid-phase parallel synthesis. The author's laboratory has found that existing libraries can be utilized to generate a diverse range of mixture-based heterocyclic libraries through the transformation of peptide and peptidomimetic libraries using the "libraries from libraries" approach (38). Such heterocyclic compounds have dramatically different physical and biological properties from the peptide libraries used as starting materials. Figures 2 and 3 illustrate a number of the transformations we have successfully carried out. The average library generated for the compound classes shown contains more than 50,000 compounds. We have recently generated a variation of the bicyclic guanidine library shown in Figure 2 (26), which is composed of more than 1.2 million bicyclic guanidines. It should be noted that each of the compounds illustrated in Figure 2 can be further transformed into other pharmacophores.

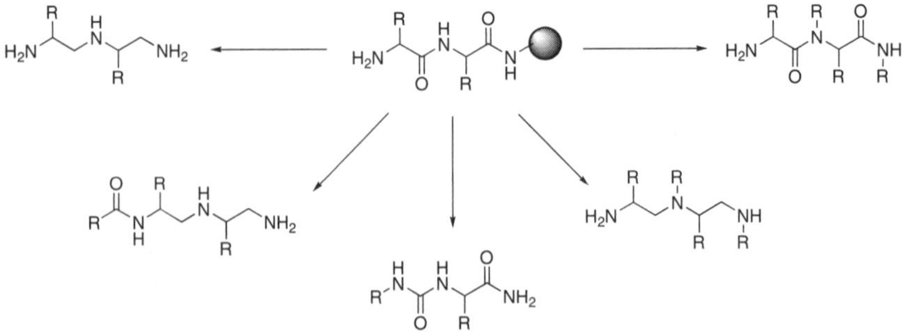

Figure 2 Solid-phase synthesis of acyclic compounds using dipeptides as starting material.

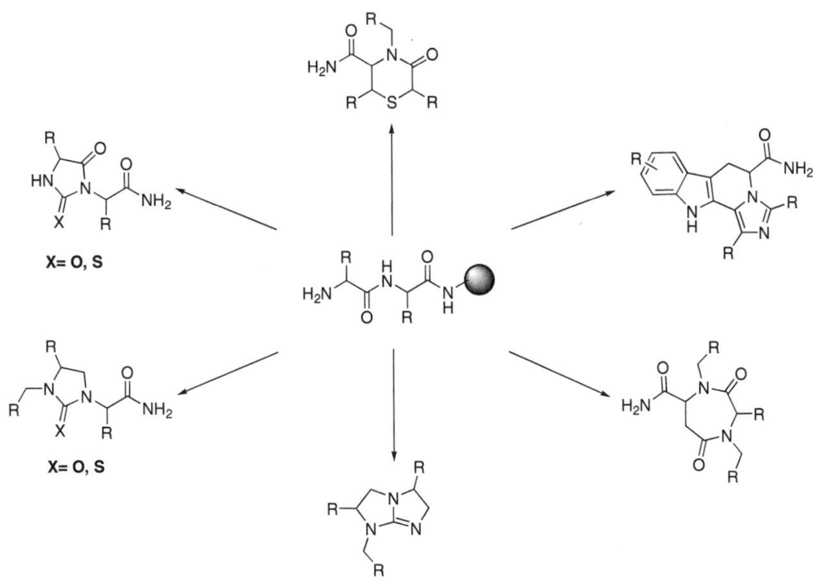

Figure 3 Solid-phase synthesis of heterocyclic compounds using dipeptides and acylated dipeptides as starting material.

CONCLUSIONS

Extensive studies on the use of mixture-based combinatorial libraries carried out by this laboratory (reviewed in 32) and others have enabled the rapid, cost-effective identification of highly active and specific individual compounds. These methods are extremely effective and broadly applicable, and have shown that there is nothing inherently unique about peptides or other oligomers that permits their successful use in mixture-based library formats as compared to heterocycles. Thus, the use of massive parallel synthesis in conjunction with classic high throughput screening methods versus the use of mixture-based combinatorial libraries must be tied to the balance between the need for complete data acquisition versus the pragmatic and rapid gathering of compound information for lead development. The use of extremely large mixture-based combinatorial libraries offers unique advantages that are simply not possible with other approaches.

Combinatorial chemistry, in all its manifestations over the past 15 years, has fundamentally changed synthetic chemistry in all areas of basic research and drug discovery. When coupled with methods such as computer-assisted design and molecular biology, combinatorial chemistry can be expected to enhance and continually increase the speed and thoroughness of drug discovery into the next millennium.

ACKNOWLEDGMENTS

The author's work is based on long-term collaborations with a number of scientific colleagues over the past 15 years. He would like to thank: John Ostresh for the development of a number of synthetic approaches, including "libraries from libraries"; Clemencia Pinilla and Jon Appel for their work in developing the positional scanning deconvolution approach and the use of combinatorial libraries in immunological systems; Sylvie Blondelle for her work in identifying antibacterial and other highly active compounds from libraries; Colette Dooley for the development of radioreceptor screening assays and the identification of highly active opioid compounds; Jutta Eichler for the development of cyclic libraries; Barbara Dörner for the development of peralkylated peptidomimetic libraries; Adel Nefzi for heterocyclic chemistry; and Darcy Wilson for his T-cell immunology expertise.

Visit the Annual Reviews home page at www.AnnualReviews.org.

LITERATURE CITED

1. Geysen HM, Meloen RH, Barteling SJ. 1984. Use of a peptide synthesis to probe viral antigens for epitopes to a resolution of a single amino acid. *Proc. Natl. Acad. Sci. USA* 81:3998–4002
2. Houghten RA. 1985. General method for the rapid solid-phase synthesis of large numbers of peptides: specificity of antigen-antibody interaction at the level of individual amino acids. *Proc. Natl. Acad. Sci. USA* 82:5131–35
3. Merrifield RB. 1963. Peptide synthesis. I. The synthesis of a tetrapeptide. *J. Am. Chem. Soc.* 85:2149–54
4. Wong JY, Leznoff CC. 1973. The use of polymer supports in organic synthesis. II. The syntheses of monoethers of symmetrical diols. *Can. J. Chem.* 51:2452–56
5. Leznoff CC, Wong JY. 1973. The use of polymer supports in organic synthesis. III. Selective chemical reactions on one aldehyde group of symmetrical dialdehydes. *Can. J. Chem.* 51:3756–64
6. Crowley JI, Rapoport H. 1976. Solid-phase organic synthesis: novelty or fundamental concept? *Acc. Chem. Res.* 9:135–44
7. Bunin BA, Ellman JA. 1992. A general and expedient method for the solid-phase synthesis of 1,4-benzodiazepine derivatives. *J. Am. Chem. Soc.* 114:10997–98
8. Cuervo JH, Rodriguez B, Houghten RA. 1988. The magainins: sequence factors relevant to increased antimicrobial activity and decreased hemolytic activity. *Pept. Res.* 1:81–86
9. Suto MJ, Girten BE, Houghten RA, Loullis CC, Tuttle RR. 1995. Cytokine restraining agents. *U.S. Patent No. 5,420,109*
10. Pinilla C, Appel JR, Blondelle SE, Dooley CT, Eichler J, et al. 1994. Versatility of positional scanning of synthetic combinatorial libraries for the identification of individual compounds. *Drug Dev. Res.* 33:133–45
11. Eichler J, Appel JR, Blondelle SE, Dooley CT, Dörner B, et al. 1995. Peptide, peptidomimetic and organic synthetic combinatorial libraries. *Med. Res. Rev.* 15:481–96

12. Merrifield RB. 1986. Solid phase synthesis. *Science* 232:341–47

13. Stewart JM, Young JD. 1984. *Solid Phase Peptide Synthesis.* Rockford, IL: Pierce Chem. Co. 2nd ed.

14. Atherton E, Sheppard RC. 1989. *Solid Phase Peptide Synthesis—A Practical Approach.* Oxford, UK: IRL Press

15. Giannis A, Kolter T. 1993. Peptidomimetics for receptor ligands—discovery, development, and medical perspectives. *Angew. Chem. Int. Ed. Engl.* 32:1244–67

16. Liskamp RMJ. 1994. A new application of modified peptides and peptidomimetics: potential anticancer agents. *Angew. Chem. Int. Ed. Engl.* 33:305–7

17. Dörner B, Husar GM, Ostresh JM, Houghten RA. 1996. The synthesis of peptidomimetic combinatorial libraries through successive amide alkylation. *Bioorg. Med. Chem.* 4:709–15

18. Gersuk VH, Rose TM, Todaro GJ. 1995. Molecular cloning and chromosomal localization of a pseudogene related to the human acyl-CoA binding protein/diazepam binding inhibitor. *Genomics* 25:469–76

19. Ostresh JM, Blondelle SE, Dörner B, Houghten RA. 1996. Generation and use of nonsupport-bound peptide and peptidomimetic combinatorial libraries. *Methods Enzymol.* 267:220–34

20. Smythe ML, Huston SE, Marshall GR. 1993. Free energy profile of a 3_{10}- to α-helical transition of an oligopeptide in various solvents. *J. Am. Chem. Soc.* 115:11594–95

21. Fruchtel JS, Jung G. 1996. Organic chemistry on solid supports. *Angew. Chem. Int. Ed. Engl.* 35:17–42

22. Douglas SP, Whitfield DM, Krepinsky JJ. 1995. Polymer supported solution synthesis of oligosaccharides using a novel versatile linker for the synthesis of D-mannopentose, a structural unit of D-mannose of pathogenic yeasts. *J. Am. Chem. Soc.* 117:2116–17

23. Schuster M, Wang P, Paulson JC, Wong C. 1994. Solid-phase chemical-enzymatic synthesis of glycopeptides and oligosaccharides. *J. Am. Chem. Soc.* 116:1135–36

24. Frecht JM, Schuerch C. 1971. Solid phase synthesis of oligosaccharides. I. Preparation of the solid support. poly[p-(1-propen-3-ol-1-yl)styrene]. *J. Am. Chem. Soc.* 93:492–96

25. Nefzi A, Ostresh JM, Houghten RA. 1997. The current status of heterocyclic combinatorial libraries. *Chem. Rev.* 97:449–72

26. Ostresh JM, Schoner C, Hamashin VT, Nefzi A, Meyer JP, et al. 1998. The solid phase synthesis of tri-substituted bicyclic guanidines via cyclization of reduced N-acylated dipeptides. *J. Org. Chem.* 63:8622–23

27. Houghten RA, Pinilla C, Blondelle SE, Appel JR, Dooley CT, et al. 1991. Generation and use of synthetic peptide combinatorial libraries for basic research and drug discovery. *Nature* 354:84–86

28. Lam KS, Salmon SE, Hersh EM, Hruby VJ, Kazmierski WM. 1991. A new type of synthetic peptide library for identifying ligand binding activity. *Nature* 354:82–84

29. Furka A, Sebestyen F, Asgedom M, Dibo G. 1991. General method for rapid synthesis of multicomponent peptide mixtures. *Int. J. Pept. Protein Res.* 37:487–93

30. Geysen HM, Rodda SJ, Mason TJ. 1986. A priori delineation of a peptide which mimics a discontinuous antigenic determinant. *Mol. Immunol.* 23:709–15

31. Ostresh JM, Winkle JH, Hamashin VT, Houghten RA. 1994. Peptide libraries: determination of relative reaction rates of amino acids in competitive couplings. *Biopolymers* 34:1681–89

32. Houghten RA, Pinilla C, Appel JR, Blondelle SE, Dooley CT, et al. 1999. Mixture-based synthetic combinatorial libraries. *J. Med. Chem.* 42:3743–78

33. Pinilla C, Appel JR, Blanc P, Houghten

RA. 1992. Rapid identification of high affinity peptide ligands using positional scanning synthetic peptide combinatorial libraries. *Biotechniques* 13:901–5

34. Konings DAM, Wyatt JR, Ecker DJ, Freier SM. 1996. Deconvolution of combinatorial libraries for drug discovery: theoretical comparison of pooling strategies. *J. Med. Chem.* 39:2710–19

35. Wilson-Lingardo L, Davis PW, Ecker DJ, Hebert N, Acevedo O, et al. 1996. Deconvolution of combinatorial libraries for drug discovery: experimental comparison of pooling strategies. *J. Med. Chem.* 39:2720–26

36. Dooley CT, Ny P, Bidlack JM, Houghten RA. 1998. Selective ligands for the mu, delta and kappa opioid receptors identified from a single tetrapeptide positional scanning combinatorial library. *J. Biol. Chem.* 273:18848–56

37. Hemmer B, Pinilla C, Appel J, Pascal J, Houghten RH, et al. 1998. The use of soluble synthetic peptide combinatorial libraries to determine antigen recognition of T cells. *J. Pept. Res.* 52:338–45

38. Ostresh JM, Husar GM, Blondelle SE, Dörner B, Weber PA, et al. 1994. Libraries from libraries: chemical transformation of combinatorial libraries to extend the range and repertoire of chemical diversity. *Proc. Natl. Acad. Sci. USA* 91:11138–42

Annu. Rev. Pharmacol. Toxicol. 2000. 40:283–94

PHARMACOLOGY OF SELECTIN INHIBITORS IN ISCHEMIA/REPERFUSION STATES

David J. Lefer

Department of Molecular and Cellular Physiology, Louisiana State University Medical Center, Shreveport, Louisiana 71130; e-mail: dlefer@lsumc.edu

Key Words P-selectin, sialyl Lewis^x, myocardial injury, endothelium, coronary circulation

■ **Abstract** Recently, the selectin family of glycoprotein adhesion molecules (P-selectin, E-selectin, and L-selectin) has been implicated in the pathogenesis of a number of inflammatory disease states. The selectins modulate the early adhesive interactions between circulating neutrophils and the endothelium. Both P-selectin and E-selectin can be expressed on the surface of endothelial cells following stimulation by a number of inflammatory mediators. In contrast, L-selectin is constitutively expressed on the surface of neutrophils at very high levels. In addition, neutrophils also express ligands for the endothelial selectins, including the carbohydrate sialyl Lewis^x and the high-affinity ligand P-selectin glycoprotein ligand 1, which facilitate neutrophil-endothelial interactions. Selectins have been extensively investigated in ischemia/reperfusion injury states. The study of selectin involvement in ischemia/reperfusion injury has been facilitated by the development of highly specific selectin antagonists, including monoclonal antibodies, carbohydrates, small molecule inhibitors, and soluble forms of P-selectin glycoprotein ligand 1. This article reviews the results of current studies of selectin antagonists in experimental models of ischemia/reperfusion injury.

INTRODUCTION

The selectins are a family of glycoproteins that play a significant role in the regulation of cell adhesion as well as in cell signalling. Selectins are expressed on the cell surface of key cell types. There are three members of the selectin family: L-selectin, P-selectin, and E-selectin. The nomenclature is based on (*a*) the fact that there is a lectin domain in their structure, hence the name selectin (1), and (*b*) the cell types on which the selectin is expressed. Thus, L-selectin is found on leukocytes, E-selectin is expressed on the surface of endothelial cells, and P-selectin is expressed on platelets and endothelial cells.

L-selectin is constitutively expressed on several select types of monocytes, lymphocytes, and neutrophils. L-selectin exists on the tips of the pseudopods of these white blood cells and can be shed from these cell surfaces upon their acti-

0362–1642/00/0415–0283$14.00

vation (2). P-selectin, however, exists internally in Weibel-Palade bodies of endo-thelial cells and α-granules of platelets (3). P-selectin can be translocated to the cell surface by activation with thrombin, histamine, hydrogen peroxide, and inhib-itors of nitric oxide synthase (3). This process peaks in 10–20 min. In contrast, E-selectin is expressed on endothelial cells only after de novo synthesis following activation of endothelial cells, a process requiring 4–6 h (4). Activators of E-selectin include the cytokines—tumor necrosis factor alpha,—interleukin 1β, and bacterial lipopolysaccharide (endotoxin).

All three selectins play a key role in the cell adhesion cascade of inflammation. Basically, the selectins initiate leukocyte rolling along the endothelium (5), the first step in leukocyte recruitment. The most important selectin in regulating leu-kocyte rolling in ischemia/reperfusion and other shock-like states is P-selectin (6). This rolling, or "capture," effectively slows the velocity of leukocyte move-ment in the microcirculation and enables many of these leukocytes to proceed to the second step, firm adhesion to the endothelium. Some of the adherent leuko-cytes will undergo transendothelial migration and thus congregate at the site of infection or inflammation (7).

In ischemia/reperfusion, the first step in reperfusion injury, an inflammatory process, is the loss of endothelium-derived nitric oxide, resulting in a rapid (i.e. within 2–5 min) endothelial dysfunction (8). The second step in the reperfusion injury process is up-regulation of P-selectin on the endothelial surface of the affected area 10–20 min following reperfusion (9). This leads to increased adhe-sion of neutrophils [polymorphonuclear leukocytes (PMNs)] to the dysfunctional/selectin up-regulated endothelium (10). At this point, the process slows down and a gradual infiltration of PMNs occurs, which at 180 minutes postreperfusion becomes significant. Finally, reperfusion injury with its resultant tissue necrosis occurs to a marked extent by 270 min (i.e. in the case of the ischemic/reperfused heart, myocardial necrosis) (11). Thus, key players in the process linking the endothelial dysfunction to the PMN involvement are the selectins, particularly P-selectin. In addition to the translocation of P-selectin to the surface of endothelial cells and platelets, new P-selectin expression occurs via up-regulation of such transcription factors as NF-κB (12, 13), a process that may amplify the role of P-selectin, by invoking a second peak of activation later in time following the early translocation of P-selectin to the cell surface. In contrast to P- and L-selectin, E-selectin does not apparently play a major role in reperfusion injury, at least during the first 4 h postreperfusion.

TYPES OF SELECTIN INHIBITORS

There are a variety of approaches that can be taken to inhibit or block one or more of the selectin family members. These are listed in Table 1. The earliest inhibitors of the selectins were monoclonal antibodies (mAbs) directed against a specific selectin molecule. These mAbs have the advantage of a high degree of

TABLE 1 Various selectin antagonists that have been investigated in ischemia/reperfusion injury states

Selectin antagonist	Antagonist type	Cellular target	Dose range	References(s)
PB 1.3 (CY-1747)[a]	Monoclonal antibody	P-selectin	1–2 mg/kg	17–24, 26
DREG-200[b]	Monoclonal antibody	L-selectin	1 mg/kg	27–29
CL-2[b]	Monoclonal antibody	E-selectin	1 mg/kg	31
CY-1787[a]	Monoclonal antibody	E-selectin	1 mg/kg	9
SLe[x]-OS (CY-1503)[a]	Carbohydrate	E-selectin, P-selectin	5–40 mg/kg	14, 36–44
TBC-1269[c]	Small molecule	E-selectin, P-selectin	25 mg/kg	47
sPSGL-1 and rsPSGL-1-Ig[d]	Peptide analog	P-selectin	5 μg/rat–1 mg/kg	50–53, 56

[a]Cytel Corporation, San Diego, CA. Sle[x]-OS, Sialyl Lewis[x] oligosaccharide.
[b]Boehringer Ingelheim, Ridgefield, CT.
[c]Texas Biotechnology, Houston, TX.
[d]Genetics Institute, Cambridge, MA. sPSGL-1, Soluble P-selectin glycoprotein ligand-1; rsPSGL, recombinant analog of sPSGL-1; Ig, immunoglobulin.

specificity, but they cross-react with only a few species. Most of the early mAbs cross-reacted with human selectin molecules but had limited actions among other mammalian species. However, many of these mAbs did cross-react with cat tissues. All mAbs were effective at doses of 1–2 mg/kg.

Once it became known that the three members of the selectin family recognize a common carbohydrate ligand (i.e. sialyl Lewis^x) (13), the race was on to develop analogs of sialyl Lewis^x (SLe^x) that acted as a soluble selectin blocker and blocked the actions of the selectins. The enormous difficulty and cost of synthesizing these carbohydrate analogs delayed progress for a while, but with the synthesis of a SLe^x-oligosaccharide (SLe^x-OS) known as CY-1503, great progress was made. This substance was effective at 10–20 mg/kg in a variety of mammalian species, and it blocked all selectins (14). Unfortunately, it had a circulating $t_{1/2}$ of only 10–30 min. A variety of small-molecule SLe^x-mimetics have been developed and studied as selectin antagonists. These are either sulfatide analogs, manosylated biphenyl derivatives, or dipeptides, and they are discussed later. Several years later, the high-affinity ligand for P-selectin, P-selectin glycoprotein ligand-1 (PSGL-1) (15), was discovered. Although PSGL-1 is a ligand primarily for P-selectin, it can serve as a ligand for all the selectins (16). Recently, a soluble form of PSGL-1 (sPSGL-1) has been used as a functional inhibitor of selectin actions in vivo. Finally, nitric oxide (NO) and NO donors have been found to be effective selectin antagonists (6, 11).

PROTECTIVE ACTIONS OF SELECTIN INHIBITORS IN ISCHEMIA/REPERFUSION

Monoclonal Antibodies Directed Against Selectins

Monoclonal antibodies neutralizing P-selectin were the first significant anti-selectin blockers available. The leading anti–P-selectin mAb is PB1.3, produced by the Cytel Corporation of San Diego, California. This antibody, also known as CY-1747, is an immunoglobulin (Ig) G$_1$ antibody raised against human P-selectin. However, it cross-reacts with feline, canine, rabbit, and rat P-selectin. Not only is it an effective P-selectin–neutralizing antibody in these species, it also recognizes only surface-expressed P-selectin and, thus, is a very valuable reagent for immunocytochemistry and immunolocalization of P-selectin expressed on the surface of endothelial cells (17). PB1.3 at a dose of 1–2 mg/kg was found to be effective in myocardial ischemia/reperfusion (MI/R) injury when given intravenously at the time of reperfusion (17). Not only was cardiac necrosis reduced by 58%, a highly significant finding ($P < 0.01$), but a comparable degree of coronary vascular endothelial preservation and reduced PMN adhesion to the coronary endothelium was also observed (17). Cardioprotection by PB1.3 was also observed following MI/R in dogs, which also confirmed that PB1.3 attenuated PMN infiltration into the reperfused myocardium (18–20).

Not only does PB1.3 protect the ischemic-reperfused myocardium in rats, it also protects against reperfusion injury in the splanchnic region by reducing intestinal injury (21) and by reducing mesenteric microvascular leakiness to albumin (22, 23). Furthermore, PB1.3 was found to attenuate reperfusion injury to the rabbit ear (24) and concomitantly reduce PMN adherence to the ischemic-reperfused endothelium. This reduced necrosis was also confirmed in the rabbit ear with a different antibody against P-selectin, a P-selectin–IgG chimera (25). In all cases, the P-selectin antibodies did not significantly induce any circulating leukopenia.

Finally, PB1.3 was also effective in total body I/R (i.e. hemorrhage-reinfusion) in rabbits (26). PB1.3 protected the microvasculature from fluid loss and maintained cardiac output and arterial blood pressure.

Monoclonal antibodies have also been produced against L-selectin. One of these, DREG-200, an IgG1 antibody, effectively blocks L-selectin on leukocytes (27). DREG-200 was found to significantly attenuate myocardial reperfusion injury in cats (28) by limiting cardiac necrosis, reducing endothelial dysfunction, and attenuating neutrophil infiltration. On the basis of these results, a humanized form of DREG-200 was prepared and tested in this same feline model of MI/R (29). This Hu DREG-200 attenuated postreperfusion cardiac necrosis by 52% compared with 60% for the nonhumanized form of DREG-200. Moreover, in addition to preserving coronary endothelial function and limiting PMN infiltration, Hu DREG-200 was found to significantly reduce left ventricular contractile dysfunction occurring in the first few hours of reperfusion (29). Employing another mAb against L-selectin, Ramasworthy et al (30) reported salutary effects in rabbits subjected to total body hemorrhage for 2 h followed by reinfusion of shed blood. As with the other L-selectin studies, there was no significant change in circulating leukocyte counts in antibody-treated animals.

With regard to mAbs directed against E-selectin, only a few reports have been published, presumably because of the lack of positive effects of these mAbs in several models of I/R injury. The first such report was published by Winquist et al (31), who showed that CL-2, an anti–E-selectin mAb, did not reduce infarct size in cynomolgus monkeys in a model of MI/R injury in which at 4 h postreperfusion an anti–intercellular adhesion molecule-1 mAb (R6.5) had been effective. Moreover, Weyrich et al (9) found a similar lack of effectiveness of an E-selectin mAb (CY-1787) in the same feline model of MI/R, in which both P-selectin and L-selectin mAbs were effective. Similarly, Kurose et al (32) found that CL-3, another anti–E-selectin mAb, was ineffective in splanchnic I/R in rats, although PB1.3 was effective in this same model system. One is forced to conclude that E-selectin does not play a significant role in reperfusion injury, at least during the first 4–6 h postreperfusion. This may be related to the important regulatory role of P-selectin on leukocyte rolling following acute tissue trauma, with a lesser role for L-selectin and virtually no influence on rolling by E-selectin (33).

Sialyl Lewis^x Analogs in Reperfusion Injury

The earliest information on the selectin ligand indicated that is was a carbohydrate structure (34). This led to the notion that sialyl Lewis^x was the selectin ligand (35). The first available chemical substance that was able to block the selectin ligand was a sialyl Lewis^x oligosaccharide (SLe^x-OS). SLe^x-OS (CY-1503) was first tested in an I/R model by Buerke et al (36). SLe^x-OS protected against reperfusion injury–induced cardiac necrosis by 83%, a value significantly greater than that observed with any single anti-selectin mAb. Moreover, CY-1503 also preserved cat coronary endothelium and markedly inhibited PMN adhesion to the endothelium, while not influencing circulating leukocyte counts. In an effort to determine whether these cardioprotective effects resulted in improved cardiac performance, the maximum velocity of the rise in left ventricular pressure, dP/dt$_{max}$, was assessed. CY-1503–treated cats subjected to MI/R exhibited 100% recovery of dP/dt$_{max}$ compared with 71% recovery for MI/R cats receiving either saline or a nonsialylated Lewis^x oligosaccharide (Le^x-OS). A similar cardioprotective effect of CY-1503 was observed in MI/R dogs reperfused for 4.5 h (37). This study also was the first to show that in vivo endothelial preservation by CY-1503 is an important component of the cardioprotection. One of the problems with SLe^x-OS is the short half-life and the need to use a dose of approximately 5–10 mg/kg. This was partially overcome by using a liposome-conjugated SLe^x-OS (38). This study indicated that the liposome-conjugated SLe^x-OS at 400 µg/kg was as effective as 10 mg/kg of the nonliposomal compound in cat MI/R, an increase in potency of 25-fold. In order to answer the important question of whether SLe^x-OS significantly protects the ischemic-reperfused myocardium or whether it merely delays injury, Flynn et al (39) studied dogs subjected to MI/R for 48 h treated with CY-1503. CY-1503 treatment reduced infarct size by 55% after 48 h of reperfusion, which correlated with a 55% reduction in PMN infiltration. Others also confirmed a cardioprotective effect of CY-1503 in dogs subjected to MI/R (40), but these investigators employed an extremely large dose (40 mg/kg). The only reports that failed to show a protective effect of CY-1503 in MI/R were those of Birnbaum et al (41), who treated rabbits with the SLe^x-OS, and Gill et al (42), who treated dogs with CY-1503. In contrast, Yamada et al (43) demonstrated that CY-1503 exerted a cardioprotective effect in rabbits subjected to MI/R. No obvious explanation exists for the differences in the studies of CY-1503 in rabbits and dogs. The SLe^x-OS clearly protected rats against I/R injury because CY-1503 was found to exert several beneficial effects in traumatic shock in rats, a form of whole body I/R (44), and in MI/R injury (45).

In the interval after the clear-cut effects of CY-1503 were reported, other small-molecule selectin inhibitors have been studied in I/R states. Seko et al (46) showed that synthetic oligopeptides corresponding to portions of the N-terminal lectin domain of human selectins significantly attenuated infarct size in rats subjected to MI and to 48 h of reperfusion, consistent with the report by Flynn et al in dogs (39). Other small-molecule anti-selectin agents are also effective in I/R models. Thus, TBC-1269, a synthetic mannosylated-biphenyl analog, was effective in hepatic I/R (47), and a SLe^x-mimetic (a serine-glutamic acid peptide analog) protected mice subjected to a form of cutaneous I/R. Similar results in mice skin were reported by Rao et al (48) using a glucaronic acid substituted analog of glycyrrhizin.

PSGL-1 Analogs in Reperfusion Injury

One of the great achievements in selectin research was the discovery of the high-affinity ligand for the selectins by Moore and coworkers (16). This substance isolated from human neutrophils was termed P-selectin glycoprotein ligand-1 (PSGL-1). PSGL-1 serves as a high-affinity ligand for P-selectin (and to a lesser extent L-selectin and E-selectin) because it displays oligosaccharide sequences recognized by the calcium-dependent lectin domain of the selectins. PSGL-1 is 10,000 times more potent than SLe^x in binding to P-selectin (49). Leukocyte trafficking is mediated by selectin–PSGL-1 interactions and is a key molecule responsible for recruitment of neutrophils into areas of inflammation (50).

Recently, peptide analogs of PSGL-1 have been constructed. A soluble form of PSGL-1 (sPSGL-1) has been found to be effective in I/R. This sPSGL-1 was reported to markedly protect against renal I/R (51) at doses of 5–50 μg in rats. sPSGL-1 significantly protected against renal necrosis due to PMN infiltration. More recently, a recombinant analog of sPSGL-1, rsPSGL-1-Ig, exerted remarkable cardioprotective effects at 1 mg/kg in intact cats subjected to MI/R (52) and in isolated, PMN-perfused rat hearts at 200–500 μg/kg (53) subjected to global I/R. The rsPSGL-1–Ig attenuated feline myocardial necrosis by 62% in cat heart and preserved myocardial contractility by 55% in isolated rat heart. In both cases, there was dramatic attenuation of infiltrated PMNs. A low-affinity mutant of rsPSGL-1–Ig was inactive in all cases (52, 53), whereas a tetramer form of rs-PSGL-1–Ig exhibited a potency twice that of the native form. In addition, a metalloproteinase isolated from cobra venom (i.e. mocarhagin) has been shown to cleave a decapeptide from the N terminus of the PSGL-1 receptor (54). Mocharagin also shows significant cardioprotective effects at 200 ng/mL in the same PMN-perfused rat heart model of I/R as reported for rsPSGL-1-Ig (55). PSGL-1–Ig also works in hemorrhage/reinfusion in mice subjected to hemorrhagic shock (56), a form of total body I/R.

It is becoming evident that interference with PSGL-1, the high-affinity ligand for the selectins or its receptor, offers an effective strategy for counteracting tissue necrosis and other effects of reperfusion injury. Moreover, using PSGL-1 as the target rather than SLe^x allows the use of doses two orders of magnitude lower than those required to block with SLe^x.

Nitric Oxide

The lipid-soluble low-molecular-weight gas, NO among its many actions, also inhibits the adherence of leukocytes to the endothelium (57, 58). NO exerts this antiadhesion effect to a large extent by inhibiting the up-regulation of P-selectin

(58). Moreover, NO releasing agents (i.e. NO donors) have been found to markedly inhibit P-selectin up-regulation in the mesenteric microvasculature in rats subjected to splanchnic I/R (59). The inverse relationship between NO and P-selectin has been reviewed in detail elsewhere (60).

P-Selectin Gene-Deficient Animals

One of the most exciting developments in recent years is the generation of specific gene deletions in mice. These so-called gene-knockout mice represent a valuable tool in that they lack a specific endogenous protein. These gene deletion animals therefore do not require receptor antagonists, synthesis inhibitors, or any other modulator of the protein of interest. Moreover, the "blockade" is lifelong, usually commencing during the prenatal development of the animal. Thus, it was exciting to have P-selectin–deficient mice available several years ago. These mice, developed by several investigators (61), are devoid of leukocyte rolling along the microvascular endothelium despite an elevation in the number of circulating neutrophils. These mice were found to be protected from postischemic endothelial dysfunction characterized by a loss of vasorelaxant effect to endothelium-dependent dilators (62). These findings serve to validate the earlier reports that there is a reciprocal relationship between endothelium-derived NO and endothelial cell P-selectin expression.

Early studies on the properties of P-selectin–deficient ($-/-$) mice were soon followed by studies in which P-selectin $-/-$ mice were observed to exhibit a very mild response to platelet activating factor at doses that usually produce intestinal necrosis and death (63). Survival was 100% in the P-selectin $-/-$ mice. Following up on these seminal investigations, Scalia et al (56) showed that P-selectin $-/-$ mice experienced a mild reaction to hemorrhage to a 40 mmHg for 45 min followed by reinfusion of all shed blood. Leukocyte rolling and adhesion were absent in response to the total body I/R, and few leukocytes infiltrated into splanchnic tissues. Moreover, the mean arterial blood pressure was well maintained postreperfusion in P-selectin $-/-$ animals. In addition, it has also been demonstrated recently that mice deficient in P-selectin are protected against the effects of MI/R injury induced by coronary artery occlusion and reperfusion (64). Myocardial infarct size and neutrophil accumulation in the myocardium were dramatically reduced in P-selectin null animals compared with wild-type controls (64). These results point to the vital role of P-selectin in mediating the pathophysiology of I/R. Other gene deletions (i.e. E-selectin) are now available and will provide interesting insights in further understanding the role of selectins in I/R injury.

SUMMARY

This brief review has attempted to evaluate and summarize the current evidence for the role of the selectin family of adhesion glycoproteins in ischemia/reperfusion (I/R) disease states. The overwhelming evidence points to an important role of the selectins in mediating the early phase of leukocyte-endothelium interaction in reperfusion injury. This mediation is exemplified by the stimulation of leukocyte rolling along the postcapillary venular endothelium triggering an inflammatory cascade, which eventually leads to neutrophil infiltration into ischemic/reperfused tissues, whereupon these neutrophils release a variety of cytotoxic mediators that contribute in a major way to the tissue injury and necrosis that is observed in reperfusion injury.

The selectins may also play a role in cell signaling among various cell types in orchestrating responses to I/R. P-selectin plays a preeminent role among the selectins as the major contributor involved in leukocyte rolling and probably is the key selectin mediator of reperfusion injury. L-selectin appears to play a significant role in the early phase of reperfusion injury, but E-selectin does not appear to be involved in the early phases. However, E-selectin may be active in responses that occur much later than 6 h postreperfusion. Finally, anti-selectin agents remain an important target for design of drugs to treat reperfusion injury states.

Visit the Annual Reviews home page at www.AnnualReviews.org.

LITERATURE CITED

1. Bevilacqua M, Nelson RM. 1993. Selectins. *J. Clin. Invest.* 91:379–87
2. McEver RP. 1991. GMP-140: a receptor for neutrophils and monocytes on activated platelets and endothelium. *J. Cell. Biochem.* 45:156–61
3. Lorant DE, Patel KD, McIntyre TM, McEver RP, Prescott SM, Zimmerman GA. 1991. Co-expression of GMP-140 and PAF by endothelium stimulated by histamine or thrombin: a juxtacrine system for adhesion and activation of neutrophils. *J. Cell. Biol.* 115:223–34
4. Bevilacqua MB, Stengelin S, Gimbrone MA Jr, Seed B. 1989. Endothelial leukocyte adhesion molecule molecule-1: an inducible receptor for neutrophils related to complement regulatory proteins and lectins. *Science* 243:1160–65
5. Butcher EC. 1991. Leukocyte-endothelial cell recognition: three (or more) steps to specificity and diversity. *Cell* 67:1033–36
6. Lefer AM, Lefer DJ. 1996. The role of nitric oxide and cell adhesion molecules on the microcirculation in ischaemia-reperfusion. *Cardiovasc. Res.* 32:743–51
7. Weiss SJ. 1989. Tissue destruction by neutrophils. *N. Engl. J. Med.* 320:365–76
8. Tsao PS, Aoki N, Lefer DJ, Johnson G, Lefer AM. 1990. Time course of endothelial dysfunction and myocardial injury during myocardial ischemia and reperfusion in the cat. *Circulation* 82:1402–12
9. Weyrich AS, Buerke M, Albertine KH, Lefer AM. 1995. Time course of coronary vascular endothelial molecule expression during reperfusion of the ischemic feline myocardium. *J. Leuk. Biol.* 57:45–55
10. Ma XL, Weyrich AS, Lefer DJ, Lefer AM. 1993. Diminished basal nitric oxide release after myocardial ischemia and reperfusion promotes neutrophil adherence to the coronary endothelium. *Circ. Res.* 72:403–12
11. Armstead VE, Minchenko AG, Schuhl RA, Hayward R, Nossuli TO, Lefer AM. 1997. Regulation of P-selectin expres-

sion in human endothelial cells by nitric oxide. *Am. J. Physiol.* 273: H740–46

12. De Caterina R, Libby P, Peng HB, Thannickal VJ, Rajavashisth TB, et al. 1995. Nitric oxide decreases cytokine-induced endothelial activation. Nitric oxide selectively reduces endothelial expression of adhesion molecules and proinflammatory cytokines. *J. Clin. Invest.* 96:60–68

13. Foxall CS, Watson SR, Dowbenko D, Fennie C, Lasky LA, et al. 1992. The three members of the selectin receptor family recognize a common carbohydrate epitope; the sialyl Lewis^x oligosaccharide. *J. Cell Biol.* 117:895–902

14. Mulligan MS, Lowe JB, Larsen RD, Paulson J, Zheng Z-L, et al. 1993. Protective effects of sialylated oligosaccharides in immune complex-induced acute lung injury. *J. Exp. Med.* 178:623–31

15. Moore KL, Varki A, McEver RP. 1991. GMP-140 binds to a glycoprotein receptor on human neutrophils: evidence for a lectin-like interaction. *J. Cell. Biol.* 112:491–99

16. Moore KL, Eaton SF, Lyons DE, Lichtenstein HS, Cummings RD, McEver RP. 1994. The P-selectin glycoprotein ligand from human neutrophils displays, sialylated, fucosylated, O-linked poly-N-acetyllactosamine. *J. Biol. Chem.* 269: 22318–27

17. Weyrich AS, Ma XL, Lefer DJ, Albertine KH, Lefer AM. 1993. In vivo neutralization of P-selectin protects feline heart and endothelium in myocardial ischemia and reperfusion injury. *J. Clin. Invest.* 91:2620–29

18. Chen LY, Nichols WW, Hendricks JB, Yang BC, Mehta JL. 1994. Monoclonal antibody to P-selectin (PB1.3) protects against myocardial reperfusion injury in the dog. *Cardiovasc. Res.* 28:1414–22

19. Lefer DJ, Flynn DM, Buda AJ. 1996. Effects of a monoclonal antibody directed against P-selectin after myocardial ischemia and reperfusion. *Am. J. Physiol.* 270:H88–98

20. Lefer DJ, Flynn DM, Anderson DC, Buda AJ. 1996. Combined inhibition of P-selectin and ICAM-1 reduces myocardial injury following ischemia and reperfusion. *Am. J. Physiol.* 271:H2421–29

21. Davenpeck KL, Gauthier TW, Albertine KH, Lefer AM. 1994. Role of P-selectin in microvascular leukocyte-endothelial interaction in splanchnic ischemia-reperfusion. *Am. J. Physiol.* 267:H622–30

22. Kurose I, Kubes P, Wolf R, Anderson DC, Paulson J, et al. 1993. Inhibition of nitric oxide production: mechanisms of vascular albumin leakage. *Circ. Res.* 73:164–71

23. Kurose I, Yamada T, Wolf R, Granger DN. 1994. P-selectin-dependent leukocyte recruitment and intestinal mucosal injury induced by lactoferrin. *J. Leuk. Biol.* 55:771–77

24. Winn RK, Liggitt D, Vedder NB, Paulson JC, Harlan JM. 1993. Anti-P-selectin monoclonal antibody attenuates reperfusion injury to the rabbit ear. *J. Clin. Invest.* 92:2042–47

25. Lee WP, Gribling P, de Guzman L, Ehsani N, Watson SR. 1995. A P-selectin immunoglobulin G chimera is protective in a rabbit ear model of ischemia-reperfusion. *Surgery* 117:458–65

26. Winn RK, Paulson JC, Harlan JM. 1994. A monoclonal antibody to P-selectin ameliorates injury associated with hemorrhagic shock in rabbits. *Am. J. Physiol.* 267:H2391–397

27. Kishimoto TK, Jutila MA, Butcher EC. 1990. Identification of a human peripheral lymph node homing receptor: a rapidly down-regulated adhesion molecule. *Proc. Natl. Acad. Sci. USA* 87:2244–48

28. Ma X-L, Weyrich AS, Lefer DJ, Buerke M, Albertine KH, et al. 1993. Monoclonal antibody to L-selectin attenuates neutrophil accumulation and protects ischemic reperfused cat myocardium. *Circulation* 88:649–58

29. Buerke M, Weyrich AS, Murohara T,

Queen C, Klingbeil CK, Lefer AM. 1994. Humanized monoclonal antibody DREG-200 directed against L-selectin protects in feline myocardial reperfusion injury. *J. Pharmacol. Exp. Ther.* 271:134–42

30. Ramasworthy C, Sharar SM, Harlan JM, Tedder TF, Winn RK. 1996. Blocking L-selectin function attenuates reperfusion injury following hemorrhagic shock in rabbits. *Am. J. Physiol.* 271: H1871–77

31. Winquist RJ, Frei PF, Letts G, Van GY, Andrews LK, et al. 1992. Monoclonal antibody to intercellular adhesion molecule-1, but not to endothelial-leukocyte adhesion molecule-1, protects against myocardial ischemia/reperfusion damage in anesthetized monkeys. *Circulation* 86:I79 (Abstr.)

32. Kurose I, Anderson DC, Miyasaks M, Tamatani T, Paulson JC, et al. 1994. Molecular determinants of reperfusion-induced leukocyte adhesion and vascular protein leakage. *Circ. Res.* 74:336–43

33. Ley K, Bullard DC, Arbones ML, Bosse R, Vestwebwer D, et al. 1995. Sequential contribution of L- and P-selectin to leukocyte rolling *in vivo. J. Exp. Med.* 181:669–95

34. Brandley BK. 1991. Cell surface carbohydrates in cell adhesion. *Semin. Cell Biol.* 2:281–87

35. Varki A. 1992. Selectins and other mammalian sialic acid-binding lectins. *Curr. Opin. Cell Biol.* 4:257–66

36. Buerke M, Weyrich AS, Zheng Z, Gaeta FCA, Forrest MJ, Lefer AM. 1994. Sialyl Lewis[x]-containing oligosaccharide attenuates myocardial reperfusion injury in cats. *J. Clin. Invest.* 93:1140–48

37. Lefer DJ, Flynn DM, Phillips L, Ratliffe M, Buda AJ. 1994. A novel sialyl Lewis[x] analog attenuates neutrophil accumulation and myocardial necrosis after ischemia and reperfusion. *Circulation* 90: 2390–401

38. Murohara T, Margiotta J, Phillips LM, Paulson JC, DeFrees S, et al. 1995. Car-

dioprotection by liposome-conjugated sialyl Lewis[x] oligosaccharide in myocardial ischaemia and reperfusion injury. *Cardiovasc. Res.* 30:965–74

39. Flynn DM, Buda AB, Jeffords PR, Lefer DJ. 1996. A sialyl Lewis[x] containing carbohydrate reduces infarct size: role of selectins in reperfusion injury. *Am. J. Physiol.* 271:H2086–96

40. Silver MJ, Sutton JM, Hook S, Lee P, Malycky JL, et al. 1995. Adjunctive selectin blockade successfully reduces infarct size beyond thrombolysis in the electrolytic canine coronary artery model. *Circulation* 92:492–99

41. Birnbaum Y, Patterson M, Kloner RA. 1997. The effect of CY-1503, a sialyl Lewis[x] analog blocker of the selectin adhesion molecules, on infarct size and "no-relow" in the rabbit model of acute myocardial infarction/reperfusion. *J. Mol. Cell Cardiol.* 29:2013–25

42. Gill EA, Yingong K, Horwitz LD. 1996. An oligosaccharide sialyl-Lewis[x] analogue does not reduce myocardial infarct size after ischemia and reperfusion in dogs. *Circulation* 94:542–46

43. Yamada K, Tojo SJ, Hayashi M, Morooka S. 1998. The role of P-selectin, sialyl Lewis[x] and sulfatide in myocardial ischemia and reperfusion injury. *Eur. J. Pharmacol.* 346:217–25

44. Tojo SJ, Yokota S, Koike H, Schultz J, Hamazume Y, et al. 1996. Reduction of rat myocardial ischemia and reperfusion injury by sialyl Lewis[x] oligosaccharide and anti-rat P-selectin antibodies. *Glycobiology* 6:463–69

45. Skirk C, Buerke M, Guo J-P, Paulson J, Lefer AM. 1994. Sialyl Lewis[x] oligosaccharide exerts beneficial effects in murine traumatic shock. *Am. J. Physiol.* 267:H2124–31

46. Seko T, Enokawa Y, Tamatani T, Jannagi R, Yagita H, et al. 1996. Expression of sialyl Lewis[x] in rat heart with ischaemia/reperfusion injury by a monoclonal anti-

body against sialyl Lewis[x]. *J. Pathol.* 180:305–10

47. Palma-Vargas JM, Toledo-Pereyra L, Dean RE, Harkema JM, Dixon RAF, Kogan TP. 1997. Small molecule selectin inhibitor protects against liver inflammatory response after ischemia and reperfusion. *J. Am. Coll. Surg.* 185:365–72

48. Rao BNN, Anderson MB, Musser JH, Gilbert JG, Schaefer ME, et al. 1994. Sialyl Lewis[x] mimics derived from a pharmacophore search are selectin inhibitors with anti-inflammatory activity. *J. Biol. Chem.* 269:19663–66

49. McEver RP, Moore KL, Cummings RD. 1995. Leukocyte trafficking mediated by selectin-carbohydrate interactions. *J. Biol. Chem.* 270:11025–28

50. Borges E, Eytner R, Moll T, Steegmaier M, Campbell MA, et al. 1997. The P-selectin ligand-1 is important for recruitment of neutrophils into inflamed mouse peritoneum. *Blood* 90:1934–42

51. Takada M, Naseau KC, Shaw GD, Marquette KA, Tilney NL. 1997. The cytokine-adhesion cascade in ischemia/reperfusion injury of the rat kidney. *J. Clin. Invest.* 99:2682–90

52. Hayward R, Campbell B, Shin YK, Scalia R, Lefer AM. 1999. Recombinant soluble P-selectin glycoprotein ligand-1 protects against myocardial ischemic reperfusion injury in cats. *Cardiovasc. Res.* 41:65–76

53. Lefer AM, Campbell B, Scalia R, Lefer DJ. 1998. Synergism between platelets and neutrophils in provoking cardiac dysfunction after ischemia and reperfusion: role of selectins. *Circulation* 98:1322–28

54. DeLuca M, Dunlop LC, Andrews RK, Flannery JV Jr, Ettling R, et al. 1995. A novel cobra venom metalloproteinase, mocarhagin, cleaves a 10-amino acid peptide from the mature N-terminus of P-selectin/glycoprotein ligand receptor. *J. Biol. Chem.* 270:26734–37

55. Lefer AM, Campbell B, Shin Y-K. 1998. Effects of a metalloproteinase that truncates P-selectin glycoprotein ligand on neutrophil-induced cardiac dysfunction in ischemia/reperfusion. *J. Mol. Cell Cardiol.* 30:2561–66

56. Scalia R, Armstead VE, Minchenko AG, Lefer AM. 1999. Essential role of P-selectin in the initiation of the inflammatory response induced by hemorrhage and reinfusion. *J. Exp. Med.* 189:931–38

57. Kubes P, Suzuki M, Granger DN. 1991. Nitric oxide: an endogenous modulator of leukocyte adhesion. *Proc. Natl. Acad. Sci. USA* 88:4651–55

58. Davenpeck KL, Gauthier TW, Lefer AM. 1994. Inhibition of endothelial-derived nitric oxide promotes P-selectin expression and actions in the rat microcirculation. *Gastroenterology* 107:1050–58

59. Gauthier TW, Davenpeck KL, Lefer AM. 1994. Nitric oxide attenuates leukocyte-endothelial interaction via P-selectin in splanchnic ischemia-reperfusion. *Am. J. Physiol.* 267:G562–68

60. Lefer AM, Lefer DJ. 1996. The role of nitric oxide and cell adhesion molecules on the microcirculation in ischaemia-reperfusion. *Cardiovasc. Res.* 32:743–51

61. Mayadas TN, Johnson RC, Rayburn H, Hynes RO, Wagner DD. 1993. Leukocyte rolling and extravasation are severely compromised in P-selectin-deficient mice. *Cell* 74:541–54

62. Banda MA, Lefer DJ, Granger DN. 1997. Postischemic endothelium-dependent vascular reactivity is preserved in adhesion molecule-deficient mice. *Am. J. Physiol.* 273:H2721–25

63. Sun X, Rozenfeld RA, Qu X, Huang W, Gonzalez-Crussi F, Hsueh W. 1997. P-selectin–deficient mice are protected from PAF-induced shock, intestinal injury, and lethality. *Am. J. Physiol.* 273:G56–61

64. Palazzo AJ, Jones SP, Anderson DC, Granger DN, Lefer DJ. 1998. Coronary endothelial P-selectin in the pathogenesis of myocardial ischemia-reperfusion injury. *Am. J. Physiol.* 275:H1865–72

Annu. Rev. Pharmacol. Toxicol. 2000. 40:295–317

A NOVEL MEANS OF DRUG DELIVERY: Myoblast-Mediated Gene Therapy and Regulatable Retroviral Vectors

Clare R. Ozawa, Matthew L. Springer, and Helen M. Blau

Department of Molecular Pharmacology, Stanford University School of Medicine, Stanford, California 94305–5332; e-mail: cozawa@stanfordalumni.org, springer@cmgm.stanford.edu, hblau@cmgm.stanford.edu

Key Words   muscle, inducible, tetracycline, angiogenesis, secreted factors

■ **Abstract**   A potentially powerful approach to drug delivery in the treatment of disease involves the use of cells to introduce genes encoding therapeutic proteins into the body. Candidate genes for delivery include those encoding secreted factors that could have broad applications ranging from treatment of inherited single-gene deficiencies to acquired disorders of the vasculature or cancer. Myoblasts, the proliferative cell type of skeletal muscle tissues, are potent tools for stable delivery of a gene of interest into the body, as they become an integral part of the muscle into which they are injected, in close proximity to the circulation. The recent development of improved tetracycline-inducible retroviral vectors allows for fine control of recombinant gene expression levels. The combination of ex vivo gene transfer using myoblasts and regulatable retroviral vectors provides a powerful toolbox with which to develop gene therapies for a number of human diseases.

INTRODUCTION

Gene therapy is a natural outcome of landmark developments witnessed in the past few decades: the emergence of recombinant DNA technology and methods for identifying and characterizing an array of human genes implicated in disease. Since the first federally approved gene therapy protocol began in 1990 (1), the number of clinical trials underway worldwide has burgeoned into the hundreds. Initially, gene therapy was thought to be best applicable for replacing or correcting single defective genes, such as those implicated in various metabolic disorders. Although efforts aimed at treating single-gene defects are currently in progress, growing attention is being directed toward treatment of multi-gene disorders, including cancer and vascular diseases. In such disorders, expression of recombinant genes may complement genetic defects and alleviate or correct the disease

0362–1642/00/0415–0295$14.00

pathophysiology. Whereas classical pharmacotherapy relies on delivering to the patient a chemical manufactured outside of the body, gene therapy strategies utilize the therapeutic transgene as the template of the drug and harness the patient's own cellular machinery to produce the drug.

A number of preclinical gene therapy approaches have employed skeletal muscle as a platform to treat both muscle- and non–muscle-related disorders. Skeletal muscle has a number of advantages for genetic manipulation over other tissue types, as is discussed below. The strategies for gene delivery into muscle fall into two categories: (*a*) in vivo approaches, in which a vector (of either viral or nonviral origin) harboring a therapeutic transgene is introduced directly into muscle tissue, and (*b*) ex vivo approaches, in which cells removed from the body are genetically engineered in culture and introduced into the patient, where they become integrated into preexisting tissue. Many of the features of skeletal muscle make it ideally suited for in vivo adenoviral, adeno-associated viral, lentiviral, and naked DNA delivery. However, the primary focus of this chapter is the use of muscle as a target tissue for ex vivo gene delivery, together with approaches for regulating gene expression to avoid toxic levels and achieve pulsatile drug delivery when desired. Ex vivo strategies for gene transfer into muscle surpass most other current methods, as they lead to long-term, stable delivery into the circulation of therapeutic proteins at physiological levels. Moreover, problematic immunological effects currently associated with most other methods can be avoided with ex vivo approaches by transplantation of autologous cells.

In this article we highlight the advances in cellular and molecular biology that have enabled gene transfer via myoblasts. We illustrate several potential applications of genetically engineered myoblasts to the treatment of human diseases. Because of the vast literature in this field, only a subset of references have been included.

EX VIVO GENE DELIVERY USING MYOBLASTS

Features and Advantages of Skeletal Muscle

Skeletal muscle has a number of properties that distinguish it from other tissue types. First, the in-depth knowledge accumulated over the years on this tissue provides insights for developing strategies of gene delivery and for assessing and controlling therapeutic protein expression. Skeletal muscle makes up approximately 10% of the total human body mass and is easily accessible for the delivery of recombinant genes. Myofibers—the typical striated differentiated cells found in skeletal muscle—are multinucleated, allowing delivery of multiple genes encoding products that can interact inside the cell. In addition, because myofibers are long-lived, they provide a stable environment for long-term expression of recombinant transgenes. Finally, although not widely recognized as a secretory tissue, genetically altered skeletal muscle tissue is surprisingly efficient at producing and delivering recombinant gene products to the circulation. All these advantages make skeletal muscle an optimal target tissue for genetic manipulation in various gene therapy strategies.

Transplantation studies conducted by Partridge and coworkers (2–7) showed that donor myoblasts could coexpress exogenous genes together with host genes in myofibers. These experiments employed isoforms of the enzyme glucose-6-phosphate isomerase as markers for distinguishing between donor and host myoblast contributions to myofibers. Following allografts of minced muscle tissue (2) and pieces of intact muscle (3), or injection of muscle precursor cells (4–7), hybrid fibers expressing isoforms containing subunits derived from donor and host were observed. These observations indicated that muscle precursor cells of one genotype injected into muscle of another genotype fuse to form hybrid myofibers, which are capable of coexpressing donor and host genes.

Myofibers contain many nuclei because they are formed during development by the fusion of mononucleated precursor cells known as myoblasts. Myoblasts continue to fuse to neighboring mature myofibers throughout adult life, aiding in regeneration following injury to muscle tissue (8), and are retained in mature muscle as satellite cells that persist between the plasma membrane of the myofiber and the surrounding extracellular matrix (9). Myoblasts can fuse randomly with all fiber types encountered and adopt the pattern of myogenic gene expression characteristic of the host muscle fiber, as was demonstrated through several experiments. Studies of the generation of patterns of slow and fast fiber types within mammalian muscle have shown that although intrinsic properties and lineage clearly play a role (10, 11), extrinsic factors are important in the creation of fiber patterning. For example, myoblasts taken from different stages of early muscle development give rise to clones expressing slow myosin heavy chain upon differentiation in culture, even if only a small percentage of fibers in vivo express the protein at the developmental stage being examined (12).

In studies of cell fate during development in which vectors encoding the marker bacterial *lacZ* gene were injected directly into muscles of rats, labeled single satellite cells gave rise to clusters of labeled fibers (13). Migration of these satellite cells into multiple fibers did not appear to be hindered by the presence of the basal lamina, a connective sheath surrounding each myofiber. Additional experiments demonstrated that myoblast clones could give rise to both slow and fast muscle fiber types in their vicinity in vivo (14). Thus, in contrast with other cell types, myoblasts become an integral part of the muscle into which they are injected and adapt to local signals in their immediate environment. Moreover, the fused cells continued to express a transgene, the marker *lacZ* gene. These studies provided the rationale for utilizing myoblasts for gene transfer into mature muscle.

Primary Myoblasts as Gene Delivery Tools for Muscle

Primary myoblasts from a range of species, including human, can be readily isolated from muscle and expanded in tissue culture. The development of this process constituted a major advance, as in early studies only established myogenic cell lines were available for use. Primary myoblasts can now be purified, genetically engineered, and extensively characterized in vitro; they then can be reimplanted back into muscle, where they fuse with preexisting muscle fibers of mice, rats, or humans. Primary mouse myoblasts stably express recombinant genes following transduction. Myoblasts that have been retrovirally transduced with the *lacZ* gene and injected into mouse skeletal muscle fuse with myofibers and express high levels of β-galactosidase for at least 6 months (15). Other studies have demonstrated stable levels of recombinant protein production via myoblast-mediated gene transfer for at least 10 months (16). Myoblasts genetically engineered to express a recombinant gene can thus be employed for long-term delivery of the gene-encoded protein within the body (Figure 1) (17).

Although not widely viewed as a secretory tissue, skeletal muscle is well-vascularized and recombinant proteins secreted from myoblasts readily gain access to the circulation. This was first demonstrated using a mouse myoblast cell line genetically engineered to express human growth hormone (hGH) (18, 19). hGH was chosen as the gene of interest because the protein has a very short half-life in mouse serum (4 min) (20), providing a stringent test for sustained production and secretion into the circulation over time. Following injection of genetically engineered myoblasts into mouse muscle, stable physiological levels of hGH

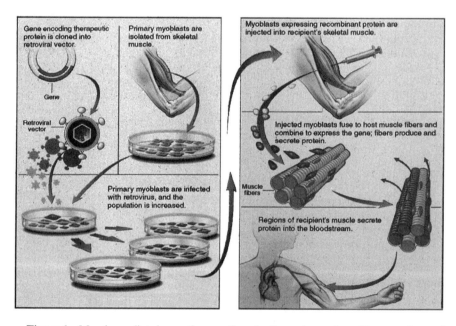

Figure 1   Muscle-mediated gene therapy. Genetically engineered myoblasts can be used for delivery of diverse therapeutic proteins either directly to muscle or, as shown, to the systemic circulation. From Reference 17 (copyright © 1995 Mass. Med. Soc. All rights reserved).

could be detected for at least 3 months (Figure 2). Moreover, muscle has also been demonstrated to be capable of carrying out posttranslational modifications normally performed by other tissue types (such as gamma carboxylation, essential for production of functional coagulation factors in the liver) (21–24). Thus, skeletal muscle may be enlisted as a "factory" for production of a range of secreted proteins for the treatment of nonmuscle disorders. These recombinant nonmuscle gene products are biologically active even when produced by muscle.

The ease of isolating myoblasts from both mouse and human muscle and purifying, growing, and transducing them in vitro is a major advantage of using myoblasts rather than other cell types for gene transfer. Primary myoblasts can be isolated from any mouse strain, including strains harboring genetic mutations or transgenic strains (25, 26), providing a broad array of genotypes either for study in tissue culture or for transplantation. Established myogenic cell lines, such as the C2 cell line, may also be implanted; however, these cells can proliferate and form tumors when implanted into mice (15). In contrast, although they exhibit an impressive capacity to proliferate in culture, primary myoblasts do not form tumors when injected into mouse muscle (15). In human myoblasts, senescence has been observed but transformation has not (27).

Myoblasts can be isolated from tissues of any age, but both the yield and number of doublings tend to be higher when obtained from younger donors. Primary cultures are derived from postnatal muscle using mechanical or enzymatic dissociation methods (15, 28) and are readily obtained from human biopsy

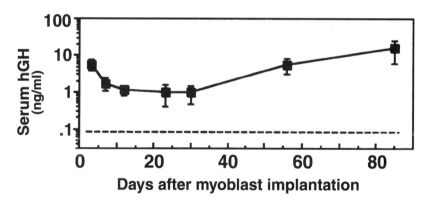

Figure 2 Persistent expression of human growth hormone (hGH) by virus-transduced myoblasts implanted into mouse muscle in vivo. C2C12 myoblasts were retrovirally transduced with hGH and injected into hind limbs of 24 C3H mice, and serum hGH levels were monitored for 85 days by radioimmunoassay of tail blood. More than 90% of the implanted cells expressed and secreted hGH, as determined by clonal analysis in culture. (*Points*) The mean ± standard deviation for 4–24 mice; (*dashed line*) the mean for serum samples from five uninjected control mice. Reprinted with permission from Science, 1991, 254 (5037):1509–12 (Reference 18) (copyright © 1991 Am. Assoc. Advance. Sci.).

or autopsy tissue (29, 30). Further purification to obtain myoblasts free from contaminating cell types can be accomplished using cell culture conditions that favor myoblast growth at the expense of other cell types, yielding a pure population of mouse myoblasts within 2 weeks of normal growth (15, 31). Alternatively, primary cells have been isolated by fluorescence-activated cell sorting using antibodies directed against $\alpha7$ integrin for mouse (W Blanco-Bose, C Yoo, R Kramer, HM Blau, manuscript in preparation) and rat (32) cultures, or against the muscle surface antigen NCAM in human-derived cultures (28). Human cells isolated by fluorescence-activated cell sorting can undergo at least 40 cell doublings without differentiating (28), implying that a kilogram of cells for use in transplantation could theoretically be derived from a 5-mm^3 biopsy. Recombinant genes can be introduced into myoblasts by lipofection, by calcium-mediated transfection, or (more readily) by retroviral infection. Optimized conditions for retroviral infection of myoblasts at high efficiency enables >99% of primary myoblasts in culture to be transduced without a selectable marker (33). Thus, primary myoblasts can be genetically engineered with relative ease, and genetic alteration does not reduce the ability of myoblasts to mature and differentiate into myofibers.

CLINICAL APPLICATIONS

The many studies establishing myoblasts as potent vehicles for delivering donor genes into host muscle led to the concept of applying myoblast-mediated gene transfer to the treatment of disease. Implanted myoblasts are integrated into preexisting muscle tissue that is highly vascularized and, thus, can be used to deliver genes encoding both muscle-specific and circulatory proteins. This section briefly summarizes the clinical applications that have been tested using myoblast-mediated gene delivery.

Delivery of Genes Encoding Muscle Structural Proteins

The first studies applying myoblast transplantation to the treatment of disease used allografts of normal myoblasts to insert donor nuclei, containing a normal genome, into genetically abnormal muscle. Although technically not gene therapy because donor myoblasts were not genetically altered in any way, these "cell therapy" experiments were important in demonstrating the validity of myoblast-mediated gene delivery, and they are the only studies involving myoblast transplantation that have been translated into human clinical trials. Duchenne muscular dystrophy (DMD), the most common of heritable human muscular dystrophies, was the first disorder to which this therapeutic approach was applied. This disease causes progressive muscle weakness beginning in childhood and is caused by mutations in the *dystrophin* gene (34). Studies on mdx dystrophin-deficient mice, the mouse model of the disorder, showed that implantation of normal myoblasts containing an intact *dystrophin* could counteract the cycle of muscle fiber degeneration and regeneration characteristic of mdx muscle (7, 35).

Clinical trials in which donor myoblasts taken from normal human muscle were introduced into DMD patients were initiated at multiple institutions (36–42). All these studies demonstrated that myoblast implantation into humans has no adverse effects. However, all but one group (36) reported the disappointing finding that only a very small percentage of host myofibers began to express *dystrophin*. Definitive evidence that donor *dystrophin* transcripts were being synthesized was first provided by polymerase chain reaction by Gussoni and colleagues (37). Recent studies employing fluorescent in situ hybridization together with immunohistochemistry to localize both the dystrophin protein and donor nuclei at the same time showed that for at least one of these studies, a large proportion of donor myoblasts did successfully integrate into host myofibers in almost every subject, because donor nuclei were interspersed and aligned with host nuclei (43, 44). Thus, viability and access were not problems. Indeed, in half of the patients tested, more than 10% of the injected nuclei were estimated to gain access to the human host fibers, a remarkable result. Furthermore, because the antibodies used in these studies were specific to the product for the deleted gene regions in the recipients, these experiments demonstrated that increased dystrophin protein production observed in recipient muscle was contributed by the donor nuclei. The dystrophin produced by a single nucleus spanned regions including 20–30 nuclei. The unresolved question at this point is why only a subset of transduced myofibers expressed *dystrophin*. Possible variables include factors specific to the DMD disease state itself, such as increased fibrosis with patient age, which could have created an environment in which the newly introduced nuclei remained transcriptionally inactive in fiber regions undergoing degeneration. An alternative hypothesis is that myoblasts are heterogeneous (45) and only a subset are capable of activating and expressing the *dystrophin* gene.

Treatment of DMD by cell therapy remains an ambitious undertaking, as it requires that a large proportion of muscle fibers be transduced in order to produce a beneficial outcome. In addition, all muscles must be implanted with myoblasts, including those that are difficult to access, such as the diaphragm or the heart. It is the failure of these two muscles that is often the cause of death in patients with DMD. For targeting a high percentage of muscle in humans, delivery of viral vectors or naked DNA encoding either full-length or truncated *dystrophin* genes (46–48), or up-regulation or delivery of the ubiquitous *utrophin* gene (49), may prove to be most effective.

Delivery of Genes Encoding Secretable Factors

Lysosomal storage diseases are a subset of disorders caused by a single-gene defect that may be amenable to gene therapy (50, 51). These recessive disorders, which are due to a single missing or defective lysosomal enzyme, result in the detrimental accumulation of lysosomal enzyme substrates within affected tissues.

Missing lysosomal enzymes manufactured by muscle and delivered to the serum can be internalized by distant tissues and appropriately targeted to lysosomes via mannose 6-phosphate receptors (52). Implantation of genetically engineered primary myoblasts encoding β-glucuronidase, a lysosomal enzyme, into muscle led to in vivo expression of the recombinant protein in adult β-glucuronidase–deficient mice (53). Production and secretion of the missing lysosomal enzyme by muscle in this case corrected phenotypic abnormalities in the liver and spleen of treated animals.

Hemophilia B, a bleeding disorder caused by a deficiency of clotting factor IX, is another single-gene defect well-suited for ex vivo gene therapy (54). Gene therapy may provide a safer and more convenient alternative to conventional protein replacement therapies that necessitate frequently repeated treatments and, for plasma-derived factors, run the risk of transmitting blood-borne pathogens (55). Implantation of C2C12 myoblasts transduced with a gene encoding human factor IX in mice led to a peak expression of recombinant protein (1 µg/ml) at day 12 and a subsequent decline back to basal levels thereafter (21). The drop in human factor IX expression was shown to be due to production of specific antibodies targeted against the protein in wild-type mice. Other experiments (22–24) have demonstrated that in immunodeficient mice, primary myoblasts engineered to constitutively express factor IX led to stable, low-level production of the protein for many months. Use of a β-actin promoter with muscle creatine kinase enhancers led to stable production of human factor IX at therapeutic levels in SCID mice for at least 8 months (16). Problems with immunogenicity are likely to affect only a percentage of hemophiliacs, because some are not null mutations but have reduced levels of factor IX (56). Of importance, recombinant factor IX manufactured in muscle undergoes the gamma carboxylation typical of liver that is required for functional activity of the protein (21–24). Future preclinical gene therapy studies should be facilitated by the recent creation of a mouse model for hemophilia B (57).

Erythropoietin (Epo)-responsive anemias, such as those associated with end-stage renal disease, are another class of disorders currently under study for muscle-mediated gene therapy. Delivery of recombinant Epo, a mammalian hormone controlling production of erythrocytes (58), has been employed as a successful treatment for anemias (59, 60). Treatments using recombinant Epo, however, require frequent hospital visits by patients and are costly. Muscle-mediated delivery of the protein could eliminate the need for multiple treatments. Implantation of primary or C2 myoblasts expressing Epo into mice led to an elevated hematocrit, a direct measure of Epo production, for 3 months (53, 61). Three months after implantation, myoblasts were shown to have fused and fully differentiated into myofibers (61). Additional experiments using implantation of human Epo-secreting C2 myoblasts and a mouse model of renal failure in which anemia is induced by nephrectomy led to reversal of the anemic phenotype (62). Levels of serum Epo, detected by ELISA, remained elevated for 2 months following myoblast implantation. Thus, myoblast-mediated expression of Epo appears to be a potential treatment for certain types of anemias. As with other gene therapies, the ability to regulate expression of Epo may be desirable so that the amount of circulating hormone may be appropriately tailored to the individual patient.

An example that particularly illustrates this point is the delivery of genes encoding angiogenic factors. Therapeutic angiogenesis—the concept of using factors to stimulate new vessels to grow as treatments for ischemic diseases, including stroke, peripheral arterial disease, and myocardial infarction—has been a subject of much recent attention. Vascular endothelial growth factor (VEGF), a potent mitogen that stimulates growth of endothelial cells and increases permeability in vascular endothelium (hence its other designation, vascular permeability factor) (63–67), is the angiogenic factor that has received the most attention. VEGF plays an important role in the induction of angiogenesis by tumors (68), in the angiogenic response of normal tissue to decreased oxygen availability, and as a critical signal during vasculogenesis, the de novo growth of blood vessels from precursor cells during embryonic development (69, 70). Thus, VEGF is a crucial regulator of development of the vasculature pre- and postnatally.

Much effort has been devoted in recent years to investigating the clinical benefits of VEGF delivery to inadequately vascularized tissues as a means of stimulating new blood vessel growth. Injection of VEGF protein has resulted in angiogenic sprouting of vessels in ischemic muscle (71–73). However, presumably because of vascular permeabilizing and/or vasodilating properties, bolus injections of the protein have been reported to cause hypotension (74, 75). As a result, recent studies have examined the feasibility of localized delivery of VEGF using plasmid DNA or adenoviral vector-mediated gene transfer. Although these two delivery methods lead to only transient production of recombinant VEGF, angiogenic sprouting from preexisting vessels was observed in matrigel in vitro (76, 77) and in adipose tissues in vivo (78), as well as in ischemic skeletal or cardiac muscle (79–82).

Using myoblast-mediated gene transfer, the effects of long-term stable production of VEGF were recently investigated (83). Myoblasts transduced with murine cDNA encoding $VEGF_{164}$ were injected into the muscles of immunodeficient SCID mice, leading to an unexpected physiological response to VEGF. At day 11 postimplantation, although mice appeared outwardly normal, histological analysis of frozen muscle sections revealed that implanted VEGF-expressing myoblasts, but not control myoblasts, were invariably associated with regions of infiltrating mononuclear cells identified by fluorescent antibody staining as endothelial cells and macrophages. By days 44–47, large hemangiomas composed of vascular channels and pools of blood appeared in all legs injected with VEGF myoblasts, whereas control legs appeared normal (Figure 3). These studies highlight the potency of myoblast-mediated VEGF gene delivery, and the results suggest that this single growth factor can lead to a cascade of events resulting in the formation of complex tissues of multiple cell types. This study was also the first to show a physiological response to VEGF in nonischemic muscle and demon-

Uninjected leg   **Injected leg**

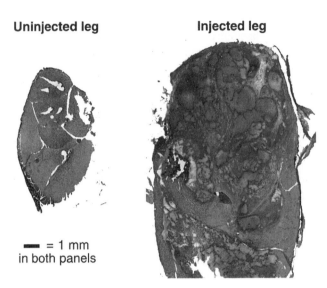

━ = 1 mm
in both panels

Figure 3 Large vascular structures developed in normal adult skeletal muscle implanted with vascular endothelial growth factor (VEGF)-expressing primary myoblasts. Histological analysis of hindlimb muscles was conducted at day 44–47 following implantation of myoblasts expressing the murine $VEGF_{164}$ gene, using hematoxylin/eosin staining of cryostat sections. Control legs that did not receive VEGF were normal in size and in morphology (*left*), whereas VEGF-injected legs were more than twice the diameter of control legs and consisted primarily of hemangioma and pools of blood (*right*). The two panels are shown at the same magnification. Adapted and reprinted with permission from Reference 83 (copyright is held by Cell Press).

strated that expression of VEGF at high levels or long duration can have deleterious effects. This latter point is of importance, as clinical trials of plasmid or adenoviral-mediated VEGF gene delivery are underway.

In contrast to studies aimed at promoting new blood vessel growth, other ongoing studies attempt to block blood vessel growth as a treatment for cancer. Both tumor growth and metastasis require persistent new blood vessel growth (84, 85); thus, therapies targeted at blocking vessel growth may arrest tumor development. The recent identification of anti-angiogenic factors such as angiostatin and endostatin may facilitate the development of such therapies. These proteolytic products of plasminogen and collagen XVIII, respectively, were isolated from fractions taken from serum and urine that were capable of inhibiting endothelial cell proliferation in vitro and metastatic tumor growth in vivo (86, 87). One recent study demonstrated that administration of plasmid DNA encoding endostatin into muscle could inhibit tumor growth and the development of metastatic lesions (88). An interesting therapy for cancer could be to engineer myoblasts to express these proteins, such that their secretion may inhibit metastases, or growth of tumors at distant sites. It will be critical to confirm that desired blood vessel synthesis at sites of injury, for example, is not impaired. Because angiostatin and endostatin are difficult to produce in adequate amounts in bacteria, gene therapy protocols will be invaluable for discerning their biological function and possible application as anti-cancer agents in vivo.

GENE REGULATION USING TETRACYCLINE-REGULATABLE RETROVIRAL VECTORS

Most gene therapy studies have relied on constitutive expression of the introduced gene. However, as is made abundantly clear in the studies of myoblast-mediated transfer of the VEGF gene into normal adult muscle (83), regulation of gene expression is extremely important. Both the ability to increase expression levels if an insufficient amount of a recombinant protein is being produced and the option to intentionally reduce or cease expression are likely to be necessary for the health of the patient in many cases.

Regulation theoretically allows timing of gene expression and levels of the gene product to be optimized on a case-by-case basis. An advantage of using retrovirally transduced myoblasts for implantation is that they allow localized delivery of a recombinant gene at sustained levels; addition of inducible elements to retroviral vectors provides a mechanism for fine-tuning gene expression to the levels required for therapy. An ideal regulatable system should display five characteristics: specificity, efficiency, dose dependency, lack of immunogenicity, and lack of toxicity. The regulatable system should not require endogenous factors for activation, nor should it interfere with cellular regulatory pathways. The system should demonstrate inducibility from low basal levels to high levels of gene expression, and the potential for repression back to uninduced levels. The system also should respond to its inducer by modulating gene expression in a sensitive and homogeneous manner. Lastly, none of its components should elicit a host immune response or be toxic to the tissues or organism as a whole. To date, the four regulatable systems displaying some or most of these characteristics are the ecdysone, RU486, FK506/rapamycin, and tetracycline-inducible systems (for review, see 89, 90). This section focuses on the attributes and recent advances of the tetracycline system, which has been extensively studied by our laboratory and has already been incorporated into myoblast gene transfer strategies.

The tetracycline-inducible system originally developed by Bujard and colleagues (91, 92) has become one of the most widely used methods of regulating gene expression. Because most elements of the system are prokaryotic and are not endogenous to mammalian cells, pleiotropic effects and endogenous ligands are avoided. In addition, the inducer becomes an integral part of the transactivator directly responsible for turning on gene expression, allowing a direct correlation between the amount of transcription factor capable of binding DNA and the concentration of exogenous inducer (tetracycline or its synthetic analog doxycycline).

Tetracycline has been used for decades in humans and animals, and adverse effects from its use have only been seen at doses higher than those required for induction of transgenes.

The original tetracycline-inducible system incorporated a tetracycline transactivator (tTA), a hybrid factor composed of a bacterial tet repressor (tetR), and the viral transactivator domain VP16 (91). When bound to tetracycline or doxycycline, tTA cannot bind to tetracycline operator sequences juxtaposed to a minimal promoter, and gene expression is not turned on. When the inducer is absent, however, tTA is free to bind to the promoter and gene expression is induced. A variation of the system allows for induction of gene expression in the presence of inducer rather than its absence (92). In this second system, a chimeric protein containing a mutated version of tetR, designated reverse tTA (rtTA), binds to tetracycline operator sequences in the presence of tetracycline. Both tTA and rtTA efficiently regulate expression in tissue culture, fruit flies, and mice (93–96).

In the past year, two additional advancements of the tetracycline system have been made. The tetR transcriptional elements are modular; the VP16 transactivator domain of tTA, for instance, may be replaced with the KRAB transrepressor domain to create a tetracycline-regulated repressor of transcription (97). A problem with expressing two tetracycline modulators within the same cell, however, is that nonfunctional heterodimers may form because modulators have identical dimerization domains (Figure 4a) (98). Using sequence information and known crystal structures of tetR as well as mutational analysis (99–101), mutually distinct dimerization domains deriving from separate classes of gram-negative bacteria have been identified (102, 103). The use of tetracycline modulators harboring specific dimerization domains allows activators and repressors to be expressed within the same cell without formation of nonfunctional heterodimers. This system, designated RetroTet-ART (activators and repressors expressed together) (102), allows gene expression to be completely extinguished or induced in a fully dose-dependent manner, resulting in a greatly enhanced dynamic range of gene expression (up to five or six orders of magnitude) (Figure 4b). This improvement is of significant advantage in applications where basal expression from the inducible promoter must be negligible or totally absent. The RetroTet-ART system has been shown to be effective in reversibly silencing expression of p16, a growth arrest protein (102).

A second variation of the tetracycline system incorporates an altered DNA binding domain of tetR that interacts with a modified tetracycline operator sequence (103). tTA and rtTA proteins harboring distinct dimerization domains were engineered with the adapted and original DNA binding sequences. By placing two separate genes under control of old and new tetracycline operator sequences and expressing both of the modified tTA and rtTA proteins, Baron and colleagues (103) were able to either repress expression of both genes or express either gene alone simply by changing the doxycycline concentration (Figure 4c). The activity of two different genes could thus be reversibly controlled in a mutually exclusive manner. However, a means of turning both genes on at once has yet to be achieved.

The application of retroviruses was a major advance in broadening the utility of the tetracycline system, because retroviral gene delivery is much more rapid and efficient than transfection with plasmids. Genes can be introduced into tens of thousands of myoblasts at high efficiency, generating polyclonal populations within a week (33), an advantage over the few stable clones routinely obtained. In addition, retroviral vectors do not form concatemers and therefore should not form a repressive chromatin environment sometimes associated with plasmids (104). For these reasons, retroviruses are well suited for delivery of tetracycline-inducible systems to primary cells. The first studies with tetracycline-regulatable cassettes in retroviruses, however, met with problems. In one case, inclusion of an autoregulatory feedback loop required high background levels of expression in order to "jumpstart" the system (105). In other instances, overcomplexity of transcription and translation units led to low viral titers (106–110). These problems were first overcome using simplified retroviral vectors in which necessary elements were dispersed over more than one retroviral vector (111). In this setup, one retrovirus encoded rtTA, whereas the other contained an inducible Epo cassette. Primary myoblasts exhibited levels of induction approximating 200-fold following multiple rounds of infection. When the engineered myoblasts were transplanted into mice, Epo expression could be repetitively turned on and off over a 5-month period by controlling levels of doxycycline in drinking water. A further improvement of this approach was the inclusion of a selectable marker such as GFP, allowing purification of regulatable populations of cells by flow cytometry (96).

To summarize, tetracycline-regulatable retroviral vectors are powerful tools for regulating gene expression in a fully inducible manner both in vitro and in vivo. Moreover, when the rtTA protein was delivered to mice using myoblasts, an immune response to foreign elements was not observed (111). Retroviruses provide an efficient means of delivering tetracycline-regulatable vectors to large numbers of primary cells, such as myoblasts. Thus, tetracycline-regulatable retroviral systems, in conjunction with myoblast-mediated gene delivery, are powerful tools for fundamental in vivo studies of gene expression as well as for gene therapy.

FUTURE PROSPECTS

Circulating Muscle Precursor Cells (Stem Cells)

A problem in using myoblasts for gene delivery in the treatment of inherited myopathies, as noted earlier, is the difficulty of targeting a large enough proportion of muscle tissue in order for treatment to be effective. Histochemical staining and enzymatic activity assays of muscle transplanted with β-galactosidase–

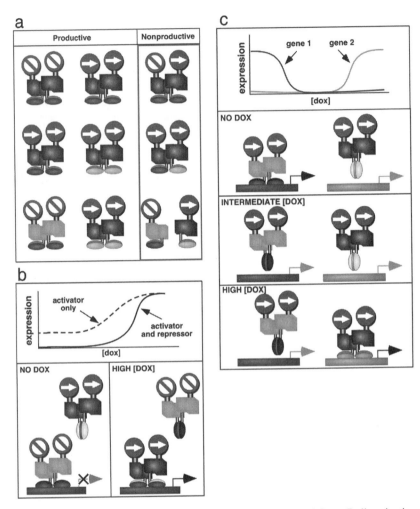

Figure 4 Improved tetracycline-regulatable systems. (*a*) The need for tetR dimerization specificity. Coexpression of tetR fusion proteins with different functional domains, such as repressor domains (represented by the "do not enter" sign) and activator domains (represented by the "go" sign), or DNA binding domains with distinct specificity (symbolized in the *middle row* by the light gray and dark gray "feet"), leads to formation of both functional homodimers and nonfunctional heterodimers. Nonfunctional heterodimers can be eliminated by engineering distinct dimerization domains into the tetR portion of the tet modulators (symbolized by the dark gray and light gray midsections in the *bottom row*). (*b*) Increasing the dynamic range of the tetracycline system. A repressor and an activator that respond oppositely to doxycycline (dox) and that do not heterodimerize because of different dimerization domains can be coexpressed within the same cell. The result is a reduction in the basal expression level of genes under tetracycline control, without affecting the fully induced level. (*c*) Independent expression of two different genes.

expressing myoblasts have shown that fusion of myoblasts into myofibers is maximal in the region of the injection site; the number of fibers to which genes are delivered by intramuscular injection decreases with increasing distance from the site (112). For a sufficiently large percentage of fibers to be treated, many closely spaced injections would be necessary. Isolation of a myoblast population that can efficiently migrate to damaged or degenerated muscle appears to be the most promising solution for effectively treating a large percentage of muscle tissue.

One method of accomplishing this goal may be to introduce genetically engineered muscle precursor cells into the circulation, where they can reach muscles throughout the entire body. Recently, the observation that bone marrow–derived cells can become incorporated into areas of damaged muscle has suggested that these cells can travel through the circulation and from there enter into skeletal muscle tissue (113). Another study examined the feasibility of intraarterial delivery of genetically labeled, immortalized L6 myoblasts to skeletal muscle (114). Infusion of these cells into the arterial circulation led to a small number of labeled fibers in skeletal leg muscle, demonstrating that the circulation may be capable of delivering muscle precursor cells to differentiated myofibers, although some were also found in the lung. A powerful approach to targeting many muscle fibers may be to isolate muscle stem cells of the bone marrow, genetically engineer them ex vivo, and inject them back into the patient where they could serve as a continual pool of circulating cells harboring vectors for the treatment of myopathies.

Several lines of evidence have suggested the existence of a muscle stem cell. Populations of cells that are capable of self-renewal and remain undifferentiated when cultured in conditions designed to induce terminal differentiation have been identified both in the myogenic C2 cell line (115) and in clones of human myoblasts (116). A recent study has also shown that only a discrete minority of transplanted myoblasts participate in regeneration of host muscle, using two genetic markers with different modes of inheritance to examine the fate of myoblasts transplanted into skeletal muscle (45). The small population of cells identified in this study appeared to divide slowly in vitro, but they proliferated rapidly when transplantated into regenerating muscle (45). Methods for characterizing and isolating this muscle stem cell population would be a great boon to the development of ex vivo therapies for a number of inherited myopathies.

Figure 4   (Continued) By coexpressing two tetR-based activators that contain DNA binding domains with distinct specificity, that respond oppositely to doxycycline, and that do not heterodimerize, two independent genes can be regulated by the same inducer. In this system, the expression of each gene can be turned off at an intermediate concentration of doxycycline and activated at markedly different doxycycline concentrations. From Reference 98 (republished with permission of the Proc. Natl. Acad. Sci. USA, 2101 Constitution Ave., NW, Washington DC 20418 and by permission of the publisher via Copyright Clearance Center, Inc).

Encapsulation for Immunoprotection

Although myoblast-mediated gene delivery has proven effective for long-term secretion of recombinant proteins into the circulation, a major hurdle limiting its utility in the therapeutic realm is the requirement for using syngeneic (genetically identical) cells for transplantation in order to avoid immunological rejection (117). Myoblasts may be both isolated from and implanted back into the same individual; however, these procedures are both time intensive and costly. Alternatively, myoblasts can be encapsulated into an immuno-isolated environment prior to implantation to prevent immune cells from coming into contact with implanted cells. Encapsulation of cells within a matrix, for example one made of alginate (although other materials may be used), allows secreted proteins to leave the capsules while obviating the necessity of a genetically identical cell donor. Encapsulated myoblasts have been shown to be effective in delivering genes encoding mouse growth hormone (118) and human factor IX (119) intraperitoneally. The encapsulated cells were retrievable for as long as 213 days postimplantation and even at that point were found to be fully viable and capable of secreting recombinant proteins ex vivo at undiminished rates (119). More recently, encapsulated primary myoblasts were used to deliver VEGF to mice subcutaneously and intraperitoneally, leading to an angiogenic response (ML Springer, G Hortelano, D Bouley, J Wong, PE Kraft, HM Blau, manuscript submitted). This technology is a promising method for nonautologous gene therapy, in which universal donor cells can be created simply by encapsulation in a benign, immunoprotected environment. Myoblasts may be the cell type of choice for this mode of gene therapy, as cell types such as fibroblasts that are encapsulated overgrow and die, whereas myoblasts do not.

CONCLUSIONS

Myoblast-mediated gene delivery is a method that may be well suited for treatment of a number of disorders, not only for diseases caused by single-gene defects but also for complex multi-gene disorders such as cardiovascular diseases and cancer. Gene delivery using myoblasts offers a number of advantages. Genetically altered myoblasts may be fully characterized in vitro before in vivo injection to ensure secretion of recombinant products of correct size and function at pharmacologically useful levels. Moreover, isolated myoblasts are genetically engineered outside of the body, a process that (a) generally assures that only the proper cell type is transduced and (b) avoids inadvertent low-level transduction of cells other than those being targeted, for example cells of the germline. The recent development of improved tetracycline-inducible retroviral vectors provides a powerful means of controlling recombinant gene expression levels. Recent studies suggest that major limitations to ex vivo gene delivery, such as the difficulty in targeting a large proportion of muscle tissue and the requirement that syngeneic myoblasts isolated from one patient be reinjected into that same patient to avoid rejection of cells by the immune system, may be overcome. Identification of a muscle stem cell could lead to methods of gene delivery to muscle throughout the body, allowing for treatment of myopathies using myoblasts. Encapsulation of myoblasts may obviate the requirement for a "tailor made" therapy, allowing allogeneic cells that are invisible to the immune system to be used, theoretically creating universal donor cells derived from muscles of a single patient that could be implanted at ectopic sites in different patients for delivery of diverse products. All these advantages make ex vivo gene delivery via myoblasts an attractive candidate for human gene therapy in the future.

Visit the Annual Reviews home page at www.AnnualReviews.org.

LITERATURE CITED

1. Blaese RM, Culver KW, Miller AD, Carter CS, Fleisher T, et al. 1995. T lymphocyte-directed gene therapy for ADA-SCID: initial trial results after 4 years. *Science* 270:475–80
2. Partridge TA, Grounds M, Sloper JC. 1978. Evidence of fusion between host and donor myoblasts in skeletal muscle grafts. *Nature* 273:306–8
3. Watt DJ, Morgan JE, Clifford MA, Partridge TA. 1987. The movement of muscle precursor cells between adjacent regenerating muscles in the mouse. *Anat. Embryol.* 175:527–36
4. Watt DJ, Lambert K, Morgan JE, Partridge TA, Sloper JC. 1982. Incorporation of donor muscle precursor cells into an area of muscle regeneration in the host mouse. *J. Neurol. Sci.* 57:319–31
5. Watt DJ, Morgan JE, Partridge TA. 1984. Use of mononuclear precursor cells to insert allogeneic genes into growing mouse muscles. *Muscle Nerve* 7:741–50
6. Morgan JE, Watt DJ, Sloper JC, Partridge TA. 1988. Partial correction of an inherited biochemical defect of skeletal muscle by grafts of normal muscle precursor cells. *J. Neurol. Sci.* 86:137–47
7. Partridge TA, Morgan JE, Coulton GR, Hoffman EP, Kunkel LM. 1989. Conversion of mdx myofibres from dystrophin-negative to -positive by injection of normal myoblasts. *Nature* 337:176–79
8. Campion DR. 1984. The muscle satellite cell: a review. *Int. Rev. Cytol.* 87:225–51
9. Mauro A. 1961. Satellite cell of skeletal muscle fibers. *J. Biophys. Biochem. Cytol.* 9:493–95
10. Hughes SM, Cho M, Karsch-Mizrachi I, Travis M, Silberstein L, et al. 1993. Three slow myosin heavy chains sequentially expressed in developing mammalian skeletal muscle. *Dev. Biol.* 158:183–99
11. Blau HM, Dhawan J, Pavlath GK. 1993. Myoblasts in pattern formation and gene therapy. *Trends Genet.* 9:269–74
12. Cho M, Webster SG, Blau HM. 1993. Evidence for myoblast-extrinsic regulation of slow myosin heavy chain expression during muscle fiber formation in embryonic development. *J. Cell Biol.* 121:795–810
13. Hughes SM, Blau HM. 1990. Migration of myoblasts across basal lamina during skeletal muscle development. *Nature* 345:350–53
14. Hughes SM, Blau HM. 1992. Muscle fiber pattern is independent of cell lineage in postnatal rodent development. *Cell* 68:659–71
15. Rando TA, Blau HM. 1994. Primary

mouse myoblast purification, characterization, and transplantation for cell-mediated gene therapy. *J. Cell Biol.* 125:1275–87

16. Wang JM, Zheng H, Blaivas M, Kurachi K. 1997. Persistent systemic production of human factor IX in mice by skeletal myoblast-mediated gene transfer: feasibility of repeat application to obtain therapeutic levels. *Blood* 90:1075–82

17. Blau HM, Springer ML. 1995. Muscle-mediated gene therapy. *N. Engl. J. Med.* 333:1554–56

18. Dhawan J, Pan LC, Pavlath GK, Travis MA, Lanctot AM, et al. 1991. Systemic delivery of human growth hormone by injection of genetically engineered myoblasts. *Science* 254:1509–12

19. Barr E, Leiden JM. 1991. Systemic delivery of recombinant proteins by genetically modified myoblasts. *Science* 254:1507–9

20. Peeters S, Friesen HG. 1977. A growth hormone binding factor in the serum of pregnant mice. *Endocrinology* 101:1164–83

21. Yao SN, Kurachi K. 1992. Expression of human factor IX in mice after injection of genetically modified myoblasts. *Proc. Natl. Acad. Sci. USA* 89:3357–61

22. Yao SN, Smith KJ, Kurachi K. 1994. Primary myoblast-mediated gene transfer: persistent expression of human factor IX in mice. *Gene Ther.* 1:99–107

23. Dai Y, Roman M, Naviaux RK, Verma IM. 1992. Gene therapy via primary myoblasts: long-term expression of factor IX protein following transplantation in vivo. *Proc. Natl. Acad. Sci. USA* 89:10892–95

24. Roman M, Axelrod JH, Dai Y, Naviaux RK, Friedmann T, et al. 1992. Circulating human or canine factor IX from retrovirally transduced primary myoblasts and established myoblast cell lines grafted into murine skeletal muscle. *Somat. Cell. Mol. Genet.* 18:247–58

25. Charlton CA, Mohler WA, Radice GL,

Hynes RO, Blau HM. 1997. Fusion competence of myoblasts rendered genetically null for N-cadherin in culture. *J. Cell Biol.* 138:331–36

26. Yang JT, Rando TA, Mohler WA, Rayburn H, Blau HM, et al. 1996. Genetic analysis of alpha 4 integrin functions in the development of mouse skeletal muscle. *J. Cell Biol.* 135:829–35

27. Webster C, Blau HM. 1990. Accelerated age-related decline in replicative lifespan of Duchenne muscular dystrophy myoblasts: implications for cell and gene therapy. *Somat. Cell. Mol. Genet.* 16:557–65

28. Webster C, Pavlath GK, Parks DR, Walsh FS, Blau HM. 1988. Isolation of human myoblasts with the fluorescence-activated cell sorter. *Exp. Cell Res.* 174:252–65

29. Blau HM, Kaplan I, Tao TW, Kriss JP. 1983. Thyroglobulin-independent, cell-mediated cytotoxicity of human eye muscle cells in tissue culture by lymphocytes of a patient with Graves' ophthalmopathy. *Life Sci.* 32:45–53

30. Blau HM, Webster C. 1981. Isolation and characterization of human muscle cells. *Proc. Natl. Acad. Sci. USA* 78:5623–27

31. Springer ML, Rando TA, Blau HM. 1997. Gene delivery to muscle. In *Current Protocols in Human Genetics,* ed. AL Boyle, pp. 13.4.1–19. New York: Wiley

32. Kaufman SJ, Foster RF. 1988. Replicating myoblasts express a muscle-specific phenotype. *Proc. Natl. Acad. Sci. USA* 85:9606–10

33. Springer ML, Blau HM. 1997. High-efficiency retroviral infection of primary myoblasts. *Somat. Cell. Mol. Genet.* 23:203–9

34. Hoffman EP, Brown RH Jr, Kunkel LM. 1987. Dystrophin: the protein product of the Duchenne muscular dystrophy locus. *Cell* 51:919–28

35. Morgan JE, Hoffman EP, Partridge TA. 1990. Normal myogenic cells from new-

born mice restore normal histology to degenerating muscles of the mdx mouse. *J. Cell Biol.* 111:2437–49

36. Law PK, Bertorini TE, Goodwin TG, Chen M, Fang QW, et al. 1990. Dystrophin production induced by myoblast transfer therapy in Duchenne muscular dystrophy. *Lancet* 336:114–15

37. Gussoni E, Pavlath GK, Lanctot AM, Sharma KR, Miller RG, et al. 1992. Normal dystrophin transcripts detected in Duchenne muscular dystrophy patients after myoblast transplantation. *Nature* 356:435–38

38. Huard J, Bouchard JP, Roy R, Malouin F, Dansereau G, et al. 1992. Human myoblast transplantation: preliminary results of 4 cases. *Muscle Nerve* 15:550–60

39. Karpati G, Ajdukovic D, Arnold D, Gledhill RB, Guttmann R, et al. 1993. Myoblast transfer in Duchenne muscular dystrophy. *Ann. Neurol.* 34:8–17

40. Mendell JR, Kissel JT, Amato AA, King W, Signore L, et al. 1995. Myoblast transfer in the treatment of Duchenne's muscular dystrophy. *N. Engl. J. Med.* 333:832–38

41. Morandi L, Bernasconi P, Gebbia M, Mora M, Crosti F, et al. 1995. Lack of mRNA and dystrophin expression in DMD patients three months after myoblast transfer. *Neuromuscul. Disord.* 5:291–95

42. Miller RG, Sharma KR, Pavlath GK, Gussoni E, Mynhier M, et al. 1997. Myoblast implantation in Duchenne muscular dystrophy: the San Francisco study. *Muscle Nerve* 20:469–78

43. Gussoni E, Wang Y, Fraefel C, Miller RG, Blau HM, et al. 1996. A method to codetect introduced genes and their products in gene therapy protocols. *Nat. Biotechnol.* 14:1012–16

44. Gussoni E, Blau HM, Kunkel LM. 1997. The fate of individual myoblasts after transplantation into muscles of DMD patients. *Nat. Med.* 3:970–77

45. Beauchamp JR, Morgan JE, Pagel CN,

Partridge TA. 1999. Dynamics of myoblast transplantation reveal a discrete minority of precursors with stem cell-like properties as the myogenic source. *J. Cell Biol.* 144:1113–22

46. Ragot T, Vincent N, Chafey P, Vigne E, Gilgenkrantz H, et al. 1993. Efficient adenovirus-mediated transfer of a human minidystrophin gene to skeletal muscle of mdx mice. *Nature* 361:647–50

47. Kochanek S, Clemens PR, Mitani K, Chen HH, Chan S, et al. 1996. A new adenoviral vector: replacement of all viral coding sequences with 28 kb of DNA independently expressing both full-length dystrophin and beta-galactosidase. *Proc. Natl. Acad. Sci. USA* 93:5731–36

48. Kumar-Singh R, Chamberlain JS. 1996. Encapsidated adenovirus minichromosomes allow delivery and expression of a 14 kb dystrophin cDNA to muscle cells. *Hum. Mol. Genet.* 5:913–21

49. Tinsley J, Deconinck N, Fisher R, Kahn D, Phelps S, et al. 1998. Expression of full-length utrophin prevents muscular dystrophy in mdx mice. *Nat. Med.* 4:1441–44

50. Akli S, Guidotti JE, Vigne E, Perricaudet M, Sandhoff K, et al. 1996. Restoration of hexosaminidase A activity in human Tay-Sachs fibroblasts via adenoviral vector-mediated gene transfer. *Gene Ther.* 3:769–74

51. Svensson EC, Tripathy SK, Leiden JM. 1996. Muscle-based gene therapy: realistic possibilities for the future. *Mol. Med. Today* 2:166–72

52. Pfeffer S. 1991. Targeting of proteins to the lysosome. *Curr. Top. Microbiol. Immunol.* 170:43–63

53. Naffakh N, Pinset C, Montarras D, Li Z, Paulin D, et al. 1996. Long-term secretion of therapeutic proteins from genetically modified skeletal muscles. *Hum. Gene Ther.* 7:11–21

54. Kay MA. 1995. Hepatic gene therapy for hemophilia B. *Adv. Exp. Med. Biol.*

386:229–34

55. Chuah MK, Collen D, VandenDriessche T. 1998. Gene therapy for hemophilia: hopes and hurdles. *Crit. Rev. Oncol. Hematol.* 28:153–71

56. Hedner U, Davie E. 1989. Introduction to homeostasis and the vitamin K-dependent coagulation factors. In *The Metabolic Basis of Inherited Disease,* ed. C Scriver, AL Beaudet, WS Sly, D Valle, pp. 2107–34. New York: McGraw-Hill. 6th ed.

57. Wang L, Zoppe M, Hackeng TM, Griffin JH, Lee KF, et al. 1997. A factor IX-deficient mouse model for hemophilia B gene therapy. *Proc. Natl. Acad. Sci. USA* 94:11563–66

58. Koury MJ, Bondurant MC. 1992. The molecular mechanism of erythropoietin action. *Eur. J. Biochem.* 210:649–63

59. Evans RW. 1991. Recombinant human erythropoietin and the quality of life of end-stage renal disease patients: a comparative analysis. *Am. J. Kidney Dis.* 18:62–70

60. Naffakh N, Danos O. 1996. Gene transfer for erythropoiesis enhancement. *Mol. Med. Today* 2:343–48

61. Hamamori Y, Samal B, Tian J, Kedes L. 1994. Persistent erythropoiesis by myoblast transfer of erythropoietin cDNA. *Hum. Gene Ther.* 5:1349–56

62. Hamamori Y, Samal B, Tian J, Kedes L. 1995. Myoblast transfer of human erythropoietin gene in a mouse model of renal failure. *J. Clin. Invest.* 95:1808–13

63. Leung DW, Cachianes G, Kuang WJ, Goeddel DV, Ferrara N. 1989. Vascular endothelial growth factor is a secreted angiogenic mitogen. *Science* 246:1306–9

64. Plouet J, Schilling J, Gospodarowicz D. 1989. Isolation and characterization of a newly identified endothelial cell mitogen produced by AtT-20 cells. *EMBO J.* 8:3801–6

65. Conn G, Soderman DD, Schaeffer MT, Wile M, Hatcher VB, et al. 1990. Purification of a glycoprotein vascular endothelial cell mitogen from a rat glioma-derived cell line. *Proc. Natl. Acad. Sci. USA* 87:1323–27

66. Senger DR, Galli SJ, Dvorak AM, Perruzzi CA, Harvey VS, et al. 1983. Tumor cells secrete a vascular permeability factor that promotes accumulation of ascites fluid. *Science* 219:983–85

67. Ferrara N, Henzel WJ. 1989. Pituitary follicular cells secrete a novel heparin-binding growth factor specific for vascular endothelial cells. *Biochem. Biophys. Res. Commun.* 161:851–58

68. Hanahan D, Folkman J. 1996. Patterns and emerging mechanisms of the angiogenic switch during tumorigenesis. *Cell* 86:353–64

69. Pardanaud L, Yassine F, Dieterlen-Lievre F. 1989. Relationship between vasculogenesis, angiogenesis and haemopoiesis during avian ontogeny. *Development* 105:473–85

70. Risau W, Flamme I. 1995. Vasculogenesis. *Annu. Rev. Cell Dev. Biol.* 11:73–91

71. Takeshita S, Pu LQ, Stein LA, Sniderman AD, Bunting S, et al. 1994. Intramuscular administration of vascular endothelial growth factor induces dose-dependent collateral artery augmentation in a rabbit model of chronic limb ischemia. *Circulation* 90:II228–34

72. Takeshita S, Zheng LP, Brogi E, Kearney M, Pu LQ, et al. 1994. Therapeutic angiogenesis. A single intraarterial bolus of vascular endothelial growth factor augments revascularization in a rabbit ischemic hind limb model. *J. Clin. Invest.* 93:662–70

73. Bauters C, Asahara T, Zheng LP, Takeshita S, Bunting S, et al. 1995. Site-specific therapeutic angiogenesis after systemic administration of vascular endothelial growth factor. *J. Vasc. Surg.* 21:314–24

74. Hariawala MD, Horowitz JR, Esakof D, Sheriff DD, Walter DH, et al. 1996. VEGF improves myocardial blood flow

but produces EDRF-mediated hypotension in porcine hearts. *J. Surg. Res.* 63:77–82

75. Horowitz JR, Rivard A, van der Zee R, Hariawala M, Sheriff DD, et al. 1997. Vascular endothelial growth factor/vascular permeability factor produces nitric oxide-dependent hypotension. Evidence for a maintenance role in quiescent adult endothelium. *Arterioscler. Thromb. Vasc. Biol.* 17:2793–800

76. Mesri EA, Federoff HJ, Brownlee M. 1995. Expression of vascular endothelial growth factor from a defective herpes simplex virus type 1 amplicon vector induces angiogenesis in mice. *Circ. Res.* 76:161–67

77. Muhlhauser J, Merrill MJ, Pili R, Maeda H, Bacic M, et al. 1995. VEGF165 expressed by a replication-deficient recombinant adenovirus vector induces angiogenesis in vivo. *Circ. Res.* 77: 1077–86

78. Magovern CJ, Mack CA, Zhang J, Rosengart TK, Isom OW, et al. 1997. Regional angiogenesis induced in nonischemic tissue by an adenoviral vector expressing vascular endothelial growth factor. *Hum. Gene Ther.* 8:215–27

79. Isner JM, Pieczek A, Schainfeld R, Blair R, Haley L, et al. 1996. Clinical evidence of angiogenesis after arterial gene transfer of phVEGF165 in patient with ischaemic limb. *Lancet* 348:370–74

80. Takeshita S, Weir L, Chen D, Zheng LP, Riessen R, et al. 1996. Therapeutic angiogenesis following arterial gene transfer of vascular endothelial growth factor in a rabbit model of hindlimb ischemia. *Biochem. Biophys. Res. Commun.* 227:628–35

81. Tsurumi Y, Takeshita S, Chen D, Kearney M, Rossow ST, et al. 1996. Direct intramuscular gene transfer of naked DNA encoding vascular endothelial growth factor augments collateral development and tissue perfusion. *Circulation* 94:3281–90

82. Mack CA, Patel SR, Schwarz EA, Zanzonico P, Hahn RT, et al. 1998. Biologic bypass with the use of adenovirus-mediated gene transfer of the complementary deoxyribonucleic acid for vascular endothelial growth factor 121 improves myocardial perfusion and function in the ischemic porcine heart. *J. Thorac. Cardiovasc. Surg.* 115:168–76

83. Springer ML, Chen AS, Kraft PE, Bednarski M, Blau HM. 1998. VEGF gene delivery to muscle: potential role for vasculogenesis in adults. *Mol. Cell* 2:549–58

84. Gimbrone MA Jr, Leapman SB, Cotran RS, Folkman J. 1972. Tumor dormancy in vivo by prevention of neovascularization. *J. Exp. Med.* 136:261–76

85. Brem S, Brem H, Folkman J, Finkelstein D, Patz A. 1976. Prolonged tumor dormancy by prevention of neovascularization in the vitreous. *Cancer Res.* 36:2807–12

86. O'Reilly MS, Holmgren L, Shing Y, Chen C, Rosenthal RA, et al. 1994. Angiostatin: a novel angiogenesis inhibitor that mediates the suppression of metastases by a Lewis lung carcinoma. *Cell* 79:315–28

87. O'Reilly MS, Boehm T, Shing Y, Fukai N, Vasios G, et al. 1997. Endostatin: an endogenous inhibitor of angiogenesis and tumor growth. *Cell* 88:277–85

88. Blezinger P, Wang J, Gondo M, Quezada A, Mehrens D, et al. 1999. Systemic inhibition of tumor growth and tumor metastases by intramuscular administration of the endostatin gene. *Nat. Biotechnol.* 17:343–48

89. Rossi FM, Blau HM. 1998. Recent advances in inducible gene expression systems. *Curr. Opin. Biotechnol.* 9:451–56

90. Harvey DM, Caskey CT. 1998. Inducible control of gene expression: prospects for gene therapy. *Curr. Opin. Chem. Biol.* 2:512–18

91. Gossen M, Bujard H. 1992. Tight control

of gene expression in mammalian cells by tetracycline-responsive promoters. *Proc. Natl. Acad. Sci. USA* 89:5547–51

92. Gossen M, Freundlieb S, Bender G, Muller G, Hillen W, et al. 1995. Transcriptional activation by tetracyclines in mammalian cells. *Science* 268:1766–69

93. Mayford M, Bach ME, Huang YY, Wang L, Hawkins RD, et al. 1996. Control of memory formation through regulated expression of a CaMKII transgene. *Science* 274:1678–83

94. Kistner A, Gossen M, Zimmermann F, Jerecic J, Ullmer C, et al. 1996. Doxycycline-mediated quantitative and tissue-specific control of gene expression in transgenic mice. *Proc. Natl. Acad. Sci. USA* 93:10933–38

95. Bello B, Resendez-Perez D, Gehring WJ. 1998. Spatial and temporal targeting of gene expression in Drosophila by means of a tetracycline-dependent transactivator system. *Development* 125:2193–202

96. Kringstein AM, Rossi FM, Hofmann A, Blau HM. 1998. Graded transcriptional response to different concentrations of a single transactivator. *Proc. Natl. Acad. Sci. USA* 95:13670–75

97. Deuschle U, Meyer WK, Thiesen HJ. 1995. Tetracycline-reversible silencing of eukaryotic promoters. *Mol. Cell. Biol.* 15:1907–14

98. Blau HM, Rossi FM. 1999. Tet B or not tet B: advances in tetracycline-inducible gene expression. *Proc. Natl. Acad. Sci. USA* 96:797–99

99. Hillen W, Berens C. 1994. Mechanisms underlying expression of Tn10 encoded tetracycline resistance. *Annu. Rev. Microbiol.* 48:345–69

100. Kisker C, Hinrichs W, Tovar K, Hillen W, Saenger W. 1995. The complex formed between Tet repressor and tetracycline-Mg2+ reveals mechanism of antibiotic resistance. *J. Mol. Biol.* 247:260–80

101. Schnappinger D, Schubert P, Pfleiderer K, Hillen W. 1998. Determinants of pro-

tein-protein recognition by four helix bundles: changing the dimerization specificity of Tet repressor. *EMBO J.* 17:535–43

102. Rossi FM, Guicherit OM, Spicher A, Kringstein AM, Fatyol K, et al. 1998. Tetracycline-regulatable factors with distinct dimerization domains allow reversible growth inhibition by p16. *Nat. Genet.* 20:389–93

103. Baron U, Schnappinger D, Helbl V, Gossen M, Hillen W, et al. 1999. Generation of conditional mutants in higher eukaryotes by switching between the expression of two genes. *Proc. Natl. Acad. Sci. USA* 96:1013–18

104. Garrick D, Fiering S, Martin DI, Whitelaw E. 1998. Repeat-induced gene silencing in mammals. *Nat. Genet.* 18:56–59

105. Hofmann A, Nolan GP, Blau HM. 1996. Rapid retroviral delivery of tetracycline-inducible genes in a single autoregulatory cassette. *Proc. Natl. Acad. Sci. USA* 93:5185–90

106. Hwang JJ, Scuric Z, Anderson WF. 1996. Novel retroviral vector transferring a suicide gene and a selectable marker gene with enhanced gene expression by using a tetracycline-responsive expression system. *J. Virol.* 70:8138–41

107. Lindemann D, Patriquin E, Feng S, Mulligan RC. 1997. Versatile retrovirus vector systems for regulated gene expression in vitro and in vivo. *Mol. Med.* 3:466–76

108. Paulus W, Baur I, Boyce FM, Breakefield XO, Reeves SA. 1996. Self-contained, tetracycline-regulated retroviral vector system for gene delivery to mammalian cells. *J. Virol.* 70:62–67

109. Hoshimaru M, Ray J, Sah DW, Gage FH. 1996. Differentiation of the immortalized adult neuronal progenitor cell line HC2S2 into neurons by regulatable suppression of the v-myc oncogene. *Proc. Natl. Acad. Sci. USA* 93:1518–23

110. Sah DW, Ray J, Gage FH. 1997. Bipotent progenitor cell lines from the human CNS. *Nat. Biotechnol.* 15:574–80

111. Bohl D, Naffakh N, Heard JM. 1997. Long-term control of erythropoietin secretion by doxycycline in mice transplanted with engineered primary myoblasts. *Nat. Med.* 3:299–305

112. Rando TA, Pavlath GK, Blau HM. 1995. The fate of myoblasts following transplantation into mature muscle. *Exp. Cell Res.* 220:383–89

113. Ferrari G, Cusella-De Angelis G, Coletta M, Paolucci E, Stornaiuolo A, et al. 1998. Muscle regeneration by bone marrow-derived myogenic progenitors. *Science* 279:1528–30

114. Neumeyer AM, DiGregorio DM, Brown RH Jr. 1992. Arterial delivery of myoblasts to skeletal muscle. *Neurology* 42:2258–62

115. Yoshida N, Yoshida S, Koishi K, Masuda K, Nabeshima Y. 1998. Cell heterogeneity upon myogenic differentiation: down-regulation of MyoD and Myf-5 generates 'reserve cells.' *J. Cell Sci.* 111:769–79

116. Baroffio A, Hamann M, Bernheim L, Bochaton-Piallat ML, Gabbiani G, et al. 1996. Identification of self-renewing myoblasts in the progeny of single human muscle satellite cells. *Differentiation* 60:47–57

117. Chang PL. 1996. Microencapsulation—an alternative approach to gene therapy. *Transfus. Sci.* 17:35–43

118. al-Hendy A, Hortelano G, Tannenbaum GS, Chang PL. 1995. Correction of the growth defect in dwarf mice with non-autologous microencapsulated myoblasts—an alternate approach to somatic gene therapy. *Hum. Gene Ther.* 6:165–75

119. Hortelano G, al-Hendy A, Ofosu FA, Chang PL. 1996. Delivery of human factor IX in mice by encapsulated recombinant myoblasts: a novel approach towards allogeneic gene therapy of hemophilia B. *Blood* 87:5095–103

Annu. Rev. Pharmacol. Toxicol. 2000. 40:319–34

5-HT$_6$ Receptors as Emerging Targets for Drug Discovery

Theresa A. Branchek and Thomas P. Blackburn
Synaptic Pharmaceutical Corporation, 215 College Road, Paramus, New Jersey 07652;
e-mail: tbranchek@synapticcorp.com, tblackburn@synapticcorp.com

Key Words serotonin, GPCR, adenylate cyclase, antisense, cognition

■ **Abstract** 5-ht$_6$ receptors are the latest serotonin receptors to be identified by molecular cloning. Their high affinity for a wide range of drugs used in psychiatry, coupled with their intriguing distribution in the brain, has stimulated significant interest. Antisense oligonucleotides, antipeptide antibodies, selective radioligands, knockout mice, and selective antagonists of the 5-ht$_6$ receptor have recently become available. Surprisingly, 5-ht$_6$ receptors appear to regulate cholinergic neurotransmission in the brain, rather than the expected interaction as modulators of dopaminergic transmission. This interaction predicts a possible role for 5-ht$_6$ receptor antagonists in the treatment of learning and memory disorders. Furthermore, polymorphisms in the sequence of the 5-ht$_6$ receptor gene may provide a genetic tool to further our understanding of the differential responses of patients to antipsychotic medications.

INTRODUCTION

The multiplicity of actions of serotonin has been known for decades (1). Although the pharmacology of these responses suggested the likelihood of receptor subtypes (2, 3), the first identification of a discreet molecular species of known (deduced) amino acid composition came only a decade ago (4). This discovery presaged an explosion in the number of genetically identified receptors for serotonin (5). Attendant to the relatively fast pace of molecular discovery has been the slower pace of receptor characterization using nucleotide probes, radioligands, known chemical entities, and biochemical functional assays. More recently, the development of newly created probes such as selective antibodies, selective agonists and antagonists, knockout animals, and genetic linkages studies has been essential to further our understanding of the functions of individual serotonin receptor subtypes. Although our knowledge is far from complete, there is now substantial progress in the elucidation of functions of the most recently discovered serotonin receptor, 5-ht$_6$, and its possible therapeutic roles.

0362–1642/00/0415–0319$14.00

MOLECULAR BIOLOGY OF 5-HT$_6$ RECEPTORS

The first cloning of the rat 5-ht$_6$ receptor reported a sequence predicted to encode a protein of 436 amino acids (6, 7). This sequence has been re-evaluated, and the receptor is now deduced to form a protein of 438 amino acids. The human homologue contains 440 amino acids (8). The human and rat amino acid sequences are 89% identical. Structural elements of this receptor sequence include a relatively short third intracellular loop (50 amino acids, rat; 57 amino acids, human) and a long carboxyl tail (120 amino acids), both of which are common to some other GPCRs that couple to adenylate cyclase stimulation (9). The 5-ht$_6$ receptor has a single glycosylation site in the amino terminus and multiple potential phosphorylation sites for protein kinase C in the cytoplasmic domains. The sequence also contains a leucine zipper motif in transmembrane (TM) III (7). The sequence has the highest amino acid identity (37%) to the *Drosophila melanogaster* cyclase stimulatory serotonin receptor (10) and the histamine H$_2$ receptor (11); lower identities are observed with 5-ht$_5$ and 5-HT$_7$ receptors. The rat and human sequences each contain two introns, one in the third intracellular loop and the other in the third extracellular loop (8). The intron in the third cytoplasmic loop appears at the same location as that described for the 5-ht$_{5a}$ and 5-ht$_{5b}$ receptors, as well as the dopamine D$_2$ and D$_3$ receptors (8). No additional subtypes have been cloned, and no functional splice variants have been identified. However, a truncated variant of the 5-ht$_6$ receptor, first noted by Monsma et al (6), was presumed to occur as a mis-splicing event and delete the seventh TM VII domain (12). Subsequently, Olsen and coworkers (13) showed that the human 5-ht$_6$ gene could give rise to an alternate splicing of the first intron, which produced a truncated variant of the receptor containing the amino terminus through TM IV. This variant is transcribed, and the transcripts are expressed in a limited subset of the brain regions (substantia nigra and caudate) occupied by mRNA for the full-length receptor.

The gene for the human 5-ht$_6$ receptor maps to chromosome region 1p35–p36, thus overlapping with the gene locus for the 5-HT$_{1D\alpha}$ receptor (8). The 5-ht$_6$ receptor sequence contains a Rsa1 restriction fragment–length polymorphism in the first extracellular loop (C267T).

MOLECULAR PHARMACOLOGY OF 5-HT$_6$ RECEPTORS

The 5-ht$_6$ receptor can be radiolabeled with [^{125}I]lysergic acid diethylamide (LSD) and couples to the stimulation of adenylate cyclase (6, 7). The distinctive properties of the pharmacology of the cloned rat 5-ht$_6$ receptor are its high affinity for a series of antipsychotic compounds, including clozapine and loxapine, as well as affinity for a number of tricyclic antidepressants such as amoxipine, clomipramine, and amitryptyline (6, 14, 15). A new potential antipsychotic compound, BIMG 80, also has moderate affinity for the 5-ht$_6$ receptor (16). Analysis of binding studies using [^{125}I] LSD as a radioligand gives the rank order of affinities: methiothepin > 5-MeOT > 5-HT > tryptamine > 5-CT > sumatriptan >> 8-OH-DPAT. The affinity of 5-HT to the 5-ht$_6$ receptor is relatively low compared with other serotonin receptors. A similar receptor profile has been reported in N8TG2 cells, a neuroblastoma line. It displays a rank order of agonist potency in both radioligand binding and cAMP assays: 5-MeOT > 5-HT > tryptamine > 2-methyl tryptamine > 5-CT > α-methyl-5-HT (17). Responses to 5-HT in this cell line are antagonized by clozapine. Affinities of compounds for the human cloned 5-ht$_6$ receptor are equivalent to those determined for the rat, with the exception of four compounds: methiothepin (4-fold higher affinity for the human receptor), metergoline, and the atypical antipsychotics, tiopyrone and amperozide (>10-fold higher affinity for the rat receptor). Clozapine is a high-affinity antagonist at both human and rat 5-ht$_6$ receptors. The rank order of binding affinities for antagonists is methiothepin > clozapine = olanzapine > ritanserin >> risperidone. A nonconserved amino acid substitution of threonine (rat) for leucine (human) in TM III may contribute to the differences in binding affinities observed between the species homologues.

   The primary signal transduction pathway of the 5-ht$_6$ receptor is the stimulation of adenylate cyclase (AC) activity. The rank order of both agonist and antagonist potencies, as well as their quantitative values, determined from AC stimulation matches closely with those determined in parallel using radioligand binding (15, 18). There are multiple isoforms of AC; for example, AC5 is a G$_s$-sensitive AC. It is highly localized in the striatum and nucleus accumbens, two major areas of 5-ht$_6$ localization. In contrast, AC1 and AC8 are calmodulin-stimulated ACs and are not activated by G$_s$ proteins in vivo. AC1 and AC8 are neural-specific cyclases. AC1 is expressed in hippocampus, and AC8 is expressed in hippocampus and hypothalamus. The 5-ht$_6$ receptor, expressed in HEK 293 cells, interacts specifically with AC5 but not with AC1 or AC8 (19).

   A limited number of mutations have been made experimentally to probe the binding pocket of the 5-ht$_6$ receptor. In TM V of many monoamine receptors, there are two "conserved" serine residues that are responsible for hydrogen bonding of hydroxyl groups of the cognate neurotransmitter (20, 21). In the many 5-HT receptors, the second serine is replaced by an alanine, and this replacement affects the binding of compounds such as N-1–substituted ergolines and tryptamines (22, 23). In the 5-ht$_6$ receptor, a threonine, rather than the "expected" alanine, occupies this position. Mutation of this residue to alanine (T196A) results in a decrease in the affinity of the mutant for LSD, 5-HT, and other N-1 unsubstituted ergolines (24). The magnitude of this change is consistent with a disruption of a hydrogen bond. In contrast, the N-1–methylated ergolines showed unchanged or enhanced affinity. Mutations were also made in TM III and TM VI (25, 26). In TM III, mutation of the conserved aspartic acid to asparagine (D106N) resulted in a loss of [^{3}H]LSD binding, although AC stimulation could still be elicited with both LSD and 5-HT. The potencies, however, were right shifted by 500-fold for LSD and 3600-fold for 5-HT (25). This change in affinity is consistent with the loss of a charge-charge interaction. In contrast, mutation of the conserved tryptophan one helical turn upstream of this mutation (W102F) resulted in only a small (two- to sixfold) reduction of affinity for most test compounds. Finally, two adjacent residues near the distal end of TM VI were probed (A287L, N288S) as doubled mutants (25). This mutant displayed an elevated affinity for tryptamine derivatives with large substitutions on the 5′ position, as well as for ergopeptine ligands with large substituents on the 2′ position, possibly consistent with formation of a new hydrogen bond to Ser288. Studies such as these will aid molecular modeling approaches used in the design of selective ligands for this receptor.

REGULATION OF 5-HT$_6$ RECEPTORS

Since 5-ht$_6$ receptors may be important mediators of some of the beneficial actions of psychiatric drugs, it would be interesting to know if 5-ht$_6$ receptors act as autoreceptors. To investigate this possibility, Gerard et al (27) evaluated the impact of selective lesioning of the serotonergic system on the distribution of 5-ht$_6$ receptors by using 5,7-dihydroxytryptamine. Three weeks after administration of the toxin by microinfusion, only 10% of the serotonin transporter, a marker of serotoninergic neurons, remained in the anterior raphe region. In contrast, 5-ht$_6$ mRNA levels were unchanged. This observation indicates that 5-ht$_6$ receptors are not located on serotoninergic neurons, and therefore are not autoreceptors. In addition, the postsynaptic target cells of the serotoninergic projections do not up- or down-regulate their 5-ht$_6$ mRNA levels in response to the lesion, at the time point examined.

Glucocorticoids are known to affect serotoninergic systems and to be related to depression (28). Blockade of glucocorticoid synthesis, with metyrapone and aminogluthethimide, increases 5-ht$_6$ mRNA levels in the CA1 regions of the hippocampus (29). This effect can be partially reversed with corticosterone replacement. Metyrapone and aminogluthethimide have both been used in resistant depression, which has led to speculation that increases in receptor number with these treatments may enhance the effect of antidepressant ligand (29).

The developmental expression of mRNA for the 5-ht$_6$ receptor has been studied using RT-PCR. Expression of these transcripts first appeared on embryonic day 12 (E12), coincident with the appearance of the first serotonergic cell bodies of brain neurons, suggesting a possible role of the 5-ht$_6$ receptor in growth factor properties of 5-HT (30). Expression increased through postnatal day 15 and then stabilized through adult at the same level.

Selective Agonists and Antagonists for 5-ht$_6$ Receptors

At present, there are no fully selective agonists. However, a careful structure-affinity analysis of 5-HT derivatives has been presented (31). The most selective agonist is 2-methyl-5-HT. Modifications on the 5 position indicate that the hydroxyl group is relatively unimportant for 5-HT binding. The conformation of the side chain that the 5-ht$_6$ receptor prefers for binding is that adopted by ergolines. An intact indole nucleus is favored for binding. Secondary and tertiary amines are preferred over the primary amine or the quaternary amine, whereas large dialkyl substitutions reduce affinity.

It was previously shown that many known antidepressants and antipsychotics are antagonists of the 5-ht$_6$ receptor (14). However, none was selective for this receptor. They typically have affinity for dopamine receptors, other 5-HT receptors, monoamine oxidase, and many other sites. Great strides have been made recently in the development of selective antagonists of the 5-ht$_6$ receptor.

The first reported 5-ht$_6$ antagonists were Ro-04–6790 [4-amino-N-(2,6 bis-methylamino-pyrimidin-4-yl)-benzene sulphonamide] and Ro-63–0563 [4-amino-N-(2,6 bis-methylamino- pyridin-4-yl)-benzene sulphonamide] (32). They are both relatively high-affinity (pK$_i$ = 7.3 and 7.9, respectively), selective competitive antagonists (pA$_2$ = 6.75 and 7.10), as evaluated in transfected cells. There are no significant differences in their affinities for rat compared with human 5-ht$_6$ receptors. Ro-04–6790 can be administered i.p. and is CNS penetrant. Ro-63–0563 can be administered i.v. and is also CNS penetrant. The preferred compound for in vivo use is Ro-04–6790, although neither compound achieves high brain levels.

These structures were evaluated for use as radioligands. [^{3}H]Ro 63–0563 was synthesized and had a specific activity of 29 Ci/mmol (33). It was used in membrane binding studies in rat striatal membranes. The measured dissociation constant was 11.7 nM and the B_{max} was 175 fmol/mg protein. However, poor levels of specific binding were observed (10–30%). In transfected cells, the ligand had a dissociation constant of 5 nM for human 5-ht$_6$ and 6.8 nM for rat 5-ht$_6$, and a better specific binding level was obtained (70%). The pharmacological profile of the 5-ht$_6$ receptor as determined using this radioligand was not significantly different from that measured with [^{3}H]LSD as a radioligand. The high nonspecific binding in native tissues limits its use as a radioligand for autoradiographic studies.

The next selective antagonist was SB-271046 (34). The initial hit from a high throughput screen was 4-bromo-N-[4-methoxy-3-(4-methylpiperazin-1-ylphenyl] benzenesulfonamide. It had a pK$_i$ of 8.3 nM and was 50-fold selective over other binding sites. This compound was moderately brain penetrant but was rapidly cleared from the blood and therefore had low oral bioavailability. A series of bisaryl sulfonamides was prepared and evaluated. The 5-chloro-3-methylbenzothiophene derivative had a subnanomolar affinity but was metabolized by N-dealkylation in the rat to yield the corresponding NH-piperazine. Synthesis of this metabolite, which was detected at a high level in blood, resulted in a 5-ht$_6$ antagonist with high affinity (pK$_i$ = 8.9 nM) and potency (pA$_2$ = 8.7 nM) and excellent selectivity. The compound was found to be moderately CNS penetrant (10%) and to have a low blood clearance, good half-life (4.8 h in rat), and 80% oral bioavailability. As such, 5-chloro-N-(4-methoxy-3-piperazin-1-yl-phenyl)-3-

methyl-2-benzothiophenesulfonamide (SB-271046) is a significant new tool for the study of 5-ht$_6$ receptor function.

In addition, another compound from the series {5-iodo-N-[4-methoxy-3-(4-methylpiperazin-1-yl-phenyl]benezenesulfonamide} has been radioiodinated to form [^{125}I]SB-258585 and evaluated for use as a radioligand (35). [^{125}I]SB-258585 had a specific activity of 2000 Ci/mmol. In binding assays on membranes derived from human 5-ht$_6$–transfected cells, a K_d = 0.8 nM was determined and 95% specific binding was obtained. Subsequent studies in native tissue homogenates (36) indicate that there is high specific binding (60–68%) in rat and pig striatal membranes and in human caudate-putamen membranes. The K_d in rat and porcine tissues was 2.8 nM with a B_{max} of 180 fmol/mg protein. In human caudate the K_d was 1.3 nM with a B_{max} of 215 fmol/mg protein. The rank order of affinities for a discriminating set of ligands was comparable to that previously determined for the cloned receptors and also by using alternate radioligands, thereby validating this as a new tool for the study of 5-ht$_6$ receptors. In addition, this ligand is useful for autoradiographic mapping studies (37) (see below).

IN VITRO STUDIES

Localization of mRNA for the 5-ht$_6$ Receptor

The distribution of mRNA encoding the 5-ht$_6$ receptor has been determined by Northern blot analysis in the rat brain and peripheral tissues (6). The highest expression was detected in the striatum with lower-density signals detected in the amygdala, cerebral cortex, and olfactory tubercle. mRNA was undetectable in cerebellum, hippocampus, hypothalamus, medulla, olfactory bulb, pituitary, retina, thalamus, and a number of peripheral tissues (heart, lung, kidney, liver, spleen, pancreas, skeletal muscle, smooth muscle, stomach, ovary, prostate, and testes). A second group observed 5-ht$_6$ mRNA signals in the hippocampus, hypothalamus, adrenal, and stomach (7). Initial in situ hybridization studies in the rat brain demonstrated high levels of mRNA in the striatum and olfactory tubercles (7). Other labeled structures included the nucleus accumbens, olfactory bulb, and hippocampus. Using in situ hybridization, Ward et al (38) have completed a detailed examination of the mRNA distribution for the 5-ht$_6$ receptor in the rat brain. Their study confirmed the high abundance of message in the olfactory tubercle, striatum, nucleus accumbens, dentate gyrus, and CA1, CA2, and CA3 fields of the hippocampus. Lower intensity labeling was found in the cerebellum, some diencephalic nuclei, amygdala, and several cortical layers (layers 2, 3, 4, and 6). In the striatum, the 5-ht$_6$ mRNA is extensively co-localized with enkephalin (68%), substance P (79%), and dynorphin (59%) output (39). Similar co-localization was detected in the substantia nigra. In the striatum, the 5-ht$_6$ transcripts are homogeneously distributed between the patch and matrix components as well as between cells projecting to the two major outflow pathways.

The distribution of the human 5-ht$_6$ mRNA has been evaluated by Northern blot analysis (8). It parallels the distribution shown in the rat brain, with the highest expression levels detected in the caudate. In the human brain, lower expression levels of 5-ht$_6$ mRNA were found in the hippocampus, amygdala, and thalamus.

Localization of the 5-ht$_6$ Receptor Protein

Immunohistochemistry   The pattern of protein expression for the 5-ht$_6$ receptor has been determined using selective antibodies to a carboxyl-terminal domain of the receptor sequence (27). Receptor protein was abundant in the plexiform layer of the olfactory tubercle and in the frontal and entorhinal corticies, nucleus accumbens, striatum, hippocampus (striata oriens and radiatum of CA1 and molecular layer of the dentate gyrus), and molecular layer of the cerebellum. A moderate degree of immunoreactivity was found in the thalamus, the substantia nigra, the superficial layer of the superior colliculus, the motor trigeminal nucleus, and the facial nucleus (27). This pattern is consistent with that seen from determination of the mRNA distribution, indicating that the protein is close to the site of synthesis, as in dendrites or somata. Dendritic localization in the striatum and dentate gyrus has been visualized by immuno-electronmicroscopy. The strong distribution of the receptor protein in the extrapyramidal and limbic areas led to the suggestion that the 5-ht$_6$ receptor may control motor function and mood-dependent behaviors. Gerard et al (27) further suggested that the 5-ht$_6$ receptors may be on the target cells of dopaminergic neurons (but see below), which might explain part of the antipsychotic activity of clozapine.

Autoradiography   Radioligand binding is an alternative to immunohistochemistry to map receptor protein in the rat brain. The first experiment used [^{3}H]clozapine as a label for 5-ht$_6$ receptors in membranes (40). Forty percent of the sites that Glatt et al (40) detected exhibited a 5-ht$_6$ profile. There were no differences in the density of these sites between cerebral cortex, striatum, and hippocampus. The [^{3}H]clozapine binding is consistent with data from in situ hybridization studies. Future studies using [^{3}H]clozapine for receptor autoradiography could provide a detailed map of 5-ht$_6$ receptors. Methiothepin is a ligand that has even higher affinity for the 5-ht$_6$ receptor. It has previously been radiolabeled with tritium, but it has not been found to be a suitable radioligand in the brain (41), as a result of its physico-chemical properties (e.g. lipophilicity) and poor receptor subtype selectivity.

Recently, a new radioligand, [^{125}I]SB-258582, has been introduced that is selective for the cloned 5-ht$_6$ receptor (35). Subsequent studies (37) indicate that there is high specific binding in native tissues and that this ligand is useful for autoradiographic mapping studies. In rat, high densities of sites were found in the cerebral cortex, nucleus accumbens, caudate-putamen, and CA1 and dentate gyrus of the hippocampus. A moderate density of labeling was detected in the thalamus and substantia nigra. Furthermore, after lesioning with 6-hydroxydopamine (6-OHDA) to the median forebrain bundle, no changes in the levels of binding were found, although there was a complete loss of tyrosine hydroxylase immunoreactivity in the striatum and nigra. This indicates that the 5-ht_6 receptors may be on cholinergic or GABAergic interneurons in the caudate putamen or on striatal GABAergic neurons or on their terminal fields in the nigra.

c-fos Activation   Neuronal activation had been monitored using antibodies to the immediate early gene c-fos after drug treatment. Typical and atypical antipsychotic compounds give characteristic distribution patterns of c-fos activation (42, 43). The high affinity of antipsychotic compounds at the 5-ht_6 receptor implies that part of their actions may be due to their action on this receptor. The selective 5-ht_6 antagonist SB-271046 was administered to rats for four days, and the brains were processed for c-fos immunoreactivity (44). Rats treated with clozapine or haloperidol were run in parallel for comparison. Clozapine enhanced c-fos levels in the median prefrontal cortex and nucleus accumbens, and haloperidol enhanced levels in the caudate putamen and nucleus accumbens. No enhancement was seen in the SB-271046–treatment group (although the caudate putamen was not examined). These data indicate that activity of clozapine as monitored in this assay is not primarily the result of its action at the 5-ht_6 receptor.

FUNCTIONS OF THE 5-HT_6 RECEPTOR

Cellular Responses

There are several early reports of "atypical" 5-HT receptors in cells lines, particularly NCB.20 cells. This cell line was created by fusing a mouse neuroblastoma line, N18TG2, and an embryonic hamster brain explant (45). In this cell line, 5-HT, 5-MeOT, and methysergide all stimulated cAMP production. Clozapine and spiperone were antagonists. This response was reinvestigated using the newer tools for characterization (46, 47). cAMP stimulation was inhibited by metergoline ($K_b = 50$ nM), but not by ICS 205–930 (47), consistent with a 5-ht_6 but not a 5-HT_4 or 5-HT_7 response profile. The parental mouse cell line (N18TG2) was also evaluated (17). 5-HT stimulates cAMP responses with a pharmacological profile similar to that of the cloned 5-ht_6 receptor. The rank order of agonist potency in both radioligand binding and second messenger assays was 5-MeOT > 5-HT > tryptamine > 2-Me-5-HT >> 5-CT > α-Me-5-HT. In binding assays methiothepin showed higher affinity than clozapine, while in second-messenger assays the antagonists methiothepin, clozapine, and mianserin exhibited similar potencies ($pA_2 = 6.5$). A molecular analysis of the N18TG2 cell line to evaluate the presence of mRNA for 5-HT receptor subtypes has not been reported.

In primary neurons, stimulatory AC responses mediated via a 5-ht$_6$–like receptor have also been described (48). In cultured mouse striatal neurons, the rank order of agonist potencies to stimulate cAMP production was 5-HT > LSD > 5-MeOT > 5-CT. The serotoninergic agonists 8-OH-DPAT, sumatriptan, and cisapride were inactive. This response was antagonized by methiothepin, nortriptyline, clozapine, and amitriptyline. In combination with high distribution of mRNA in the striatum, this pharmacological profile indicates that these were 5-ht$_6$ responses in native neurons.

Furthermore, mRNA for 5-ht$_6$ receptors has been detected in an immortalized serotoninergic cell line from rat raphe nuclei (49). This may serve as an interesting model system for future studies of 5-ht$_6$ receptor regulation in a neuronal context.

TISSUE RESPONSES

Potential functional correlates of 5-ht$_6$ receptors have also been observed in vitro (50). A study of glycogenesis in tissue slices from rat cortex may reflect a 5-ht$_6$–like profile. In this preparation, 5-HT, 5-MeOT, and tryptamine stimulated glycogen hydrolysis. Tricyclic antidepressants were among the most potent competitive antagonists of the response. Methiothepin was weaker than expected for a 5-ht$_6$ response in antagonizing the glycogen hydrolysis response; physicochemical properties of the compound may have limited its efficacy. N,N-dimethyltryptamine (N,N-DMT) also antagonized this response, but its efficacy was greater than methiothepin. At the human 5-ht$_6$ receptor, N,N-DMT was equipotent with 5-HT (pK$_i$ = 7.2).

In pig caudate membranes (51), a rank order of agonist potencies similar to that determined for 5-ht$_6$ was observed: 5-HT = 5-MeOT > 5-CT. The agonists 8-OH-DPAT, sumatriptan, and renzapride were inactive. The antagonist rank order was methiothepin > clozapine >> ketanserin. Neither of these receptor profiles derived from striatal preparations exactly matches the rank order of potencies in the N18TG2 cell line or the rank order of binding affinities from the cloned rat receptor. However, cross species comparisons or methodological differences may obscure the true relationships.

Electrophysiology

At present, there are no available reports of electrophysiological studies on the 5-ht$_6$ receptor.

IN VIVO STUDIES OF 5-HT$_6$ RECEPTOR FUNCTION

Molecular Approaches to Function In Vivo

Antisense Oligonucleotides   The first behavioral studies of possible 5-ht$_6$–mediated function have been attempted using antisense oligonucleotides (AOs) targeted to the 5-ht$_6$ receptor subtype (52). In these studies, the rats exhibited a behavioral phenotype consisting of an increased number of yawns and stretches. This behavior was blocked by atropine, suggesting a role of the 5-ht$_6$ receptor in the control of cholinergic neurotransmission. If so, then a 5-ht$_6$ antagonist might be useful in the treatment of depression, anxiety, and/or memory disorders (52).

Using a similar approach, Yoshioka and colleagues (53) evaluated the effect of AOs in a conditioned fear stress paradigm (CFS). After seven days of AO administration to the lateral ventricle, the 5-ht$_6$ receptor number decreased by 30%. In these animals, but not the sense oligonucleotide controls, the CFS-induced 5-HT release was suppressed, although freezing behavior was unaffected. This result suggests a potential role for the 5-ht$_6$ receptor in some forms of anxiety.

Finally, a preliminary report has appeared linking the 5-ht$_6$ receptor to memory acquisition and feeding (54). Again using AOs applied i.c.v., rats were treated for six days and evaluated in the Morris water maze test. AO-treated rats had no differences in visual acuity or swim speed, but they had a shorter average latency and longer time spent on the learned platform than controls. In addition, they had a lower body weight. Confirmation of these fascinating results is awaited.

Knockout Mice   Targeted gene disruption has served as a useful probe for receptor function (55). A constitutive knockout animal lacking functional 5-ht$_6$ receptors has been produced and evaluated in several tests. At present, the only detectable difference from the wild-type animals has been an increase in anxiety-like behavior in the elevated zero maze (56). Additional studies are required to fully probe the changes in behavior and physiology in this knockout mouse.

Selective Antagonist Studies of 5-ht$_6$ Receptor Function

The selective 5-ht$_6$ receptor antagonist Ro 04–6790 was administered to rats by systemic injection. The compound induced a behavioral syndrome that included a dose-dependent increase in yawning, stretching, and chewing and was similar to that seen with the antisense treatment (32). The maximal effect was obtained at a dose that gave a cerebrospinal fluid concentration sufficient to occupy more than 70% of the 5-ht$_6$ receptors. Further exploration of this syndrome revealed that the stretching component was dose dependent and statistically significant (57). Pretreatment with muscarinic antagonists inhibited the stretching induced by Ro 04–6790. A non-CNS penetrant muscarinic antagonist was unable to inhibit the behavior, indicating a central mechanism. In addition, haloperidol had no effect. As with the antisense treatment, the 5-ht$_6$ antagonists produced a stretching behavior that is likely to be mediated by an increase in cholinergic, but not dopaminergic, neurotransmission. In contrast, the yawning was neither dose dependent nor statistically significant. This was in contrast to the effect of AO treatment on yawning. A number of explanations are possible, but further studies are required to evaluate them.

The distribution and pharmacology of the 5-ht$_6$ receptor suggest a link with dopaminergic function. mRNA for the 5-ht$_6$ receptor is preferentially down-regulated in rats in certain brain regions after a two-week treatment with clozapine or haloperidol (58). Bourson and colleagues (59) investigated the effects of Ro 04–6790 on dopaminergic function. Ro 04–6790 did not induce catalepsy and had no effect on haloperidol or SCH 23390–induced catalepsy. It did not elicit rotational behavior in rat with unilaterally lesion of the median forebrain bundle induced by 6-OHDA. Ro 04–6790 had no effect on L-Dopa or amphetamine-induced rotational behavior. In contrast, antagonism of the 5-ht$_6$ receptor inhibited rotational behavior in the lesioned rats in response to cholinergic antagonists such as scopolamine and atropine. Therefore, consistent with previous reports using oligonucleotides, 5-ht$_6$ receptors are involved in cholinergic but not dopaminergic neurotransmission.

Using a second and more highly brain penetrant 5-ht$_6$ antagonist, Routledge et al (60) demonstrated that SB-271046 significantly potentiated physostigmine-induced yawning. It was also tested in two models of cognition enhancement (61). SB-271046 improved retention in the water maze test of spatial learning and memory. The compound also produced a significant improvement in performance of aged rats in an operant-delayed alternation task. These results all suggest that the 5-ht$_6$ receptor is implicated in the control of central cholinergic function and may be an interesting avenue for the treatment of cholinergic defects in cognitive dysfunctions such as Alzheimer's disease. Taken in the context of the 6-OHDA lesioning studies along with autoradiography, functional 5-ht$_6$ receptors may be on cholinergic or GABAergic interneurons in the caudate putamen or on striatal GABAergic neurons or their terminal fields in the nigra. This distribution is consistent with the proposal that 5-ht$_6$ receptors may regulate motor function and control memory and mood (37).

POTENTIAL THERAPEUTIC INDICATIONS FOR 5-HT$_6$ RECEPTORS

The distribution of the 5-ht$_6$ receptor, as well as its affinity for antipsychotic compounds, has led to significant efforts to understand its possible role in psychiatry. Mapping and lesioning studies so far indicate that there is no direct involvement of 5-ht$_6$ receptors in dopaminergic neurotransmission. However, two genetic association studies have been recently reported with respect to the 5-ht$_6$ receptor gene. The first looked at association between the 5-ht$_6$ receptor gene and schizophrenia (62) in a Japanese population. Three hundred subjects were genotyped for the biallelic variation (267C/T); half were schizophrenic and half were healthy controls. No significant difference in allele frequencies was detected between the schizophrenic patients and the healthy controls. This suggested that the 5-ht$_6$ receptor gene may not contribute directly to schizophrenia. However, a second study evaluated the relationship between the C267T polymorphism and the clinical response of schizophrenic patients, who were refractory to typical antipsychotics and to the atypical antipsychotic compound clozapine (63). Ninety-nine chlorpromazine-resistant patients of the same ethnic Chinese background were genotyped and their response to clozapine after a minimum of eight weeks was determined. The distribution of the three possible genotypes was in Hardy-Weinberg distribution. There were no differences in baseline scores. In 60.6% of patients, the Brief Psychiatric Rating Score (BPRS) decreased by over 20% from baseline after clozapine treatment. Patients with the 267T/T genotype had a significantly better response to clozapine than the other two groups. Although the group size was small, the results were significant. The changes in general symptoms were also close to significance. This parameter reflects somatic concern, anxiety, guilt, tension, and depressed mood, i.e. the emotional control systems. These results are particularly interesting since C267T is a silent mutation that does not change the amino acid sequence. It may, however, affect parameters such as RNA stability or translational efficiency. Although a larger study is needed to confirm these observations, they may suggest that the 5-ht$_6$ genotype may help predict patients' responses to clozapine.

A surprising outcome of the antisense studies, confirmed by the antagonist experiments, is the role of 5-ht$_6$ receptors in the control of central cholinergic function (59, 61). This is also supported by localization and lesion studies. Although the antagonist data have appeared in preliminary form only, it is exciting that the 5-ht$_6$ antagonists may have a role in the treatment of cognitive dysfunction. Other possible avenues presently under investigation are the link to depression and anxiety (53) and the effect on body weight (54). As the new pharmacological tools become more widely available, the larger picture of 5-ht$_6$ receptor function will be sketched.

ACKNOWLEDGMENTS

The authors would like to thank Mary Johnson for her expert assistance in preparing the manuscript.

Visit the Annual Reviews home page at www.AnnualReviews.org.

LITERATURE CITED

1. Erspamer V. 1966. 5-Hydroxytryptamine and related indolealkylamines. In *Handbook of Experimental Pharmacology,* ed. V Erspamer, 19:132–81. New York: Springer-Verlag
2. Gaddum JH, Picarelli ZP. 1957. Two kinds of tryptamine receptor. *Br. J. Pharm. Chemother.* 12:323–28
3. Peroutka SJ, Snyder SH. 1979. Multiple serotonin receptors: differential binding of ^{3}H 5-hydroxytryptamine, ^{3}H lysergic acid diethylamide and ^{3}H spiroperidol. *Mol. Pharmacol.* 16:687–99
4. Fargin A, Raymond JR, Lohse MJ, Kobilka BK, Caron MC, Lefkowitz RJ. 1988. The genomic clone G-21 which resembles a β-adrenergic receptor sequence encodes the 5-HT$_{1A}$ receptor. *Nature* 335:358–60
5. Hartig PR. 1997. Molecular biology and

transductional characteristics of 5-HT Receptors. In *Handbook of Experimental Pharmacology,* ed. HG Baumgarten, M Göthert, 129:175–212. Berlin: Springer-Verlag

6. Monsma FJ Jr, Shen Y, Ward RP, Hamblin MW, Sibley DR. 1993. Cloning and expression of a novel serotonin receptor with high affinity for tricyclic psychotropic drugs. *Mol. Pharmacol.* 43:320–27

7. Ruat M, Traiffort E, Arrang J-M, Tardivel-Lacombe J, Diaz J, et al. 1993. A novel rat serotonin (5-HT$_6$) receptor: molecular cloning, localization, and stimulation of cAMP accumulation. *Biochem. Biophys. Res. Commun.* 193:268–76

8. Kohen R, Metcalf MA, Khan N, Druck T, Huebner K, et al. 1996. Cloning, characterization, and chromosomal localization of a human 5-HT6 serotonin receptor. *J. Neurochem.* 66:47–56

9. Lefkowitz RJ, Caron MG. 1988. Adrenergic receptors. Models for the study of receptors coupled to guanine nucleotide regulatory proteins. *J. Biol. Chem.* 263:4993–96

10. Witz P, Amlaiky N, Plassat JL, Maroteaux L, Borrelli E, Hen R. 1990. Cloning and characterization of a Drosophila serotonin receptor that activates adenylate cyclase. *Proc. Natl. Acad. Sci. USA* 87:8940–44

11. Ruat M, Leurs R, Schartz JC, Traiffort E, Arrang JM. 1991. Cloning and tissue expression of a rat histamine H2-receptor gene. *Biochem. Biophys. Res. Commun.* 179:1470–78

12. Hamblin MW, Guthrie CR, Kohen R, Heidmann DE. 1998. Gs protein-coupled serotonin receptors: receptor isoforms and functional differences. *Ann. NY Acad. Sci.* 861:31–37

13. Olsen MA, Nawoschik SP, Schurman BR, Schmitt HL, Burno M, et al. 1999. Identification of a human 5-HT6 receptor variant produced by alternative splicing. *Brain Res. Mol. Brain Res.* 64:255–63

14. Roth BL, Craigo SC, Choudray MS, Uluer A, Monsma FJ Jr, et al. 1994. Binding of typical and atypical antipsychotic agents to 5-hydroxytryptamine-6 and 5-hydroxytryptamine-7 receptor. *J. Pharmacol. Exp. Ther.* 268:1403–10

15. Boess FG, Monsma FJJ, Carolo C, Meyer V, Rudler A, et al. 1997. Functional and radioligand binding characterization of rat 5-HT6 receptors stably expressed in HEK293 cells. *Neuropharmacology* 36:713–20

16. Volonte M, Monferini E, Cerutti M, Fodritto F, Borsini F. 1997. BIMG 80, a novel potential antipsychotic drug: evidence for multireceptor actions and preferential release of dopamine in prefrontal cortex. *J. Neurochem.* 69:182–90

17. Unsworth CD, Molinoff PB. 1994. Characterization of a 5-hydroxytryptamine receptor in mouse neuroblastoma N18TG2 cells. *J. Pharmacol. Exp. Ther.* 269:246–55

18. Zgombick JM, Butkerait P, Raddatz R, Peters J, Pu X, Branchek TA. 1998. Functional characterization of the recombinant human 5-HT$_6$ receptor coupled to elevations of intracellular cAMP: modulation by 5-HT and PMA. *IUPHAR Satellite Meet. on Serotonin, 4th, Rotterdam.* Abstr. PP86

19. Baker LP, Nielsen MD, Impey S, Metcalf MA, Poser SW, et al. 1998. Stimulation of type 1 and type 8 Ca2 +/calmodulin-sensitive adenylyl cyclases by the Gs-coupled 5-hydroxytryptamine subtype 5-HT7A receptor. *J. Biol. Chem.* 273:17469–76

20. Strader C, Candelore M, Hill W, Sigal I, Dixon R. 1989. Identification of two serine residues involved in agonist activation of the β-adrenergic receptor. *J. Biol. Chem.* 264:13572–78

21. Cox B, Henningsen A, Spanoyannis A, Neve R, Neve K. 1992. Contributions of conserved serine residues to the interactions of ligands with dopamine D$_2$ receptors. *J. Neurochem.* 59:627–35

22. Kao H-T, Adham N, Olsen MA, Wein-

shank RL, Branchek TA, Hartig PR. 1992. Site-directed mutagenesis of a single residue changes the binding properties of the serotonin 5-HT$_2$ receptor from a human to a rat pharmacology. *FEBS Lett.* 307:324–28

23. Johnson MP, Loncharich RJ, Baez M, Nelson DL. 1994. Species variations in transmembrane region V of the 5-hydroxytryptamine type 2A receptor alter the structure-activity relationship of certain ergolines and tryptamines. *Mol. Pharmacol.* 45:277–86

24. Boess FG, Monsma FJJ, Meyer V, Zwingelstein C, Sleight AJ. 1997. Interaction of tryptamine and ergoline compounds with threonine 196 in the ligand binding site of the 5-hydroxytryptamine$_6$ receptor. *Mol. Pharmacol.* 52:515–23

25. Boess FG, Monsma FJJ, Sleight AJ. 1998. Identification of residues in transmembrane regions III and VI that contribute to the ligand binding site of the serotonin 5-HT6 receptor. *J. Neurochem.* 71:2169–77

26. Boess FG, Monsma FJJ, Bourson A, Zwingelstein C, Sleight AJ. 1998. Residues in transmembrane regions III and VI contribute to the 5-ht6 receptor ligand binding site. *Ann. NY Acad. Sci.* 861:242–43

27. Gerard C, Martres MP, Lefevre K, Miquel MC, Verge D, et al. 1997. Immuno-localization of serotonin 5-HT6 receptor-like material in the rat central nervous system. *Brain Res.* 746:207–19

28. Martin JB, Reichlin S, Brown GM. 1977. *Clinical Neuroendocrinology.* Philadelphia: Davis

29. Yau JL, Noble J, Widdowson J, Seckl JR. 1997. Impact of adrenalectomy on 5-HT6 and 5-HT7 receptor gene expression in the rat hippocampus. *Brain Res. Mol. Brain Res.* 45:182–86

30. Grimaldi B, Bonnin A, Fillion MP, Ruat M, Traiffort E, Fillion G. 1998. Characterization of 5-ht6 receptor and expression of 5-ht6 mRNA in the rat brain

during ontogenetic development. *Naunyn Schmiedebergs Arch. Pharmacol.* 357:393–400

31. Glennon RA, Bondarev M, Roth BL. 1999. 5-HT$_6$ serotonin receptor binding of indolealkylamines: a preliminary structure-affinity investigation. *Med. Chem. Res.* 9:108–17

32. Sleight AJ, Boess FG, Bos M, Levet-Trafit B, Riemer C, Bourson A. 1998. Characterization of Ro 04–6790 and Ro 63–0563: potent and selective antagonists at human and rat 5-HT$_6$ receptors. *Br. J. Pharmacol.* 124:556–62

33. Boess FG, Riemer C, Bos M, Bentley J, Bourson A, Sleight AJ. 1998. The 5-hydroxytryptamine$_6$ receptor-selective radioligand [^{3}H]Ro 63–0563 labels 5-hydroxytryptamine receptor binding sites in rat and porcine striatum. *Mol. Pharmacol.* 54:577–83

34. Bromidge SM, Brown AM, Clarke SE, Dodgson K, Gager T, et al. 1999. 5-Chloro-N-(4-methoxy-3-piperazin-1-yl-phenyl)-3-methyl-2-benzothiophene-sulfonamide (SB-271046): a potent, selective, and orally bioavailable 5-HT$_6$ receptor antagonist. *J. Med. Chem.* 42:202–5

35. Hirst WD, Minton JAL, Bromidge SM, Routledge C, Middlemiss DN, Price GW. 1999. [^{125}I]SB-258585—A selective antagonist radioligand for 5-HT$_6$ receptors. *Br. J. Pharmacol. Suppl.* In press

36. Minton JAL, Hirst WD, Bromidge SM, Routledge C, Middlemiss DN, Price GW. 1999. Characterisation of [^{125}I]SB-258585 binding to 5-ht$_6$ receptors in native tissues. *BPS Meet., Nottingham.* Abstr. P111

37. Roberts JC, Hirst WD, Reavill C, Patel S, Routledge C, Leslie RA. 1999. Autoradiographic localisation of the 5-HT$_6$ receptor in the CNS of the rat using [125I]SB-258585. *BPS Meet., Nottingham.* Abstr. P110

38. Ward RP, Hamblin MW, Lachowicz JE,

Hoffman BJ, Sibley DR, Dorsa DM. 1995. Localization of serotonin subtype 6 receptor messenger RNA in the rat brain by *in situ* hybridization histochemistry. *Neuroscience* 64:1105–11

39. Ward RP, Dorsa DM. 1996. Colocalization of serotonin receptor subtypes 5-HT2A, 5-HT2C, and 5-HT6 with neuropeptides in rat striatum. *J. Comp. Neurol.* 370:405–14

40. Glatt CE, Snowman A, Sibley DR, Snyder SH. 1995. Clozapine: selective labeling of sites resembling 5-HT$_6$ serotonin receptors. *Mol. Med.* 1:398–406

41. Nelson DL, Herbet A, Pichat L, Glowinski J, Hamon M. 1997. *In vitro* and *in vivo* disposition of ^{3}H-methiothepin in brain tissues: relationship to the effects of acute treatment with methiothepin on central serotonergic receptors. *Naunyn Schmiedebergs Arch. Pharmacol.* 310:25–33

42. Robertson GS, Fibiger HC. 1996. Effects of olanzapine on regional c-fos expression in rat forebrain. *Neuropsychopharmacology* 14:105–10

43. Arnt J, Skarsfeldt T. 1998. Do novel antipsychotics have similar pharmacological characteristics? A review of the evidence. *Neuropsychopharmacology* 18:63–101

44. Ireland MD, Cilia J, Jones DNC, Routledge C, Leslie RA. 1999. C-fos expression patterns induced in the rat brain by clozapine, haloperidol and the selective 5-HT$_6$ receptor antagonist SB-271046. *BPS Meet., Nottingham.* Abstr. P113

45. Berry-Kravis E, Dawson G. 1983. Characterization of an adenylate cyclase-linked serotonin (5-HT$_1$) receptor in a neuroblastoma x brain explant hybrid cell line (NCB-20). *J. Neurochem.* 40:977–85

46. Connor DA, Mansour TE. 1990. Serotonin receptor-mediated activation of adenylate cyclase in the neuroblastoma NCB.20: a novel 5-hydroxytryptamine receptor. *Mol. Pharmacol.* 37:742–51

47. Cossery JM, Mienville J-M, Sheehy PA, Mellow AM, Chuang D-M. 1990. Characterization of two distinct 5-HT receptors coupled to adenylate cyclase activation and ion current generation in NCB-20 cells. *Neurosci. Lett.* 108:149–54

48. Sebben M, Ansanay H, Bockaert J, Dumuis A. 1994. 5-HT$_6$ receptors positively coupled to adenylyl cyclase in striatal neurones in culture. *NeuroReport* 5:2553–57

49. Jackson ZE, Stringer BM, Foster GA. 1997. Identification of 5-HT receptor sub-types in a homogeneous population of presumptive serotoninergic neurones. *Neuropharmacology* 36:543–48

50. Quach TT, Rose C, Duchemin AM, Schartz JC. 1982. Glycogenolysis induced by serotonin in brain: identification of a new class of receptor. *Nature* 298:373–75

51. Schoeffter P, Waeber C. 1994. 5-Hydroxytryptamine receptors with a 5-HT$_6$ receptor-like profile stimulating adenylyl cyclase activity in pig caudate membranes. *Naunyn Schmiedebergs Arch. Pharmacol.* 350:356–60

52. Bourson A, Boroni E, Austin RH, Monsma FJ Jr, Sleight AJ. 1995. Determination of the role of the 5-ht$_6$ receptor in rat brain: a study using antisense oligonucleotides. *J. Pharmacol. Exp. Ther.* 274:173–80

53. Yoshioka M, Matsumoto M, Togashi H, Mori K. 1998. Central distribution and function of 5-ht$_6$ receptor subtype in the rat brain. *Ann. NY Acad. Sci.* 861:244

54. Bentley JC, Sleight AJ, Marsden CA, Fone KC. 1997. 5-HT6 antisense oligonucleotides i.c.v. affects rat performance in the water maze and feeding. *J. Psychopharmacol.* 11:864

55. Murphy DL, Wichems C, Li Q, Heils A. 1999. Molecular manipulations as tools for enhancing our understanding of 5-HT neurotransmission. *Trends. Pharmacol. Sci.* 20:246–52

56. Tecott LH, Chu H-M, Brennan TJ. 1998.

Neurobehavioral analysis of 5-HT$_6$ receptor null mutant mice. *IUPHAR Satellite Meet. on Serotonin, 4th, Rotterdam.* Abstr. S1.2

57. Bentley JC, Bourson A, Boess FG, Fone KCF, Marsden CA, et al. 1999. Investigation of stretching behaviour induced by the selective 5-HT$_6$ receptor antagonist, Ro 04–6790, in rats. *Br. J. Pharmacol.* 126:1537–42

58. Frederick JA, Lopez JF, Meador-Woodruff JH. 1995. Effects of clozapine and haloperidol on expression of 5-HT$_6$ and 5-HT$_7$ receptors. *Soc. Neurosci. Abstr.* 21:1857

59. Bourson A, Boess FG, Bos M, Sleight AJ. 1998. Involvement of 5-HT6 receptors in nigro-striatal function in rodents. *Br. J. Pharmacol.* 125:1562–66

60. Routledge C, Bromidge SM, Moss SF, Newman H, Riley G, et al. 1999. Characterisation of SB-271046: a potent and selective 5-HT6 receptor antagonist. *Br. J. Pharmacol. Suppl.* 127:21P

61. Rogers DC, Robinson CA, Quilter AJ, Hunter C, Routledge C, Hagan JJ. 1999. Cognitive enhancement effects of the selective 5-HT6 antagonist SB-271046. *Br. J. Pharmacol. Suppl.* 127:22P

62. Shinkai T, Ohmori O, Kojima H, Terao T, Suzuki T, Abe K. 1999. Association study of the 5-HT6 receptor gene in schizophrenia. *Am. J. Med. Genet.* 88:120–22

63. Yu YWY, Tsai S-J, Lin C-H, Hsu C-P, Yang K-H, Hong C-J. 1999. Serotonin-6 receptor variant (C267T) and clinical response to clozapine. *NeuroReport* 10:1231–33

Annu. Rev. Pharmacol. Toxicol. 2000. 40:335–52

THE IMPACT OF GENOMICS-BASED TECHNOLOGIES ON DRUG SAFETY EVALUATION

Jeffrey F. Waring and Roger G. Ulrich

Strategic and Exploratory Sciences, Abbott Laboratories, Abbott Park, Illinois 60064–6123; e-mail: jeff.waring@abbott.com, roger.ulrich@abbott.com

Key Words molecular toxicology, microarrays, high throughput, real-time PCR, drug screening

■ **Abstract** Determining the potential toxicity of compounds early in the drug discovery process can be extremely beneficial in terms of both time and money conservation. Because of the speed of modern chemical synthesis and screening, to accurately evaluate the large number of compounds being produced, toxicology assays must have both high-fidelity and high-throughput capabilities. In addition, assays must be performed using limited amounts of compound. In the past decade, several new and innovative techniques have been developed that not only allow for high-throughput screening but can also provide detailed information concerning the molecular mechanisms behind toxic effects. Techniques such as hybridization microarrays, real-time polymerase chain reaction, and large-scale sequencing are some of the methods that have been or are starting to be used routinely in pharmaceutical companies. This review examines the contributions of these and related techniques toward toxicity evaluation of potential drug candidates and their future role in the discovery of new therapeutics.

INTRODUCTION

In the pharmaceutical industry, drug safety evaluation laboratories are currently charged with two distinct functions: aiding in discovery of lead selection and conducting human risk assessment. As part of the drug discovery process, assessment of toxic potential is used to select compounds that are more likely to succeed during preclinical development (lead selection and enhancement). Determining the potential liabilities of compounds early in the drug discovery process can save development time and money by focusing resources on compounds that are more likely to succeed. The success of toxicity screening in drug discovery depends both on the speed or turnaround time of evaluation and on the reliability of results. In order to keep up with high-throughput screening hits or chemical syntheses (chemists usually outnumber biologists several times over), toxicology assays must have sufficient throughput to be able to handle relatively high volumes of compounds and, hence, must be of relatively low fidelity, usually measuring a

0362–1642/00/0415–0335$14.00 **335**

single parameter focused on a single toxicity issue. The reliability of an assay depends on the relatedness of the parameter measured to the actual mechanism of toxicity for the lead or template compound; nonspecific cell viability or lysis assays are of limited value because all chemicals will kill cells at some concentration. As with any screen for high throughput, toxicity assays must also be economical to conduct. Screening results from mechanism-based assays are generally used to prioritize compounds for subsequent examination rather than eliminate compounds from further consideration.

During drug development, toxicology is charged with determining or predicting potential adverse effects in humans (risk or safety assessment). Risk assessment is used both to establish a dose that is safe to administer to humans during clinical development and to evaluate risk due to prolonged exposure. Drug toxicity is conventionally determined by conducting animal studies and examining for changes in serum chemistry parameters and histopathology; human risk is determined by extrapolation from animal study results. Toxicity evaluation from animal studies is thorough, though fidelity decreases when comparing animal species or extrapolating results to human risk assessment. For a detailed discussion of risk assessment, see the recent review by Brecher (1). Here, too, the reliability of risk assessment depends on the relationship between the parameters measured and the actual mechanism of toxicity of the drug candidate, particularly when extrapolating to humans from animal species used in the laboratory.

Determining the mechanism of toxicity for a xenobiotic requires a diversity of investigative techniques, sufficient time, and a degree of serendipity [for a review, see Ulrich & Slatter (2)]. Although some problems can be readily solved, others may require the dedication of more resources than a company is prepared to risk. Investigative techniques can yield quite useful results, however; structure-toxicity relationships can be used to guide chemical synthesis toward less toxic analogues or problem structures can be eliminated from development. Mechanistic data can also aid in the interpretation of animal toxicology findings and help clarify their significance in human risk assessment. However, most mechanistic toxicology is conducted retrospectively in an attempt to salvage a discovery program or clinical candidate. A more useful approach would be to generate mechanistic data early so as to predict animal and human toxicities prior to conducting expensive developmental studies. This is the challenge currently faced by toxicologists and it is formidable. In order to meet the demands of drug discovery teams, toxicity assessment must be rapid, accurate, and modest in terms of drug requirements (usually <100 mg, though for particularly interesting compounds a chemist can generally synthesize gram quantities). For high-throughput toxicology screening, assays must also be simple in design and even more compound sparing (<1 mg). The application of genomics-associated tools to toxicity or safety assessment holds the promise of meeting these demands.

The past decade has seen an explosion in the number and variety of techniques available for molecular analysis of toxicological effects, and the emphasis has begun to sway toward molecular toxicology as an early assessment of chemical effects. These techniques focus on determining changes in gene expression at the level of transcription. This article reviews several of these techniques and their current application in toxicity assessment, including differential display, subtractive hybridization, serial analysis of gene expression (SAGE), hybridization microarrays, real-time polymerase chain reaction (PCR), scintillation proximity, and branched-DNA (bDNA) signal amplification. These techniques can be roughly divided into two categories: high-fidelity, low-throughput techniques and low-fidelity, high-throughput techniques (see Figure 1). Large-scale hybridization techniques such as microarrays and sequencing techniques such as SAGE produce a detailed picture of gene responses that can bridge the entire expressed genome.

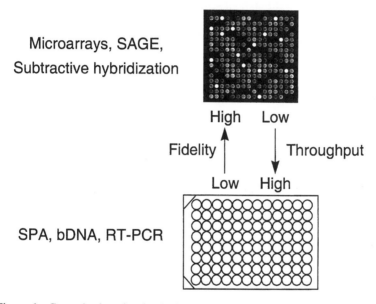

Figure 1 Genomics-based technologies that have an application in toxicity assessment. Microarrays, serial analysis of gene expression (SAGE), or subtractive hybridization can be used to comprehensively characterize or "fingerprint" responses. These techniques are of high fidelity in that they generate a considerably detailed image of a response to a particular compound. Because of the amount of information generated, the amount of mRNA required, the number of steps involved, and the costs, these techniques are not high throughput but can be used to identify specific markers to be used in other assay formats. Scintillation proximity (SPA), branched-DNA (bDNA), and real-time polymerase chain reaction (RT-PCR) assays are used to follow responses in one or a few genes and can be constructed as high-throughput screens using cultured cells. A toxicology screening assay using one of these techniques is low in fidelity, however, because only a single parameter is evaluated compared with the large number of possible responses. Hence, a degree of caution must be used when extrapolating from results because the accuracy and reliability of these assays decreases even further when they are applied outside of a chemical analogue series or to a different species.

Microarrays in particular have generated a lot of excitement in toxicology because it is now possible to generate a comprehensive image of cell and tissue responses to a compound without the time and labor investment or subjectivity of traditional analyses such as histopathology. This new capability has been the subject of several recent reviews and perspectives (3–7). However, these techniques are expensive and require a relatively large amount of mRNA (much more than can be generated from a 96-well plate) and, hence, are most appropriate for individual compound studies rather than for screening of chemical libraries. Real-time PCR, scintillation proximity, and branched-DNA technologies are designed to follow single endpoints (changes in expression levels for an individual gene), or small sets of endpoints, and require small amounts of mRNA. These assays can be automated for high-throughput screening of compound sets.

DIFFERENTIAL DISPLAY

Differential display was developed by Liang & Pardee (8) and has been modified several times since its inception. RNA is isolated from two different cell populations and then subjected to reverse transcription using four different sets of oligo(dT) primers. The oligo(dT) primers have the sequence T_NAB, where N represents the number of thymidines in the primer, usually 10 or 12; A can be guanine, adenine, or cytosine and B can be guanine, adenine, cytosine, or thymidine. The resulting cDNA is then amplified using the same oligo(dT) primer and a random primer at the 5' end. The amplified PCR products represent different subpopulations, which are defined by the oligo(dT) primer, and they should represent most of the mRNA species in a cell. The PCR products from two or more different cell populations are then run on a denaturing polyacrylamide gel, and differentially expressed RNA samples can be identified, isolated, and amplified.

For analyzing gene responses during toxic reactions, differential display has several advantages over other high-throughput techniques. One strength is that mRNA samples from several cells can be analyzed at the same time; this is not possible with other techniques, such as subtractive hybridization. In addition, differential display has the ability to identify previously unknown genes that may be regulated during a toxic response, which is not possible using hybridization microarray assays.

Differential display has been used by several researchers to identify genes whose expression is regulated by certain toxins. One toxin that has been studied fairly extensively using differential display is TCDD (2,3,7,8-tetrachlorodibenzo-*p*-dioxin). For example, Wang et al (9) treated Hep G2 cells with TCDD for 24 h and then analyzed gene expression changes using differential display. Using this method, four clones were isolated that were shown to be regulated by TCDD treatment. Two of the clones were fibrinogen and plastin, both of which were down-regulated with TCDD treatment. The other two clones were induced with TCDD treatment and their sequences did not match with any known genes in the database (9). Fibrinogen is important for the formation of fibrin clots, which suggests that TCDD may play a role in hemostasis, whereas plastin may indicate a role for TCDD in tumorigenesis. Significantly, neither fibrinogen or plastin was previously known to be regulated by TCDD, demonstrating how techniques such as differential display can reveal dimensions that could not be predicted by other standard methods. In 1996, Selmin et al (10) used differential display with total liver mRNA from rats that had been treated with acute or chronic levels of TCDD. Approximately 30 potential responsive genes were isolated. Of these 30 genes, 13 were shown to be not regulated by TCDD, indicating that the method can have a high rate of false positives. However, Selmin et al (10) did isolate a novel gene that was consistently up-regulated in response to both chronic and acute TCDD treatment and that was shown to be related by amino acid sequence to the interleukin (IL)-6 receptor. Other researchers have also used differential display to examine TCDD-induced gene expression changes in rat prostate (11) and in mouse lung (12). In both of these cases, genes were identified that were not previously known to be regulated by TCDD.

Differential display has been used to identify genes regulated by other known toxins as well. The results from Muhlenkamp & Gill (13) show how methods such as differential display can identify different molecular mechanisms of compounds that seem to have the same phenotypic effect. Both clofibrate and diethylhexylphthalate (DEHP) are known peroxisomal proliferators (14). Differential display showed that the gene GRP58, a carnitine palmitoyl transferase, is down-regulated by DEHP. Subsequent work showed that clofibrate also can down-regulate GRP58, but to a much smaller extent than DEHP, indicating that although these two compounds both cause peroxisomal proliferation, they may do so by different mechanisms (13). In a different study, Ye et al (15) used differential display to identify another gene regulated by DEHP, cytochrome 450 *Cyp2f2*, a naphthalene hydroxylase (15). Other investigators have used differential display to study the genetic changes induced by chloroform (16), phenobarbitol (6), and liver regeneration (17). In all these cases, genes were identified that were not previously known to be regulated by these agents.

SUBTRACTIVE HYBRIDIZATION

Subtractive hybridization is another high-throughput technique that allows one to isolate and clone mRNA species unique to a cell population. Its main advantage over differential display is that generally it yields a lower number of false positives. However, it can only compare two populations at a time. There are different methods of subtractive hybridization; one of the most common was pioneered by Sive & St. John (18) in 1988 and modified by Wang & Brown (19) in 1991. For this method, mRNA from two different cell populations is harvested and reverse transcribed to make cDNA using oligo(dT) primers. Following this, the cDNA is digested with a restriction enzyme to make short fragments, and the two sets of cDNA samples have different adapters ligated to their ends. The samples are then amplified by PCR. One set of cDNA is designated "driver" and the other set is designated "tracer." The tracer population is radioactively labeled, and the driver population is labeled with biotin. The two populations are then denatured and hybridized to each other at a ratio of 20:1 driver to tracer. This ensures that any cDNA present in the tracer population will anneal to its complement in the driver population, if it is present. Following this, biotin-labeled cDNA species are removed by streptavidin. Any cDNA in the tracer population that is unique will not hybridize to the driver population and will not be removed by streptavidin. The hybridization steps need to be repeated several times to fully enrich for unique mRNA species (18, 19).

A study was conducted whereby primary hepatocyte cultures from male Fischer rats were treated with aflatoxin B_1, a known hepatotoxin in both rats and humans (20, 21). In order to identify genes that are regulated by aflatoxin, three different methods were used: differential display and two variations on subtractive hybridization, one called representational difference analysis (22) and the other suppression subtractive hybridization (23). It is interesting to note that the three methods all identified different genes, and no gene was identified in more than one assay. In this study, differential display had the highest rate of false positives identified, 93%, followed by representational difference analysis at 30% and lastly by suppression subtractive hybridization, which did not identify any false positives. The three methods identified several genes, such as cytochrome P450 4F1 and 3A1, transferrin, and serum amyloid A, that may shed light on molecular mechanisms underlying aflatoxin B_1 toxicity (24).

Subtractive hybridization has also been successfully used to identify genes that are involved in the molecular mechanism of toxicity caused by the neurotoxin trimethyltin (TMT). Toggas et al (25) used subtractive hybridization to isolate genes that cause some neural cells to be sensitive to TMT. They identified a gene they called *stannin*, which was expressed only in neurons sensitive to TMT (25). Subsequent work with antisense oligonucleotides directed against *stannin* strongly suggests that the expression of *stannin* is necessary for TMT toxicity (26). Chen & Safe also used subtractive hybridization to look for genes regulated by TCDD. They identified several genes, among them estradiol-induced genes that were down-regulated by TCDD (27).

HYBRIDIZATION MICROARRAYS

By far, the greatest excitement in genomics-based techniques in the past few years has been the development of microarrays. Hybridization on microarrays is a relatively new technique and has seen widespread application only in the past 2–3 years. Because of this, there are relatively few papers in peer-reviewed journals utilizing hybridization microarray techniques in toxicology. Thus, much of the work reviewed in this section has only recently been submitted for publication or is available only in abstract form. Nonetheless, the potential benefits of hybridization microarrays for the field of toxicology are enormous, and in a very short time it has become a standard method for studying the molecular mechanisms of toxicology.

Hybridization microarrays are basically an extension of techniques that have been available to molecular biologists for decades, specifically northern blotting and dot blotting assays. There are different types of hybridization microarrays, but they fall essentially into two catagories: cDNA spotted onto a solid surface, such as glass slides or nylon membranes, and oligonucleotides synthesized onto a solid surface (an example is the Affymetrix chip).

Membrane-based microarray assays are the forerunner of current hybridization microarrays. An advantage of membrane-based over other methods of hybridization microarrays is that they are reasonably affordable. Membrane filters containing numerous genes that encode for proteins involved in various aspects of cell regulation are available from several companies, including Clontech (http://www.clontech.com/), Research Genetics (http://www.resgen.com/), and Genome Systems (http://www.genomesystems.com/). The disadvantage of doing membrane-based microarray analysis is that to compare two mRNA species, one has to use duplicate filters. In addition, the cDNA is labeled with radioactivity as opposed to fluorescence, which is not as sensitive (28).

The mechanism of how the filters are made and used in microarray analysis is summarized by Cheung et al (29). A high-precision robot is used to spot hundreds to several thousands of cDNA sequences into set quadrants on two identical nylon membranes. mRNA from two different cell populations is then reverse transcribed and radioactively labeled. The two sets of radioactively labeled cDNA are then hybridized to the two filters overnight and washed, in much the same way as a southern blot is done. The blots are developed against X-ray film or a phosphoimager screen, and the two filters are compared for intensity of hybridization.

Membrane-based hybridization microarrays have been used to study the molecular mechanisms of toxicity caused by carbon tetrachloride. The human hepatoma cell line HepG2 was treated with carbon tetrachloride (CCl_4) or with dimethyl formamide (DMF), a chemical that does not cause liver damage (PR Holden, personal communication). RNA from the two populations was harvested, reverse transcribed, labeled, and hybridized to a microarray (Atlas Human cDNA expression array). The results showed that 47 genes appeared to be either up- or down-regulated by CCl_4 compared with DMF. These genes included genes involved in apoptosis, cell cycle regulation, and gene expression. Two genes were selected for further investigation. These were IL-8, which appeared to be upregulated 7.5-fold by CCl_4, and prohibitin, an antiproliferative gene that appeared to be down-regulated 5.3-fold by CCl_4. Further analysis of the gene expression by northern blot analysis could not confirm the prohibitin down-regulation; however, both northern blotting assays and ELISA assays showed that CCl_4 does up-regulate IL-8 at both the mRNA and protein levels (PR Holden, personal communication). The finding that CCl_4 regulates IL-8 expression is a novel discovery and has many implications for molecular mechanisms of CCl_4 toxicity.

Although microarray analysis using filter membranes is a useful tool, the next generation of microarray technology has the potential to provide even faster and more efficient methods of studying molecular toxicology. Microarray analysis on glass slides is similar to analysis using membrane filters, but it has several key improvements. First, the cDNA is spotted onto a glass slide coated with poly-lysine or amino silanes instead of a nitrocellulose or nylon membrane (30). This surface is less porous than nitrocellulose or nylon membranes, which enhances hybridization, washing, and visualization (31). Another advantage of hybridization microarray on a glass slide over microarray analysis on membrane filters is that the cDNA from two cell populations is labeled with fluorescent probes Cye3 or Cye5-dUTP instead of with radioactivity. This allows one to hybridize the cDNA from both populations to the same slide, which makes the comparison of the two cell populations more accurate. The glass slide is then scanned by a fluorescent scanner, which quantitates the ratio of the Cye3 to Cye5 signal (30). Companies that provide custom-made or commercially available glass slides are listed elsewhere (28).

In our laboratory, we have used hybridization microarray on glass slides to study the effects of various drugs or chemicals on mRNA regulation in cultured human hepatocytes; two examples are illustrated here. The first example is with the drug efivirenz, a reverse transcriptase inhibitor with minimal hepatic toxicity. The drug in the second example (designated CpdR) produced hepatotoxicity in rats; the mechanism is unknown. Studies in rats showed CpdR to produce significant increases in liver weight and severalfold induction in serum levels of alkaline phosphatase, alanine amino transferase, and aspartate amino transferase following 3 days of administration. Human hepatocytes from organ donor tissue were isolated by using a two-step liver perfusion method (32). Cultured cells were either vehicle treated (DMSO) or treated with noncytolytic concentrations of efivirenz or CpdR for 24 h, followed by RNA isolation. cDNA was prepared, labeled, and hybridized to the Human UniGem V chip from Incyte Pharmaceuticals. This chip contains approximately 7000 genes from the human database. Treating human hepatocytes with efivirenz caused a low number of genes to have a greater than twofold change in expression. The results are shown in Figure 2. Two of the genes that were up-regulated were cyp3A7 and aminolevulinate delta-synthase 1. Cytochrome P450 3A7 is a major fetal cytochrome P450 that is normally not expressed in adults. However, the gene sequences of cyp3A7 and cyp3A4 (the major cytochrome P450 in adults) are very similar so it is possible that cross hybridization occurred and efivirenz actually up-regulated cyp3A4. Aminolevulinate is an intermediary in heme synthesis, and up-regulation of aminolevulinate delta-synthase 1 could be associated with the increased cytochrome P450 expression.

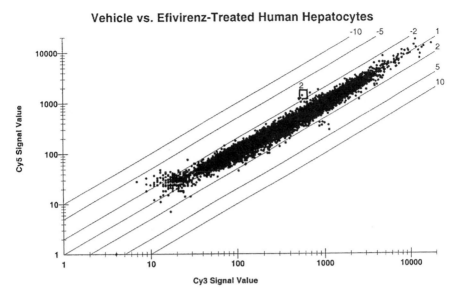

Figure 2 Changes in gene expression levels in cultured human hepatocytes treated with reverse transcriptase inhibitor, efivirenz. Hepatocytes were treated with the vehicle DMSO or with efivirenz. The mRNA was harvested, reverse transcribed, and labeled with Cy3 (vehicle-treated cells) or with Cy5 (efivirenz-treated cells). The labeled cDNA was hybridized to the UniGemV microarray chip (Incyte Pharmaceuticals). The results are displayed on the graph as a ratio of Cy5 versus Cy3 signal. (*Square*) The location of the genes cyp3A7 and aminolevulinate delta synthase 1.

In contrast to the results with efivirenz, several genes were shown to be changed in expression in cultured human hepatocytes when treated with the hepatotoxic CpdR. The results are shown in Figure 3. The gene that showed the greatest change in expression level was phospholipase A2, which showed an increase in mRNA levels of over eightfold. Phospholipase A2 (PLA2) is an enzyme that hydrolyzes the acyl bond of phospholipids, resulting in the release of arachidonic acid and lysophospholipid. PLA2 is also present in many different types of snake venom, including that of elapids, vipers, crotalids, and colubrids (33). PLA2 has also been shown to be up-regulated with CCl_4 treatment of rat hepatocytes and has been directly linked to the mechanism of toxicity of CCl_4 (34–36). Up-regulation of PLA2 in human hepatocytes by treatment with CpdR suggests a role for increased arachidonic acid in the mechanism of hepatic toxicity for this compound. Additonal useful observations were made from these and other studies. First, DMSO produced no changes in gene expression observable after 24 h of exposure. This is important because this is the most commonly used solvent in drug discovery research. Second, attempts to hybridize liver cDNA libraries from rats treated with CpdR to human cDNA chips were not successful;

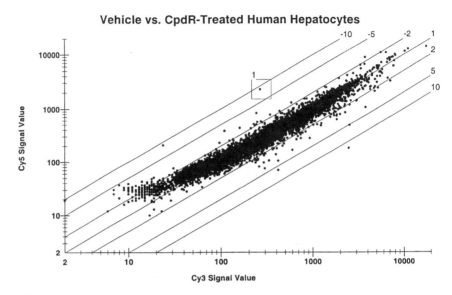

Figure 3   Changes in gene expression levels in cultured human hepatocytes treated with DMSO (Cy3) or CpdR (Cy5). (*Square*) The location of the phospholipase A2 gene.

no significant changes in gene expression were observed. This stresses the need to conduct analyses using same-species arrays.

Studies were done on the genetic expression changes that occur in HT29 colon tumor cells when treated with the DNA methylation inhibitor 5-aza-2'deoxy-cytidine (5-Aza-CdR) (DA Jones, personal communication). The microarray slide contained 4608 randomly selected cDNAs from the Unigene set. HT29 cells were exposed to 5-Aza-CdR for 9 days, whereupon RNA from the cells was harvested and hybridized to the microarray slide. It is interesting to note that all 19 genes induced by 5-Aza-CdR were also inducible with interferon. This result led to the further observation that STAT (signal transducers and activators of transcription) factors 1, 2, and 3 were transcriptionally activated by 5-Aza-CdR. These results are potentially significant because STAT 1 expression is often depressed in certain metastatic melonama cell lines, and these tumor cell lines often respond poorly to interferon treatment (DA Jones, personal communication). These results again demonstrate how techniques such as hybridization microarray can direct research down pathways that had not been previously anticipated.

Schena et al (37) used hybridization microarray analysis to identify genes that are regulated during heat shock or by phorbol ester in human T-cells. Jurkat cells were incubated at 37°C for control and then were either incubated at 43°C for 4 h or were treated with phorbol ester. The mRNA from the cell populations was harvested, reverse transcribed, labeled, and hybridized to a microarray glass slide containing a total of 1056 cDNAs. The microarray results showed 17 genes that were regulated during heat shock, all of which were confirmed by dot blotting assays. Of the 17 genes identified, many encoded for proteins involved in protein degradation or factors that function as molecular chaperones, which is consistent with mechanisms of heat shock induction. Six genes were identified as being regulated by phorbol ester, one of which, NF-κB1, is a known target gene of phorbol ester regulation. It is interesting to note that several unknown genes were identified that may be important for understanding the molecular mechanisms of phorbol ester and heat shock cellular regulation (37).

High-density synthetic oligonucleotide slides are another powerful tool that has greatly transformed molecular analysis of toxicology and will continue to do so. With this method, oligonucleotides are synthesized directly onto a glass substrate. The major company that markets synthetic oligonucleotide microarray slides is Affymetrix. However, other companies will no doubt start to market other microarray chips. (For updates on microarray technology, consult the following website: http://www.mpiz-koeln.mpg.de/%7Eweisshaa/Adis/DNA-array-links.html.)

Affymetrix chips are constructed using a photolithographic method. A glass substrate is coated with covalent linker molecules that terminate with a photolabile protecting group. Light is directed through a mask that exposes selected portions of the probe array to ultraviolet light. This removes the photolabile protecting group, which allows nucleotides to couple to the unprotected sites. This process is repeated using different filters until a complete set of oligonucleotides is synthesized on the glass slide. The Affymetrix chips contain hundreds of thousands of genes on an area 1.28 × 1.28 cm on each array. The oligonucleotides are generally 20 bp long, and every gene is represented by multiple oligonucleotides of different sequences that will hybridize to the same mRNA. In addition, mutated oligonucleotides, containing a single base pair change, are present for every perfect oligonucleotide sequence. By using multiple oligonucleotides for the same gene, and by having the mutated sequences present, the number of false positive signals is vastly reduced (38). Another difference between Affymetrix chips and microarray chips with cDNA spotted onto glass slides is that mRNA from individual cell populations is hybridized to an individual chip. This is done because the Affymetrix chips give a quantitative level of expression of mRNA from each cell; the data are not displayed as a ratio of the expression of one mRNA population over the other. This has certain advantages because once a cell population has been hybridized to an Affymetrix chip, the gene expression results can be compared to those from other cell populations without the need for multiple hybridizations. (More information on the Affymetrix chip is available at the following website: http://www.affymetrix.com/.)

The genetic changes induced in *Saccharomyces cerevisiae* when treated with the alkylating agent methyl methanesulfonate (MMS) were studied. MMS has been shown to cause DNA damage and to activate DNA repair genes (39). Yeast cells were treated with a low dose of MMS, which induces DNA-repair genes while causing minimal cell death. The mRNA was harvested from the cells and hybridized to Affymetrix chips containing 6218 open reading frame (ORF) yeast sequences. The results showed that of the 6218 genes present on the chip, 325 showed a more than fourfold induction in transcript level compared with the control group, and 75 of the ORF sequences were down-regulated more than threefold. To confirm these results, 50 of the ORF sequences that were either up- or down-regulated were chosen for further confirmation by northern blot analysis. The northern blotting results showed that 48 out of the 50 ORF sequences chosen were indeed changed in expression by MMS, and the amount of induction or repression as shown by Affymetrix or northern blotting analysis was very similar. Of the genes that were shown to be regulated by MMS, many fell into the category of genes that would be expected to be activated in case of DNA damage, such as DNA repair, cell wall biogenesis, membrane transport, and signal transduction genes. In addition, 91 of the 143 known protein degradation genes were induced, which is interesting considering the dosage level of MMS was relatively nontoxic. Overall, Jelinsky & Samson (40) showed 15-fold more genes than had previously been thought to be induced by a DNA-damaging agent. In addition, the study suggested several new mechanisms that cells may utilize to protect against chemicals that induce DNA damage (40).

Oligonucleotide microarrays have been and are being used in many different areas of biological research as well, such as polymorphism analysis and genotyping (41), disease management (42), and cell signaling (43). Because oligonucleotide microarray analysis is a relatively new technique, there is not a great deal of literature on its use in toxicology. This will undoubtedly change as more pharmaceutical companies begin exploiting its vast potential.

SERIAL ANALYSIS OF GENE EXPRESSION

SAGE analysis was first described in 1995 by Velculescu et al (44). Similar to differential display or subtractive hybridization, this method allows one to compare the expression profiles of genes between different cell populations. Unlike the aforementioned techniques, however, SAGE actually quantitates the level of RNA in each individual cell population. In this regard, SAGE is similar to oligonucleotide microarrays. Unlike microarrays, however, SAGE allows for the identification of unknown gene sequences. SAGE is based on the principle that a short gene sequence has enough information to identify a transcript. RNA is isolated from a cell population and reverse transcribed using a poly(dT) primer. Following this, the cDNA is cleaved with a frequent restriction enzyme cutter, termed the anchoring enzyme; the 3' end of the cDNA is captured and isolated using streptavidin-coated magnetic beads. The cDNA is then split into two populations, and each population has ligated onto it via the anchoring restriction site and a linker (A or B) containing a site for a type IIS restriction enzyme (tagging enzyme). The tagging enzyme is then used to release a 9-bp fragment of the cDNA. The two populations are then ligated together and amplified with primers specific for linkers A and B. The linkers are then released using the anchoring enzyme, and the resulting cDNA fragments are ligated together, forming concatemers of many different 9-bp fragments. The concatemers are then cloned and sequenced to identify each fragment. The number of times a given fragment appears is a direct measure of the quantity of that RNA species in the original cell population (44, 45).

SAGE has been used to study the expression levels in a variety of systems, such as the transcriptional changes induced by p53 expression in human colorectal cancer cells (46, 47), to study gene expression profiles in normal and cancer cells (48), and to characterize the yeast transcriptome (49). (For more information concerning SAGE, consult the following website: http://www.genzyme.com/sage.) A similar system has been developed by Perkin Elmer GenScope, called GeneTag™ (http://www.genscope.com). Though no published reports utilizing SAGE or GeneTag™ specifically for toxicology studies could be found, this will likely change as these techniques becomes more widely used.

REAL-TIME PCR, BRANCHED-DNA, AND SCINTILLATION PROXIMITY ASSAYS

Real-time PCR, branched-DNA (bDNA), and scintillation proximity assays (SPA) are examples of high-throughput, low-fidelity techniques available to toxicology. These techniques are similar in that unlike the previous techniques reviewed in this article, which give in one experiment the expression changes for thousands of genes regulated by one compound, real-time PCR, bDNA, and SPA can potentially give information on expression changes for one gene using many different compounds in an experiment. These three methods are extremely useful for confirming and expanding upon information gained from other high-throughput techniques, such as hybridization microarrays. Thus, far from being exclusive, real-time PCR, bDNA, and SPA are complementary to other high-throughput methods.

Real-time PCR kinetics was pioneered in 1993, when Higuchi et al (50) constructed a system that detected the accumulating levels of double-stranded DNA by monitoring the increase in the fluorescence of ethidium bromide that binds to duplex DNA. By calculating the number of cycles necessary to detect a signal, it is possible to determine the starting levels of a certain gene present in the cell population. The method has been subsequently improved on to allow detection using a specific probe rather than ethidium bromide. The current method for real-time PCR detection is as follows. A probe is designed that hybridizes specifically to the gene of interest. This probe hybridizes between the forward and reverse primers and contains both a reporter fluorescent dye and a quencher dye attached to it. If the probe is intact, the proximity of the quencher strongly reduces the fluorescence emitted by the reporter. When the probe is cleaved by the 5' nuclease activity of the DNA polymerase, the reporter dye is separated from the quencher, and a signal is generated. This signal is monitored by a fluorescence reader. The starting copy number of the gene of interest can then be determined based on the cycle at which the PCR signal is first detected (51). The PCR reaction is done in a 96-well plate, thus making it possible to test numerous compounds or conditions in the same experiment.

The principal company offering a real-time PCR system is Perkin Elmer Applied Biosystems, which markets the ABI Prism 7700 PCR® technology. Bio-Rad also markets a real-time PCR system, the iCycler. (For more information on these systems, see the following websites: http://www.pebio.com/ab/about/pcr/sds and http://www.discover.bio-rad.com.)

SPA is similar to real-time PCR in that many different conditions or compounds can be tested in the same experiment for the regulation of a target gene. Cells are plated directly onto Cytostar-T™ 96-well scintillating microplates, into which solid scintillants have been incorporated. Cultured cells are treated, then fixed in the wells. Radiolabeled probes are added, and the cells are RNase treated and washed. Bound radioactive probes are then quantitated on a scintillation counter (7, 52). Harris et al (52) used this method to detect the levels of *c-fos* in quiesced rat smooth muscle cells with or without induction of platelet-derived growth factor. The results were compared against those from a northern blotting assay. Both assays gave the same results, but SPA was found to be 20-fold more sensitive and easier to perform (52). (More information can be obtained at the website for Amersham Pharmacia Biotech: http://www.apbiotech.com.)

Branched DNA is similar to real-time PCR in that it is extremely sensitive. However, unlike real-time PCR, which amplifies the starting material, bDNA amplifies the signal. This is accomplished by the use of probes specific for the gene, which are attached to alkaline phosphatase conjugated labels. Cells are plated in 96-well plates and treated. Following this, the medium is aspirated off, and cell lysis buffer containing the alkaline phosphatase labeled probes are added. The cell lysate is then transferred to a bDNA assay plate, which captures the mRNA of interest. The level of expression is assayed by adding a chemiluminescent substrate, and the light emission is measured using a luminometer (7). An example from our own laboratory is shown in Figure 4. In this example, cultured rat hepatocytes were treated with either the peroxisome proliferator activated receptor alpha (PPARα) agonist bezafibrate or the PPARγ agonist pioglitazone. The endpoint for the assay was quantitation of mRNA expression for acyl-coenzyme A oxidase, a marker gene for peroxisomal proliferation, as compared with the "housekeeping" gene glyceraldehyde phosphate dehydrogenase. The bDNA technique clearly differentiates between the responses generated by these two compounds: a robust response for the peroxisome proliferator bezafibrate and a mild response for the relatively weak PPARα agonist pioglitazone. In our hands, results from bDNA evaluation for this gene response are similar or identical to those from SPA.

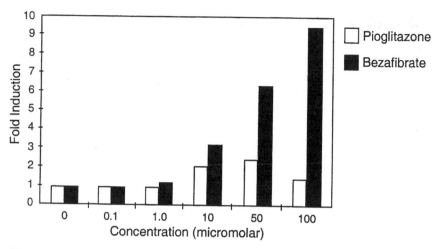

Figure 4 Changes in acyl-coenzyme A oxidase gene expression in cultured rat hepatocytes treated with either the peroxisome proliferating drug bezafibrate or the thiazolidinedione pioglitazone. Hepatocytes were treated overnight with the compounds, and specific mRNA was quantified by using the branched-DNA signal amplification method. Glyceraldehyde phosphate dehydrogenase gene expression was used as a control (not shown).

DISCUSSION

In this review we discussed several genomics-based tools that are currently available for use in toxicity evaluation. The advent of these technologies and their application in drug safety research represents a change in approach, if not in paradigm, from histopathology to molecular pathology/toxicology. Microarrays offer the promise of identifying liabilities and mechanisms in a short amount of time. In addition to evaluation responses due to single-compound exposure, these technologies may be used to assess complications due to interactions between drugs, assessing the contribution of each compound as well as the combined effects. Enthusiasm for microarray technologies is certainly justifiable but needs to be tempered; microarrays are too new for their full value or potential to be understood (in fact, no reports showing the use of microarrays specifically for safety or risk assessment appear in the peer-reviewed literature).

Of more practical current value is the application of these tools to toxicology applied at the early drug discovery level. Gene response targets, identified by microarray or sequencing analysis, can be used to develop toxicology screens with techniques such as real-time PCR or bDNA. As with any single endpoint assay, however, a degree of caution must be used when extrapolating from results because the fidelity of these assays decreases even further when applied outside of a chemical analogue series or to a different species.

Application of genomic-based technologies in day-to-day safety evaluation, and particularly in regulated studies and other studies required for product registration, will likely require the development of large databases. It remains a challenge for the pharmaceutical and vendor industries to cooperate in developing shared databases that can be queried by other companies and by regulatory agencies; this is important for reducing product liability and ensuring consumer safety. Clearly, the new tools available to the toxicologist have opened a new age of discovery.

Visit the Annual Reviews home page at www.AnnualReviews.org.

LITERATURE CITED

1. Brecher RW. 1997. Risk assessment. *Toxicol. Pathol.* 25:23–31
2. Ulrich RG, Slatter JG. 1997. The role of investigative techniques in toxicity evaluation. In *Toxicity Testing and Evaluation Comprehensive Toxicology,* ed. P Williams, G Hottenforf, pp. 203–25. New York: Elsevier Sci. 2nd ed.
3. Gerhold D, Rushmore T, Caskey CT. 1999. DNA chips: promising toys have become powerful tools. *Trends Biochem. Sci.* 24:168–73
4. Medlin JF. 1999. Timely toxicology. *Environ. Health Perspect.* 107:A256–58
5. Nuwaysir EF, Bittner M, Trent J, Barrett JC, Afshari CA. 1999. Microarrays and toxicology: the advent of toxicogenomics. *Mol. Carcinog.* 24:153–59
6. Rodi CP, Bunch RT, Curtiss SW, Kier LD, Cabonce MA, et al. 1999. Revolution through genomics in investigative and discovery toxicology. *Toxicol. Pathol.* 27:107–10
7. Todd MD, Ulrich RG. 1999. Emerging technologies for accelerated toxicity evaluation of potential drug candidates. *Curr. Opin. Drug Discov. Dev.* 2:58–68
8. Liang L, Pardee AB. 1992. Differential display of eukaryotic messenger RNA by means of the polymerase chain reaction. *Science* 257:967–71
9. Wang X, Harris PKW, Ulrich RG, Voorman RL. 1996. Identification of dioxin-responsive genes in Hep G2 cells using differential mRNA display RT-PCR. *Biochem. Biophys. Res. Commun.* 220: 784–88
10. Selmin O, Lucier GW, Clark GC, Tritscher AM, Vanden Heuvel JP, et al. 1996. Isolation and characterization of a novel gene induced by 2,3,7,8-tetrachlorodibenzo-*p*-dioxin in rat liver. *Carcinogenesis* 17:2609–15
11. Roman BL, Peterson RE. 1998. *In utero* and lactational exposure of the male rat to 2,3,7,8-tetrachlorodibenzo-*p*-dioxin impairs prostate development. *Toxicol. Appl. Pharmacol.* 150:240–53
12. Donat S, Abel J. 1998. Analysis of gene expression in lung and thymus of TCDD treated C57BL/6 mice using differential display RT-PCR. *Chemosphere* 37:1867–72
13. Muhlenkamp CR, Gill SS. 1998. A glucose-regulated protein, GRP58, is downregulated in C57B6 mouse liver after diethylhexyl phthalate exposure. *Toxicol. Appl. Pharmacol.* 148:101–8
14. Green S. 1992. Peroxisome proliferators: a model for receptor mediated carcinogenesis. *Cancer Surv.* 14:221–32
15. Ye X, Lu L, Gill SS. 1997. Suppression of cytochrome P450 *Cyp2f2* mRNA levels in mice by the peroxisome proliferator diethylhexylphthalate. *Biochem. Biophys. Res. Commun.* 239:660–65
16. Kegelmeyer AE, Sprankle CS, Horesov-

sky GJ, Butterworth BE. 1997. Differential display identified changes in mRNA levels in regenerating livers from chloroform-treated mice. *Mol. Carcinog.* 20:288–97

17. Kar S, Carr BI. 1995. Differential display and cloning of messenger RNAs from the late phase of rat liver regeneration. *Biochem. Biophys. Res. Commun.* 212: 21–26

18. Sive HL, St. John T. 1988. A simple subtractive hybridization technique employing photoactivatable biotin and phenol extraction. *Nucleic Acids Res.* 22:10937

19. Wang Z, Brown DD. 1991. A gene expression screen. *Proc. Natl. Acad. Sci. USA* 88:11505–9

20. Wogan GN, Newberne PM. 1967. Dose-response characteristics of aflatoxin B1 carcinogenesis in the rat. *Cancer Res.* 27:2370–76

21. Groopman JD, Cain LG, Kensler TW. 1988. Aflatoxin exposure in human populations: measurement and relationship to cancer. *Crit. Rev. Toxicol.* 19:113–45

22. Lisitsyn N, Lisitsyn N, Wigler M. 1993. Cloning the differences between two complex genomes. *Science* 259:946–51

23. Diatchenko L, Lau YC, Campbell AP, Chenchik A, Moqadam F, et al. 1996. Suppression subtractive hybridization: a method for generating differentially regulated or tissue-specific cDNA probes and libraries. *Proc. Natl. Acad. Sci. USA* 93:6025–30

24. Harris AJ, Shaddock JG, Manjanatha MG, Lisenbey JA, Casciano DA. 1998. Identification of differentially expressed genes in aflatoxin B1-treated cultured primary rat hepatocytes and Fischer 344 rats. *Carcinogenesis* 19:1451–58

25. Toggas SM, Krady JK, Billingsley ML. 1992. Molecular neurotoxicology of trimethyltin: identification of stannin, a novel protein expressed in trimethyltin-sensitive cells. *Mol. Pharmacol.* 42:44–56

26. Thompson TA, Lewis JM, Dejneka NS,

Severs WB, Polavarapu R, Billingsley ML. 1996. Induction of apoptosis by organotin compounds in vitro: neuronal protection with antisense oligonucleotides directed against stannin. *J. Pharmacol. Exp. Ther.* 276:1201–16

27. Chen I, Safe S. 1999. Identification of estrogen-induced genes downregulated by 2,3,7,8-tetrachlorodibenzo-*p*-dioxin (TCDD) by suppression subtractive hybridization. *Toxicol. Sci.* 48(1-S):1007 (Abstr.)

28. Bowtell DDL. 1999. Options available—from start to finish—for obtaining expression data by microarray. *Nat. Genet. Suppl.* 21:25–32

29. Cheung VG, Morley M, Aguilar F, Massimi A, Kucherlapati R, Childs G. 1999. Making and reading microarrays. *Nat. Genet. Suppl.* 21:15–19

30. Duggan DJ, Bittner M, Chen Y, Meltzer P, Trent JM. 1999. Expression profiling using cDNA microarrays. *Nat. Genet. Suppl.* 21:10–14

31. Southern E, Mir K, Shchepinov M. 1999. Molecular interactions on microarrays. *Nat. Genet. Suppl.* 21:5–10

32. Ulrich RG, Cramer CT, Sun EL, Bacon JA, Petrella DK. 1998. A protocol for isolation, culture and cryopreservation of hepatocytes from human liver. *In Vitro Mol. Toxicol.* 11:23–33

33. Goldstein RS, Schnellmann RG. 1996. Toxic responses of the kidney. In *Casarett & Doull's Toxicology: The Basic Science of Poisons,* ed. CD Klaassen, 5:417–43. New York/St. Louis: McGraw-Hill. 1111 pp.

34. Horton AA, Wood JM. 1989. Effects of inhibitors of phospholipase A2, cyclooxygenase and thromboxane synthetase on paracetamol hepatotoxicity in the rat. *Eicosanoids* 2:123–29

35. Chiarpotto E, Biasi F, Comoglio A, Leonarduzzi G, Poli G, Dianzani MU. 1990. CCl4-induced increase of hepatocyte free arachidonate level: pathogene-

sis and contribution to cell death. *Chem. Biol. Interact.* 74:195–206

36. Glende EA, Recknagel RO. 1991. An indirect method demonstrating that CCl₄-dependent hepatocyte injury is linked to a rise in intracellular calcium ion concentration. *Res. Commun. Chem. Pathol. Pharmacol.* 73:41–52

37. Schena M, Shalon D, Heller R, Chai AO, Brown P, Davis R. 1996. Parallel human genome analysis: microarray-based expression monitoring of 1000 genes. *Proc. Natl. Acad. Sci. USA* 93:10614–19

38. Lipshutz RJ, Fodor SPA, Gingeras TR, Lockhart DJ. 1999. High density synthetic oligonucleotide arrays. *Nat. Genet. Suppl.* 21:20–25

39. Chen J, Derfler B, Samson L. 1990. *Saccharomyces cerevisiae* 3-methyladenine DNA glycosylase has homology to the AlkA glycosylase of *E. coli* and is induced in response to DNA alkylation damage. *EMBO J.* 9:4569–75

40. Jelinsky SA, Samson LD. 1999. Global response of *Saccharomyces cerevisiae* to an alkylating agent. *Proc. Natl. Acad. Sci. USA* 96:1486–91

41. Hacia JG, Fan JB, Ryder O, Jin L, Edgemon K, et al. 1999. Determination of ancestral alleles for human single-nucleotide polymorphisms using high-density oligonucleotide arrays. *Nat. Genet.* 22:164–67

42. Kozal MJ, Shah N, Shen N, Yang R, Fucini R, et al. 1996. Extensive polymorphisms observed in HIV-1 clade B protease gene using high-density oligonucleotide arrays. *Nat. Med.* 2:753–59

43. Der SD, Zhou A, Williams BR, Silver-man RH. 1998. Identification of genes differentially regulated by interferon alpha, beta, or gamma using oligonucleotide arrays. *Proc. Natl. Acad. Sci. USA* 95:15623–28

44. Velculescu VE, Zhang L, Vogelstein B, Kinzler KW. 1995. Serial analysis of gene expression. *Science* 270:484–87

45. Bertelsen AH, Velculescu VE. 1998. High-throughput gene expression analysis using SAGE. *Drug Discov. Today* 3:152–59

46. Polyak K, Xia Y, Zweler JL, Kinzler KW, Vogelstein B. 1997. A model for p53-induced apoptosis. *Nature* 389:300–5

47. Madden SL, Galella EA, Zhu J, Bertelsen AH, Beaudry GA. 1997. SAGE transcript profiles for p53-dependent growth regulation. *Oncogene* 15:1079–85

48. Zhang L, Zhou W, Velculescu VE, Kern SE, Hruban RH, et al. 1997. Gene expression profiles in normal and cancer cells. *Science* 276:1268–72

49. Velculescu VE, Zhang L, Zhou W, Vogelstein J, Basrai MA, et al. 1997. Characterization of the yeast transcriptome. *Cell* 88:243–51

50. Higuchi R, Fockler C, Dollinger G, Watson R. 1993. Kinetic PCR analysis: real-time monitoring of DNA amplification reactions. *Biotechnology* 11:1026–30

51. Gibson UE, Heid CA, Williams PA. 1996. A novel method for real time quantitative PCR. *Genome Res.* 6:995–1001

52. Harris DW, Kenrick MK, Pither RJ, Anson JG, Jones DA. 1996. Development of a high-volume in situ mRNA hybridization assay for the quantification of gene expression utilizing scintillating microplates. *Anal. Biochem.* 243:249–56

Annu. Rev. Pharmacol. Toxicol. 2000. 40:353–88

MITOCHONDRIAL TARGETS OF DRUG TOXICITY

K. B. Wallace and A. A. Starkov

Department of Biochemistry and Molecular Biology, University of Minnesota School of Medicine, Duluth, Minnesota 55812; e-mail: kwallace@d.umn.edu, astarkov@d.umn.edu

Key Words   oxidative phosphorylation, uncouplers, bioenergetics, permeability transition, redox cycling

■ **Abstract**   Mitochondria have long been recognized as the generators of energy for the cell. Like any other power source, however, mitochondria are highly vulnerable to inhibition or uncoupling of the energy harnessing process and run a high risk for catastrophic damage to the cell. The exquisite structural and functional characteristics of mitochondria provide a number of primary targets for xenobiotic-induced bioenergetic failure. They also provide opportunities for selective delivery of drugs to the mitochondrion. In light of the large number of natural, commercial, pharmaceutical, and environmental chemicals that manifest their toxicity by interfering with mitochondrial bioenergetics, it is important to understand the underlying mechanisms. The significance is further underscored by the recent identification of bioenergetic control points for cell replication and differentiation and the realization that mitochondria play a determinant role in cell signaling and apoptotic modes of cell death.

INTRODUCTION

At the dawn of history, our single-celled glycolytic ancestors welcomed a new inhabitant, an oxygen-utilizing primitive proteobacteria. These newcomers would bring final relief to the eukaryotic community from the ever-increasing energy demands of ongoing evolution. Eventually, eukaryotic hosts completely integrated their new inhabitants, turning them into specialized energy-producing organelles, which we refer to as mitochondria. Mitochondria are present in almost all types of modern eukaryotic cells, their chief (but not their only) function being energy production for the benefit of the host cell.

In the long run, however, infection with mitochondria brought with it additional vulnerabilities. As with any power source, malfunctioning mitochondria present a hazard to the host cells. Insufficient energy production is an obvious but not the only consequence of mitochondrial poisoning; a great deal of harm at the cellular level arises from mitochondria-catalyzed side reactions, such as exothermic oxygen combustion and free radical emission. There is also an emerging

0362–1642/00/0415–0353$14.00

353

appreciation for the important role that mitochondria play in metabolic cell signaling pathways and in the regulation of cell morphology, mobility, multiplication, and apoptosis. Accordingly, pharmacologists and toxicologists have recently addressed mitochondria as an important intracellular target in the manifestation of a variety of both beneficial and adverse biological activities.

What are mitochondria, how do they produce energy, and what features render them vulnerable to chemical-induced malfunction? This treatise addresses these questions, with a focus on better understanding the critical characteristics that determine the biological activities of mitochondrial poisons.

Energy Production in Mitochondria: An Overview

Mitochondria are intracellular organelles, varying in both shape and size. They may be spherical or elongated, or even branched, and the number may vary from 6–12 small discrete organelles per rat thymus lymphocyte, to a massive and dynamically fluctuating network composed of an indefinable number of single interconnected mitochondria in a typical human fibroblast. Despite the wide variability in number and morphology, all mitochondria share several fundamental properties regardless of the cell type.

All mitochondria are bound by two lipid bilayer membranes. The outer membrane is permeable to ions and solutes up to 14 kDa. It is rich in cholesterol and contains embedded or attached enzymes that interface the mitochondrion with the rest of the cellular metabolic network. The inner membrane encloses a water-containing compartment, the so-called matrix, where mitochondrial DNA and various soluble enzymes, such as those of the tricarboxylic acid cycle and the β-oxidation pathway, are located. This membrane is not freely permeable to ions and metabolites, but instead contains special membrane proteins that transport selected metabolites across the membrane. This feature, the protein-mediated and -regulated permeability of the inner membrane, is of vital importance for the morphological and functional integrity of the mitochondrion: It is also the most common target for mitochondrial toxicants. Many foreign chemicals damage mitochondria either by increasing the permeability of the inner membrane or by inhibiting transport proteins embedded within it. The lipid composition of the inner membrane is unique in that it contains large amounts of cardiolipin and virtually no cholesterol. The presence of cardiolipin represents a second important feature: Many drugs (e.g. adriamycin-like anthraquinones) have a very high affinity for cardiolipin and thereby preferentially bind to and concentrate in the inner mitochondrial membrane.

The inner membrane also contains many different proteins that participate in various metabolic activities, including the production of energy. It also contains a mobile electron carrier, ubiquinone, dissolved in the lipid phase of the membrane. The primary form of energy generated in mitochondria is the so-called electrochemical proton gradient ($\Delta\bar{\mu}_H+$) that is produced by three respiratory chain complexes, which are sophisticated protein ensembles composed of varying numbers of polypeptide subunits. The electrochemical proton gradient furnishes the energy required to produce ATP and to support other activities of the mitochondria, such as the electrophoretic or protonophoric transport of ions, metabolic substrates, and proteins destined for the mitochondrial matrix. Several reviews on energy production and transformation in mitochondria are available [1; for a textbook devoted entirely to bioenergetics, see also Skulachev (36)]. Here, we briefly summarize the major features of mitochondrial energy production. This summary provides the basis for understanding the selective actions of mitochondria-targeted toxicants.

The mitochondrial respiratory chain catalyzes the oxidation of various substrates by oxygen. Substrates dissolved in the aqueous matrix space are oxidized by their specific dehydrogenases, which use the released energy to reduce NAD^+ or the ubiquinone of the inner membrane. Reduced NADH and ubiquinol are then oxidized by the respiratory chain complexes. NADH is oxidized by complex I (NADH:ubiquinone reductase) and the released energy is used to reduce a ubiquinone molecule and to generate $\Delta\bar{\mu}_H +$. The majority of substrates are oxidized by this route, meaning that this is the main entry point for channeling electrons toward the final electron acceptor, molecular oxygen. Because of this, inhibition of NADH:ubiquinone electron flow blocks most of the oxidative metabolic reactions conducted by mitochondria. The second entry point of the respiratory chain is complex III (ubiquinol:cytochrome c reductase), which is also known as the bc_1-complex. This complex oxidizes the reduced ubiquinol. It also generates $\Delta\bar{\mu}_H +$ and reduces the third member of the respiratory chain, cytochrome c. The latter is a mobile protein attached to the cytosolic (intermembrane space) side of the inner mitochondrial membrane. It serves as an electron carrier between complex III and complex IV, which is the terminal cytochrome c oxidase. Complex IV directly reduces molecular oxygen to water and generates $\Delta\bar{\mu}_H +$. It is obvious that inhibition of complex III or complex IV completely blocks all of the energy production in mitochondria. In situations of partial inhibition of complex III or cytochrome oxidase, the electrons supplied by substrates may be diverted to the bulk production of toxic reactive oxygen species by the respiratory chain.

The $\Delta\bar{\mu}_H +$ is generated by means of electrogenic pumping of protons from the mitochondrial matrix to the cytosol (intermembrane space), which is catalyzed by the membrane-spanning respiratory chain complexes. Proton pumping is ultimately coupled to electron flow so that there is no respiration without proton pumping and vice versa. The generated $\Delta\bar{\mu}_H +$ consists of two components, the electrical membrane potential and the pH gradient across the inner mitochondrial membrane. The electrical potential represents the major component of $\Delta\bar{\mu}_H +$. However, it is interchangeable with the pH gradient in such a way that, to some degree, a decrease in membrane potential alone results in an increase in the pH gradient with no changes in $\Delta\bar{\mu}_H +$. Similarly, dissipation of the pH gradient results in a slight hyperpolarization of the membrane. The inner mitochondrial membrane is anisotropic, the matrix side being negatively charged and slightly alkaline; membrane potential is typically in the range of -180 to -220 mV with a ΔpH of 0.4–0.6 U. This charge and pH anisotropy represents the third important feature of mitochondria that contributes to their vulnerability. Because of this feature, mitochondria can accumulate large amounts of positively charged lipophilic compounds and some acids. In the case of a positively charged compound such as 1-methyl-4-phenylpyridium ion or ethidium bromide, the concentration in the mitochondrial matrix can exceed that of the cytosol by several orders of magnitude, providing a strong basis for selective poisoning of mitochondria.

The overall rate of electron transport in the respiratory chain of mitochondria is regulated by the amplitude of $\Delta\tilde{\mu}_H+$, a phenomenon known as respiratory control. When $\Delta\tilde{\mu}_H+$ is high, respiration rate is low. Conversely, a decrease in $\Delta\tilde{\mu}_H+$ causes an immediate stimulation of oxygen consumption. Under physiological conditions, the decrease in $\Delta\tilde{\mu}_H+$ is due to the metabolic work performed in mitochondria, so the rate of respiration is tightly coupled to the rate of metabolism. It is obvious that the permeability of the inner mitochondrial membrane to protons and other charged species must be exquisitely low and that the dissipation of $\Delta\tilde{\mu}_H+$ must be mechanistically coupled with the performance of work. This coupling occurs by means of enzymes of the inner membrane that are capable of converting the energy stored in the form of $\Delta\tilde{\mu}_H+$ into the desirable kind of work (e.g. protein transport or ATP synthesis). A nonspecific increase in permeability of the inner membrane or a decrease in the degree of coupling of the protonomotive and phosphorylative complexes will dissipate $\Delta\tilde{\mu}_H+$ nonproductively in the form of heat emission. Such a malfunction in mitochondrial bioenergetics instantaneously transforms the mitochondrion from an essential powerhouse of the cell into a molecular furnace, efficiently wasting the metabolic energy of substrates. This is the most common mechanism of mitochondrial poisoning; literally hundreds of different toxicants damage mitochondria by increasing the permeability of the inner membrane to protons and other ions. In the following sections, we consider the major groups of mitochondria-specific toxicants, with particular attention to their mechanisms of action.

Enveloped within the mitochondrial membranes are a number of soluble enzyme activities related to the generation of reducing equivalents for the membrane-embedded electron transport chain. Among these soluble enzyme activities are the fatty acid β-oxidation and tricarboxylic acid oxidation pathways. Although there are many examples of chemicals that interfere with specific enzymatic steps within these pathways that lead to bioenergetic deficits within the cell, the focus of this article is the activity and turnover of membrane-associated bioenergetic functions, such as electron transport and respiration.

BIOENERGETIC POISONS

There are two means by which chemicals can affect mitochondrial bioenergetics, either by interfering with the generation of $\Delta\tilde{\mu}_H^+$ or by causing its dissipation. Acute poisoning with inhibitors of electron transporting complexes cause symptoms such as muscle weakness, easy fatigability, hypotension, headache, facial flushing, nausea, confusion, and aggravation of latent myocardial angina. This inability to utilize oxygen is manifested as a cytotoxic hypoxia wherein the chemicals cause a metabolic acidosis and hyperpnea, despite the normal pA_{O2} and absence of cyanosis. Inhibitors of the supply of reducing substrates for the respiratory chain, such as the fluoroacetates and acetamides, cause a remarkably similar metabolic syndrome that is difficult to distinguish from inhibitors of the electron transport chain.

Contrast this to poisons that dissipate $\Delta\tilde{\mu}_H+$, which likewise cause ATP deficits and metabolic acidosis and hyperpnea, but also induce excessive oxygen consumption, as reflected by the lower pA_{O2} and cyanosis. The free energy of substrate oxidation is liberated as heat causing fever in individuals poisoned by such agents. Examples of this latter group of chemicals include agents that increase membrane permeability to individual ions, such as channel-forming proteins, ionophores, uncouplers of oxidative phosphorylation, and inducers of the permeability transition of the mitochondrial membrane. The next several paragraphs summarize the characteristics of each of these classes of chemicals.

Inhibitors of Respiratory Chain

Inhibitors of Complex I   Mitochondrial NADH:ubiquinone oxidoreductase (complex I; EC 1.6.5.3) is the first in the series of membrane-associated proton pumps of the mitochondrial respiratory chain (Figure 1A). The details of the path of electron transfer through components of complex I, the exact stoichiometry of proton pumping, and the mechanism of proton pumping are not clear. However, significant progress is being made and several excellent recent reviews are available (3–5). This enzyme is the most vulnerable of the respiratory chain complexes to chemical-induced malfunction. More than 60 different types of natural and synthetic compounds are known to inhibit mitochondrial complex I activity. Characteristics of the various inhibitors of this complex, the mechanisms of inhibition, and structure-activity relationships for major classes of potent inhibitors of complex I are all reviewed in a recent series of papers (5–8). The list of inhibitors of complex I includes pesticides; neuroleptics and natural neurotoxins; antihistaminic, antianginal, and antiseptic drugs; rodenticides; phenolic pollutants; fluorescent dyes; and myxobacterial and other antibiotics. The large number and structural diversity of inhibitors of complex I is in excellent agreement with the summation by Degli Esposti (5) that a "potent . . . inhibitor of complex I has a modular similarity with ubiquinone, with a cyclic 'head' . . . and a hydrophobic 'tail'."

All of the inhibitors can be classified into one of three categories based on their specificity toward complex I. The first group includes compounds that inhibit at the level of the NADH-flavin interaction, such as rhein. Such compounds are not specific to complex I because they also affect a variety of other dehydrogenases. The second category is represented by quinole antagonists, which are inhib-

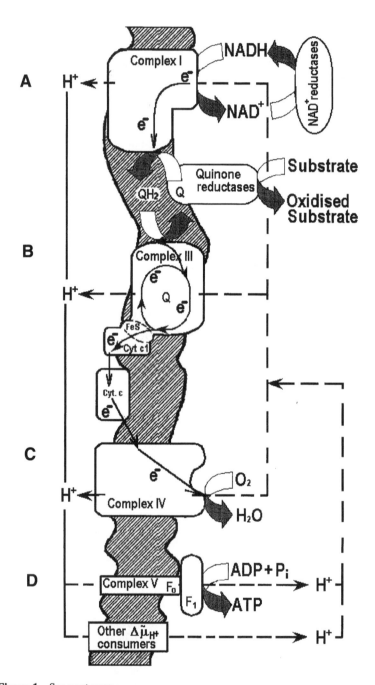

Figure 1   See next page.

itory for both complex I and the bc_1-complex. Examples of this group include myxothiazol and the quinolone aurachins produced by *Pseudomonas aeruginosa* and *Stigmatella aurantiaca*. These compounds interfere with quinol binding and some are twice as potent as rotenone in inhibiting mammalian mitochondrial NADH:ubiquinone oxidoreductase (5). The third group of inhibitors consists of compounds that seem to be specific and potent inhibitors of complex I, acting at concentrations low enough to have no effect on other respiratory chain complexes. Among this group is the classical inhibitor rotenone, which is a member of the rotenoid family of naturally occurring isoflavonoids produced by Leguminosae

Figure 1 Mitochondrial respiratory chain. (*A*) Mitochondrial NADH:ubiquinone oxido-reductase (complex I; EC 1.6.5.3) catalyzes the oxidation of NADH generated by NAD-linked dehydrogenases within the mitochondrial matrix. The enzyme reduces ubiquinone to the ubiquinol and generates $\Delta\bar{\mu}_H+$ across the inner membrane of the mitochondria. Complex I is the largest and most sophisticated enzyme of the respiratory chain. It is composed of several polypeptide subunits encoded both by mitochondrial and nuclear DNA, and it contains FMN and several FeS centers. (*B*) Complex III (bc_1-complex, ubiquinol:cytochrome *c* oxidoreductase, EC 1.10.2.2) oxidizes ubiquinol, reduces cyto-chrome *c*, and generates $\Delta\bar{\mu}_H+$. Mammalian complex III is composed of 11 subunits, including cytochrome *b*, having both a low and a high potential heme group (b_L and b_H), Rieske iron-sulfur protein containing a single Fe_2S_2 cluster, cytochrome *c*1 with a cova-lently bound heme *c*, and eight polypeptide subunits whose functions are unclear. Complex III subunits are encoded both by nuclear and mitochondrial DNA (12, 13). The bc_1-com-plex works through a Q-cycle mechanism. It contains two separate ubiquinone-binding sites, a quinol-oxidizing site Q_o, and a quinone-reducing site Q_i. Reduced ubiquinol dis-solved in the inner mitochondrial membrane is oxidized in a bifurcated reaction. The first electron is transferred via the Rieske protein and cytochrome *c*1 to cytochrome *c*. This leaves an ubisemiquinone at center Q_o, which is unstable and quickly donates the remain-ing electron to heme b_L and b_H and to a ubiquinone or a stable ubisemiquinone anion bound in the Q_i site. The oxidation of one molecule of ubiquinol to ubiquinone yields two reduced molecules of cytochrome *c*, two protons are consumed on the negative (matrix) side of the membrane, and four protons are released on the positive (cytoplasmic) side. (*C*) Cytochrome c oxidase (complex IV; EC 1.9.3.1) is a heme/copper terminal oxidase that uses cytochrome *c* as electron donor. It catalyzes the four-electron reduction of O_2 to water, coupled to the generation of $\Delta\bar{\mu}_H+$ across the inner mitochondrial membrane in which it is embedded. The mammalian enzyme contains 13 polypeptide subunits, two iron centers, heme *a* and heme a_3, and two copper centers, Cu_A and Cu_B. Subunit I of COX contains the heme *a* and the oxygen-binding site, which is composed of the heme a_3 and Cu_B. The binuclear Cu_A center is contained within subunit II of the complex. (*D*) H^+-ATP synthetase (complex V, EC 3.6.1.34) uses the $\Delta\bar{\mu}_H+$ to produce ATP from ADP and phosphate. The enzyme consists of several polypeptide subunits that are encoded both in the cell nucleus and in mitochondria. The part of the enzyme that is located in the mito-chondrial matrix forms soluble ATPase or so-called F_1-ATPase; if separated from the rest of enzyme, it can hydrolyze ATP. F_1-ATPase is connected by the stalk to the membrane-buried part, which is termed F_0. This part participates in proton conduction. For more details, two well-written reviews are recommended (87, 88).

plants. In isolated beef heart or liver mitochondria, the median inhibitory concentration (IC_{50}) for rotenone is 0.07 nmol/mg of protein with a K_i of 4 nM. The most powerful and specific inhibitor is rolliniastatin-1, which belongs to the family of acetogenins produced by Annonaceae plants. For complex I, it has an IC_{50} of 0.03 nmol/mg of protein with a K_i of 0.3 nM (5).

Although complex I is present in all eukaryotic organisms possessing mitochondria and in many bacteria, the structure of this enzyme and its sensitivity toward inhibitors is vastly different in different species. In general, insect and fish mitochondria are the most sensitive to complex I inhibition whereas plant and fungi mitochondria are fairly resistant. In mammalians, neuronal mitochondria tend to be most sensitive to inhibitors of complex I.

Inhibitors of Complex III   Complex III (bc_1-complex, ubiquinol:cytochrome c oxidoreductase, EC 1.10.2.2) is the second membrane-spanning, proton-translocating complex of the mitochondrial electron transport chain. The mechanism of proton pumping is not clear, however the overall reaction sequence in this segment of the respiratory chain is well understood (9–11) (Figure 1*B*). The minimal sufficient structure of the bc_1-complex consists of only three subunits, as in bacteria *Paracoccus denitrificans,* and there is considerable variability in the structure of complex III in mitochondria from different species. The sensitivity of various species to a particular inhibitor of the bc_1 complex also varies greatly (12–16), which allows relatively safe practical application of some of these compounds as fungicides and as antimalarial, antiprotozoan, and anticancer drugs (17–24).

The major inhibitors of the bc_1-complex have been reviewed by von Jagow & Link (25), who classified them in four groups according to the site of action and the part of electron transfer within the bc_1-complex that is blocked by a particular inhibitor. Group I includes compounds of natural origin, such as myxothiazol, strobilurines, and oudemansins. These quinol antagonists contain a β-methoxyacrylate group that resembles part of the structure of ubiquinone. As a result, they block ubiquinol oxidation at center Q_o. Myxothiazol, which is produced by the myxobacterium *Myxococcus fulvus,* is the most tightly binding and potent inhibitor. In beef heart mitochondria, 0.58 molecule of myxothiazol per bc_1-complex produces 50% inhibition of respiration (26).

Group II inhibitors also resemble ubiquinone in that they contain a 6-hydroxyquinone fragment as a common structural element. They block electron transfer between the Rieske Fe_2S_2 center and cytochrome $c1$, thereby inhibiting the reduction of cytochrome b_L. This group includes undecylhydroxydioxobenzothiazole (UHDBT), undecylhydroxynaphtoquinone (UHNQ), and similar compounds (25).

Group III includes inhibitors acting at center Q_i. The antibiotics antimycin A, funiculosin, and quinolones such as heptylhydroxyquinoline-N oxide (HHQNO) inhibit electron transfer from heme b_H to a quinone or semiquinone molecule bound at center Q_i. The herbicide 2,4-dichlorophenoxyacetic acid (2,4-D) may also belong to this class of inhibitors of complex III (27). The most frequently used inhibitor of this group is antimycin, which is produced by various *Streptomyces* species and has the highest affinity for the bc_1-complex among all the other inhibitors ($K_d = 3.2 \times 10^{-11}$ M). The structural factors required for inhibition were studied with synthetic antimycin analogues (28). Mitochondria are not the only targets of antimycin in a cell, however. Antimycin also inhibits peroxisomal β-oxidation by inhibiting acyl-coenzyme A oxidase (29) and interferes with thyroid hormone transport in the cell nucleus (30). However, all such effects require much higher concentrations of antimycin than are necessary to completely inhibit mitochondrial respiration.

In mitochondria, inhibition of the respiratory chain by group III inhibitors is not the only harmful effect. The generation of superoxide and hydrogen peroxide (reactive oxygen species) contributes to both the cellular and tissue toxicity of antimycin, funiculoside, and HHQNO (31–33). The mechanism of reactive oxygen species generation consists of one-electron reduction of oxygen by a semiquinone, which is normally formed at center Q_o but which is rapidly oxidized by b_L:b_H (see above). In the presence of group III inhibitors, the transfer of electrons from b_H to center Q_i is blocked, which increases the probability of one electron reduction of molecular oxygen by the ubisemiquinone at center Q_o (34).

Two more classes of complex III inhibitors of toxicological importance should be considered, namely substituted phenols, including those with uncoupling capability, and metal cations. Many phenolic uncouplers partially inhibit complex III. This can be easily observed in experiments with isolated mitochondria; a curve of the dependence of respiration rate on uncoupler concentration is typically bell-shaped both with NADH-dependent substrates and with succinate (in the former case because of the inhibition of both complex I and III). The structure-activity relationships of inhibition of the bc_1-complex by phenolic uncouplers and by a series of substituted nitrophenols have been studied (35); however, no simple conclusions were made.

Zinc ions are also known to inhibit mitochondrial electron transport at complex III (36, 37). Zn^{2+} (5 μM; $K_i = 10^{-7}$ at pH 7.0) induces practically complete inhibition of activity of the bc_1-complex isolated from beef heart mitochondria; zinc ions bind reversibly and with high affinity to a single site that Link & von Jagow (37) suggested is part of the proton channel at center Q_o. With isolated mitochondria, 2 μM of Zn^{2+} inhibits succinate:O_2 activity by 40%, whereas more than 400 μM is required to achieve 90% inhibition. Among 20 other di- and trivalent metal cations tested, Hg^{2+}, Ag^+, Cu^{2+}, and Cd^{2+} were all found to be inhibitory of complex III, but less effective (37).

Inhibitors of center Q_i such as antimycin, funiculosin, and HQNO (hydroxyquinoline-N-oxide) are specific for the bc_1 complex, whereas naturally occurring center Q_o inhibitors, which possess ubiquinone-like structure, are less specific and inhibit complex I as well (38, 39). It should be noted, however, that the concentrations at which Q_o center inhibitors affect complex I activity are substantially higher than is necessary to completely block the bc_1 complex (39).

Inhibitors of Complex IV, Cytochrome c Oxidase   Complex IV, cytochrome c oxidase (COX) (EC 1.9.3.1) is a heme/copper terminal oxidase that uses cytochrome c as electron donor (Figure 1*C*). According to the classification by Nicholls & Chance (40), COX inhibitors fall into four categories: (*a*) heme-binding inhibitors that are noncompetitive with both O_2 and cytochrome c (e.g. azide, cyanide, and sulfide), (*b*) inhibitors competitive with oxygen, such as carbon monoxide (CO) and nitric oxide (NO), (*c*) inhibitors competitive with cytochrome c (polycations); and (*d*) noncompetitive inhibitors not affecting the heme groups, such as phosphate ions and alkaline pH.

Noncompetitive Heme-Binding Inhibitors   Cyanide and azide are the oldest known and the most frequently used inhibitors of COX. Both react with heme a_3 noncompetitively with oxygen [for a review, see Nicholls & Chance (40)]. Contrary to the wide-spread belief, cyanide is neither a specific nor a selective inhibitor of COX. It inhibits other heme-containing enzymes (e.g. peroxidases, cytochrome c) with the same or even greater potency. The pattern of inhibition of mitochondrial respiration by azide is unique in that state 3 respiration is much more sensitive to inhibition ($IC_{50} \sim 60\ \mu M$) than state 4 respiration ($\geq 300\ \mu M$ azide), and the inhibition of state 3 can be released by various protonophoric uncouplers (41). These features can be explained by the well-known inhibitory effect of azide on ATP synthase and uncoupling of oxidative phosphorylation.

Hydrogen sulfide (H_2S) is a naturally occurring toxic compound [the toxicity of sulfide has been reviewed (42)]. Inhalation of high concentrations (50–400 ppm) of gaseous H_2S inhibits COX activity in mitochondria of rat lungs both in vivo and ex vivo (43). Brain cytochrome c oxidase activity was reported to be particularly sensitive to inhibition (IC_{50} for $H_2S = 0.13\ \mu M$) (44). Like cyanide, sulfide is not a specific inhibitor of COX; it inhibits other hemoproteins as well (e.g. superoxide dismutase, glutathione peroxidase, glutathione reductase, and catalase (45)).

Formic acid (HCOOH) is a natural by-product of metabolism of methanol, methyl ethers, esters, and amides. Its toxicity is due primarily to inhibition of mitochondrial respiration resulting in histotoxic hypoxia [for a review, see Liesivuori & Savolainen (46)]. Formate inhibits COX with a K_i depending on the degree of oxidase reduction and varying from 30 mM (100% reduction) to 1 mM (100% oxidation) at pH 7.4. The apparent affinity increases with acidification. The formic acid (HCOOH) molecule binds to ferric heme iron of cytochrome a_3, thus preventing its reduction by cytochrome c. In isolated mitochondria, formate also inhibits succinate–cytochrome c reductase activity in a reaction competitive with succinate.

Hydroxylamine (NH_2OH), a naturally occurring product of cellular metabolism, exerts various toxic effects [some of the biological activities of hydroxylamine are reviewed elsewhere (47)]. At millimolar concentrations, hydroxylamine inhibits mitochondrial respiration with an azide–like pattern, state 3 being particularly sensitive. Hydroxylamine can form complexes with copper and iron, and it also can generate NO, a potent COX inhibitor.

O2 Competitive Inhibitors   Inhibition of COX by CO or NO is competitive toward oxygen. Binding of CO to cytochrome oxidase is reversible; dissociation of the complex is strongly promoted by light. There are several reports indicating the significance of CO inhibition of COX in vivo (48, 49). CO–induced inhibition of COX could also be a mechanism of toxicity of some xenobiotics, such as dichloromethane (methylene chloride), which liberates CO as a product of its metabolism by cytochrome P4502E1 (50).

NO is a naturally occurring metabolite that exerts a number of important biological activities. It has long been known that NO binds reversibly to COX. However, the inhibition of mitochondrial respiration by NO was shown only recently (see 51 and references therein). This inhibition shows competition with oxygen, the K_i being lower at low oxygen concentrations. Although the exact mechanism of inhibition is not clear, it probably involves the reaction of NO with oxidized Cu_B of the COX binuclear center, leading to the reduction of this metal center and formation of nitrite.

Cytochrome c Competitive Inhibitors   Polycations represent a different type of inhibition of COX activity that does not involve direct binding to heme. High-molecular-weight polylysine, histones, cationic lysosomal proteins, protamine, and some other high-molecular-weight synthetic and natural polycations are known to inhibit mitochondrial respiration as well as isolated COX activity (52). The inhibition is competitive toward cytochrome *c*. These compounds bind to anionic sites of mitochondrial membranes and COX with high affinity, thus decreasing the mobility of the cytochrome and/or preventing the proper orientation of the cytochrome *c* molecule toward its reduction and oxidation sites. A polycationic type of inhibition was also suggested for the inhibitory effect of adriamycin–Fe^{3+} complexes, where COX was competitively inhibited by the complex with a K_i of 12 μM, whereas free adriamycin was without effect (53).

Other Inhibitors   Local anesthetics such as dibucaine, lidocaine, and tetracaine are widely used in clinical practice. In vitro, these compounds inhibit mitochondrial respiration at the level of COX. Because of the correlation between hydrophobicity and inhibitory potency, it is proposed that this activity reflects the nonspecific interaction of anesthetics with the lipid phase in which COX is embedded (54). Others (55), however, have shown that dibucaine inhibits the oxidase activity by interacting with cytochrome *a* and its associated copper. However, significant inhibition is observed only at millimolar concentrations of anesthetics.

Hydrophobic metal chelators inhibit COX activity as well, most probably by chelating a copper atom of the binuclear center. The inhibition occurs at relatively low concentrations; bathocuproine at 14 μM inhibits oxidase activity by 75% both in mitochondria and in solubilized enzyme (56). However, the physiological significance of this class of inhibitors is not clear.

Psychosine (galactosylsphingosine), a cytotoxic lipid that is accumulated in brain cells of some animals and humans with Krabbe disease, is a powerful inhibitor of complex IV. In vitro, it produces 50% inhibition at concentrations of 0.1 μg/mg of mitochondria (57).

Recently, it was found that 4-hydroxynonenal, a major product of lipid peroxidation, can inhibit COX activity. This establishes a potential direct link between oxidative stress and inhibition of respiration, which may represent a primary mechanism of oxidative stress–induced damage to mitochondria (58).

Inhibitors of ATP-Synthetase

H^+-ATP synthetase (complex V, EC 3.6.1.34) uses the $\Delta\tilde{\mu}_H+$ to synthesize ATP from ADP and phosphate (Figure 1D). It is the major source of ATP in aerobic cells [for recent reviews, see Junge et al (59), Boyer (60)]. The enzyme is reversible. Under some conditions it can work as an ATPase to hydrolyze ATP and generate $\Delta\tilde{\mu}_H+$. Evolutionarily, the mitochondrial ATP synthetase is a well-conserved protein, and it is not surprising that many of its known inhibitors are of natural, mostly fungal, origin. These antibiotics were intensively searched for, isolated, and studied because of their selective and potent toxicity against other fungi. Examples of mycotoxins possessing significant ATPase inhibiting activity are the aurovertins A-E, leucinostatins A and B, venturicidin and ossamycin, efrapeptin, and the classic inhibitors of mitochondrial ATPase, oligomycins A-D. Consumption of rice contaminated with the mycotoxin citreoviridin, which also inhibits mitochondrial ATPase, causes symptoms of acute cardiac beri-beri (convulsions, vomiting, ascending paralysis, and respiratory arrest) in humans and experimental animals. Injection of oligomycin to rats causes a marked inhibition of oxygen consumption and severe lactic acidemia with no change in arterial pO_2 (61). The mechanisms of inhibition of ATPase by the mycotoxins involve binding the F^1 subunit or to the F^0 subunit of the enzyme to block proton conduction. With isolated mitochondria, the range of IC_{50} values for ATPase inhibition for all mycotoxins is 0.1–5.0 nmol/mg of protein (62–64). The acute 50% lethal dose (LD_{50}) values (intraperitoneally, and subcutaneously) are on the order of 1–10 mg/kg in rats and mice (64–67).

Although mycotoxins are the most powerful inhibitors of mitochondrial ATP synthetase, many other compounds and classes of compounds share this same activity. Examples include naturally occurring flavonoids (68), a commonly used beta-adrenergic receptor antagonist propranolol (69), local anesthetics (70), the herbicide paraquat (71), several pyrethroid insecticides (72) and possibly DDT and parathion (73, 74), diethylstilbestrol (75), several cationic dyes (76), and organotin compounds (64, 77).

Uncouplers of Oxidative Phosphorylation

A wide variety of compounds indispensable to our everyday activities are uncouplers of mitochondrial oxidative phosphorylation. The most abundant are compounds used as drugs or pesticides. Uncoupling activity is considered to be a common characteristic of antiinflammatory agents with an ionizable group (78); nonsteroidal antiinflammatory drugs (diclofenac, aspirin, nimesulide, meloxicam, piroxicam, and indomethacin) exert an uncoupling effect both in isolated mitochondria and in perfused rat liver at concentrations that correspond to the pharmacological doses employed in antipyretic and antiinflammatory treatments (79, 80). Antipsychotic and antidepressant drugs (81, 82), some of the antitumor drugs (83, 84), a number of plasticizers, lipid-lowering drugs and other peroxisome proliferators (85–88), antimycotics (89, 90), drugs used to treat trypanosomiasis and leishmaniasis (91), numerous antihelmintics (92–94), antispermatogenic drugs (95), agents that are implicated in causing Reye's syndrome (96), and various herbicides and insecticides (27, 97–99) are all reported to uncouple isolated mitochondria.

In the mitochondria-related literature, the term uncoupler is traditionally suffixed with the words "of oxidative phosphorylation," which emphasizes the impact of these compounds on mitochondrial ATP production. Uncouplers are compounds that decrease the efficiency of ATP production. Unfortunately, such a definition implicitly blurs the fundamental fact that all of the other known energy-dependent metabolic functions of mitochondria are equally affected by all of the known uncouplers of oxidative phosphorylation (perhaps, with the only exception being the so-called decouplers, which are not considered here due to the highly debatable nature of the subject). In this treatise, the term uncoupling is taken to mean any energy-dissipating process competing for energy with routine mitochondrial functions, thus inducing a metabolically futile wasting of energy. This then explains the hyperpyresis that is characteristic of intoxication with mitochondrial uncouplers. Under such a definition, any xenobiotic-induced enhancement of any energy-consuming mitochondrial function (such as ion, metabolite, or protein transport across the inner membrane) would also be considered uncoupling.

The following sections review some of the properties of representative uncouplers of different chemical classes that we believe to be most important to the fields of pharmacology and toxicology on the basis of abundance and use characteristics (Figures 2–5). Critical reviews are cited where available, which can be consulted for more detailed information on a particular class of uncouplers. Some additional types of uncouplers and uncoupling mechanisms are listed in Figure 2.

Lipophilic Weak Acids The majority of compounds possessing protonophoric activity are lipophilic weak acids (Figure 2) with a pK_a in the range of 5–7. Generally, structural requirements for uncoupling activity include the presence of

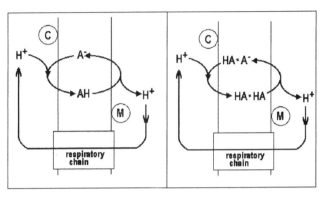

Figure 2   Lipophilic weak acids: proton shuttling. All the known uncouplers of this type can selectively increase the permeability of natural and artificial lipid membranes to protons. Numerous studies with artificial bilayer membranes reveal two major mechanisms of proton translocation. According to the first model, a molecule of a lipophilic weak acid (HA) penetrates the lipid core of the membrane both in the protonated H form and in the ionized A$^-$ form. This model describes the proton shuttling mechanism of potent uncouplers such as FCCP, CCCP, S-13, and SF6847. In mitochondria, an undissociated uncoupler molecule dissolves in the lipid of the inner mitochondrial membrane, crosses it, and releases the proton into the mitochondrial matrix (M), which is slightly more alkaline than the external medium. This discharges the ΔpH; in turn, the ionized negatively charged molecule diffuses across the membrane, down the gradient of electric field, and discharges the membrane potential. At the cytoplasmic side of the membrane (C), it can again bind a proton and complete the cycle. The second model of proton shuttling differs in that the charged molecule of an uncoupler crosses the membrane as a HA$_2{}^-$ dimer, a complex of the protonated (HA) and anionic (A$^-$) forms of the weak acid. This mechanism describes the proton translocation by uncouplers similar to 2,4-dinitrophenol and substituted benzimidazoles. Both mechanisms result in the net transport of protons catalyzed by cyclic movement of an uncoupler molecule, which dissipates $\Delta\tilde{\mu}_H+$ [for a review, see Mc-Laughlin & Dilger (101)].

an acid-dissociable group, bulky lipophilic groups, and a strong electron-withdrawing moiety [for reviews, see Terada (100), McLaughlin & Dilger (101)]. These properties determine the important features of proton-transporting lipophilic weak acids that affect their uncoupling efficiency, such as the solubility in lipid membranes, the stability of the ionized form in the membrane, and the ability to release and bind a proton. The most representative uncouplers of this class are substituted phenols, trifluoromethylbenzimidazoles, salicylanilides, and carbonyl cyanide phenylhydrazones.

2,4-Dinitrophenol and Other Substituted Phenols   Substituted phenols are the best represented and studied class of mitochondrial poisons. Some of these compounds, such as 2,4-dinitrophenol (DNP) have a long and curious history. There were times when DNP was considered to be a miracle drug, a new hope in an

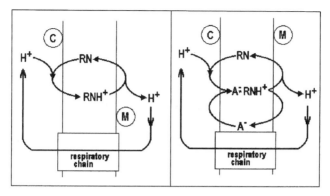

Figure 3 Local anesthetics: lipophilic ion pairs. Uncoupling by a mechanism involving an electrophoretic H^+ uniport does not necessarily require the compound to be a proton-ophore. A concerted action of some compounds exerting no protonophoric activity can significantly increase membrane permeability to protons. Many pharmacologically active amines with local anesthetic properties are known to exert various effects on mitochondria, including uncoupling (see 102 and references therein). It was shown that uncoupler-like activity of amine local anesthetics could be fully explained by their ability to form lipophilic ion pairs with certain anions. Electrophoretic H^+ uniport and uncoupling results from transmembrane cycling of neutral amine, charged anion, and neutral ion pair (102, 103). More lipid-soluble local anesthetics, such as bupivacaine, can uncouple mitochondria even in the absence of pair–forming lipophilic anions (103). General anesthetics: changes in fluidity of the inner membrane. Millimolar concentrations of the general anesthetics chloroform and halothane inhibit ATP synthesis in rat liver mitochondria, stimulate mito-chondrial ATPase activity, and reduce the respiratory control and ADP:O ratio. The same concentrations of halothane and chloroform increase the fluidity of the inner mitochondrial membrane (104). An increase in membrane fluidity potentiates the intrinsic proton per-meability of lipid bilayer, the so-called proton leak. In addition, it may affect the func-tioning of proteins embedded in the membrane, such as ATP synthetase and proton pumps, decreasing the degree of coupling between electron transport and proton pumping, thus decreasing overall efficiency of energy conservation.

everlasting fight of humankind against obesity. These hopes died in the 1930s along with those unlucky patients who had received the "miracle drug" (cf 119). However, the wide-spread use of DNP and compounds such as the phenolic her-bicides and insecticides has sustained the interest in this mode of toxicity. In man, the syndrome of DNP poisoning "consists of lassitude, malaise, headache, increased perspiration, thirst, and dyspnea which may progress to hyperpyrexia, profound weight loss, respiratory failure, and death" (120). In mice, the LD_{50} for DNP is 141 μmol/kg (121). The uncoupling efficiency of substituted phenols (expressed as the concentration inducing 50% uncoupling) varies from 30–100 μM for relatively inefficient uncouplers like dicoumarol and DNP, to 5–10 nM for SF6847 [2,6-di-tert-butyl-4-(2',2'-dicyanovinyl)phenol]. The latter compound is the most powerful uncoupler known, and the "turnover number" of the SF6847

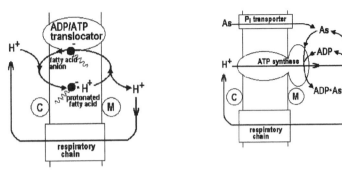

Figure 4   Long-chain free fatty acids: protein–mediated uncoupling. The phenomenology of long-chain free fatty acids–induced uncoupling resembles that of classical protonophores such as 2,4-dinitrophenol. The protonophoric action requires that fatty acids (FAs) cross the membrane in both the protonated and the anionic forms. Protonated long-chain FAs are sufficiently hydrophobic and easily penetrate lipid membranes. However, in a deprotonated form they cannot cross the hydrophobic barrier because of the strong negative charge. The mechanism of apparent protonophoric action of FA remained a mystery for about 40 years [for a review, see Wojtczak & Schonfeld (105)]. Recently, it was shown that ATP/ADP translocase, an integral protein of the inner mitochondrial membrane, facilitates FA anion transport across the hydrophobic core of the inner membrane, thus allowing net H^+ cycling (106). It has also been suggested that the aspartate/glutamate antiporter, which is another membrane protein of the same family, participates in FAs–induced uncoupling (107). Uncouplers acting at the level of ATP synthetase. It has long been known that arsenate uncouples oxidative phosphorylation and releases state 4 respiration of isolated mitochondria, the effects being completely inhibited by oligomycin (108). The sensitivity to this highly specific (109) antibiotic and the well–known ability of arsenate to participate in phosphorylation reactions points to the involvement of ATP synthase in the mechanism of arsenate's action. It was shown that arsenate uncouples oxidative phosphorylation by a mechanism involving intramitochondrial synthesis of ADP-arsenate, followed by its rapid nonenzymatic hydrolysis (110). The formation of ADP-arsenate in an ATP synthetase–catalyzed reaction at the expense of the protonmotive force and its rapid hydrolysis establishes a futile energy-dissipating cycle in the matrix of a mitochondrion. This cycle abolishes energy conservation and turns normally functioning ATP synthetase into an energy-burning furnace. Strictly speaking, it is not correct to term this kind of energy-dissipating mechanism as uncoupling. The oxidation of substrates is well coupled with phosphorylation, but the product of the phosphorylation is unstable and cannot serve to conserve energy. However, we use the term uncoupling to emphasize the futile nature of this pathway.

molecule in mitochondrial membranes is close to the theoretical maximum according to Brownian motion of the uncoupler molecule (122). Structure-activity studies with various substituted phenols (123–125) confirmed the protonophoric mechanism of their action in mitochondria and revealed important correlations between the uncoupling activity and physicochemical properties such as hydro-

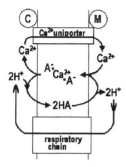
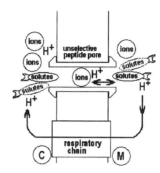

Figure 5   A23187-mediated uncoupling: Ca^{2+} cycling and other mechanisms. The mechanism consists of A23187-mediated ΔpH–dissipating release of cations from the organelle followed by reuptake of Ca^{2+}, which is mediated by an electrogenic Ca^{2+} uniporter of the inner mitochondrial membrane. The uptake of Ca^{2+} by the uniporter decreases the membrane potential, thus completing the energy-dissipating cycle (111). Another mitochondria-specific mechanism of A23187-mediated uncoupling is related to the ability of this ionophore to bind and transport Mg^{2+}. It was reported that A23187 can severely deplete mitochondria of endogenous Mg^{2+}. In the presence of physiological concentrations of K^+, the Mg^{2+} depletion activates a latent K^+ uniport pathway in the mitochondrial membrane. This, in turn, induces electrogenic uptake of potassium ions, which is accompanied by membrane depolarization and stimulation of respiration (112, 113). The protein conferring the K^+ uniport activity was not identified; however, the participation of Ca^{2+} uniporter was proposed (114). The Me^+ uniport pathway activated in mitochondria by Mg^{2+} depletion can be a more universal mechanism of divalent ionophore–induced uncoupling. Another *Streptomyces* antibiotic, oleficin, was shown to uncouple liver mitochondria, the features being similar to the divalent cationophoric mechanism of A23187–induced K^+ uniport (115). A23187–mediated uncoupling has been demonstrated in isolated mitochondria and may also occur in situ, in tissue, and in isolated cells. However, taking into account the high concentrations of Ca^{2+} in biological fluids and the high activity of the mitochondrial Ca^{2+} uniporter, it is probable that exposure to A23187 specifically uncouples mitochondria in situ even without interacting directly with organelles. Flooding of cellular cytosol with Ca^{2+} would stimulate continuous electrogenic uptake of the cation into mitochondria, which will compete with other energy-dependent processes and induce osmotic swelling and damage of organelles. Membrane-active peptides. Various short peptides (especially of fungal origin) are known to increase the conductance of lipid bilayer membranes. Such peptides are usually amphipathic, 15–20 amino acids long, and enriched in α-aminoisobutyric acid. They form channels of various sizes in bilayer lipid membranes, thus inducing high permeability to normally impermeable ions and solutes. Alamethicin is the most widely studied peptide of this class; it forms voltage-gated pores and exerts numerous biological activities (116, 117). Structural requirements for uncoupling activity were studied with synthetic derivatives of alamethicin A. It was shown that a minimum peptide chain length of 13 residues is necessary for uncoupling activity. Peptide esters were more potent than the corresponding acid forms, and in general the structural requirements for uncoupling activity were similar to those for ionophoretic activity in liposomes (118).

phobicity, acidity, and the stability of ionized intermediate in the lipid phase of a membrane [for a review, see Terada (122)].

Trifluoromethylbenzimidazoles   2-Trifluoromethylbenzimidazoles (TFBs) were introduced in the early 1960s as a new class of potent herbicidal and insecticidal compounds. The high toxicity of these compounds to animals was immediately evident, and much effort has been aimed at the synthesis of derivatives in an attempt to obtain an "acceptably safe and yet active herbicide" (126). In mitochondria, many of these compounds act similar to DNP (Figure 2); however, their efficiency is significantly higher. The most active uncoupler of this class is 4,5,6,7-tetrachloro-2-trifluoromethylbenzimidazole (TTFB), which produces 50% uncoupling of oxidative phosphorylation (measured as ATP synthesis) at 8 x 10^{-8} M in isolated liver mitochondria (127) (compared with 8 × 10^{-6} M for DNP under the same experimental conditions). Similar to other acidic uncouplers, the efficiency of TFB derivatives increases with the acidity of the dissociable -NH- group (128, 129).

The toxicity of a number of substituted TFBs in mice, houseflies, and honeybees was compared with their uncoupling efficiency in isolated mitochondria (130). In this study, the LD_{50} in mice for a number of TFBs and other uncouplers, such as salicylanilide, dinitrophenol, and phenylhydrazone type, was plotted against their uncoupling activity in isolated mouse liver and brain mitochondria. A reasonably good correlation was obtained; generally, the toxicity increased with the increase in uncoupling efficiency. In the same study, it was also found that with some of the TFB derivatives, brain mitochondria were three to five times more sensitive than liver mitochondria. The principal manifestations of toxicity of injected TFBs were dyspnea, occasional salivation, weakness, and death in an extended position with immediate rigor mortis (126, 130), which is typical for other mitochondrial uncouplers as well.

Salicylanilides   Salicylanilide   (2-hydroxy-N-phenylbenzamide)   derivatives have been shown to possess bacteriostatic, fungicidal, and molluscicidal activity; some of the members of this class are widely used as anticestodal, antitrematodal, and antihelmintic drugs. Many of these chemicals are protonophoric uncouplers of mitochondrial oxidative phosphorylation (127, 128). The most efficient uncoupler of this class is S-13, 2',-5-dichloro-4'-nitro-3-tert-butyl-salicylanilide, which induces complete uncoupling at only 0.2 molecule per cytochrome oxidase heme *aa*3 (which is about 42 pmol of uncoupler per mg of mitochondrial protein). The mechanism of the uncoupling action is similar to that of other A⁻ protonophores (129). Structure-activity relationships with 28 derivatives substituted at both the salicylic acid moiety and the aniline moiety revealed that both hydrophobicity and electron-withdrawing power were necessary for uncoupling activity (130).

Carbonyl Cyanide Phenylhydrazones   Carbonyl cyanide *p*-trifluromethoxy-phenyl-hydrazone (FCCP) and carbonyl cyanide *meta*-chlorophenylhydrazone

(CCCP) are probably the most frequently used uncouplers in experimental biology. In mice, FCCP and CCCP induce rapid rigor mortis at death after intraperitoneal injection (131, 132), with LD_{50}s of 32 and 40 μmol/kg, respectively. These compounds were introduced in the early 1960s by Heytler & Prichard (133, 134) and since that time have remained among the most powerful commercially available protonophoric uncouplers. The uncoupling activity of these phenylhydrazones correlates well with their protonophoric activity (135), and the requirements for maximal uncoupling efficiency are a lipophilicity (octanol/buffer partition coefficient) above 2×10^3 and a pKa (in diluted aqueous solution) between 4.5 and 5.5 (136).

The protonophoric activity, however, may not be the only mechanism by which these compounds interact with mitochondria. FCCP can form stable complexes with other mitochondria-active compounds, such as lipophilic amine local anesthetics and K^+-valinomycin. FCCP, CCCP, and other carbonyl cyanide phenylhydrazone ring-substituted analogs readily react with mitochondrial thiols and aminothiols (cysteine, glutathione), yielding corresponding N-(substituted phenyl)-N'-(alkylthiodicyano)-methylhydrazine derivatives. The reactivity of carbonyl cyanide phenylhydrazone with thiols is comparable to the reactivity of phenyl isothiocyanate and N-ethylmaleimide (134, 137), well-known SH-group modifiers. Thiols are known to protect and reverse the FCCP uncoupling effects in mitochondria (138) in vitro.

Other Types of Uncouplers

Protein–Mediated Uncoupling by Free Fatty Acids   Endogenous and exogenous long-chain free fatty acids (FFA) (Figure 4) have long been known to be efficient uncouplers of mitochondrial oxidative phosphorylation both in situ (e.g. in perfused liver) and in vitro (105). Studies over the past decade reveal that adenine nucleotide translocase, an integral protein of the inner mitochondrial membrane, is involved in the uncoupling action of long chain FFAs (106). Adenine nucleotide translocase—mediated uncoupling of mitochondria represents an important mechanism of FFA toxicity because many pathologies are associated with the accumulation of free long-chain FFA in the affected tissues. It should be expected that an increase in FFA would preferentially affect mitochondrial energetics, wasting energy at first and inhibiting respiration at higher concentrations. In mitochondria-rich tissue, the effect of excessive FFA accumulation can be devastating, strongly increasing local temperature and oxygen consumption at the expense of oxidizable substrates [e.g. as is the case in malignant muscle hyperthermia (139)]. Other fatty acid–like compounds, such as perfluorodecanoic acid, sulfuramide, and methyl-substituted hexadecanedioic acid, uncouple mitochondria apparently by the same mechanism (88, 140, 141).

Ionophores   Ionophores are compounds of various chemical structures that are capable of transporting small ions across a lipid membrane. There are hundreds of such compounds of both natural and synthetic origin. Physical and chemical properties of various ionophores, mechanisms of ion transport, and their numerous biological activities have been thoroughly reviewed (e.g. see 142, 143). Here, we mention only the most general properties of ionophores that render them efficient uncouplers of mitochondrial oxidative phosphorylation.

Ionophores can be divided into two general groups based on the mechanism of ion transport: a carrier type or a channel type. The latter is typical of short amphiphilic peptides that form channels of various sizes in lipid membranes (Figure 5). These channels can be selective toward small ions such as protons or K^+, depending on the particular peptide, the membrane structure, and the experimental conditions. Gramicidins (gramicidin A, D, and S) are the most studied antibiotics of this type and are powerful uncouplers of energy transduction in mitochondria. The short, linear gramicidins A and D assume helical conformation to form a channel whereas the cyclic gramicidin S forms a β-sheet structure, which disturbs lipid packing in the membrane. The resulting increase in membrane permeability toward protons and K^+ efficiently collapses $\Delta\tilde{\mu}_H+$ in mitochondria, due either to proton cycling or to electrophoretic K^+ transport (144, 145).

Carrier–type ionophores are able to form neutral or charged lipid-soluble complexes with an ion to facilitate its electrophoretic transport (uniport) or electroneutral exchange with protons (antiport) across a hydrophobic membrane. Depending on the chosen experimental conditions, these ionophores may or may not uncouple isolated mitochondria in vitro; Me^+/H^+ exchangers like nigericin can, by collapsing the ΔpH, actually hyperpolarize mitochondrial membranes. However, under in vivo conditions, alkali cations such as K^+ and penetrating anions such as inorganic P_i are present in high concentrations and mitochondrial membranes are energized to approximately 180 mV. This means that electrophoretic transport of a cation such as K^+ facilitated by valinomycin or a similar ionophore will proceed down the gradient of membrane potential, collapsing $\Delta\tilde{\mu}_H+$ and uncoupling the mitochondria. Moreover, because of the presence of P_i and the P_i/H^+ symporter in mitochondrial membranes, a significant amount of K^+ can be accumulated, which will induce osmotic swelling of the organelle and physical damage to the coupling membrane. This phenomenon is evidenced by the common experimental use of valinomycin to selectively eliminate mitochondria from cultured cells.

At high concentrations, even electroneutral Me^+/H^+ ionophores can uncouple mitochondria. For example, the K^+/H^+ exchanger nigericin at concentrations higher then 1 µM increases the conductance of black lipid membranes by forming a mobile dimer with both molecules of nigericin protonated and complexed with one K^+. If formed in the mitochondrial membrane, such a charge-transferring complex can indeed cause uncoupling due to electrophoretic cation transfer (146).

Ionophores that are selective to Ca^{2+} or Mg^{2+} can uncouple mitochondria by several different mechanisms. Some of these mechanisms are very specific because they involve intrinsic mitochondrial proteins, as with the divalent cation ionophore A23187 (calcimycin). This carboxylic polyether antibiotic is produced by *Streptomyces chartreusensis*. It forms a lipid-soluble 2:1 ionophore:Me^{2+} complex and transports divalent cations across lipid membranes by means of electroneutral $Me^{2+}/2H^+$ exchange. The induction of such cation transport per se cannot uncouple mitochondria. However, by dissipating the calcium gradient, A23187 establishes a futile, energy–dissipating cyclic flux of Ca^{2+}, which is responsible for the uncoupling activity of this compound (Figure 5).

Some of carrier–type ionophores are far more efficient in mitochondrial membranes than in other cellular membranes. For example, the valinomycin-K^+ complex turnover number is about 100 times higher in mitochondrial membranes than in erythrocytes. There is also evidence that valinomycin and nigericin increase the ionic conductivity of the inner mitochondrial membrane, but not that of the plasma membrane of intact lymphocytes (147) or yeast cells (148). What factors besides membrane potential may contribute to this membrane selectivity have yet to be identified.

Cationic Uncouplers   Several cationic compounds uncouple mitochondria by increasing membrane permeability to ions (Figure 3). The uncoupling action of compounds such as cyanine dye tri-S-$C_4(5)$, Cu^{2+}-(*o*-phenanthroline)$_2$ complex, and pentamidine requires the presence of inorganic phosphate and can be efficiently prevented by inhibiting the mitochondrial $P_i:H^+$ symporter. The molecular mechanism of uncoupling action of these compounds is obscure; however, it most likely is that all such P_i-dependent compounds affect the physical integrity of mitochondrial membranes. Indeed, it was recently shown that tri-S-$C_4(5)$ and Cu^{2+}-(*o*-phenanthroline)$_2$ uncouple by inducing the mitochondrial permeability transition pore (149).

Membrane-Active Peptides   Membrane-active peptides (Figure 5) can form channels, which are more or less selective to alkaline cations and/or protons, or they can form large pores allowing permeation of high-molecular-weight (>100 Da) solutes. Pore-forming peptides such as alamethicin possess a high affinity toward mitochondrial membranes because insertion of the peptide into the membrane and/or pore formation is driven by the electrical potential. These peptides induce nonspecific permeability changes, which results in oncotic swelling and disruption of the charged organelles.

Many short amphipathic peptides (especially of fungal origin) are known to uncouple oxidative phosphorylation in mitochondria at submicromolar concentrations by rendering the inner mitochondrial membrane permeable to various solutes (118, 150, 151). However, membrane–active peptides can also uncouple mitochondria in a much more specific manner. Mastoparan, an amphipathic peptide from wasp bee venom, induces the opening of a Ca^{2+}-dependent cyclosporine A–sensitive mitochondrial permeability transition pore. At higher concentrations, mastoparan depolarizes the mitochondrial inner membrane by acting on the lipid phase with no apparent involvement of the permeability transition pore (152).

Under certain circumstances, positively charged signal peptides, whose normal function is the targeting of newly synthesized proteins to mitochondria, can uncouple mitochondria (153, 154). The effect of the peptides on mitochondrial integrity was shown to be dependent on concentration. At low peptide/mitochondria ratios, signaling peptides induce a gradual lysis of the outer membrane and a release of enzymes from the intermembrane space. At higher peptide/mitochondria ratios, the permeability of the inner membrane increases, leading to complete uncoupling of respiration and dissipation of the membrane potential (155). Signal peptide–induced uncoupling is of great interest and importance for several reasons. These peptides are synthesized inside the cell and they are naturally and selectively targeted to the mitochondria by their very structure. In the case of malfunctioning of the protein import machinery, such peptides may accumulate within mitochondria, discharging the membrane potential and eliminating damaged organelles. Recently, signaling peptides have been explored as prototypes for creating new drugs selectively targeted to mitochondria within the cell (156).

Alternate Electron Acceptors   Mitochondrial electron carriers are distributed randomly within the inner membrane, but functionally they are arranged according to their respective redox potential. "Respiratory chain" refers to the sequence of electron and proton-transferring reactions. The efficiency of conversion of chemical energy from the oxidation of substrates into a useful form of $\Delta\bar{\mu}_H+$ depends on how precisely electrons follow their "prescribed" pathways through the ordered sequence of electron acceptors in the respiratory chain. In all known cases, any alternate pathway of electron transfer greatly diminishes the efficiency of energy conversion, speeding up the oxidation of substrates and diverting the excess energy to wasteful heat production (i.e. uncoupled oxidative phosphorylation). Technically, at least two kinds of alternate electron pathways can be distinguished. The first group are terminal electron acceptors, which are compounds capable of being reduced by an electron carrier of respiratory complex, thereby competing with the natural acceptor for this carrier. These compounds intercept electron flow and divert it toward their own reduction. In theory, these compounds can participate in so-called futile redox cycling, where a compound is reduced by the respiratory chain at the expense of energy derived from substrates and then oxidized back in a side reaction. Side reactions may include direct univalent reduction of oxygen, or reacting with protein thiols or glutathione. In either case, the net reaction is a stimulation of cyanide-insensitive respiration and consumption of both oxygen and reducing substrates with no net metabolism of the parent compound. As with all other uncouplers, this mitochondrial combustion leads to rapid dissipation of all transmembrane gradients, including the $\Delta\bar{\mu}_H+$.

The second group of alternate electron acceptors are so-called electron shunts, which accept electrons and feed them back to the respiratory chain at some higher redox potential. This allows electrons to bypass a portion of a respiratory complex or a whole segment of respiratory chain, excluding it from energy generation (see Figure 6). In these cases, the secondary electron acceptor that completes the redox cycle is a terminal complex of the mitochondrial electron transport chain, not molecular oxygen. Accordingly, such compounds do not generate oxygen free radicals or stimulate cyanide-insensitive respiration to the same extent as the redox cycling electron acceptors.

There are several examples of compounds that act as redox cycling alternate electron acceptors to uncouple mitochondrial oxidative phosphorylation. They include adriamycin, paraquat, and variously substituted naphthoquinones and N-nitrosoamines (157–159). The essence of their activity is the instability of the univalently reduced free radical intermediate, which under physiological conditions autooxidizes at the expense of reducing molecular oxygen to superoxide anion free radicals. Associated with this is a dramatic stimulation of oxygen

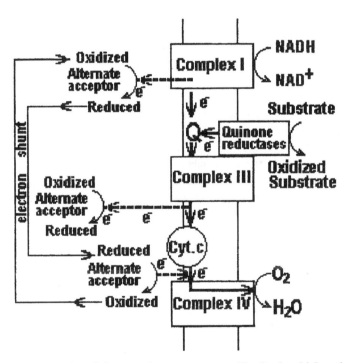

Figure 6   Interaction of alternate electron acceptors with mitochondrial respiratory chain. Alternate terminal electron acceptors are capable of being reduced by an electron carrier of the respiratory complex, thus competing with a natural acceptor of this carrier. These compounds intercept electron flow and divert it toward their own reduction. Electron shunts can be both reduced and oxidized by the respiratory chain, thus allowing electrons to bypass a portion of a respiratory complex or a whole segment of respiratory chain and excluding it from energy generation.

consumption and substrate oxidation, both of which are insensitive to inhibition by cyanide. Such chemicals stimulate the liberation of oxygen free radicals from isolated mitochondria, which most likely accounts for their observed cytotoxicity.

The antineoplastic agent doxorubicin (DXR) (adriamycin) represents a classic example of a compound that redox cycles on the mitochondrial electron transport chain [for a recent, thorough review, see Wallace (160)]. With a redox potential of approximately -320 mV, DXR is a good alternate electron acceptor for the mitochondrial respiratory chain. Incubation of DXR with cardiac mitochondria stimulates state 4 respiration and decreases the respiratory control ratio, as would be expected for an alternate electron acceptor. DXR accepts electrons exclusively from complex I of the mitochondrial respiratory chain to generate the univalently reduced semiquinone free radical intermediate (160, 161). This intermediate is highly unstable and rapidly autooxidizes to the parent quinone at the expense of reducing molecular oxygen to the superoxide anion free radical. Because the rate-limiting step in this redox cycle is the univalent reduction of the parent quinone, the overall reaction is controlled by the redox state of complex I; inhibitors of complexes III and IV, which increase the reduction state of complex I, stimulate the rate of DXR-induced oxygen consumption and free radical production (160, 161). The oxidation of mitochondrial glutathione (162), induction of the mito-chondrial permeability transition (163), and cardioselective oxidation of mito-chondrial DNA in vivo (164, 165) attest to the importance of mitochondrial redox cycling as a critical pathway in the mechanism of DXR-induced cardiotoxicity (160).

The aromatic amine 2-nitrosofluorene and its reduced hydroxylamine, N-hydroxy-aminofluorene, are metabolites of the carcinogen 2-acetylaminofluorene. 2-Nitrosofluorene is reduced at the level of complex I and complex III, and the reduced N-hydroxy-aminofluorene can be oxidized directly by oxygen to liberate oxygen free radicals, which appear to be central in mediating the pathogenic response (166, 167).

Naphthoquinones, both substituted and unsubstituted, represent another impor-tant class of alternate electron acceptors that redox cycle of the mitochondrial respiratory chain. Like DXR, naphthoquinones are reduced by complex I to their corresponding semiquinones, which autooxidize in aerobic solutions to the parent quinone and, in the process, generate superoxide anion free radicals from molec-ular oxygen. Structure-activity studies indicate that a univalent redox potential of -170 mV to $+50$ mV is the primary determinant of whether naphthoquinones are good alternate electron acceptors for the mitochondrial respiratory chain (168, 169). Furthermore, the rates of free radical generation correlate with the degree of mitochondrial dysfunction and the extent of cytotoxicity, implicating mito-chondrial dysfunction and free radical generation as critical factors in the mech-anism of cell killing by redox-active naphthoquinones (159, 170–174).

Not all naphthoquinones are pure terminal electron acceptors, however. Men-adione (vitamin K_3, 2-methyl-1,4-naphthoquinone) is a classical alternate electron acceptor that possesses a mixed chemical reactivity. It both redox cycles on the mitochondrial respiratory chain to generate oxygen free radicals and it is also a soft electrophile, which accounts for its arylation of critical cellular nucleophiles. Its cytotoxicity correlates with the depletion of ATP in hepatocytes (175, 176), which can be circumvented by providing glycolytic substrates (177). Like all redox-active naphthoquinones, menadione stimulates oxygen consumption in cell cultures (178). However, rather than reducing molecular oxygen, menadione serves as an electron shunt. It accepts electrons from complex I and feeds them back to complex IV, bypassing a portion of the electron transport chain (179). Some hepatotoxic fungal naphthoquinones, such as xanthomegnin and viomellein, act similarly to menadione (65). Another example of alternate electron shunts are the p-phenylenediamines (e.g. N,N,N',N'- tetramethyl-p-phenylenediamine), which are widely used industrial and household chemicals (180). A number of these compounds cause necrosis in cardiac and skeletal muscle tissues, with a concomitant decrease in respiratory control and ADP:O ratios (180).

Although terminal electron acceptors that redox cycle on the mitochondrial electron transport chain to generate oxygen free radicals are toxic and offer no benefit to the cell, electron shunts have been used therapeutically to combat certain bioenergetic disorders. The therapeutic rationale is that disorders associated with the inhibition or malfunction of complex III of the respiratory chain can be overcome by shuttling electrons from complex I to complex IV, bypassing the dysfunctional portion of the chain. The best example of this therapeutic strategy is the use of menadione to treat mitochondrial encephalomyopathies (181–183). This disorder is characterized by a functional deficiency in the bc_1 complex (complex III) and involves multiple organ systems, particularly those rich in mitochondria, such as nerve and muscle. Symptoms include ataxia and disorientation, muscle cramps and weakness, depressed phosphocreatine and ATP levels, and lactic acidosis. Administration of menadione to these individuals resolves many of the bioenergetic deficiencies (lactic acidosis and low phosphocreatine and ATP), with significant improvement in both neurological and muscular performance. This is an important demonstration that not all xenobiotics that interact with the mitochondrial respiratory chain are toxic and that it is possible to harness the energy of the electron transport chain to improve the bioenergetic well-being of the individual.

SIGNIFICANCE OF MITOCHONDRIAL-MEDIATED PATHOGENESIS

In this article, we review the various mechanisms by which xenobiotics (both therapeutics and toxicants) interact with the mitochondrial respiratory chain to alter the efficiency and/or capacity of oxidative phosphorylation. We also point out the major distinction in symptomology of poisoning by the two major classes of compounds that directly affect mitochondrial bioenergetics, inhibitors and uncouplers of mitochondrial respiration. The significance of these mechanisms of cytotoxicity is underscored by the hundreds of commonly used products and byproducts that are known to interfere with the mitochondrial electron transport chain. However, there are many additional modes by which chemicals can be cytotoxic wherein the mitochondrial bioenergetic deficit is secondary to another critical target, and perhaps intermediary in the ultimate expression of toxicity (184).

Examples of secondary bioenergetic deficiencies include exposures to agents that interfere with mitochondrial biogenesis, gene expression, or protein synthesis, or compounds that inhibit essential membrane transporters. There are numerous examples of chemicals that inhibit each of these active processes, all of which cause a secondary mitochondrial bioenergetic deficit that is not easily distinguished from a primary mitochondrial dysfunction on the basis of clinical features. Although these modes of toxicity are not covered in this review, the reader is cautioned to be mindful of these potential pathways of mitochondrial dysfunction.

Finally, mitochondrial dysfunction is not always manifested as a classical bioenergetic failure; lactic acidosis, neurological impairment, and incoordination and muscle fatigue are the classic symptoms. In deed, there is a burgeoning of recent evidence demonstrating a primary role for mitochondria in the apoptogenic process, integral to activation of the caspase enzyme cascade (cf 185–189). It is widely accepted that mitochondria play a critical role in determining necrotic versus apoptotic cell death and that mitochondrial bioenergetics plays a defining role in regulating cell cycling and differentiation. For example, mitochondrial dysfunction may trigger a premature apoptotic cell death, thereby preventing the clonal expansion of bioenergetically compromised cells. Failure of this mitochondrially regulated program of controlled cell death may be a critical event in the pathogenesis of hyperplastic disorders, including carcinogenesis. This is an explosive area of current research and is only recently yielding promising opportunities for therapeutic interventions (24, 190–192). Armed with this understanding of the important features of mitochondrial bioenergetics, we are now on the verge of developing more selective pesticides and new therapeutic strategies for treating the debilitating metabolic disorders associated with genetic defects or exposures to the numerous agents that selectively interfere with normal mitochondrial bioenergetics.

Visit the Annual Reviews home page at www.AnnualReviews.org.

LITERATURE CITED

1. Skulachev VP. 1994. Chemiosmotic concept of the membrane bioenergetics: What is already clear and what is still waiting for elucidation? *J. Bioenerg. Biomembr.* 26:589–98

2. Skulachev VP. 1988. *Membrane Bioenergetics.* New York: Springer-Verlag
3. Vinogradov AD. 1998. Catalytic properties of the mitochondrial NADH-ubiquinone oxidoreductase (complex I) and

the pseudo-reversible active/inactive enzyme transition. *Biochim. Biophys. Acta* 1364:169–85

4. Finel M. 1998. Organization and evolution of structural elements within complex I. *Biochim. Biophys. Acta* 1364: 112–21

5. Degli Esposti M. 1998. Inhibitors of NADH-ubiquinone reductase: an overview. *Biochim. Biophys. Acta* 1364:222–35

6. Miyoshi H, Ohshima M, Shimada H, Akagi T, Iwamura H, McLaughlin JL. 1998. Essential structural factors of annonaceous acetogenins as potent inhibitors of mitochondrial complex I. *Biochim. Biophys. Acta* 1365:443–52

7. Miyoshi H. 1998. Structure-activity relationships of some complex I inhibitors. *Biochim. Biophys. Acta* 1364:236–44

8. Lummen P. 1998. Complex I inhibitors as insecticides and acaricides. *Biochim. Biophys. Acta* 1364:287–96

9. Iwata S, Lee JW, Okada K, Lee JK, Iwata M, et al. 1998. Complete structure of the 11 subunit bovine mitochondrial cytochrome bc_1 complex. *Science* 281:64–71

10. Crofts AR, Berry EA. 1998. Structure and function of the cytochrome bc_1 complex of mitochondria and photosynthetic bacteria. *Curr. Opin. Struct. Biol.* 8:501–9

11. Trumpower BL. 1990. The protonmotive Q cycle. Energy transduction by coupling of proton translocation to electron transfer by the cytochrome bc_1 complex. *J. Biol. Chem.* 265:11409–12

12. Kraiczy P, Haase U, Gencic S, Flindt S, Anke T, et al. 1996. The molecular basis for the natural resistance of the cytochrome bc_1 complex from strobilurin-producing basidiomycetes to center Qp inhibitors. *Eur. J. Biochem.* 235:54–63

13. Vaidya AB, Lashgari MS, Pologe LG, Morrisey J. 1993. Structural features of *Plasmodium* cytochrome b that may underlie susceptibility to 8-aminoquinolines and hydroxynaphthoquinones. *Mol. Biochem. Parasitol.* 58:33–42

14. Ghelli A, Crimi M, Orsini S, Gradoni L, Zannotti M, et al. 1992. Cytochrome b of protozoan mitochondria: relationships between function and structure. *Comp. Biochem. Physiol. B* 103:329–38

15. Degli Esposti M, Ghelli A, Crimi M, Baracca A, Solaini G, et al. 1992. Cytochrome b of fish mitochondria is strongly resistant to funiculosin, a powerful inhibitor of respiration. *Arch. Biochem. Biophys.* 295:198–204

16. Degli Esposti M, Ghelli A, Butler G, Roberti M, Mustich A, Cantatore P. 1990. The cytochrome b of the sea urchin *Paracentrotus lividus* is naturally resistant to myxothiazol and mucidin. *FEBS Lett.* 263:245–47

17. Wiggins TE, Jager BJ. 1994. Mode of action of the new methoxyacrylate antifungal agent ICIA5504. *Biochem. Soc. Trans.* 22:68S

18. Ueki M, Taniguchi M. 1997. The mode of action of UK-2A and UK-3A, novel antifungal antibiotics from *Streptomyces* sp. 517–02. *J. Antibiot.* 50:1052–57

19. Fry M, Pudney M. 1992. Site of action of the antimalarial hydroxynaphthoquinone, 2-[trans-4-(4'-chlorophenyl) cyclohexyl]-3-hydroxy-1,4-naphthoquinone (566C80). *Biochem. Pharmacol.* 43:1545–53

20. Buxton D. 1998. Protozoan infections (*Toxoplasma gondii, Neospora caninum* and *Sarcocystis* spp.) in sheep and goats: recent advances. *Vet. Res.* 29:289–310

21. Williams RB. 1997. The mode of action of anticoccidial quinolones (6-decyloxy-4-hydroxyquinoline-3-carboxylates) in chickens. *Int. J. Parasitol.* 27:101–11

22. Fry M, Hudson AT, Randall AW, Williams RB. 1984. Potent and selective hydroxynaphthoquinone inhibitors of mitochondrial electron transport in *Eimeria tenella* (Apicomplexa: Coccidia). *Biochem. Pharmacol.* 33:2115–22

23. Wang CC. 1975. Studies of the mitochondria from *Eimeria tenella* and inhibition of the electron transport by

quinolone coccidiostats. *Biochim. Biophys. Acta* 396:210–19

24. Schulz P, Link TA, Chaudhuri L, Fittler F. 1990. Role of the mitochondrial bc_1-complex in the cytotoxic action of diethylstilbestrol-diphosphate toward prostatic carcinoma cells. *Cancer Res.* 50:5008–12

25. von Jagow G, Link TA. 1986. Use of specific inhibitors on the mitochondrial bc_1 complex. *Methods Enzymol.* 126: 253–71

26. Thierbach G, Reichenbach H. 1981. Myxothiazol, a new inhibitor of the cytochrome bc_1 segment of the respiratory chain. *Biochim. Biophys. Acta* 638:282–89

27. Palmeira CM, Moreno AJ, Madeira VM. 1994. Interactions of herbicides 2,4-D and dinoseb with liver mitochondrial bioenergetics. *Toxicol. Appl. Pharmacol.* 127:50–57

28. Miyoshi H, Tokutake N, Imaeda Y, Akagi T, Iwamura H. 1995. A model of antimycin A binding based on structure-activity studies of synthetic antimycin A analogues. *Biochim. Biophys. Acta* 1229:149–54

29. Vamecq J, Schepers L, Parmentier G, Mannaerts GP. 1987. Inhibition of peroxisomal fatty acyl-CoA oxidase by antimycin A. *Biochem. J.* 248:603–7

30. Valdivielso L, Bernal J. 1987. Inhibition of nuclear binding of triiodothyronine by antimycin A in cultured human fibroblasts. *Biochem. Biophys. Res. Commun.* 147:1241–44

31. Loschen G, Azzi A, Flohe L. 1973. Mitochondrial H_2O_2 formation at site II. *Hoppe Seylers Z. Physiol. Chem.* 354: 791–94

32. Ksenzenko M, Konstantinov AA, Khomutov GB, Tikhonov AN, Ruuge EK. 1983. Effect of electron transfer inhibitors on superoxide generation in the cytochrome bc_1 site of the mitochondrial respiratory chain. *FEBS Lett.* 155:19–24

33. Boveris A, Chance B. 1973. The mitochondrial generation of hydrogen peroxide. General properties and effect of hyperbaric oxygen. *Biochem. J.* 134: 707–16

34. Turrens JF. 1997. Superoxide production by the mitochondrial respiratory chain. *Biosci. Rep.* 17:3–8

35. Miyoshi H, Saitoh I, Iwamura H. 1993. Quantitative analysis of electron transport inhibition of rat-liver mitochondrial cytochrome bc_1 complex by nitrophenols. *Biochim. Biophys. Acta* 1143:23–28

36. Skulachev VP, Chistyakov VV, Jasaitis AA, Smirnova EG. 1967. Inhibition of the respiratory chain by zinc ions. *Biochem. Biophys. Res. Commun.* 26:1–6

37. Link TA, von Jagow G. 1995. Zink ions inhibit the Qp center of bovine heart mitochondria bc_1 complex by blocking a protonable group. *J. Biol. Chem.* 270:25001–6

38. Degli Esposti M. 1998. Inhibitors of NADH-ubiquinone reductase: an overview. *Biochim. Biophys. Acta* 1364:222–35

39. Degli Esposti M, Ghelli A, Crimi M, Estornell E, Fato R, Lenaz G. 1993. Complex I and complex III of mitochondria have common inhibitors acting as ubiquinone antagonists. *Biochim. Biophys. Res. Commun.* 190:1090–96

40. Nicholls P, Chance B. 1974. Cytochrome c oxidase. In *Molecular Mechanisms of Oxygen Activation,* ed. O Hayaishi, pp. 479–534. New York: Academic

41. Wilson DF, Chance B. 1966. Reversal of azide inhibition by uncouplers. *Biochem. Biophys. Res. Commun.* 23:751–56

42. Beauchamp RO, Bus JS, Popp JA, Boreiko CJ, Andjelkovich DA. 1984. A critical review of the literature on hydrogen sulfide toxicity. *CRC Crit. Rev. Toxicol.* 13:25–97

43. Khan AA, Schuler MM, Prior MG, Yong S, Coppock RW, et al. 1990. Effects of hydrogen sulfide exposure on lung mito-

chondrial respiratory chain enzymes in rats. *Toxicol. Appl. Pharmacol.* 103:482–90

44. Nicholson RA, Roth SH, Zhang A, Zheng J, Brookes J, et al. 1998. Inhibition of respiratory and bioenergetic mechanisms by hydrogen sulfide in mammalian brain. *Toxicol. Environ. Health* 54:491–507

45. Khan AA, Schuler MM, Coppock RW. 1987. Inhibitory effects of various sulfur compounds on the activity of bovine erythrocyte enzymes. *J. Toxicol. Environ. Health* 22:481–90

46. Liesivuori J, Savolainen H. 1991. Methanol and formic acid toxicity: biochemical mechanisms. *Pharmacol. Toxicol.* 69:157–63

47. Gross P. 1985. Biologic activity of hydroxylamine: a review. *Crit. Rev. Toxicol.* 14:87–99

48. Miro O, Casademont J, Barrientos A, Urbano-Marquez A, Cardellach F. 1998. Mitochondrial cytochrome c oxidase inhibition during acute carbon monoxide poisoning. *Pharmacol. Toxicol.* 82:199–202

49. Brown SD, Piantadosi CA. 1990. In vivo binding of carbon monoxide to cytochrome c oxidase in rat brain. *J. Appl. Physiol.* 68:604–10

50. Lehnebach A, Kuhn C, Pankow D. 1995. Dichloromethane as an inhibitor of cytochrome c oxidase in different tissues of rats. *Arch. Toxicol.* 69:180–84

51. Brown GC. 1995. Nitric oxide regulates mitochondrial respiration and cell functions by inhibiting cytochrome oxidase. *FEBS Lett.* 369:136–39

52. Mochan BS, Elliott WB, Nicholls P. 1973. Patterns of cytochrome oxidase inhibition by polycations. *J. Bioenerg.* 4:329–45

53. Hasinoff BB, Davey JP. 1988. The iron(III)-adriamycin complex inhibits cytochrome c oxidase before its inactivation. *Biochem. J.* 250:827–34

54. Casanovas AM, Nebot MFM, Courriere P, Oustrin J. 1983. Inhibition of cytochrome oxidase activity by local anesthetics. *Biochem. Pharmacol.* 32:2715–19

55. Stringer BK, Harmon HJ. 1990. Inhibition of cytochrome oxidase by dibucaine. *Biochem. Pharmacol.* 40:1077–81

56. Harmon HJ, Crane FL. 1974. Inhibition of cytochrome c oxidase by hydrophobic metal chelators. *Biochim. Biophys. Acta* 368:125–29

57. Igisu H, Nakamura M. 1986. Inhibition of cytochrome c oxidase by psychosine (galactosylsphingosine). *Biochem. Biophys. Res. Commun.* 137:323–27

58. Chen J, Schenker S, Frosto TA, Henderson GI. 1998. Inhibition of cytochrome c oxidase activity by 4-hydroxynonenal (HNE). Role of HNE adduct formation with the enzyme subunits. *Biochim. Biophys. Acta* 1380:336–44

59. Junge W, Lill H, Engelbrecht S. 1997. ATP synthase: an electrochemical transducer with rotatory mechanics. *Trends Biochem. Sci.* 22:420–23

60. Boyer PD. 1997. The ATP synthase—a splendid molecular machine. *Annu. Rev. Biochem.* 66:717–49

61. Kramar R, Hohenegger M, Srour AN, Khanakah G. 1984. Oligomycin toxicity in intact rats. *Agents Actions* 15:660–63

62. Lardy HA. 1980. Antibiotic inhibitors of mitochondrial energy transfer. *Pharmacol. Ther.* 11:649–60

63. Lardy H, Reed P, Lin CHC. 1975. Antibiotic inhibitors of mitochondrial ATP synthesis. *Fed. Proc.* 34:1707–10

64. Linnett PE, Beechey RB. 1979. Inhibitors of the ATP synthethase system. *Methods Enzymol.* 55:472–518

65. Ueno Y. 1985. The toxicology of mycotoxins. *Crit. Rev. Toxicol.* 14:99–132

66. Fukushima K, Arai T, Mori Y, Tsuboi M, Suzuki M. 1983. Studies on peptide antibiotics, leucinostatins. I. Separation, physico-chemical properties and biologi-

cal activities of leucinostatins A and B. *J. Antibiot.* 36:1606–12

67. Mikami Y, Fukushima K, Arai T, Abe F, Shibuya H, Ommura Y. 1984. Leucinostatins, peptide mycotoxins produced by *Paecilomyces lilacinus* and their possible roles in fungal infection. *Zentralbl. Bakteriol. Mikrobiol. Hyg. A* 257:275–83

68. Bohmont C, Aaronson LM, Mann K, Pardini RS. 1987. Inhibition of mitochondrial NADH oxidase, succinoxidase, and ATPase by naturally occurring flavonoids. *J. Nat. Prod.* 50:427–33

69. Wei YH, Lin TN, Hong CY, Chiang BN. 1985. Inhibition of the mitochondrial Mg^{2+}-ATPase by propranolol. *Biochem. Pharmacol.* 34:911–17

70. Dabbeni-Sala F, Schiavo G, Palatini P. 1990. Mechanism of local anesthetic effect on mitochondrial ATP synthase as deduced from photolabelling and inhibition studies with phenothiazine derivatives. *Biochim. Biophys. Acta* 1026:117–25

71. Palmeira CM, Moreno AJ, Madeira VM. 1995. Mitochondrial bioenergetics is affected by the herbicide paraquat. *Biochim. Biophys. Acta* 1229:187–92

72. Rao KS, Chetty CS, Desaiah D. 1984. In vitro effects of pyrethroids on rat brain and liver ATPase activities. *J. Toxicol. Environ. Health* 14:257–65

73. Moreno AJ, Madeira VM. 1991. Mitochondrial bioenergetics as affected by DDT. *Biochim. Biophys. Acta* 1060:166–74

74. Moreno AJ, Madeira VM. 1990. Interference of parathion with mitochondrial bioenergetics. *Biochim. Biophys. Acta* 1015:361–67

75. McEnery MW, Pedersen PL. 1986. Diethylstilbestrol. A novel F0-directed probe of the mitochondrial proton ATPase. *J. Biol. Chem.* 261:1745–52

76. Mai MS, Allison WS. 1983. Inhibition of an oligomycin-sensitive ATPase by cationic dyes, some of which are atypical uncouplers of intact mitochondria. *Arch. Biochem. Biophys.* 221:467–76

77. Snoeij NJ, Penninks AH, Seinen W. 1987. Biological activity of organotin compounds—an overview. *Environ. Res.* 44:335–53

78. Mahmud T, Rafi SS, Scott DL, Wrigglesworth JM, Bjarnason I. 1996. Nonsteroidal antiinflammatory drugs and uncoupling of mitochondrial oxidative phosphorylation. *Arthritis Rheum.* 39:1998–2003

79. Petrescu I, Tarba C. 1997. Uncoupling effects of diclofenac and aspirin in the perfused liver and isolated hepatic mitochondria of rat. *Biochim. Biophys. Acta* 1318:385–94

80. Moreno-Sanchez R, Bravo C, Vasquez C, Ayala G, Silveira LH, Martinez-Lavin M. 1999. Inhibition and uncoupling of oxidative phosphorylation by nonsteroidal anti-inflammatory drugs: study in mitochondria, submitochondrial particles, cells, and whole heart. *Biochem. Pharmacol.* 57:743–52

81. Burbenskaya NM, Nartsissov YR, Tsofina LM, Komissarova IA. 1998. The uncoupling effect of some psychotropic drugs on oxidative phosphorylation in rat liver mitochondria. *Biochem. Mol. Biol. Int.* 45:261–68

82. Souza ME, Polizello AC, Uyemura SA, Castro-Silva O, Curti C. 1994. Effect of fluoxetine on rat liver mitochondria. *Biochem. Pharmacol.* 48:535–41

83. Schwaller MA, Allard B, Lescot E, Moreau F. 1995. Protonophoric activity of ellipticine and isomers across the energy-transducing membrane of mitochondria. *J. Biol. Chem.* 270:22709–13

84. Rush GF, Rinzel S, Boder G, Heim RA, Toth JE, Ponsler GD. 1992. Effects of diarylsulfonylurea antitumor agents on the function of mitochondria isolated from rat liver and GC3/c1 cells. *Biochem. Pharmacol.* 44:2387–94

85. Keller BJ, Marsman DS, Popp JA, Thurman RG. 1992. Several nongenotoxic

carcinogens uncouple mitochondrial oxidative phosphorylation. *Biochim. Biophys. Acta* 1102:237–44

86. Keller BJ, Liang D, Thurman RG. 1991. 2-Ethylhexanol uncouples oxidative phosphorylation in rat liver mitochondria. *Toxicol. Lett.* 57:113–20

87. Zhou S, Wallace KB. 1999. The effect of peroxisome proliferators on mitochondrial bioenergetics. *Toxicol. Sci.* 48:82–89

88. Schnellmann RG, Manning RO. 1990. Perfluorooctane sulfonamide: a structurally novel uncoupler of oxidative phosphorylation. *Biochim. Biophys. Acta* 1016:344–48

89. Kawai K, Watanabe R, Nozawa Y, Nozaki M, Tsurumi K, Fujimura H. 1983. A new anti-mycotic drug tioxaprofen and its uncoupling effect on isolated mitochondria. *Experientia* 39:889–90

90. Kawai K, Shiojiri H, Watanabe R, Nozawa Y. 1983. Chlorination-induced enhancement of biological activities in imidazole antimycotics. A possible explanation to the molecular mechanism for their antimycotic activities. *Res. Commun. Chem. Pathol. Pharmacol.* 40:255–65

91. Moreno SN. 1996. Pentamidine is an uncoupler of oxidative phosphorylation in rat liver mitochondria. *Arch. Biochem. Biophys.* 326:15–20

92. McCracken RO, Carr AW, Stillwell WH, Lipkowitz KB, Boisvenue R, et al. 1993. Trifluoromethanesulfonamide anthelmintics. Protonophoric uncouplers of oxidative phosphorylation. *Biochem. Pharmacol.* 45:1873–80

93. Sjogren EB, Rider MA, Nelson PH, Bingham S Jr, Poulton AL, et al. 1991. Synthesis and biological activity of a series of diaryl-substituted alpha-cyano-beta-hydroxypropenamides, a new class of anthelmintic agents. *J. Med. Chem.* 34:3295–301

94. van Miert AS, Groeneveld HW. 1969. Anthelmintics, used for the treatment of fascioliasis as uncouplers of oxidative phosphorylation in warm blooded animals. *Eur. J. Pharmacol.* 8:385–88

95. Merola AJ, Brierley GP. 1970. Inhibition of mitochondrial oxidation and uncoupling of phosphorylation by antispermatogenic bis-dichloroacetamides. *Biochem. Pharmacol.* 19:1429–42

96. Trost LT, Lemasters JJ. 1996. The mitochondrial permeability transition: a new pathological mechanism of Reye's syndrome and toxic liver injury. *J. Pharmacol. Exp. Ther.* 278:1000–5

97. Zychlinski L, Zolnierowicz S. 1990. Comparison of uncoupling activities of chlorophenoxy herbicides in rat liver mitochondria. *Toxicol. Lett.* 52:25–34

98. Pritchard JB, Krall AR, Silverthorn SU. 1982. Effects of anionic xenobiotics on rat kidney. I. Tissue and mitochondrial respiration. *Biochem. Pharmacol.* 31:149–55

99. Olorunsogo OO, Malomo SO, Bababunmi EA. 1985. Protonophoric properties of fluorinated arylalkylsulfonamides. Observations with perfluidone. *Biochem. Pharmacol.* 34:2945–52

100. Terada H. 1981. The interaction of highly active uncouplers with mitochondria. *Biochim. Biophys. Acta* 639:225–42

101. McLaughlin SG, Dilger JP. 1980. Transport of protons across membranes by weak acids. *Physiol. Rev.* 60:825–63

102. Garlid KD, Nakashima RA. 1983. Studies on the mechanism of uncoupling by amine local anesthetics. Evidence for mitochondrial proton transport mediated by lipophilic ion pairs. *J. Biol. Chem.* 258:7974–80

103. Dabadie P, Bendriss P, Erny P, Mazat JP. 1987. Uncoupling effects of local anesthetics on rat liver mitochondria. *FEBS Lett.* 226:77–82

104. Rottenberg H. 1983. Uncoupling of oxidative phosphorylation in rat liver mito-

chondria by general anesthetics. *Proc. Natl. Acad. Sci. USA* 80:3313–17

105. Wojtczak L, Schonfeld P. 1993. Effect of fatty acids on energy coupling processes in mitochondria. *Biochim. Biophys. Acta* 1183:41–57

106. Andreyev AYu, Bondareva TO, Dedukhova VI, Mokhova EN, Skulachev VP, et al. 1989. The ATP/ADP-antiporter is involved in the uncoupling effect of fatty acids on mitochondria. *Eur. J. Biochem.* 182:585–92

107. Samartsev VN, Smirnov AV, Zeldi IP, Markova OV, Mokhova EN, Skulachev VP. 1997. Involvement of aspartate/glutamate antiporter in fatty acid-induced uncoupling of liver mitochondria. *Biochim. Biophys. Acta* 1319:251–57

108. Welle HF, Slater EC. 1967. Uncoupling of respiratory-chain phosphorylation by arsenate. *Biochim. Biophys. Acta* 143:1–17

109. Lardy HA. 1980. Antibiotic inhibitors of mitochondrial energy transfer. *Pharmacol. Ther.* 11:649–60

110. Moore SA, Moennich DM, Gresser MJ. 1983. Synthesis and hydrolysis of ADP-arsenate by beef heart submitochondrial particles. *J. Biol. Chem.* 258:6266–71

111. Reed PW, Lardy HA. 1972. A23187: a divalent cation ionophore. *J. Biol. Chem.* 247:6970–77

112. Bernardi P, Angrilli A, Ambrosin V, Azzone GF. 1989. Activation of latent K^+ uniport in mitochondria treated with the ionophore A23187. *J. Biol. Chem.* 264:18902–6

113. Nicolli A, Redetti A, Bernardi P. 1991. The K^+ conductance of the inner mitochondrial membrane. A study of the inducible uniport for monovalent cations. *J. Biol. Chem.* 266:9465–70

114. Kapus A, Szaszi K, Kaldi K, Ligeti E, Fonyo A. 1990. Ruthenium red inhibits mitochondrial Na^+ and K^+ uniports induced by magnesium removal. *J. Biol. Chem.* 265:18063–66

115. Meszaros L, Hoffmann L, Konig T, Horvath I. 1980. Interaction of oleficin with the inner membrane of rat liver mitochondria. *J. Antibiot.* 33:494–500

116. Fringeli UP, Fringeli M. 1979. Pore formation in lipid membranes by alamethicin. *Proc. Natl. Acad. Sci. USA* 76:3852–56

117. Ritov VB, Tverdislova IL, Avakyan TYu, Menshikova EV, Leikin YuN, et al. 1992. Alamethicin-induced pore formation in biological membranes. *Gen. Physiol. Biophys.* 11:49–58

118. Mathew MK, Nagaraj R, Balaram P. 1981. Alamethicin and synthetic peptide fragments as uncouplers of mitochondrial oxidative phosphorylation. Effect of chain length and charge. *Biochem. Biophys. Res. Commun.* 98:548–55

119. Racker E. 1974. *A New Look at Mechanisms in Bioenergetics.* New York: Academic

120. Leftwich RB, Floro JF, Neal RA, Wood AJ. 1982. Dinitrophenol poisoning: a diagnosis to consider in undiagnosed fever. *South. Med. J.* 75:182–84

121. Ilivicky J, Casida JE. 1969. Uncoupling action of 2,4-dinitrophenols, 2-trifluoromethylbenzimidazoles and certain other pesticide chemicals upon mitochondria from different sources and its relation to toxicity. *Biochem. Pharmacol.* 18:1389–401

122. Terada H. 1981. The interaction of highly active uncouplers with mitochondria. *Biochim. Biophys. Acta* 639:225–42

123. Miyoshi H, Tsujishita H, Tokutake N, Fujita T. 1990. Quantitative analysis of uncoupling activity of substituted phenols with a physicochemical substituent and molecular parameters. *Biochim. Biophys. Acta* 1016:99–106

124. Miyoshi H, Fujita T. 1988. Quantitative analyses of the uncoupling activity of substituted phenols with mitochondria from flight muscles of house flies. *Biochim. Biophys. Acta* 935:312–21

125. Miyoshi H, Nishioka T, Fujita T. 1987.

Quantitative relationship between protonophoric and uncoupling activities of substituted phenols. *Biochim. Biophys. Acta* 891:194–204

126. Burton DE, Lambie AJ, Ludgate JC, Newbold GT, Percival A, Saggers D. 1965. T2-trifluoromethylbenzimidazoles: a new class of herbicidal compounds. *Nature* 208:1166–69

127. Jones OT, Watson WA. 1965. Activity of 2-trifluoromethylbenzimidazoles as uncouplers of oxidative phosphorylation. *Nature* 208:1169–70

128. Beechey RB. 1966. The uncoupling of respiratory-chain phosphorylation by 4,5,6,7-tetrachloro-2-trifluoromethyl-benzimidazole. *Biochem. J.* 98:284–89

129. Jones OT, Watson WA. 1967. Properties of substituted 2-trifluoromethylbenzimidazoles as uncouplers of oxidative phosphorylation. *Biochem. J.* 102:564–73

130. Ilivicky J, Casida JE. 1969. Uncoupling action of 2,4-dinitrophenols, 2-trifluoromethylbenzimidazoles and certain other pesticide chemicals upon mitochondria from different sources and its relation to toxicity. *Biochem. Pharmacol.* 18:1389–401

131. Parker VH. 1965. Uncouplers of rat-liver mitochondrial oxidative phosphorylation. *Biochem. J.* 97:658–62

132. Ilivicky J, Casida JE. 1969. Uncoupling action of 2,4-dinitrophenols, 2-trifluoromethylbenzimidazoles and certain other pesticide chemicals upon mitochondria from different sources and its relation to toxicity. *Biochem. Pharmacol.* 18:1389–401

133. Heytler PG, Prichard WW. 1962. A new class of uncoupling agents—carbonyl cyanide phenylhydrazones. *Biochem. Biophys. Res. Commun.* 2:272–75

134. Heytler PG. 1963. Uncoupling of oxidative phosphorylation by carbonyl cyanide phenylhydrazones. I. Some characteristics of m-Cl-CCP action on mitochondria and chloroplasts. *Biochemistry* 2:357–61

135. Cunarro J, Weiner MW. 1975. Mechanism of action of agents which uncouple oxidative phosphorylation: direct correlation between proton-carrying and respiratory-releasing properties using rat liver mitochondria. *Biochim. Biophys. Acta* 387:234–40

136. Balaz S, Sturdik E, Durcova E, Antalik M, Sulo P. 1986. Quantitative structure-activity relationship of carbonylcyanide phenylhydrazones as uncouplers of mitochondrial oxidative phosphorylation. *Biochim. Biophys. Acta* 851:93–98

137. Drobnica L, Sturdik E. 1979. The reaction of carbonyl cyanide phenylhydrazones with thiols. *Biochim. Biophys. Acta* 585:462–76

138. Toninello A, Siliprandi N. 1982. Restoration of membrane potential in mitochondria deenergized with carbonyl cyanide p-trifluoromethoxyphenylhydrazone (FCCP). *Biochim. Biophys. Acta* 682:289–92

139. Cheah KS, Cheah AM, Fletcher JE, Rosenberg H. 1989. Skeletal muscle mitochondrial respiration of malignant hyperthermia-susceptible patients. Ca^{2+}-induced uncoupling and free fatty acids. *Int. J. Biochem.* 21:913–20

140. Hermesh O, Kalderon B, Bar-Tana J. 1998. Mitochondria uncoupling by a long chain fatty acyl analogue. *J. Biol. Chem.* 273:3937–42

141. Langley AE. 1990. Effects of perfluoro-n-decanoic acid on the respiratory activity of isolated rat liver mitochondria. *J. Toxicol. Environ. Health* 29:329–36

142. Reed PW. 1979. Ionophores. *Methods Enzymol.* 55:435–54

143. Pressman BC, Fahim M. 1982. Pharmacology and toxicology of the monovalent carboxylic ionophores. *Annu. Rev. Pharmacol. Toxicol.* 22:465–90

144. Katsu T, Kobayashi H, Hirota T, Fujita Y, Sato K, Nagai U. 1987. Structure-activity relationship of gramicidin S analogues on membrane permeability. *Biochim. Biophys. Acta* 899:159–70

145. Luvisetto S, Azzone GF. 1989. Nature of proton cycling during gramicidin uncoupling of oxidative phosphorylation. *Biochemistry* 28:1100–8

146. Toro M, Gomez-Lojero C, Montal M, Estrada S. 1976. Charge transfer mediated by nigericin in black lipid membranes. *J. Bioenerg.* 8:19–26

147. Felber SM, Brand MD. 1982. Valinomycin can depolarize mitochondria in intact lymphocytes without increasing plasma membrane potassium fluxes. *FEBS Lett.* 150:122–24

148. Kovac L, Bohmerova E, Butko P. 1982. Ionophores and intact cells. I. Valinomycin and nigericin act preferentially on mitochondria and not on the plasma membrane of *Saccharomyces cerevisiae.* *Biochim. Biophys. Acta* 721:341–48

149. Shinohara Y, Bandou S, Kora S, Kitamura S, Inazumi S, Terada H. 1998. Cationic uncouplers of oxidative phosphorylation are inducers of mitochondrial permeability transition. *FEBS Lett.* 428:89–92

150. Das MK, Raghothama S, Balaram P. 1986. Membrane channel forming polypeptides. Molecular conformation and mitochondrial uncoupling activity of antiamoebin, an alpha-aminoisobutyric acid containing peptide. *Biochemistry* 25:7110–17

151. Takaishi Y, Terada H, Fujita T. 1980. The effect of two new peptide antibiotics, the hypelcins, on mitochondrial function. *Experientia* 36:550–52

152. Pfeiffer DR, Gudz TI, Novgorodov SA, Erdahl WL. 1995. The peptide mastoparan is a potent facilitator of the mitochondrial permeability transition. *J. Biol. Chem.* 270:4923–32

153. Gillespie LL, Argan C, Taneja AT, Hodges RS, Freeman KB, Shore GC. 1985. A synthetic signal peptide blocks import of precursor proteins destined for the mitochondrial inner membrane or matrix. *J. Biol. Chem.* 260:16045–48

154. Glaser SM, Cumsky MG. 1990. A synthetic presequence reversibly inhibits protein import into yeast mitochondria. *J. Biol. Chem.* 265:8808–16

155. Nicolay K, Laterveer FD, van Heerde WL. 1994. Effects of amphipathic peptides, including presequences, on the functional integrity of rat liver mitochondrial membranes. *J. Bioenerg. Biomembr.* 26:327–34

156. Murphy MP. 1997. Selective targeting of bioactive compounds to mitochondria. *Trends Biotechnol.* 15:326–30

157. Bironaite D, Cenas NK, Kulys JJ. 1991. The rotenone-insensitive reduction of quinones and nitrocompounds by mitochondrial NADH:ubiquinone reductase. *Biochim. Biophys. Acta* 1060:203–9

158. Doroshow JH, Davies KJ. 1986. Redox cycling of anthracyclines by cardiac mitochondria. II. Formation of superoxide anion, hydrogen peroxide, and hydroxyl radical. *J. Biol. Chem.* 261:3068–74

159. Henry TR, Wallace KB. 1995. Differential mechanisms of induction of the mitochondrial permeability transition by quinones of varying chemical reactivities. *Toxicol. Appl. Pharmacol.* 134:195–203

160. Wallace KB. 1999. Doxorubicin-induced mitochondrial cardiomyopathy. In *Mitochondria in Pathogenesis,* ed. JJ Lemasters, A-L Nieminen. New York: Plenum. In press

161. Davies KJ, Doroshow JH. 1986. Redox cycling of anthracyclines by cardiac mitochondria. I. Anthracycline radical formation by NADH dehydrogenase. *J. Biol. Chem.* 261:3060–67

162. Meredith MJ, Reed DJ. 1983. Depletion in vitro of mitochondrial glutathione in rat hepatocytes and enhancement of lipid peroxidation by adriamycin and 1,3-bis-(2-chloroethyl)-1-nitrosourea (BCNU). *Biochem. Pharmacol.* 32:1383–88

163. Solem LE, Wallace KB. 1993. Selective activation of the sodium-independent,

cyclosporin A-sensitive calcium pore of cardiac mitochondria by doxorubicin. *Toxicol. Appl. Pharmacol.* 121:50–57

164. Palmeira CM, Serrano J, Kuehl DW, Wallace KB. 1997. Preferential oxidation of cardiac mitochondrial DNA following acute doxorubicin intoxication. *Biochim. Biophys. Acta* 1321:101–6

165. Serrano J, Palmeira CM, Kuehl DW, Wallace KB. 1999. Cardioselective and cumulative oxidation of mitochondrial DNA following subchronic doxorubicin administration. *Biochim. Biophys. Acta* 44724:1–5

166. Klohn PC, Brandt U, Neumann HG. 1996. 2-Nitrosofluorene and N-hydroxy-2-aminofluorene react with the ubiquinone-reduction center (center N) of the mitochondrial cytochrome bc_1 complex. *FEBS Lett.* 389:233–37

167. Klohn PC, Neumann HG. 1997. Impairment of respiration and oxidative phosphorylation by redox cyclers 2-nitrosofluorene and menadione. *Chem. Biol. Interact.* 106:15–28

168. Powis G, Appel PL. 1980. Relationship of the single-electron reduction potential of quinones to their reduction by flavoproteins. *Biochem. Pharmacol.* 29:2567–72

169. Powis G, Svingen BA, Appel P. 1981. Quinone-stimulated superoxide formation by subcellular fractions, isolated hepatocytes, and other cells. *Mol. Pharmacol.* 20:387–94

170. Miller MG, Rodgers A, Cohen GM. 1986. Mechanisms of toxicity of naphthoquinones to isolated hepatocytes. *Biochem. Pharmacol.* 35:1177–84

171. Ross D, Thor H, Threadgill MD, Sandy MS, Smith MT, et al. 1986. The role of oxidative processes in the cytotoxicity of substituted 1,4-naphthoquinones in isolated hepatocytes. *Arch. Biochem. Biophys.* 248:460–66

172. Gant TW, Ramakrishna RDN, Mason RP, Cohen GM. 1988. Redox cycling and sulfhydryl arylation: their relative impor-

tance in the mechanism of quinone cytotoxicity to isolated hepatocytes. *Chem. Biol. Interact.* 65:157–73

173. Thor H, Mirabelli F, Salis A, Cohen GM, Bellomo G, Orrenius S. 1988. Alteration in hepatocyte cytoskeleton caused by redox cycling and alkylating quinones. *Arch. Biochem. Biophys.* 266:397–407

174. van Toxopeus C, Holstein I, Thuring JWF, Blaauboer BJ, Noordhoek J. 1993. Cytotoxicity of menadione and related quinones in freshly isolated rat hepatocytes: effects of thiohomeostasis and energy charge. *Arch. Toxicol.* 67:674–79

175. Redegeld FA, Moison RM, Barentsen HM, Koster AS, Noordhoek J. 1990. Interaction with cellular ATP generating pathways mediates menadione-induced cytotoxicity in isolated rat hepatocytes. *Arch. Biochem. Biophys.* 280:130–36

176. Redegeld FAM, Moison RMW, Koster ASJ, Noordhoek J. 1989. Alterations in energy status by menadione metabolism in hepatocytes isolated from fasted and fed rats. *Arch. Biochem. Biophys.* 273:215–22

177. Henry TR, Wallace KB. 1996. Differential mechanisms of cell killing by redox cycling and arylating quinones. *Arch. Toxicol.* 70:482–89

178. de Groot H, Noll T, Sies H. 1985. Oxygen dependence and subcellular partitioning of hepatic menadione-mediated oxygen uptake. Studies with isolated hepatocytes, mitochondria, and microsomes from rat liver in an oxystat system. *Arch. Biochem. Biophys.* 243:556–62

179. Kolesova GM, Karnaukhova LV, Iaguzhinskii LS. 1991. Interaction of menadione and duroquinone with Q-cycle during DT-diaphorase function. *Biokhimia* 56:1779–86

180. Munday R. 1992. Mitochondrial oxidation of p-phenylenediamine derivatives in vitro: structure-activity relationships and correlation with myotoxic activity in vivo. *Chem. Biol. Interact.* 82:165–79

181. Walker UA, Byrne E. 1995. The therapy

of respiratory chain encephalopathy: a critical review of the past and current perspective. *Acta Neurol. Scand.* 92: 273–80

182. Eleff S, Kennaway NG, Buist NR, Darley-Usmar VM, Capaldi RA, et al. 1984. ^{31}P NMR study of improvement in oxidative phosphorylation by vitamin K3 and C in a patient with a defect in electron transport at complex III in skeletal muscle. *Proc. Natl. Acad. Sci. USA* 81:3529–33

183. Toscano A, Fazio MC, Vita G, Cannavo S, Bresolin N, et al. 1995. Early-onset cerebellar ataxia, myoclonus and hypogonadism in a case of mitochondrial complex III deficiency treated with vitamin K3 and C. *J. Neurol.* 242:203–9

184. Wallace KB, Eells JT, Madeira VMC, Cortopassi G, Jones DP. 1997. Mitochondria-mediated cell injury. *Fund. Appl. Toxicol.* 38:23–37

185. Green DR, Reed JC. 1998. Mitochondria in apoptosis. *Science* 281:1309–12

186. Green D, Kroemer G. 1998. The central executioners of apoptosis: caspases or mitochondria? *Trends Cell. Biol.* 8:267–71

187. Cavalli LR, Liang BC. 1998. Mutagenesis, tumorigenesis, and apoptosis: Are the mitochondria involved? *Mutat. Res.* 398:19–26

188. Mignottee B, Vayssiere JL. 1998. Mitochondria and apoptosis. *Eur. J. Biochem.* 15:1–15

189. Zamzami N, Hirsch T, Dallaporta B, Petit P, Kroemer G. 1997. Mitochondrial implication in accidental and programmed cell death: apoptosis and necrosis. *J. Bioenerg. Biomembr.* 29: 185–93

190. Stacpoole PW. 1997. Lactic acidosis and other mitochondrial disorders. *Metabolism* 46:306–21

191. Taylor RW, Chinnery PF, Clark KM, Lightowlers RN, Turnbull DM. 1997. Treatment of mitochondrial disorders. *J. Bioenerg. Biomembr.* 29:195–205

192. Decaudin D, Marzo I, Brenner C, Kroemer G. 1998. Mitochondria in chemotherapy-induced apoptosis: a prospective novel target of cancer therapy. *Int. J. Oncol.* 12:141–52

Annu. Rev. Pharmacol. Toxicol. 2000. 40:389–430

MOLECULAR MECHANISMS AND REGULATION OF OPIOID RECEPTOR SIGNALING

Ping-Yee Law[1], Yung H. Wong[2], and Horace H. Loh[3]

[1]*Department of Pharmacology, University of Minnesota Medical School, Minneapolis, Minnesota 55455; e-mail: Ping@mail.ahc.umn.edu*
[2]*Department of Biology and the Biotechnology Research Institute, Hong Kong University of Science and Technology, Clear Water Bay, Kowloon, Hong Kong, China; e-mail: boyung@ust.hk*
[3]*Department of Pharmacology, University of Minnesota Medical School, Minneapolis, Minnesota 55455; e-mail: Lohxx001@tc.umn.edu*

Key Words   G proteins, signal transduction, receptor structure/activity, receptor phosphorylation, receptor genes, knockout mice

■ **Abstract**   Cloning of multiple opioid receptors has presented opportunities to investigate the mechanisms of multiple opioid receptor signaling and the regulation of these signals. The subsequent identification of receptor gene structures has also provided opportunities to study the regulation of receptor gene expression and to manipulate the concentration of the gene products in vivo. Thus, in the current review, we examine recent advances in the delineation basis for the multiple opioid receptor signaling, and their regulation at multiple levels. We discuss the use of receptor knock-out animals to investigate the function and the pharmacology of these multiple opioid receptors. The reasons and basis for the multiple opioid receptor are addressed.

INTRODUCTION

The cloning of the δ-, μ-, and κ-opioid receptors (1–7) have led to further under-standing of the molecular mechanism of opioid receptor function. From the sequence analysis of these cloned opioid receptors, it is unequivocal that the opioid receptors belong to the superfamily of G protein–coupled receptor (GPCR) and the subfamily of rhodopsin receptor. These opioid receptors all have the putative structure of seven transmembrane domains, extracellular N terminus with multiple glycosylation sites, third intracellular loop with multiple amphiphatic α-helixes, and fourth intracellular loop formed by the putative palmitoylation sites at the carboxyl tails (1–7). On the whole, these receptors are about 60% identical to each other, with the greatest identity found in the transmembrane domains (73–76%) and intracellular loops (86–100%). The greatest divergent areas were found in the N terminus (9–10%), extracellular loops (14–72%), and C terminus (14–20%) (8). These opioid receptors could regulate the same spectrum of effectors,

0362–1642/00/0415–0389$14.00

which include adenylyl cyclase (1–7), the N-type (9) and L-type (10, 11) Ca^{2+} channels, phospholipase C (12, 13), inward rectifying K^+ channels (14), and mitogen-activated protein kinases ERK1 and ERK2 (15, 16).

With these multiple effectors being regulated by the opioid receptors, the question of the molecular basis for the pharmacology of opioid agonists needs to be addressed. In order to address such an issue, the structural requirement for the receptor activation of these effectors, the G proteins, and other cellular proteins that are involved must be evaluated. The identity of the opioid receptor that mediates the specific pharmacological function of the agonist, such as analgesia, must be identified. How these receptors are being regulated cellularly must be addressed. Thus, in this review, we examine the differential regulation of the effector systems by various opioid agonists, and the subsequent cellular regulation of the receptor activities. We also review the current status of using receptor knockout mice to address the pharmacological activities of the opioid peptides and opiate alkaloids.

REGULATION OF EFFECTORS BY OPIOID RECEPTORS

Opioid receptors are prototypical "G_i/G_o-coupled" receptors because opioid signals are efficiently blocked by pertussis toxin (PTX), a bacterial toxin produced by *Bordetella pertussis* that ADP-ribosylates and inactivates the α subunits of G_i/G_o proteins ($G\alpha_{i/o}$ subunits). Like many receptors that utilize G_i subfamily members for signal transduction, the opioid receptors have long been known to inhibit adenylyl cyclases (17) and Ca^{2+} channels (18, 19), as well as to stimulate K^+ channels (20) and to increase intracellular Ca^{2+} levels (21). More recently, the opioid receptors have been shown to regulate the mitogen-activated protein (MAP) kinase cascade (15, 16, 22). One of the major advances in understanding opioid-mediated signal transduction is the unraveling of the regulatory mechanisms for these effectors.

New Insights on the Regulation of Adenylyl Cyclase Activity by Opioids

Early studies on opioid-induced inhibition of adenylyl cyclase in brain membranes and neuroblastoma cells were interpreted on the basis of our limited understanding of the complexity of the G protein—adenylyl cyclase pathway. As PTX abolished opioid inhibition of adenylyl cyclase in the neuroblastoma x glioma NG108–15 cells (23), and rat-brain opioid receptors were solubilized as a tight complex with PTX-sensitive G proteins (24), it was generally believed that opioid receptors inhibit adenylyl cyclase only via the G_i proteins. Studies with $G\alpha$-specific antibodies suggested that G_{i2} mediates the δ-opioid receptor inhibition of adenylyl cyclase activity in NG108–15 cells (25) whereas G_o mediates the μ-opioid receptor inhibition of the adenylyl cyclase activity in SHSY5Y cells and brain membrane (26). The promiscuity of the opioid receptor was demonstrated by the ability of the receptor to induce GTP binding to all the G_i/G_o α-subunits. By using either ^{32}P-azidoanilido GTP to photoaffinity label the $G\alpha$ subunits or cholera toxin to ADP-ribosylate the $G\alpha_{i/o}$ α-subunits after their dissociation from the $\beta\gamma$ subunits, authors of several reports have indicated that the μ-, δ- and κ-opioid receptors could activate the G_i/G_o proteins with equal potency (27–31, 191, 264). All three $G\alpha_i$ subtypes ($G\alpha_{i1}$, $G\alpha_{i2}$, and $G\alpha_{i3}$) were shown to inhibit the adenylyl cyclase activity (32, 33). The discovery that G_z, a PTX-insensitive member of the G_i subfamily, can also potently inhibit cAMP accumulation upon receptor activation (33) provided new perspectives on opioid signaling. The functional and structural (~66% homology) similarities between $G\alpha_z$ and $G\alpha_i$ subunits strongly suggest that $G\alpha_z$ may substitute for $G\alpha_{i/o}$ to mediate opioid-induced signals. Detailed examination of opioid-induced inhibition of adenylyl cyclase in NG108–15 cells, which are known to coexpress the δ-opioid receptor and G_z, revealed a small but significant inhibitory component that cannot be abolished by PTX (34). When G_z was coexpressed with any one of the three cloned opioid receptors in transfected mammalian cells, opioid-mediated inhibition of adenylyl cyclase became PTX-resistant (35, 36, 37). Physical association between G_z and the δ-opioid receptor was demonstrated by coimmunoprecipitation of the recombinant proteins (38). These studies lend staunch support to the notion that opioid receptors can utilize PTX-insensitive G proteins for signal transduction. There is evidence to indicate the involvement of G_z in μ-opioid receptor-induced supraspinal antinociception in mice by immunological (39), antisense (40, 41), and biochemical (42) approaches. Because G_z is primarily expressed in neuronal tissues, it may play other roles in coupling brain opioid receptors to their corresponding effectors. The recent discovery of G_z's ability to link GPCRs to inhibition of N-type Ca^{2+} channels and stimulation of G protein gated inward rectifying potassium channels (GIRK) channels in superior cervical ganglion neurons (43) suggests that G_z may indeed serve additional roles in the propagation of opioid signals.

   One of the intriguing observations in opioid signaling is that opioids and opiates can stimulate adenylyl cyclase in brain membranes (44), F-11 neuroblastoma-sensory neuron hybrid cells (45), olfactory bulb (46), and spinal cord–ganglion explants (47). At least nine isoforms of mammalian adenylyl cyclases have been cloned, and they exhibit diverse sensitivities to regulators such as G proteins, Ca^{2+}, and kinases (48). Of particular relevance here is the ability of the G-protein $\beta\gamma$ complex ($G\beta\gamma$) to stimulate type 2, 4, and 7 adenylyl cyclases. Many classical inhibitory receptors (e.g. α_2-adrenergic and dopamine-D_2 receptors) stimulate the type 2 adenylyl cyclase through the $G\beta\gamma$ released from activated PTX-sensitive G_i proteins (49, 50). In order for the $G\beta\gamma$ subunits to stimulate type 2 adenylyl cyclase, GTP-bound $G\alpha_s$ must also be present (49, 51). This requirement allows the cell to integrate extracellular signals generated through G_s and other G-protein pathways into the intracellular messenger cAMP. Provision of activated $G\alpha_s$ can indeed permit all three forms of opioid receptors to stimulate cAMP accumulation in transfected cells coexpressing the type 2 adenylyl cyclase (35–37). Under such conditions, the opioid-induced stimulation of cAMP formation is PTX-sensitive. However, if G_z is also present in the heterologous expression system, the opioid-induced stimulatory response becomes PTX-resistant (35–37). Because both type 2 and 4 adenylyl cyclases are expressed in the brain, it is conceivable that some of the central actions of opioids are mediated by these adenylyl cyclases, which act as molecular switches for the detection of coincident signals. The δ-opioid agonist-induced potentiation of the behavioral responses elicited by dopamine D_1 receptor agonists in mice may involve these kinds of coincident signals (52). An interesting twist in the tale of Gβγ-mediated stimulation of type 2 adenylyl cyclase is the replacement of the activated $G\alpha_s$ preconditioning by protein kinase C (PKC)-mediated phosphorylation (53). Activation of PKC by G_q-coupled receptors or phorbol esters leads to the phosphorylation of type 2 adenylyl cyclase, and this modification in turn allows the Gβγ interacting domain of the enzyme to become responsive. Hence, costimulation of a G_q-coupled receptor and an opioid receptor may activate type 2 adenylyl cyclase in a synergistic fashion. Endogenous cholecystokinin has been reported to enhance the analgesic potentials of opioids in the CNS (54). It remains to be determined if these synergistic actions are, in fact, processed through the type 2 adenylyl cyclase.

An alternative explanation for opioid-induced elevation of cAMP levels is a direct coupling between opioid receptors and G_s. The α_2-adrenergic receptor is typically considered a G_i-coupled receptor, yet it is capable of eliciting a weak stimulation of adenylyl cyclase via G_s when the G_i proteins are ADP-ribosylated by PTX (49). Using the Gβγ-mediated stimulation of type 2 adenylyl cyclase as an index of G-protein activation, functional interactions between the μ-opioid receptor and various G proteins have been examined (35). The μ-opioid receptor can couple to six members of the G_i subfamily (G_{i1-3}, G_{o1-2}, and G_z), but there is no evidence of its association with G_s. A conversion step may be required, as in the case for other GPCRs. The G_s-coupled vasoactive intestinal peptide and β_2-adrenergic receptors can acquire the ability to interact with G_i proteins when they are phosphorylated by cAMP-dependent protein kinases (PKA) (55). For opioid receptors, the conversion may be regulated by the GM1 ganglioside (56). In dorsal root ganglion (DRG) neurons, the action potential duration is modulated by morphine in a bimodal fashion (57) where the cAMP-dependent excitatory effects are mediated by G_s-coupled opioid receptors. Treatment with GM1 ganglioside, but not with other gangliosides, rapidly converts the opioid receptors from an inhibitory to an excitatory mode in the DRG neurons. Similar treatments with GM1 ganglioside allow the δ-opioid receptor to stimulate cAMP formation in NG108-15 (58) and CHO (59) cells. It is noteworthy that gangliosides are abundantly distributed on the surface of most neurons, and by altering the coupling specificity of opioid receptors, GM1 may modulate opioid analgesia, tolerance, and dependence (56).

The complexity and versatility of the mammalian adenylyl cyclase system allow other routes for opioids to stimulate rather than inhibit cAMP production. For instance, type 1 and 8 adenylyl cyclases are activated by Ca^{2+}/calmodulin, whereas the basal activities of type 2, 4, and 7 adenylyl cyclases are elevated upon phosphorylation of the enzyme by PKC. Given that opioid receptors are capable of stimulating phospholipase C (PLC) and mobilizing intracellular Ca^{2+} (as discussed below), it is not surprising to note that the opioid-induced elevation of basal cAMP level in SK-N-SH cells involves Ca^{2+} entry and calmodulin activation (60). With the existence of nine different adenylyl cyclases, the regulation of intracellular cAMP by opioid receptors is far more complicated than first envisaged two decades ago. Under different cellular environments, the μ-opioid receptor can inhibit the activity of type 5 adenylyl cyclase but stimulate that of the type 7 enzyme (61). Adenylyl cyclase superactivation induced by chronic exposure of cells to opioids also appears to be isozyme specific (62). Future attempts to map opioid-induced cAMP signals will undoubtedly require the identification of cell-specific molecular components in order to fully understand the functions of opioid receptors.

Opioid Receptors and Ion Channels

Opioid receptors are known to suppress the release of neurotransmitters in many pharmacological preparations by preventing Ca^{2+} influx. All three opioid receptors share the ability to inhibit different types of Ca^{2+} channels in many regions of the mammalian brain. For example, μ- and κ-opioid receptors inhibit N- and P/Q-type Ca^{2+} channels in the nucleus tractus solitarius of the rat (63), whereas Christie and co-workers (64) showed that μ-opioid receptors, but not δ- or κ-opioid receptors, are responsible for the modulation of Ca^{2+} channel currents in mouse periaqueductal grey neurons. The cloning of multiple Ca^{2+} channel subunits provided the molecular basis for a variety of voltage-gated Ca^{2+} channels (e.g. L-, N-, P/Q-, R-, and T-type), and soon it became apparent that functional regulation of Ca^{2+} channels is no less complicated than the adenylyl cyclase system (65). The number of possible subunit combinations of Ca^{2+} channels is staggering, and the subunit composition of each channel may dictate its regulatory profiles. The availability of cloned opioid receptors together with modern electrophysiological techniques provided unique opportunities to study the modulation of different Ca^{2+} channels by opioid agonists. The first step toward this endeavor involves coexpression of cloned opioid receptors and Ca^{2+} channel subunits in cellular environments amenable to electrophysiological recordings. When expressed in NG108–15 cells, the cloned rat μ-opioid receptor is functionally coupled to the ω-conotoxin-sensitive N-type Ca^{2+} channels (66). On the other hand, the cloned μ- and δ-opioid receptors inhibit voltage-activated L-type Ca^{2+} channels via G_i/G_o proteins in GH3 pituitary cells (10, 11). Functional coupling of the κ-opioid receptor to Ca^{2+} channels has also been reported. Coexpression of neuronal Ca^{2+} channel subunits with the κ-opioid receptor in *Xenopus* oocytes allows the κ-agonist, U50488H, to inhibit the depolarization-evoked Ba^{2+} current (67). At least those Ca^{2+} channels containing the α1A, α1B, or α1E subunits have been shown to be inhibited by the μ-opioid receptor (68). It is not known if Ca^{2+} channels composed of other α1 subunits can be similarly regulated by opioid receptors.

The involvement of G_o proteins in the mediation of opioid-induced inhibition of Ca^{2+} channels has been demonstrated more than a decade ago (18) and was later confirmed by the use of $Gα_o$-specific antiserum (69). It is now realized that the Ca^{2+} channel is inhibited by the $Gβγ$ rather than the $Gα_o$ subunit. Expression of $Gβγ$ in rat sympathetic neurons mimicked GPCR-induced inhibition of Ca^{2+} currents (70), and similar results were observed when $Gβγ$ was coexpressed with Ca^{2+} channel subunits in a heterologous expression system (71). Although the $Gβγ$ subunits are responsible for mediating the inhibition of Ca^{2+} channels, the $Gα_o$ subunit is indispensable for coupling the opioid receptors to this $Gβγ$-dependent effect. The most convincing evidence comes from $Gα_o$ knockout studies. In DRG neurons obtained from $Gα_o$ knockout mice, the ability of opioid agonists to inhibit Ca^{2+} channels is significantly impaired (72). It is interesting that the G_o-deficient mice are also hyperalgesic.

The regulation of Ca^{2+} channel activity is subject to multiple inputs. In neurons, activation of PKC results in the phosphorylation and stimulation of N-type Ca^{2+} channel activity and antagonizes G protein–mediated inhibition (73). Indeed, in rat DRG neurons, activation of κ- and μ-opioid receptors decreases N-type Ca^{2+} current whereas activation of PKC produces an opposite effect (74). However, inhibition of neuronal Ca^{2+} channel subunits by the κ-opioid receptor is unaffected by the actions of PKA and PKC (67). It seems reasonable to speculate that additional crosstalk between G proteins and other signaling molecules may exist. If so, they may explain why κ-agonists stimulate rather than inhibit L-type Ca^{2+} channels in the human placenta (75).

At the postsynaptic membrane, many GPCRs produce hyperpolarization by activating K^+ channels, thereby preventing excitation or propagation of the action potentials. Electrophysiological studies in the rat locus coeruleus have shown that both μ- and δ-opioid receptors can activate K_G channels via PTX-sensitive G proteins (20). However, κ-agonists are without effect in the same preparation. Intracellular recordings made from substantia gelatinosa neurons indicate that all three types of opioid receptors are capable of activating K_G currents (76, 77). Indeed, coexpression studies in *Xenopus* oocytes confirmed that the κ-opioid receptor can activate an inward rectifying K^+ channel via PTX-sensitive G proteins (14, 78). In terms of physiological relevance of the regulation of K_G channels by opioid agonists, activation of $δ_1$-opioid receptors is involved in the cardioprotective effect of ischemic preconditioning. This is supported by the observation that a $δ_1$-selective agonist, TAN-67, can significantly reduce infarct size in rats with coronary artery occlusion by activating K_G channels via G_i proteins (79). It should be noted that K_G channels can also be inhibited by opioid receptors, as seen with the κ-subtype in a catecholaminergic neuronal cell line (80).

Recent progress in the cloning of K_G channels has enabled researchers to study the structure and function relationship of these channels at the molecular level, and to elucidate the mechanism of activation by $G\beta\gamma$ subunits (81). At least 12 distinct channel subunits are responsible for the complexity and diversity of inward rectifying K^+ channels. One of the major subunits of K_G is GIRK1. There is evidence to indicate that different types of $G\beta$ interacted with GIRK1 with distinct efficacies (82). The differential abilities of different opioid receptors to activate K_G channels may therefore be due to their association with distinct G-protein heterotrimers containing different $G\beta$ subunits. However, the specificity of interaction with K_G is lost when $G\beta$ is bound to $G\gamma$, because K_G channel currents in *Xenopus* oocytes expressing GIRK1 can be activated by different combinations of $G\beta\gamma$ (83). A recent study proposed that phosphatidyl-D-myo-inositol-4,5-bisphosphate (PIP_2) is critically involved in $G\beta\gamma$-induced activation of K_G channels (84) and opens the possibility for opioid receptors to regulate K^+ channel activities indirectly via the metabolism of PIP_2.

Apart from Ca^{2+} and K^+ channels, opioid receptors may regulate the functions of other ion channels. For example, excitatory postsynaptic currents evoked by N-methyl-D-aspartate (NMDA) receptors in the hippocampal dentate gyrus are inhibited by μ-opioid agonists (85). Since intracellular application of PTX as well as activators and inhibitors of PKA can prevent and reverse the μ-opioid–induced reduction in NMDA currents, G_i/G_o proteins and PKA may be involved. It is interesting that the opioid receptors can be reciprocally modulated by NMDA. Acute incubation of NG108–15 cells with NMDA significantly attenuated the ability of the δ-opioid receptor agonist DPDPE to inhibit forskolin-stimulated cAMP production (86). The ability of DPDPE to stimulate $[^{35}S]GTP\gamma S$ binding in NG108–15 cells is also significantly suppressed by NMDA in a dose-dependent manner, and the mechanism of regulation may in part involve PKC-mediated phosphorylation of $G\alpha_{i2}$ (87). The inhibitory effect of NMDA is also observed with μ- and κ-opioid receptors in primary cultured neurons. The ability of NMDA to attenuate acute opioid-induced inhibition of adenylyl cyclase (86) suggests that other effectors of opioid receptors may be similarly affected by NMDA.

Stimulation of Phospholipase C and Ca^{2+} Mobilization

The ability of opioid receptors to regulate the phospholipase Cβ (PLCβ) pathway and Ca^{2+} mobilization was not examined seriously until it was realized that many G_i-coupled receptors can regulate these effectors without activating G_q proteins. Sure enough, activation of δ-opioid receptors in NG108–15 cells stimulates myo-inositol 1,4,5-triphosphate (IP_3) formation and subsequent Ca^{2+} mobilization (21, 88). Opioid stimulation of PLCβ and the generation of IP_3 have also been reported in the human neuroblastoma SH-SY5Y cells (89). Similar observations were noted with the cloned opioid receptors. The cloned δ-opioid receptor stimulates IP_3 production in transfected Ltk$^-$ cells (37) whereas the rat μ-opioid receptor activates PLCβ in transfected CHO cells (90). Both systems require the participation of PTX-sensitive G proteins. Since none of the PTX-sensitive Gα subunits can activate PLCβ by themselves (35), the opioid-induced stimulation of PLCβ appears to be mediated via the G$\beta\gamma$ subunits. It is well established that the activities of PLCβ1–3 are potentiated upon binding G$\beta\gamma$ subunits. The relatively high EC$_{50}$ of opioids required to stimulate IP$_3$ formation is in fact consistent with such a concept. However, other mechanisms are available for opioids to regulate the PLCβ pathway. The mechanism of activation of PLC by μ-opioids in SH-SY5Y cells does not appear to involve G$\beta\gamma$ subunits; instead, Ca^{2+} influx via the L-type Ca^{2+} channel may be involved (91). Intriguingly, a subtype of κ-opioid receptor is found to inhibit PLCβ activity in the guinea pig cerebellum via G$_{i1}$ (92). The significance of this observation is unclear, but it should be noted that the κ-opioid receptor can also produce atypical responses in the regulation of Ca^{2+} (75) as well as K$^+$ (80) channels.

The ability of different opioid receptors to stimulate PLCβ is determined in part by the availability of complementary G proteins in any particular cell type. Using antisense oligodeoxynucleotides against specific Gα subunits, it was shown (100) that the opioid-induced Ca^{2+} mobilization in ND8–47 neuroblastoma x DRG hybrid cells is specifically mediated by G$_{i2}$. In contrast, activation of PLCβ by μ- and κ-opioid appears to utilize Gα_{i1} because coinjection of Gα_{i1} RNA into *Xenopus* oocytes is required for the detection of opioid-induced Ca^{2+}-dependent chloride currents (94), whereas all three types of opioid receptors activate PLC-β3 via G$\beta\gamma$ released from G$_{i2}$ or G$_o$ in intestinal smooth muscle (95). In a human neuroblastoma cell line, SK-N-BE, δ-opioid receptors mobilize Ca^{2+} from intracellular ryanodine-sensitive stores, and the mechanism involved is independent of the PTX-sensitive G$_i$/G$_o$ proteins (96). The possibility that opioid receptors can utilize PTX-insensitive G proteins to regulate PLCβ and Ca^{2+} mobilization was demonstrated by coexpressing the μ-opioid receptor with Gα_{16} in COS-7 cells (97). Linkage to this promiscuous G protein allowed the μ-opioid receptor to stimulate PLCβ in a PTX-insensitive manner. Both δ- and κ-opioid receptors were subsequently shown to activate G$_{16}$ more efficiently than the μ-opioid receptor (98). Albeit the opioid receptors were able to stimulate PLCβ via Gα_{16}, the EC$_{50}$ values for their respective agonists were ~50-fold higher than those observed for G$_i$-mediated inhibition of adenylyl cyclase (98). This lower efficacy in opioid receptor coupling to G$_{16}$ versus G$_i$ may provide a mechanism to differentially activate the two systems by controlling the agonist concentration.

The physiological relevance of opioid-induced stimulation of PLCβ is not immediately apparent. Elevation of intracellular IP$_3$ has been associated with only a few opioid effects. PLCβ1 is implicated in the supraspinal antinociceptive effects of δ-agonists because mice treated with antisense oligodeoxynucleotides against Gα_{i2}, Gα_{i3}, Gα_{o1}, Gα_{o2}, Gα_q, Gα_{11}, or PLCβ1 exhibit impaired antinociceptive response to δ-agonists (99). Another example is the arrhythmogenic effect of κ-agonists, which is mediated via a PTX-sensitive, G protein–regulated PLC pathway in the isolated rat heart (100). Even though the mere coexpression of opioid receptors with $G\alpha_{16}$ can hardly be taken as evidence of their functional association, several reports do in fact support such a notion. In T cells, activation of the δ-opioid receptor stimulates Ca^{2+} mobilization (101) and enhances interleukin (IL)-2 secretion (102). On the contrary, both Ca^{2+} mobilization and IL-2 secretion are reduced in T cells expressing a function-deficient mutant of $G\alpha_{16}$ (103). Stimulation of PKC and Ca^{2+}-dependent protein kinases usually occur after the activation of PLCβ. PKC-mediated phosphorylation of PLCβ3 has been demonstrated to rapidly attenuate opioid-induced phosphoinositide turnover in NG108–15 cells (104). This feedback mechanism may limit the involvement of PLCβ in the chronic actions of opioids. With regard to Ca^{2+}-dependent protein kinases, the activity of Ca^{2+}/calmodulin-dependent protein kinase II (CaMK II) in the rat hippocampus is stimulated by morphine (55). Chronic morphine treatment appears to down-regulate CaMK II, whereas naloxone-induced precipitation of morphine withdrawal leads to the up-regulation of CaMK II, in particular the β isoform. It has been reported that suppression of PLC can block G_i-mediated inhibition of adenylyl cyclase activity in NG108–15 and SK-N-SH cells (105). Such an observation might be explained by the presence of the neurospecific type 1 adenylyl cyclase in these neuroblastoma cells. In the presence of Ca^{2+}/calmodulin, type 1 adenylyl cyclase is inhibited by $G\alpha_o$ as well as $G\beta\gamma$ (106). Inhibition of PLCβ activity will invariably lead to a decrease in the level of Ca^{2+}/calmodulin and thus attenuate the ability of opioids to inhibit adenylyl cyclase via $G\alpha_o$ and $G\beta\gamma$.

Links to MAPK Cascades

A large number of GPCRs regulate cellular events such as growth and differentiation by stimulating the MAP kinase cascades. There are at least three sets of mammalian MAP kinase modules. They are the extracellular-signal–regulated kinases (ERKs), the Jun N-terminal kinases (JNKs), and the p38 kinases. Mitogenic signals from GPCRs are often transmitted along the ERK pathway. Stimulation of the ERK1 and ERK2 by opioids was first demonstrated with the μ-opioid receptor in recombinant CHO cells (15). The stimulation showed ligand selectivity, agonist dose-dependency, and PTX sensitivity. Likewise, when expressed in Rat-1 fibroblasts, the δ-opioid receptor can stimulate the phosphorylation and activation of ERK1/2 (22). The involvement of G_i/G_o proteins in the activation of MAP kinase is again implicated by the ability of PTX to block this response. In fact, all three types of opioid receptors have been shown to stimulate ERK1/2 in a heterologous expression system (16), and the activation of ERKs occur through the $G\beta\gamma$ subunits in a Ras-dependent manner. An interesting twist in the tale is the recent discovery that GPCRs can stimulate ERKs via focal adhesion complexes as well as by the process of GPCR desensitization and sequestration (107). Although μ-opioid agonists have been shown to activate the focal adhesion kinase in chick embryo cortical neurons (108) and internalization of the δ-opioid receptor is required for opioid stimulation of MAP kinase (109), κ-opioid receptor internalization does not appear to be necessary for MAP kinase activation (110). Apart from linking opioid receptor activation to mitogenesis, stimulation of the MAP kinase cascade may be required for other aspects of opioid signaling. For instance, the immunomodulatory and immunosuppressive effects of morphine on human lymphocytes may be mediated in part by the activation of the MAP kinase cascade (111). Desensitization as well as internalization of μ-opioid receptors may also involve MAP kinase (112). MAP kinase activities in cortical neurons (layers II/III), median eminence, and amygdaloid and hypothalamic nuclei are diminished in rats with chronic morphine treatment (113). Acute morphine treatment has no effect on the ERK activity in these brain regions. On the other hand, morphine withdrawal produces a dramatic increase in ERK MAP kinase phosphorylation in somata and fibers of locus coeruleus, solitary tract and hypothalamic neurons. The relationship between the observed differential regulation of ERK and opioid tolerance and dependence is unclear but certainly warrants further investigation.

In the complex signaling network of MAP kinases, there are plenty of opportunities for opioids to modulate the activities of disparate pathways through the actions of Gβγ subunits. One of the many capabilities of Gβγ is the stimulation of the γ-isoform of phosphoinositide 3-kinase (PI3K) (114). Agonists of the μ-opioid receptor have been shown to stimulate three different effectors of a PI3K-dependent signaling cascade in recombinant CHO cells (115). [D-Ala^2,MePhe4,Gly^5-01]-enkephalin (DAMGO) stimulates the activity of Akt (also known as protein kinase B), a serine/threonine protein kinase downstream of PI3K, which inhibits apoptosis in neurons. Two other effectors of PI3K, the p70 S6 kinase and the repressors of mRNA translation, 4E-BP1 and 4E-BP2, are also phosphorylated upon stimulation by DAMGO. Hence, opioids may regulate neuronal development and synaptic plasticity by modulating neuronal survival and translational control. The opioid receptors can also modulate signals generated by classical growth factors. For example, chronic activation of μ- or κ-opioid receptors has been shown to attenuate the epidermal growth factor–induced stimulation of ERKs (116). Furthermore, tyrosine kinase activity appears to be stimulated upon activation of the opioid receptor in SK-N-SH cells (117), where a 58 kDa protein is phosphorylated on tyrosine residues following treatment with morphine. The tyrosine phosphorylation can be blocked by PTX treatment. In Rat-1 fibroblasts stably expressing the δ-opioid receptor, [D-Ala^2,D-Leu^5]-enkephalin (DADLE) significantly stimulates the tyrosine phosphorylation of p52 Shc adaptor protein in a PTX-sensitive manner (118). DADLE can also concentration-dependently activate the p70 and p85 S6 kinases in these Rat-1 fibroblasts (119). Collectively, the activation of MAP kinase, S6 kinase, PI3K, and Shc proteins provides a strong mitogenic signal for opioids to regulate cell growth. The μ- and δ-opioid receptors possess different abilities to potentiate growth factor–induced cell proliferation in various cell types (120). Such differences may be related to the different capacities of the opioid receptors to regulate specific mitogenic signals. Little is known with regard to the involvement of JNK or p38 kinase in opioid signaling. The ability of deltorphin to enhance the activity of NF-AT/AP-1 transcription factor in Jurkat T cells (102) suggests that at least the δ-opioid receptor may possess the capability to regulate JNK in addition to activating the ERKs. Given that all three forms of opioid receptors are capable of stimulating G_{16} (98) and that G_{16} has been shown to activate JNK (121), such an assumption is perfectly plausible.

REGULATION OF RECEPTOR ACTIVITY BY PHOSPHORYLATION

Receptor Phosphorylation and Desensitization

Being a member of the GPCR, the opioid receptor activities could be regulated similarly as those of other GPCRs. A model in which the β_2-adrenergic receptor activities can be regulated has been proposed by Lefkowitz (122). In this model, agonist binding to the receptor results in the rapid phosphorylation of the receptor by protein kinases including the G protein–coupled receptor kinases (GRKs), thereby promoting the association of the cellular protein arrestin. Not only did the association of arrestin with the receptor uncouple the receptor from the respective G protein that transduces the signal and thus blunt the receptor signaling (receptor desensitization), the arrestin also is involved in the agonist-induced, clathrin-coated vesicles–mediated receptor internalization. Arrestin itself also serves as an adapter molecule in the β_2-adrenergic receptor signaling such that a receptor-src kinase complex is formed through which activation of the MAP kinases ERK1/2 by the β_2-adrenergic receptor is accomplished (123).

In the proposed model for GPCR desensitization, the initiation step involves the phosphorylation of the receptor. Concrete demonstration of opioid receptor phosphorylation was first demonstrated by Pei et al (124) with the δ-opioid receptor and by Arden et al (125) with the μ-opioid receptor. Agonist-induced phosphorylation of the κ-opioid receptor was also reported (126). A variety of biochemical approaches have revealed a rapid, agonist-dependent phosphorylation of the receptor protein. Studies with the δ-opioid (124) and μ-opioid (127, 128) receptors suggested that the agonist-induced phosphorylation is mediated via GRKs and not by protein kinase C. Predictably, the ability of opioid ligand to induce receptor phosphorylation correlated to its efficacy (129). With the exception of morphine, agonists such as DAMGO or etorphine were all reported to induce μ-opioid receptor phosphorylation. Wang and coworkers (129) reported that morphine induces μ-opioid receptor phosphorylation in CHO cells, whereas Arden et al (125) and Zhang et al (130) reported morphine does not induce receptor phosphorylation in HEK293 cells. The fact that overexpression of GRK2 in HEK293 cells resulted in the morphine-induced phosphorylation of the μ-opioid receptor (130) suggests that the morphine-receptor complex is a poor substrate for the GRKs. Thus, the discrepancy in the ability of morphine to induce receptor phosphorylation could be due to the differences in the level of protein kinases in the CHO and HEK293 cell lines. The difference between the morphine-receptor complex and other agonist-receptor complexes was further illustrated by the ability of in vitro PKA catalytic subunit to phosphorylate the morphine-receptor complex and not the DAMGO-receptor complex (131).

Though the sites of agonist-dependent receptor phosphorylation have not yet been identified, it is apparent that the major phosphorylation sites are at the carboxyl tails of the opioid receptors. Deletion of the last 31 amino acids of the δ-opioid receptor resulted in the abolition of both GRK- and PKC-mediated agonist-dependent phosphorylation of the receptor (132). Truncation of the mouse δ-opioid receptor after Thr^{344} also blocked the ability of DPDPE to induce phosphorylation of the receptor (133). Since there are seven putative phosphorylation sites within the carboxyl tail sequence of the δ-opioid receptor, such observations suggested that the agonist must induce phosphorylation of either Thr^{352}, Thr^{353}, Thr^{358}, Thr^{361} or Ser^{363}. As for the μ- and κ-opioid receptor, the phosphorylation sites are less well defined. Our studies have indicated that the carboxyl tail is the target for the kinases. Mutation of all the Ser and Thr within the carboxyl tail to Ala resulted in a mutant μ-opioid receptor that was not phosphorylated in the presence of DAMGO (Maestri-El-Kouhen, PY Law, HH Loh, unpublished data). The exact residues that are being phosphorylated within the carboxyl tail of the μ-opioid receptor remain to be identified.

The protein kinases that participate in the agonist-induced receptor phosphorylation are most likely members of GRKs. Expression of the dominant negative mutant of GRK or overexpression of GRK5 resulted in the attenuation or potentiation of agonist-dependent phosphorylation of the δ-opioid receptor (124). Though overexpression of GRK2 in HEK293 cells could potentiate etorphine- or morphine-induced phosphorylation of the μ-opioid receptor (130), the same overexpression of GRK2 had minimal effect on the DAMGO-induced receptor phosphorylation (128). Probably, the discrepancy between these studies lies within the level of receptor being expressed in the HEK293 cells, or the morphine- or etorphine-receptor complexes represent a better substrate for the GRK2 than the DAMGO-receptor complex, or the DAMGO-receptor complex is an excellent substrate for the endogenous GRKs. Whether these ligands induced the phosphorylation of the same residues in the presence or absence of overexpressed GRK2 needs to be examined.

Some reports suggested that other protein kinases might be involved in the phosphorylation of the receptor. The candidates are Ca^{2+}/calmodulin-dependent protein kinase II, PKA, and the ERK1/ERK2. Though the agonist-dependent phosphorylation of the μ- and δ-opioid receptor is not mediated by the PKC (124, 127, 128), basal phosphorylation of the μ-opioid receptor appears to involve the CaM kinase, as indicated by CaM kinase inhibitor studies (134). Koch et al (135) reported that by mutating the two putative consensus sites (Ser^{261} and Ser^{266}) for CaM kinase II of the μ-opioid receptor to Ala, the increase in rate of receptor desensitization when the CaM kinase II is overexpressed can be blocked either in HEK293 cells or in *Xenopus* oocytes. Unfortunately, no direct phosphorylation experiment was carried out; therefore, whether the μ-opioid receptor is being phosphorylated by CaM kinase II could not be evaluated. Nevertheless, in view of the observation that the amino terminus domain of GRK5 could interact with calmodulin while the carboxyl terminus domain interacts with the Gβγ subunit (136), it is possible that CaM kinase II could be recruited to the vicinity of the μ-opioid receptor and affect the receptor activities.

Indirect evidence suggested that PKA might phosphorylate the μ-opioid receptor during chronic treatment. By carrying out back-phosphorylation studies, both Chakrabarti et al (131) and Berstein & Welch (137) reported that the treatment of neuroblastoma cells or animals with morphine resulted in a decrease in PKA-induced phosphorylation of the μ-opioid receptor. This reduction in the PKA-mediated back-phosphorylation does not indicate that during chronic morphine treatment, there is PKA phosphorylation of the receptor. Besides, chronic DAMGO treatment did not alter the ability of in vitro morphine-dependent PKA-mediated phosphorylation of the receptor (131). Since chronic treatment of the neuroblastoma cells with either DAMGO or morphine resulted in the loss of response, the lack of DAMGO effect on the back-phosphorylation studies further suggested that PKA did not participate in the agonist-induced receptor phosphorylation.

Intriguing probable kinases that might phosphorylate the μ-opioid receptor are the ERK1/2 of the MAP kinase family. Blockade of this MAP kinase pathway activation by the MAP kinase kinase (MEK) inhibitor PD98059, or the PI3K inhibitors wortmannin or LY294002, resulted in the inability of a 2-h DAMGO pretreatment to desensitize or to down-regulate the μ-opioid receptor stably expressed in CHO cells (112). Though the direct phosphorylation of the receptor was not determined in this study, the ability of MAP kinase to phosphorylate other GPCRs, such as the angiotensin AT1 receptor, has been reported (138). The μ- or κ-opioid receptor carboxyl tail sequences do not contain a consensus phosphorylation sequence recognized by MAP kinase. However, the Thr^{361} residue of the δ-opioid receptor is a putative MAP kinase phosphorylation site. ERK1/2 could probably mediate the agonist-dependent phosphorylation of the δ-opioid receptor.

There appears to be a casual relationship between δ-opioid receptor phosphorylation and desensitization. Desensitization of the δ-opioid receptor was reported to correlate with the phosphorylation of the receptor protein in the SK-N-BE cells (139). The strongest evidence in this report in support of the hypothesis is the inhibitor studies in which heparin or Zn^{2+}, inhibitors of GRKs, could block the desensitization, whereas the PKA/PKC inhibitor H7 could not. Pei et al (124) demonstrated with the dominant negative mutants of GRKs that DPDPE-induced receptor desensitization can be blocked. Overexpression of GRK2 in HEK293 cells could accelerate the DPDPE-induced δ-opioid receptor desensitization (128). Mutation of the last four Thr and Ser residues at the C terminus of the δ-opioid receptor to Ala would block the GRK- and arrestin-mediated desensitization (140). However, the δ-opioid receptor lacking the C-terminal 31 amino acids, the sites for agonist-induced phosphorylation, can be rapidly desensitized by pretreating the CHO cells with DPDPE for 10 min (141). In the same studies, the authors reported that staurosporin could block the DPDPE-induced desensitization, suggesting the involvement of protein phosphorylation by PKC.

The question of whether there is a direct correlation between μ-opioid receptor phosphorylation and desensitization has not been adequately addressed. Zhang et al (127) used two separate models to demonstrate a time course for DAMGO-induced μ-opioid receptor regulation of the GIRK1 channels' fast desensitization, as measured in *Xenopus* oocytes, and receptor phosphorylation, as measured in CHO cells. Pak et al (142) reported the T394A mutant of the μ-opioid receptor could not be desensitized by a 1-h DAMGO pretreatment. Since the mutation of the glutamic acid residues preceding the Thr^{394} also eliminated the DAMGO desensitization, these data implicated the phosphorylation of Thr^{394} by the GRKs, which are acidokinases (143). The importance of Thr^{394} in receptor desensitization was partially supported by the findings with the splice variant of μ-opioid receptor, MOR-1B. MOR-1B has sequence homology with the wild-type MOR-1 receptor up to Glu^{386}, where the sequence then differs by five amino acids and is ultimately seven amino acids shorter than MOR-1 (144). This mutant is more resistant to agonist-induced receptor desensitization than is the wild-type receptor, and the rate of desensitization could be enhanced if the inhibitor of endosome acidification, monensin, was used (145). This apparent decrease in the rate of desensitization could be attributed to the faster internalization and resensitization rates of the splice variant (146). However, the increase in the internalization rate should accelerate the fast desensitization of the MOR-1B variant. Pak et al (147) demonstrated that the agonist-induced desensitization of the μ-opioid receptor was mediated by the loss of membrane receptors. Studies by Whistler & von Zastrow (148) indicated that the overexpression of arrestin could enhance the morphine-induced receptor internalization and the fast desensitization of the μ-opioid receptor. Whether phosphorylation of Thr^{394} is a requisite for such regulation of the opioid receptor activities remains to be demonstrated.

Rapid desensitization of the μ-opioid receptor was reported only with the GTPγS binding assays, or with membrane adenylyl cyclase assays (142, 148). Even with coexpression of the μ-opioid receptor with GRK3 (β-ARK2) and β-arrestin 2 in *Xenopus* oocytes, the desensitization of the receptor required more than 2 h (140). These data are in agreement with the lack of effect on μ-opioid receptor–mediated inhibition of adenylyl cyclase activity in HEK293 cells overexpressing β-arrestin 1 (149). Taken together, these data suggested that the phosphorylation of the μ-opioid receptor might not lead to the uncoupling from the G protein by arrestin and, subsequently, receptor desensitization.

Other cellular events in addition to receptor phosphorylation might play an important role in μ-opioid receptor desensitization. This hypothesis is supported by the observation that the complete mutation of all Ser and Thr residues within the third intracellular loop and the C terminus of the μ-opioid receptor did not prevent the slow desensitization induced by DAMGO (150). Though prolonged morphine treatment could elicit a loss of response (151), morphine normally does not induce receptor phosphorylation. Thus, it is interesting to note that Koover et al (152), in a later study, reported rapid μ-opioid receptor desensitization (fewer than 20 min) in oocytes expressing GRK3 or GRK5 with β-arrestin 2 where the regulation of GIRK1/GIRK4 channel activities were measured. DAMGO fentanyl or sufentanyl but not morphine could induce such rapid desensitization. These data, in contrast to data from one of their earlier reports (140), suggested that phosphorylation of the μ-opioid receptor resulted in the rapid uncoupling to the regulation of K^+ channel. Because GRK could phosphorylate substrates other than GPCRs, and because the rapid uncoupling of the μ-opioid receptor from GIRK1 channels might not involve phosphorylation (153), it is imperative that the actual phosphorylation of the μ-opioid receptor by the exogenously expressed GRKs be demonstrated.

Role of Receptor Phosphorylation in Receptor Internalization and Down-Regulation

Agonist-induced receptor internalization and down-regulation were initially demonstrated in clonal or recombinant cell lines expressing the δ-opioid receptor (154–157). Agonist-induced internalization of the receptor via the endocytic pathway was first demonstrated in NG108–15 cells (158) and later with cell lines expressing the cloned δ-opioid receptor either with antibodies (159–161) or with fluorescent opioid peptides (162). Only agonists could induce down-regulation of the receptor; partial agonists and antagonists could not (159, 163). Morphine could not induce δ-opioid receptor down-regulation except in the presence of μ-opioid receptor (164, 165). This effect of morphine can be blocked by the μ-opioid receptor selective antagonist β-funaltrexamine (165).

Agonist-induced μ-opioid receptor down-regulation was demonstrated with the 7315C pituitary tumor cells (166), human neuroblastoma SHSY5Y cells (164, 167, 168), human neuroblastoma SK-N-SH cells (165), and human neuroblastoma NMB cells (169). Similar agonist-induced receptor down-regulation was reported with the cloned μ-opioid receptor expressed in neuroblastoma neuro2A cells (151), C6 glioma cells (170), or fibroblasts (125, 130, 159, 171). Though morphine could not induce the rapid receptor internalization (125, 130, 148, 159), it could induce μ-opioid receptor down-regulation in clonal cell lines (164, 165, 167) or in cell lines heterologously expressing the cloned μ-opioid receptor (151, 170). The mechanisms by which morphine could induce receptor down-regulation but could not promote receptor internalization remain to be determined.

Similarly, the κ-opioid receptor can be down-regulated upon agonist treatment. The down-regulation of the receptor was demonstrated in the mouse R1.1 thymoma cell line (169, 172) or in CHO cells expressing the cloned human κ-opioid receptor (173). Though the pretreatment of these two cell lines with U50,488 resulted in the decrease in antagonist binding, the agonist treatment resulted in receptor desensitization in CHO cells, as measured by the GTPγS binding assay (173), but not in R1.1 thymoma cells, as measured by agonist inhibition of the adenylyl cyclase activity (172). In the same studies, a 50% reduction in the receptor number by pretreating with the irreversible opioid antagonist, β-chlornaltrexamine, resulted in a six-fold increase in the U50,488 IC_{50} value to inhibit adenylyl cyclase activity in the R1.1 thymoma cells. Thus, it is intriguing that a similar reduction in receptor number would not alter the agonist potency in the same cell.

Trafficking of the opioid receptor in the agonist-dependent receptor internalization and down-regulation is probably mediated by the clathrin coated pits of the endocytic pathway. This is concluded from observations in which opioid receptors co-localize with the transferrin receptor after internalization (159, 161, 174) and in which this receptor internalization can be blocked by the dominant negative mutant of arrestin or dynamin (110, 130, 133, 148, 175). However, the functioning of this endocytic pathway appears to be agonist and receptor type-dependent. DAMGO, but not morphine, induced the μ-opioid receptor internalization (125, 130, 148, 159). The inability of morphine to induce receptor internalization can be rescued by the overexpression of GRK2 (130) or β-arrestin (148). This suggested that the morphine-receptor complex could be promoted into the endocytic pathway by increasing the arrestin binding to the complex either by the increase in receptor phoshorylation or by the increase in arrestin concentration. However, the inability of morphine to induce δ-opioid receptor internalization cannot be rescued by overexpression of GRK2 (176). The absolute requirement for receptor phosphorylation in the agonist-induced receptor endocytosis has not been established. Thr^{353} of the δ-opioid receptor has been initially reported to be required for agonist-induced receptor internalization and down-regulation in CHO cells (157, 160). However, though the agonist-induced receptor phosphorylation of the δ-opioid receptor truncated mutant (DOR344T) was blocked in HEK293 cells, the agonist-induced receptor endocytosis between the wild-type and mutant receptors was similar in HEK293 cells but was attenuated in CHO cells by the truncation (133). Mutation of Ser^{356} and Ser^{363} of the μ-opioid receptor could block etorphine-induced receptor down-regulation without significantly altering the agonist-induced receptor phosphorylation (177). These data suggested that mutation of putative phosphorylation sites might not alter the agonist-induced phosphorylation, but rather the interaction between receptor and cellular molecules that are involved in receptor endocytosis, such as arrestin. Moreover, there appear to be differences in the cellular regulation of the opioid receptors. The rate of the agonist-induced receptor endocytosis appears to be different, with δ- >μ- >κ-opioid receptor. Etorphine induced a rapid internalization (175) and down-regulation (178) of the δ-opioid receptor, whereas the internalization of the κ-opioid receptor expressed in the same cell (175), or the down-regulation of the μ-opioid receptor (178), was slow. The carboxyl tail of these receptors apparently was involved in these processes. Receptor chimeras containing the carboxyl tails of the δ-opioid receptors exhibited an increased rate of internalization or down-regulation (175, 178). However, caution must be used in the interpretation of such data. In view of the facts that mutation of Thr[394] of the μ-opioid receptor to Ala can enhance the recycling of the receptor (146) and truncation mutation such as the MOR354T can result in a constitutively internalizing and recycling receptor (174), the increase in the apparent rate of receptor internalization could be due to a change in the recycling rate.

In addition to being dependent on β-arrestin and dynamin, the opioid agonist-induced receptor endocytosis also appears to depend on the ability of receptor to form a high-affinity complex with G proteins independent of receptor activation. Pretreatment of cell lines with PTX resulted in the uncoupling of the δ-opioid receptor from G_i/G_o and the abolition of effector signals, but not the agonist-induced receptor down-regulation (163, 179, 180). A similar observation was reported with the ability of agonists to induce down-regulation but not activation of the receptor mutant in which Asp[95] was mutated to Ala (180). Under these conditions, a high percentage of the δ-opioid receptor remained in the high-affinity, G protein–coupled states (179, 180). The requirement of a high-affinity state was demonstrated with similar experiments with the μ-opioid receptor. Mutation of Asp[114] of the μ-opioid receptor, or pretreatment of the cells with PTX resulted in the complete uncoupling of the μ-opioid from the G proteins and blockade of the agonist-induced receptor down-regulation (180). Yabaluri & Medzihradsky (170) reported that PTX pretreatment did not block the agonist-induced receptor down-regulation of C6 glioma cells expressing the μ-opioid receptor. However, the percentage of receptors in the high-affinity state was not measured in this study. Aggregation or association of the receptor with each other or with other cellular proteins prior to internalization was supported by the clustering or capping of the receptors in the presence of agonists, but not antagonists (162, 181). Conversely, Cvejic & Devi (182) reported that the δ-opioid receptor existed as a dimer, and upon agonist binding, monomers are formed. However, receptor mutants with the last 15 amino acid residues deleted that did not exhibit agonist-induced receptor internalization did not exist as dimers. Hence, the formation of monomers appeared to be the prerequisite for agonist-induced receptor internalization. Such behavior of the δ-opioid receptor in the presence of agonist is in contrast with other GPCRs in which agonist induced the dimerization of the receptors (183–185). The role of receptor dimerization in opioid receptor endocytosis remains to be demonstrated.

REGULATION OF OPIOID RECEPTOR ACTIVITIES AT THE TRANSCRIPTIONAL LEVEL

Regulation of Opioid Receptor mRNA Levels

In addition to the phosphorylation and uncoupling of the receptor from G proteins, the activities of the opioid receptors can be regulated by the transcription of the receptor genes and subsequently the receptor levels. Though the general principle of "spare" receptor applies in the opioid receptor regulation of the second messenger systems, the agonist potency and the effector that it regulates are receptor density-dependent (22, 155). Thus the control of the expression of the opioid receptor will determine the agonist activities.

The reduction of the receptor protein during chronic agonist treatment as a probable mechanism for tolerance development has been widely reported by several laboratories. Thus, it is logical to hypothesize that the observed reduction in receptor protein is due to the inhibition of the receptor gene transcription and hence the steady state levels of the opioid receptor mRNAs. However, the majority of the studies reported the decrease in the receptor level was not accompanied by a decrease in the receptor mRNA level. Intracerebroventricular injection of [D-Ala^2]deltorphin II for 5 days resulted in the development of tolerance to the peptide without alteration in the δ-opioid receptor mRNA levels (186). Though chronic morphine or antagonist treatment could up-regulate the receptor level, such treatment did not alter the opioid receptor mRNA levels (187–189). A report with female guinea pigs suggested that morphine treatment could decrease the μ-opioid receptor mRNA levels minimally (15%) in the basal hypothalamus (190). Such action of morphine on the receptor level in the female guinea pig might be related to the estrogen regulation of the μ-opioid receptor mRNA levels in the forebrain of female rats (191). Nevertheless, one could argue that the lack of alteration in the receptor mRNA levels after chronic agonist treatment is the result of the receptor-specific agonist not being used or a relatively high steady state level of the agonist could not be maintained with the animals. Treatment of NG108–15 cells with etorphine (192) or cortical astrocytes primary cell cultures with DPDPE (193) resulted respectively in the down-regulation or up-regulation of the δ-opioid receptor mRNA. However, the ability to down-regulate the δ-opioid receptor mRNA levels in NG108–15 by etorphine treatment was not mimicked by treating the same cells with the peptide agonist, DSLET (188). Whether such discrepancy is due to the agonist used or treatment paradigm remains to be resolved.

In contrast to chronic opioid agonist treatment, the opioid receptor gene expression can be altered dramatically by the exposure to pharmacological agents such as alcohol or cocaine. In neuroblastoma cell lines, ethanol has been reported to increase δ-opioid receptor transcripts, which can be blocked by the activation of PKA activity (194–196). Because it is difficult to maintain in vivo alcohol concentration at >100 mM, it is not surprising that the induction of the δ-opioid receptor gene was not observed in animals (197, 198). But in experiments in which alcohol-preferring mice, C57BL/6, and alcohol-avoiding mice, DBA/2, were used, differential alteration of the δ- and μ-opioid receptor mRNA levels were observed in distinct brain areas such as striatum and hypothalamus (199). Cocaine treatment, either under the chronic or "binge" paradigm, resulted in the up-regulation of the μ-opioid mRNA in the nucleus accumbens (200, 201) or decrease in κ-opioid receptor mRNA in the substantia nigra (202), that might be related to the activation of the dopamine receptor (203). This alteration in the receptor mRNA levels could be caused by the alteration in the levels of growth factors or second messengers that regulate protein kinase activity. The nerve growth factor (NGF) has been reported to increase both mRNA and protein levels of the δ-opioid receptor in the rat pheochromocytoma PC12 cells (204). The κ-opioid receptor mRNA level increased in oligodendrocytes in the presence of bFGF and PDGF-BB (205). Immunocytokines such as interleukin-1, IL-1b, were reported to increase the μ-opioid receptor mRNA in the astrocytes-enriched strial-tal, cerebellar, and hippocampal primary cultures, but not in cultures derived from the cortex or hypothalamus (206, 207). IL-1 also has been observed to induce the expression of μ-opioid receptor mRNA in the neural microvascular endothelial cells (208). Opioid receptor transcription could also be induced with agents such as retinoic acid in NG108–15 cells (209) or concanavalin A in CD4$^+$ T cells from murine splenocytes (210). Despite a contradictory report from another group in which concanavalin A apparently reduced the δ-opioid receptor level (211), the control of the opioid receptor level by extracellular signals is unmistakable. Elevation in the intracellular cAMP level in NG108–15 cells has been reported to consistently decrease the opioid receptor mRNA levels, which is probably not due to increase in the degradation of the mRNA (212, 213). Increase in the intra-cellular cAMP level in astrocytes also decreased the κ-opioid receptor mRNA level (214). Hence, changes in the intracellular cAMP level during acute and chronic agonist treatment could account for the changes in the opioid receptor mRNA levels (192, 193). Increase in the PKC activity with the phorbol ester phorbol-12-myristate-13-acetate (TPA) resulted in the decrease in the μ-opioid receptor mRNA level in SHSY5Y cells (214), whereas activation of the Ca^{2+}/calmodulin-dependent kinase by membrane depolarization in NG108–15 cells resulted in the increase in the δ-opioid receptor mRNA level (215). Because the measurement of δ-opioid receptor mRNA level was not determined simultaneously with the SHSY5Y studies, it is unclear whether the increase in the various Ca^{2+}-dependent protein kinases' activities would result in differential regulation of the transcription of these two opioid receptor genes.

Opioid Receptor Gene Structures

If the regulation of the opioid receptor mRNA levels is due to the alteration in the transcriptional activities of the receptor genes, then the structure of the opioid receptor genes and the *cis-* and *trans*-elements that regulate the transcriptional activities must be determined. Though the three cloned opioid receptor genes are distributed in different chromosomes [distal part of the short arm of the chromosome 1 for DOR, distal part of the long arm chromosome 6 for MOR, and the proximal long arm of chromosome 8 for KOR (216, 217)], the three receptors all have multiple introns and they span large distances in the chromosomal DNA. The MOR-1 gene is more than 53k bp long, with exon splice junctions at the first intracellular loop (Arg^{95}), the second extracellular loop (Glu^{213}), and the cytoplasmic C-terminal region (Glu^{386}/Leu^{387}) (218), and with a splice variant at the cytoplasmic C-terminal region (219). Similarly, the DOR gene spans 32 kbp with multiple intronic structure (220). The splice junctions of the DOR gene are located at the corresponding amino acids in the first intracellular and second extracellular loop, with the exception that the splice junction at the carboxyl tail of MOR is absent in DOR. However, the multiple-exons structure of the mouse κ-opioid receptor gene is different from those of MOR and DOR. The KOR gene spans more than 16 kbp in the chromosome and has at least four exons (221). Exon I of the KOR encodes the major portion of the 5′-untranslated region and spans a distance of 334, 340, or 716 nucleotides, depending on the sites of transcription initiation. The first intron spans a distance of 371 nucleotides. Exon II of the KOR gene contains 271 nucleotides, including 14 nucleotides of the 5′-untranslated sequence and a splice site at Arg^{86}. Exon III contains 353 nucleotides and has the splice site at Val^{204}. Exon IV begins at Val^{204} and encodes the rest of the 3′ end sequence of the mouse κ-opioid receptor cDNA. The fact that the exon splice junctions of these three opioid receptor genes are at the same amino acids of the coding region suggests that they evolved from a single ancestral gene.

Using 5′RACE and RNase protection assays or primer extension studies, the multiple transcriptional start sites of these opioid receptor genes have been identified. They all have distal and proximal promoters (218, 220, 222). In most cases, transcription of the opioid receptor mRNAs is initiated from the proximal promoters. In rodent brain, the μ-opioid receptor transcripts originated from the proximal promoter (223). Reporter gene assays indicated that both μ- and δ-opioid receptor gene transcriptions are controlled by the proximal promoters (223, 224). However, the KOR gene is transcribed by both proximal and distal promoters, with the transcripts from the distal promoter being the dominant ones (222). The role of these distinct promoter regions in the transcription of the opioid receptor gene is unknown. However, it can be demonstrated that the distal promoter, as reported by Liang et al (225), is the transcriptional start site for MOR-1 and is under inhibitory control. Removal of an inhibitory regulatory region (−775 to −444 from the ATG start site) restored the distal promoter activity in a reporter gene assay (226). The distal promoter regulation sequence can be defined to center around a 34-bp negative *cis*-acting element that was demonstrated to be position- and promoter-dependent (226). Hence, the regulation of the distal promoter activity by such negative element can affect the transcription of the opioid receptor gene.

Similar to other GPCR genes, the opioid receptor genes contain no consensus TATA box within the promoter regions. Comparing the nucleotide sequences of receptor genes upstream from the ATG initiation codon with those in the Transcription Factors Database, it could be demonstrated that several putative binding sites for known transcriptional factors are present. In the 5′ upstream region of MOR-1, consensus binding sites for Sp1, AP2, AP1, glucocorticoid/mineralcorticoid response element, immune-cell-specific element Pu-1, cytokine response elements NF-IL6 and NF-GMb, and the cAMP response elements are found (218). Similarly, consensus binding sites for AP2, NF-κB, NGF–induced transcriptional activator NGFI-B, and NF-IL6 are found in the 5′ upstream regions of DOR

(220). The presence of these transcriptional binding sites could explain the observed cytokine-induced increase in the μ-opioid receptor mRNA levels in the astrocyte-enriched primary culture (206, 207), NGF induced increase in the δ-opioid receptor mRNA levels in PC12 cells (204), and the cAMP induced decrease of the opioid receptor gene transcripts (205, 212, 213). However, the direct demonstration of the involvement of these *cis*-acting elements with reporter gene assays could not be established. The putative NF-IL6 binding site of the opioid receptor genes was demonstrated to be nonfunctional, as determined by reporter gene assays in several immune cell line models (227). Reporter gene assays with the 5′ upstream sequence could not demonstrate that the transcriptional factors were involved in either the cAMP- or NGF-dependent regulation of the δ-opioid receptor mRNA levels (228). Such lack of effects could have several explanations: (*a*) The cytokines' effect on μ-opioid receptor mRNA levels with mixed cell cultures may suggest involvement of multiple cytokines. (*b*) The changes in the steady state levels of mRNAs as detected by RT-PCR could reflect the stability of the mRNAs and not the de novo transcription of the receptor gene. (*c*) The regulation of receptor gene transcription involves elements other than those that are within the proximity of the promoter regions. However, the most likely explanation is that the receptor gene is under the control of multiple transcription factors and *cis*-elements.

An excellent example of the interaction among transcriptional factors could be demonstrated with the analysis of the promoter activities of these receptor genes. Electrophoretic mobility shift assays have indicated that the nuclear proteins immunologically related to Sp1 and Sp3 are specifically bound to the iGA motif of the MOR promoter region (229). Mutation of the binding sites and the use of *Drosophila* SL2 cells which do not express Sp1 or Sp1-like proteins demonstrated that these Sp proteins have a major role in MOR promoter activity. Furthermore, the transactivation of Sp1 and Sp3 are additive (229). Hence, the ratio of Sp1 and Sp3 molecules in the cells can contribute to the μ-opioid receptor gene transcription. A similar situation is also observed with the δ-opioid receptor gene. The presence of the E box and GC box within the promoter region of the DOR gene allows the transactivation of the DOR promoter by the upstream stimulating factor (USF) and Sp families of transcriptional factors (224). Functional and physical interactions between the USF and Sp transcriptional factors can be demonstrated. Such interactions are critical for the activity of the DOR promoter. By regulating the cellular content or composition of the complex, the opioid receptor gene transcription can be controlled. The significance of these transcriptional factors' interaction on the overall spatial and temporal control of the receptor gene expression remains to be investigated.

Receptor Gene Concentration and Pharmacological Activities

The isolation of the receptor genes and the identification of their structures provided an opportunity to address the fundamental question of how a receptor's level affects the pharmacological activities of drugs. By disrupting the transcription of a specific receptor gene, the involvement of a specific opioid receptor in the in vivo activities of a drug can be determined. Using the homologous recombination method to disrupt receptor transcription, several groups have successfully generated strains of mice in which the μ-opioid receptor was "knocked-out" (230–234). A similar approach was also used to generate mice in which the κ- (235) or the δ-opioid receptor (236) was knocked out. Either by radioactive ligand binding studies, immunoflourescence studies, or quantitative autoradiographic studies (237), these receptor knockout animals exhibited the specific reduction in the receptor protein levels without the alteration of other opioid receptor types. Furthermore, the reduction in the level of receptor was proportional to the gene dosage, demonstrated by the heterozygotic mice that had 50% of the receptor level.

The overall behavior of the receptor knockout animals remains similar to that of the wild-type, with some minor behavioral changes. Changes in the locomotive activity were described in the MOR knockout animals (230, 232) but not in KOR-deficient mice (235). The KOR and MOR knockout mice did not exhibit any changes in the anxiety tests (open-field and O-maze tests). One strain of MOR knockout mice appeared to have changes in their sexual function, as shown by reduced mating activity (232). With the exception of one report with the MOR knockout (231), the lack of a single opioid receptor did not alter the nociceptive threshold after the application of thermal stimuli, either the tail-flick, tail immersion, or the hot plate tests (230, 232, 233, 235, 236), or by mechanical stimuli (238). It is interesting to note that the KOR knockout animals exhibited an increase in the writhing response with the injection of acetic acid that indicated a decrease in the nociceptive response (235). Apparently, the κ-opioid receptor is linked to the control of chemical visceral pain, as suggested by the earlier pharmacological studies.

The absence of an opioid receptor type in these receptor knockout animals enabled investigators to address the issue of which opioid receptor mediates the specific functions of the opioid agonists. In every strain of MOR knockout mice, morphine did not exhibit any antinociceptive effect after thermal stimuli, or produced lethality at high doses (230–234). Though in one report, lethality was observed with an extremely high dose of morphine (233), the cause of death was not due to the normal respiratory suppression effect of the drug. Depending on the method of generating the mutant animals, there were conflicting reports on the ability of the metabolite of morphine, morphine-6β-glucuronide (M6G), and heroin to elicit antinociceptive responses in the knockout animals. M6G and heroin did not produce antinociceptive responses in the μ-opioid receptor knockout mice generated by the deletion of exons 2 and 3 (233, 239) but retained antinociceptive activities in mice generated by an exon 1 deletion (234). Significant levels of M6G binding and the presence of mRNAs detected with the exon 2 and 3 primers were demonstrated in mutant mice with an MOR exon 1 deletion (234). These observations and others suggest the existence of a splice variant of the μ-opioid receptor that is specific for the M6G pharmacological actions. However, active receptors can be formed from two separate fragments of the rhodopsin and muscarinic receptor. In addition, formation of a putative heterodimer between δ- and κ-opioid receptors could result in a receptor complex that exhibits different pharmacological responses to the receptor selective ligands (240). Hence it is probable that the exon 1 truncated μ-opioid receptor could either scavenge or dimerize with other GPCRs to form a functional M6G receptor. The role of M6G and heroin function in the exon 1 deleted MOR knockout animals remains unclear.

The κ-opioid agonist activities were retained in the MOR knockout animals. However, there appears to be a discrepancy in the δ-opioid agonist activity among different strains of mice. The DPDPE antinociceptive effect was not altered in MOR knockout mice when the peptide was injected intracerebroventricularly (233). However, this effect was attenuated when the peptide was injected intra-thecally in the μ-opioid receptor–deficient mice (230, 241). This apparent discrepancy can probably be partially explained by the involvement of multiple opioid receptors in the DPDPE-induced analgesia. In DOR-1–deficient mice, Zhu et al (236) reported that the spinal analgesia of DPDPE was greatly attenuated whereas the supraspinal analgesia was not affected by the absence of δ-opioid receptor. The supraspinal analgesic activity of DPDPE was eliminated in the MOR and DOR double-knockout mice (J Pintar, personal communication). Such observed decrease in the DPDPE analgesic response in the MOR knockout animal could be held as genetic evidence for the existence of a μ/δ-opioid receptor complex (242). However, even with the reduction in the DPDPE analgesic activity, the in vitro activities of DPDPE were not altered in the MOR knockout (243). Thus, whether the DPDPE analgesic activity depends on the physical interaction between the μ- and δ-opioid receptor remains to be investigated.

In addition to identifying whether the μ-opioid receptor is responsible for the morphine-induced antinociceptive responses in the animals, it could be demonstrated that MOR is involved in the morphine-induced decrease in the gastrointestinal transit time but not in the basal transit time (244). The effect of morphine on lymphoid organ atrophy was not observed in the MOR knockout animals (245). Similarly, the regulation of macrophage phagocytosis and secretion of TNFα by morphine was absent in μ-opioid receptor–deficient animals (246). In both of these two studies, the immune cells' functions, such as regulating splenic and thymic cell number and mitogen-induced proliferation, or the inhibition of IL1 and IL6 secretion by macrophages, were not different between the wild-type and mutant mice. However, increase in the proliferation of granulocyte-macrophage and in erythroid and multipotential progenitor cells in both bone marrow and spleen were observed in the MOR knockout animals (232). These data indicated a probable link between hematopoiesis and the μ-opioid receptor.

As expected, the KOR-deficient mice demonstrated that KOR is critical for the U50,488-induced hypolocomotor, analgesic, and aversive activities in the animals (235). KOR was shown to be not involved in the morphine analgesia and reward. This finding substantiated the observation with the MOR knockout in which the morphine pharmacological actions were completely eliminated. Interestingly, KOR was shown to participate in the manifestation of morphine abstinence. The naloxone-precipitated morphine withdrawal syndrome was less severe in the knockout animals as compared to that in the litter mate wild-type control (235). Because the degree of tolerance to morphine was not investigated in the reported studies, it is not certain whether the diminished naloxone-precipitated withdrawal syndrome has a parallel in the tolerance development.

The role of δ-opioid receptor in the pharmacology of the receptor-selective ligands such as DPDPE or BW873U86 was not clearly defined by the DOR-deficient mice. As discussed earlier, the ability of DPDPE or [D-Ala^2,D-Glu^4]deltorphin to elicit a supraspinal analgesic response was not altered in the DOR knockout animals (236). Though the DPDPE spinal analgesic response was reduced by sixfold, the peptide can elicit maximal antinociceptive activity when injected intrathecally into the knockout animals. The complete absence of the δ-opioid receptor in these animals suggested that the DPDPE spinal analgesic response could be mediated by receptors other than the classical δ-opioid receptor. To compound the problem, the antinociceptive activity of BW873U86 was greatly potentiated in the DOR-deficient mice (236). These data suggested that a secondary analgesic pathway, unmasked in the DOR knockout mice, was responsible for the observed antinociceptive activities of these compounds.

The definite role of DOR in the development of morphine tolerance was established with the knockout studies. In previous reports with the selective δ-opioid receptor antagonist naltrindole (247) or with antisense oligonucleotides to DOR (248), partial blockade of the tolerance development to morphine was observed with the reduction of δ-opioid receptor activity. In the DOR-deficient mutant mice, chronic treatment with morphine for 10 days did not change the potency of morphine (236). The DPDPE-induced supraspinal analgesia in these knockout animals also did not develop tolerance during chronic DPDPE treatment. These data suggested not only the role of DOR in the development of morphine tolerance, but also that the receptor that manifest the supraspinal DPDPE effect in the knockout mice is regulated similarly to that of the μ-opioid receptor.

PERSPECTIVE

The opioid receptors are unique among all the GPCRs. The number of multiple receptor subtypes as defined by pharmacological or biochemical binding studies appears to far exceed the number of cloned receptors and their genes. The existence of μ_1-, μ_2-, μ_3-, δ_1-, δ_2-, κ_1-, κ_2-, and κ_3-opioid receptors has long been postulated. The presence of introns within the receptor genes allows for the generation of splice variants, and probable subtypes of the receptors. Though a splice variant of the μ-opioid receptor cDNA was isolated (144), the pharmacology of this splice variant resembled that of the wild-type MOR. With extensive low-stringency hybridization procedures, no opioid receptor type other than the cloned μ-, δ-, and κ-opioid receptors could be isolated. At best, the orphanin FQ or nociceptin receptor with high homology to the opioid receptors was cloned using this approach (249–254). One could argue that the other opioid receptor subtypes are structurally dissimilar to the cloned opioid receptors, as in the case of GABA or histamine receptor types. However, this argument was not supported by the studies with the receptor knockout animals. The disruption of an opioid receptor gene normally did not result in residual binding that could account for the existence of receptor subtypes. Though with the mice that have the first intron of MOR deleted, M6G and heroin remained active. The multiple possibilities that could cause such a phenomenon, as discussed previously, suggested that the conclusion of the existence of unique M6G binding sites may be too premature. The vast literature on the existence of multiple δ-opioid receptor subtypes was not supported by the DOR knockout. The complete absence of DPDPE binding in the DOR-deficient mice and the retention of the DPDPE-induced supraspinal analgesia in these animals suggested the observed effect of DPDPE is mediated by other opioid receptors. It is also probable that this DPDPE effect is mediated by a yet-unidentified receptor.

In the absence of identified proteins, alternative explanations must be used to account for the reported multiple opioid receptors. It is still possible that a single amino acid difference among the receptors will generate the subtype pharmacology, as it was clearly demonstrated with the single amino acid mutation in the putative fourth transmembrane serine residue could result in the phenotype of antagonist activating the receptor (255). However, the human opioid receptor polymorphism studies have not revealed such a situation. At best, the human μ-opioid receptor with a single nucleotide polymorphism binds β-endorphin with higher affinity (256). A different polymorphism in δ-opioid receptor did not reveal any pharmacological phenotype (257). Thus it is possible that the multiple opioid receptor subtypes could be generated from single nucleotide polymorphism that has eluded detection by conventional means. This could be accomplished only by detailed nucleotide sequencing of the receptor mRNAs in regions where the pharmacology of the receptor subtypes was reported. With the current sequencing technology, such a goal can be reached. Another intriguing possibility has been reported on the alteration of the pharmacological activities of the opioid receptors when they are heterodimerized (240). The inability of the receptor-selective ligands such as DPDPE or U69593 to compete for diprenorphine binding to the putative κ/δ-opioid receptors dimer provided another level of regulation of the opioid receptor activities. It is possible that the opioid receptor subtypes reported are the results of the heterodimerization of various opioid receptors. Whether the opioid receptors actually dimerized and whether receptor dimerization could generate the pharmacology reported for the various subtypes should be investigated.

With all the molecular biological tools, the fundamental question on the molecular mechanism for opioid tolerance and dependence remains to be adequately addressed. It is attractive to suggest that receptor phosphorylation is the fundamental basis for opioid tolerance. No doubt, opioid agonists could induce the phosphorylation of all the opioid receptor types. However, it is even doubtful that the receptor phosphorylation is the sole mechanism for the observed homologous desensitization to various effector systems. The noncorrelation between the time course of receptor phosphorylation and desensitization, as reported by some laboratories, could be reconciled by the dephosphorylation and resensitization of the internalized receptor. Depending on the efficacy of the receptor coupling to individual effector and the rate of receptor recycling, it is probable that the receptor activity is not altered even with a robust phosphorylation of the receptor. Phosphorylation and subsequent inactivation of the effector system could also cause homologous desensitization. Phosphorylation of the type II adenylyl cyclase in the guinea pig ileum longitudinal muscle myenteric plexus (258) and $PLC\beta_3$ in NG108–15 cells (104) after opioid receptor activation have been reported. In NG108–15 cells, the transient activation and inactivation of $PLC\beta_3$ by δ-opioid receptors correlated to the phosphorylation of the enzyme itself (104). In the case of $PLC\beta_3$ phosphorylation, the ability of other GPCR agonists, such as LPA, to induce phosphorylation of the same proteins suggested probable compartmentalization of the receptor with the $PLC\beta_3$, thus allowing homologous desensitization. Hence, homologous desensitization could occur with multiple mechanisms.

The uncoupling of the receptor from the effector, or the inactivation of a specific pool of effector, may not be the basis for opioid tolerance and dependence either. The involvement of transcriptional responses for the adaptation to long-term exposure to the drug has long been proposed. This was clearly demonstrated in mice that had the α and δ isoforms of the cAMP-responsive element binding protein (CREB) disrupted. The symptoms of morphine withdrawal were greatly attenuated in these animals (259). However, the uncoupling of the opioid receptor, CREB, and the immediate early genes might be three of the many factors that contribute to the chronic opioid responses. The involvement of other receptors in the modulation of opioid tolerance has been demonstrated. The DOR-deficient mice provided the genetic evidence for the involvement of δ-opioid receptor for morphine tolerance (236). Additionally, the participation of NMDA receptor in morphine tolerance has been established. By the concurrent administration of the NMDA antagonists, LY274614 and MK-801, morphine tolerance can be attenuated (260, 261). Thus, the regulation of multiple neuronal activities by multiple receptors could then manifest the overall response to chronic opioid treatment. The manifestation of the chronic response might be a probable reason for the evolution of the multiple opioid receptors.

The complexity in the signal transduction of the opioid receptor goes beyond the simple involvement of receptor-Gi/Go proteins and the effectors. As discussed in this review, a universal mechanism cannot be applied to all receptor agonists. The two μ-opioid receptor agonists, morphine and DAMGO, definitely elicited differential cellular responses, and their receptor complexes can be distinguished from each other. Further, the overall response to the activation of Gi/Go by opioid agonists will depend on the composition of the neurons expressing the receptor. This is best illustrated by the differential responses exhibited by the multiple adenylyl cyclase subtypes to the activation of the receptor. One can imagine that the identity and the concentration of the proteins participating in the signaling within the membrane microdomains of the receptor will greatly affect the opioid receptor signaling. The signaling through scaffold, anchoring, and adaptor proteins has been well established with many membrane receptors, in particular those of the tyrosine kinase family (262). Recognition of the phosphorylated tyrosine by proteins such as Grb2 that contain both the SH2 and SH3 domains will allow Grb2 to serve as an adaptor that recruits other cellular proteins, such as Sos, to the vicinity of the receptor and participates in the signal cascades. The recruitment of other proteins with an adaptor that has multiple docking sites will allow the amplification or modulation of the signals. An excellent example is the *Drosophila* InaD gene that codes for a protein with 5 PDZ domains (263). InaD associates through these PDZ domains with a light-activated Ca^{2+} channel (TRP), PLCβ, and PKC. The organization of these effectors by InaD allows for the efficient activation of TRP by PLCβ in response to the stimulation of rhodopsin and $Gα_q$, and the inactivation by the phosphorylation of TRP by PKC. If a similar scenario exists for the opioid receptor, the recruitment of molecules such as $PLCβ_3$ and PKC to the vicinity of the receptor could provide a rapid control mechanism for the opioid receptor signaling. The local increase in the intracellular Ca^{2+} level due to $PLCβ_3$ activation would active the PKC, which in turn could phosphorylate and inactivate the $PLCβ_3$, and thus turn off the signal. Depending on the kinetics of such a feedback cycle, the magnitude of the signals can be regulated. Hence, the immediate emphasis for the understanding of the receptor signaling should be the identification of cellular proteins that participate in the opioid receptor signaling. With the possibility that opioid receptor dimerization could affect the activity also, the formation of the signaling complexes within a microdomain could greatly affect the cellular responses to a specific pharmacological agent targeted for a particular type of opioid receptor. These signaling complexes might be the true distinction between the multiple opioid receptors.

ACKNOWLEDGMENTS

This work was supported by NIH grants DA11806, DA00564, DA01583, DA07339, DA70554, and by the A and F Stark Fund of the Minnesota Medical Foundation. This work was also supported by grants HKUST567/95M and HKUST6176/97M to YHW.

Visit the Annual Reviews home page at www.AnnualReviews.org.

LITERATURE CITED

1. Evans CJ, Keith DE, Morrison H, Magendzo K, Edwards RH. 1992. Cloning of a delta opioid receptor by functional expression. *Science* 258:1952–55
2. Kieffer BL, Befort K, Gaveriaux-Ruff C, Hirth CG. 1992. The δ-opioid receptor: isolation of a cDNA by expression cloning and pharmacological characterization. *Proc. Natl. Acad. Sci. USA* 89:12048–52

3. Chen Y, Mestek A, Liu J, Hurley JA, Yu L. 1993. Molecular cloning and functional expression of a μ-opioid receptor from rat brain. *Mol. Pharmacol.* 44:8–12

4. Fukuda K, Kato Mori SK, Hishi M, Takeshima H. 1993. Primary structures and expression from cDNAs of rat opioid receptor δ- and μ-subtypes. *FEBS Lett.* 327:311–14

5. Yasuda K, Raynor K, Kong H, Breder CD, Takeda J, et al. 1993. Cloning and functional comparison of κ and δ opioid receptors from mouse brain. *Proc. Natl. Acad. Sci. USA* 90:6736–40

6. Meng F, Xie GX, Thompson RC, Mansour A, Goldstein A, et al. 1993. Cloning and pharmacological characterization of a rat kappa-opioid receptor. *Proc. Natl. Acad. Sci. USA* 90:9954–58

7. Li S, Zhu J, Chen C, Chen YW, Deriel JK, et al. 1993. Molecular cloning and expression of a rat κ-opioid receptor. *Biochem. J.* 295:629–33

8. Chen Y, Mestek A, Liu J, Yu L. 1993. Molecular cloning of a rat κ opioid receptor reveals sequence similarities to the μ- and δ-opioid receptors. *Biochem. J.* 295:625–28

9. Tallent M, Dichter MA, Bell GI, Reisine T. 1994. The cloned kappa opioid receptor couples to an N-type calcium current in undifferentiated PC-12 cells. *Neuroscience* 63:1033–40

10. Piros ET, Prather PL, Lo HH, Law PY, Evans CJ, Hales TG. 1995. Ca^{+2} channel and adenylyl cyclase modulation by cloned μ-opioid receptors in GH3 cells. *Mol. Pharmacol.* 47:1041–49

11. Piros ET, Prather PL, Law PY, Evans CJ, Hales TG. 1996. Voltage-dependent inhibition of L-type Ca^{+2} channels by cloned μ- and δ-opioid receptors. *Mol. Pharmacol.* 50:947–56

12. Johnson PS, Wang JB, Wang WF, Uhl GR. 1994. Expressed mu opiate receptor couples to adenylate cyclase and phosphatidyl inositol turnover. *NeuroReport* 5:507–9

13. Spencer RJ, Jin W, Thayer SA, Chakrabarti S, Law PY, Loh HH. 1997. Mobilization of Ca^{+2} from intracellular stores in transfected neuro2a cells by activation of multiple opioid receptor subtypes. *Biochem. Pharmacol.* 54:809–18

14. Henry DJ, Grandy DK, Lester HA, Davidson N, Chavkin C. 1995. κ-opioid receptors couple to inwardly rectifying potassium channels when coexpressed by *Xenopus* oocytes. *Mol. Pharmacol.* 47:551–57

15. Li LY, Chang KJ. 1996. The stimulatory effect of opioids on mitogen-activated protein kinase in Chinese hamster ovary cells transfected to express μ-opioid receptors. *Mol. Pharmacol.* 50:599–602

16. Fukuda K, Kato S, Morikawa H, Shoda T, Mori K. 1996. Functional coupling of the δ-, μ- and κ-opioid receptors to mitogen-activated protein kinase and arachidonate release in Chinese hamster ovary cells. *J. Neurochem.* 67:1309–16

17. Sharma SK, Klee WA, Niremberg M. 1977. Opiate dependent modulation of adenylate cyclase activity. *Proc. Natl. Acad. Sci. USA* 74:3365–69

18. Hescheler J, Rosenthal W, Trautwein W, Schultz G. 1987. The GTP-binding protein, G_o, regulates neuronal calcium channels. *Nature* 325:445–47

19. Surprenant A, Shen KZ, North RA, Tatsumi H. 1990. Inhibition of calcium currents by noradrenaline, somatostatin and opioids in guinea-pig submucosal neurones. *J. Physiol. Lond.* 431:585–608

20. North RA, Williams JT, Surprenant A, Christie MJ. 1987. Mu and delta receptors belong to a family of receptors that couple to potassium channels. *Proc. Natl. Acad. Sci. USA* 84:5487–91

21. Jin W, Lee NM, Loh HH, Thayer SA. 1992. Dual excitatory and inhibitory effects of opioids on intracellular calcium in neuroblastoma × glioma hybrid

NG108–15 cells. *Mol. Pharmacol.* 42: 1083–89

22. Burt AR, Carr IC, Mullaney I, Anderson NG, Milligan G. 1996. Agonist activation of p42 and p44 mitogen-activated protein kinases following expression of the mouse δ-opioid receptor in Rat-1 fibroblasts: effects of receptor expression levels and comparisons with G-protein activation. *Biochem. J.* 320:227–35

23. Hsia JA, Moss J, Hewlett EL, Vaughan M. 1984. ADP-ribosylation of adenylate cyclase by pertussis toxin. Effects on inhibitory agonist binding. *J. Biol. Chem.* 259:1086–90

24. Wong YH, Demoliou-Mason CD, Barnard EA. 1989. The opioid receptor(s) in magnesium-digitonin solubilized rat brain membranes are tightly coupled to a pertussis toxin sensitive guanine nucleotide binding protein. *J. Neurochem.* 52:999–1009

25. McKenzie FR, Milligan G. 1990. δ-Opioid receptor mediated inhibition of adenylate cyclase is transduced specifically by the guanine-nucleotide-binding protein Gi2. *Biochem. J.* 267:391–98

26. Carter BD, Medzihradsky F. 1993. Go mediates the coupling of the μ opioid receptor to adenylyl cyclase in cloned neural cells and brains. *Proc. Natl. Acad. Sci. USA* 90:4062–66

27. Roerig SC, Loh HH, Law PY. 1992. Identification of three separate G-proteins which interact with the delta opioid receptor in NG108–15 neuroblastoma × glioma hybrid cells. *Mol. Pharmacol* 41:822–31

28. Prather PL, Loh HH, Law PY. 1994. Interaction of δ-opioid receptors with multiple G-proteins: a non-relationship between agonist potency to inhibit adenylyl cyclase and activation of G-proteins. *Mol. Pharmacol.* 45:997–1003

29. Prather PL, McGinn TM, Erickson LJ, Evans CJ, Loh HH, Law PY. 1994. Ability of δ − opioid receptors to interact with multiple G-proteins is independent of

receptor density. *J. Biol. Chem.* 269: 21293–302

30. Prather PL, McGinn TM, Claude PA, Liu-Chen LY, Loh HH, Law PY. 1995. Properties of κ-opioid receptor expressed in CHO cells: activation of multiple G-proteins similar to other opioid receptors. *Mol. Brain Res.* 29:336–46

31. ChakrabartiS, Prather PL, Yu L, Law PY, Loh HH. 1995. Expression of the μ-opioid receptor in CHO cells: ability of μ-opioid ligands to promote ^{32}P-α-azidoanilido GTP labeling of multiple G protein α-subunits. *J. Neurochem.* 64: 2354–543

32. Wong YH, Federman A, Pace AM, Zachary I, Evans T, et al. 1991. Mutant α subunits of G$_{i2}$ inhibit cyclic AMP accumulation. *Nature* 351:63–65

33. Wong YH, Conklin BR, Bourne HR. 1992. G$_z$-mediated inhibition of cAMP accumulation. *Science* 255:339–42

34. Selley DE, Breivogel CS, Childers SR. 1998. Opioid inhibition of adenylyl cyclase in membranes from pertussis toxin-treated NG108–15 cells. *J. Recept. Signal Transduct. Res.* 18:25–49

35. Chan JSC, Chiu TT, Wong YH. 1995. Activation of type II adenylyl cyclase by the cloned μ-opioid receptor: coupling to multiple G proteins. *J. Neurochem.* 65:2682–89

36. Lai HWL, Minami M, Satoh M, Wong YH. 1995. G$_z$ coupling to the rat κ-opioid receptor. *FEBS Lett.* 360:97–99

37. Tsu RC, Chan JSC, Wong YH. 1995. Regulation of multiple effectors by the cloned δ-opioid receptor: stimulation of phospholipase C and type II adenylyl cyclase. *J. Neurochem.* 64:2700–7

38. Law SF, Reisine T. 1997. Changes in the association of G protein subunits with the cloned mouse δ-opioid receptor on agonist stimulation. *J. Pharmacol. Exp. Ther.* 281:1476–86

39. Sanchez-Blazquez P, Juarros JL, Martinez-Pena Y, Castro MA, Garzon J. 1993. G$_{x/z}$ and G$_{i2}$ transducer proteins on μ/δ

opioid mediated supraspinal antinociception. *Life Sci.* 53:381–86

40. Sanchez-Blazquez P, Garcia-Espana A, Garzon J. 1995. In vivo injection of antisense oligodeoxynucleotides to Gα subunits and supraspinal analgesia evoked by μ and δ opioid agonists. *J. Pharmacol. Exp. Ther.* 275:1590–96

41. Standifer KM, Rossi GC, Pasternak GW. 1996. Differential blockade of opioid analgesia by antisense oligodeoxynucleotides directed against various G protein alpha subunits. *Mol. Pharmacol.* 50:293–98

42. Garzon J, Martinez-Pena Y, Sanchez-Blazquez S. 1997. Gx/z is regulated by μ but not δ opioid receptors in the stimulation of the low K_m GTPase activity in mouse periaqueductal grey matter. *J. Neurosci.* 9:1194–200

43. Jeong SW, Ikeda SR. 1998. G protein α subunit G $α_z$ couples neurotransmitter receptors to ion channels in sympathetic neurons. *Neuron* 21:1201–12

44. Puri SK, Cochin J. Volicer L. 1975. Effect of morphine sulfate on adenylate cyclase and phosphodiesterase activities in rat corpus striatum. *Life Sci.* 16:759–68

45. Cruciani RA, Dvorkin B, Morris SA, Crain SM, Makman MH. 1993. Direct coupling of opioid receptors to both stimulatory and inhibitroy guanine nucleotide-binding proteins in F-11 neuroblastoma-sensory neuron hybrid cells. *Proc. Natl. Acad. Sci. USA* 90:3019–23

46. Olianas MC, Onali P. 1995. Participation of δ opioid receptor subtypes in the stimulation of adenylyl cyclase activity in rat olfactory bulb. *J. Pharmacol. Exp. Ther.* 275:1560–67

47. Makman MH, Dvorkin B, Crain SM. 1988. Modulation of adenylate cyclase activity of mouse spinal cord-ganglion explants by opioids, serotonin and pertussis toxin. *Brain Res.* 445:303–13

48. Tang WJ, Hurley JH. 1998. Catalytic mechanism and regulation of mammalian adenylyl cyclases. *Mol. Pharmacol.* 54:231–40

49. Federman AD, Conklin BR, Schrader KA, Reed RR, Bourne HR. 1992. Hormonal stimulation of adenylyl cyclase through G_i-protein βγ subunits. *Nature* 356:159–61

50. Tsu RC, Allen RA, Wong YH. 1995b. Stimulation of type II adenylyl cyclase by formyl peptide and C5a chemoattractant receptors. *Mol. Pharmacol.* 47:835–41

51. Taussig R, Tang WJ, Hepler JR, Gilman AG. 1994. Distinct patterns of bidirectional regulation of mammalian adenylyl cyclases. *J. Biol. Chem.* 269:6093–100

52. Toyoshi T, Ukai M, Kameyama T. 1992. Combination of a δ-opioid receptor agonist but not a μ-opioid receptor agonist with the D_1-selective dopamine receptor agonist SKF 38393 markedly potentiates different behaviors in mice. *Eur. J. Pharmacol.* 213:25–30

53. Tsu RC, Wong YH. 1996. G_i-mediated stimulation of type II adenylyl cyclase is augmented by G_q-coupled receptor activation and phorbol ester treatment. *J. Neurosci.* 16:1317–23

54. Noble F, Derrien M, Roques BP. 1993. Modulation of opioid antinociception by CCK at the supraspinal level: evidence of regulatory mechanisms between CCK and enkephalin systems in the control of pain. *Br. J. Pharmacol.* 109:1064–70

55. Lou L, Zhou T, Wang P, Pei G. 1999. Modulation of Ca^{2+}/calmodulin-dependent protein kinase II activity by acute and chronic morphine administration in rat hippocampus: differential regulation of α and β isoforms. *Mol. Pharmacol.* 55:557–63

56. Crain SM, Shen KF. 1998. Modulation of opioid analgesia, tolerance and dependence by Gs-coupled, GM1 ganglioside-regulated opioid receptor functions. *Trends Pharmacol. Sci.* 19:358–65

57. Crain SM, Shen KF. 1996. Modulatory effects of Gs-coupled excitatory opioid receptor functions on opioid analgesia,

tolerance and dependence. *Neurochem. Res.* 21:1347–51

58. Wu G, Lu ZH, Alfinito P, Ledeen RW. 1997. Opioid receptor and calcium channel regulation of adenylyl cyclase, modulated by GM1, in NG108–15 cells: competitive interactions. *Neurochem. Res.* 22:1281–89

59. Wu G, Lu ZH, Ledeen RW. 1997. Interaction of the δ-opioid receptor with GM1 ganglioside: conversion from inhibitory to excitatory mode. *Mol. Brain Res.* 44:341–46

60. Sarne Y, Rubovitch V, Fields A, Gafni M. 1998. Dissociation between the inhibitory and stimulatory effects of opioid peptides on cAMP formation in SK-N-SH neuroblastoma cells. *Biochem. Biophys. Res. Commun.* 246:128–31

61. Yoshimura M, Ikeda H, Tabakoff B. 1996. μ-opioid receptors inhibit dopamine-stimulated activity of type V adenylyl cyclase but enhance dopamine-stimulated activity of type VII adenylyl cyclase. *Mol. Pharmacol.* 50:43–51

62. Avidor-Reiss T, Nevo I, Saya D, Bayerwitch M, Vogel Z. 1997. Opiate-induced adenylyl cyclase superactivation is isozyme-specific. *J. Biol. Chem.* 272:5040–47

63. Rhim H, Miller RJ. 1994. Opioid receptors modulate diverse types of calcium channels in the nucleus tractus solitarius of the rat. *J. Neurosci.* 14:7608–15

64. Connor M, Schuller A, Pintar JE, Christie MJ. 1999. μ-opioid receptor modulation of calcium channel current in periaqueductal grey neurons from C57B16/J mice and mutant mice lacking MOR-1. *Br. J. Pharmacol.* 126:1553–58

65. Randall AD. 1998. The molecular basis of voltage-gated Ca^{2+} channel diversity: Is it time for T? *J. Membr. Biol.* 161:207–13

66. Morikawa H, Fukuda K, Kato S, Mori K, Higashida H. 1995. Coupling of the cloned μ-opioid receptor with the ω-

conotoxin-sensitive Ca^{2+} current in NG 108–15 cells. *J. Neurochem.* 65:1403–6

67. Kaneko S, Fukuda K, Yada N, Akaike A, Mori Y, Satoh M. 1994. Ca^{2+} channel inhibition by κ opioid receptors expressed in *Xenopus* oocytes. *NeuroReport* 5:2506–8

68. Bourinet E, Soong TW, Stea A, Snutch TP. 1996. Determinants of the G protein-dependent opioid modulation of neuronal calcium channels. *Proc. Natl. Acad. Sci. USA* 93:1486–91

69. Moises HC, Rusin KI, MacDonald RL. 1994. μ-opioid receptor-mediated reduction of neuronal calcium current occurs via a G_o-type GTP-binding protein. *J. Neurosci.* 14:3842–51

70. Ikeda SF. 1996. Voltage-dependent modulation of N-type calcium channels by G-protein βγ subunits. *Nature* 380:225–58

71. Herlitze S, Garcia DE, Mackie K, Hille B, Scheuer T, Catterall WA. 1996. Modulation of Ca^{2+} channels by G-protein βγ subunits. *Nature* 380:258–62

72. Jiang M, Gold MS, Boulay G, Spicher K, Peyton M, et al. 1998. Multiple neurological abnormalities in mice deficient in the G protein Go. *Proc. Natl. Acad. Sci. USA* 95:3269–74

73. Zamponi GW, Bourinet E, Nelson D, Nargeot J, Snutch TP. 1997. Crosstalk between G proteins and protein kinase C mediated by the calcium channel α_1 subunit. *Nature* 385:442–46

74. King AP, Hall KE, MacDonald RL. 1999. κ- and μ-opioid inhibition of N-type calcium currents is attenuated by 4β-phorbol 12-myristate 13-acetate and protein kinase C in rat dorsal root ganglion neurons. *J. Pharmacol. Exp. Ther.* 289:312–20

75. Cemerikic B, Zamah R, Ahmed MS. 1998. Identification of L-type calcium channels associated with κ opioid receptors in human placenta. *J. Mol. Neurosci.* 10:261–72

76. Grudt TJ, Williams JT. 1993. κ-opioid

receptors also increase potassium conductance. *Neurobiology* 90:11429–32

77. Schneider SP, Eckert WA, Light AR. 1998. Opioid-activated postsynaptic, inward rectifying potassium currents in whole cell recordings in substantia gelatinosa. *J. Neurophysiol.* 80:2954–62

78. Ma GH, Miller RF, Kuznetsov A, Philipson LH. 1995. κ-opioid receptor activates an inwardly rectifying K+ channel by a G protein-linked mechanism: coexpression in *Xenopus* oocytes. *Mol. Pharmacol.* 47:1035–40

79. Schultz JJ, Hsu AK, Nagase H, Gross GJ. 1998. TAN-67, a δ 1-opioid receptor agonist, reduces infarct size via activation of $G_{i/o}$ proteins and KATP channels. *Am. J. Physiol.* 274:H909–14

80. Baraban SC, Lothman EW, Lee A, Guyenet PG. 1995. κ opioid receptor-mediated suppression of voltage-activated potassium current in a catecholaminergic neuronal cell line. *J. Pharmacol. Exp. Ther.* 273:927–33

81. Yamada M, Inanobe A, Kurachi Y. 1998. G protein regulation of potassium ion channels. *Am. Soc. Pharmacol. Exp. Ther.* 50:724–57

82. Yan K, Gautam N. 1996. A domain on the G protein β subunit interacts with both adenylyl cyclase 2 and the muscarinic atrial potassium channel. *J. Biol. Chem.* 271:17597–600

83. Lim NF, Dascal N, Labarca C, Davidson N, Lester HA. 1995. A G protein-gated K+ channel is activated via β_2-adrenergic receptors and Gβγ subunits in *Xenopus* oocytes. *J. Gen. Physiol.* 105:421–39

84. Huang CL, Feng S, Hilgemann DW. 1998. Direct activation of inward rectifier potassium channels by PIP_2 and its stabilization by Gβγ. *Nature* 391:803–6

85. Xie CW, Lewis DV. 1997. Involvement of cAMP-dependent protein kinase in μ-opioid modulation of NMDA-mediated synaptic currents. *J. Neurophysiol.* 78: 759–66

86. Cai YC, Ma L, Fan GH, Zhao J, Jiang LZ, Pei G. 1997. Activation of N-methyl-D-aspartate receptor attenuates acute responsiveness of δ-opioid receptor. *Mol. Pharmacol.* 51:583–87

87. Fan GH, Zhao J, Wu YL, Lou LG, Zhang Z, et al. 1998. N-Methyl-D-aspartate attenuates opioid receptor-mediated G protein activation and this process involves protein kinase C. *Mol. Pharmacol.* 53:684–90

88. Smart D, Lambert DG. 1996. δ-Opioids stimulate inositol 1,4,5-triphosphate formation, and so mobilize Ca^{2+} from intracellular stores, in undifferentiated NG108–15 cells. *J. Neurochem.* 66: 1462–67

89. Smart D, Smith G, Lambert DG. 1994. μ-Opioid receptor stimulation of inositol (1,4,5)trisphosphate formation via a pertussis toxin-sensitive G protein. *J. Neurochem.* 62:1009–14

90. Smart D, Hirst RA, Hirota K, Grandy DK, Lambert DG. 1997. The effects of recombinant rat μ-opioid receptor activation in CHO cell on phospholipase C, $[Ca^{2+}]_i$ and adenylyl cyclase. *Br. J. Pharmacol.* 120:1165–71

91. Smart D, Smith G, Lambert DG. 1995. μ-opioids activate phospholipase C in SH-SY5Y human neuroblastoma cells via calcium-channel opening. *Biochem. J.* 305:577–81

92. Misawa H, Udea H, Katada T, Ui M, Satoh M. 1995. A subtype of opioid κ-receptor is coupled to inhibition of Gi1-mediated phospholipase C activity in the guinea pig cerebellum. *FEBS Lett.* 36:106–10

93. Tang T, Kiang JG, Cote TE, Cox BM. 1995. Antisense oligodeoxynucleotide to the G_{i2} protein α subunit sequence inhibits an opioid-induced increase in the intracellular free calcium concentration in ND8–47 neuroblastoma × dorsal root ganglion hybrid cells. *Mol. Pharmacol.* 48:189–93

94. Ueda H, Miyamae T, Fukushima N,

Takeshima H, Fukuda K,et al. 1995. Opioid μ- and κ-receptor mediate phospholipase C activation through G_{i1} in *Xenopus* oocytes. *Mol. Brain Res.* 32:166–70

95. Murthy KS, Makhlouf GM. 1996. Opioid μ, δ, and κ receptor-induced activation of phospholipase C-β 3 and inhibition of adenylyl cyclase is mediated by G_{i2} and G(o) in smooth muscle. *Mol. Pharmacol.* 50:870–77

96. Allouche S, Polastron J, Jauzac P. 1996. The δ-opioid receptor regulates activity of ryanodine receptors in the human neuroblastoma cell line SK-N-BE. *J. Neurochem.* 67:2461–70

97. Offermanns S, Simon M. 1995. $G\alpha_{15}$ and $G\alpha_{16}$ couple a wide variety of receptors to phospholipase C. *J. Biol. Chem.* 270:15175–80

98. Lee JWM, Joshi S, Chan JSC, Wong YH. 1998. Differential coupling of μ, δ, and κ opioid receptors to Gα16-mediated stimulation of phospholipase C. *J. Neurochem.* 70:2203–11

99. Sanchez-Blazquez P, Garzon J. 1998. δ Opioid receptor subtypes activate inositol-signaling pathways in the production of antinociception. *J. Pharmacol. Exp. Ther.* 285:820–27

100. Bian JS, Zhang WM, Xia Q, Wong TM. 1998. Phospholipase C inhibitors attenuate arrhythmias induced by κ-receptor stimulation in the isolated rat heart. *J. Mol. Cell. Cardiol.* 30:2103–10

101. Sharp BM, McKean DJ, McAllen K, Shahabi NA. 1998. Signaling through δ-opioid receptors on murine splenic T cells and stably transfected Jurkat cells. *Ann. NY Acad. Sci.* 840:420–24

102. Hedin KE, Bell MP, Kalli KR, Huntoon CJ, Sharp BM, McKean DJ. 1997. δ-opioid receptors expressed by Jurkat T cells enhance 1L-2 secretion by increasing AP-1 complexes and activity of the NF-AT/AP-1-binding promoter element. *J. Immunol.* 159:5431–40

103. Zhou J, Stanners J, Kabouridis P, Han H,

Tsoukas CD. 1998. Inhibition of TCR/CD3-mediated signaling by a mutant of the hematopoietically expressed G16 GTP-binding protein. *Eur. J. Immunol.* 28:1645–55

104. Strassheim D, Law PY, Loh HH. 1998. Contribution of phospholipase C-β_3 phosphorylation to the rapid attenuation of opioid-activated phosphoinositide response. *Mol. Pharmacol.* 53:1047–53

105. Fan GH, Zhou TH, Zhang WB, Pei G. 1998. Suppression of phospholipase C blocks Gi-mediated inhibition of adenylyl cyclase activity. *Eur. J. Pharmacol.* 341:317–22

106. Tang WJ, Gilman AG. 1991. Type-specific regulation of adenylyl cyclase by G protein βγ subunits. *Science* 254:1500–3

107. Luttrell LM, Daaka Y, Lefkowitz RJ. 1999. Regulation of tyrosine kinase cascades by G-protein-coupled receptors. *Curr. Opin. Cell Biol.* 11:177–83

108. Mangoura D. 1997. μ-Opioids activate tyrosine kinase focal adhesion kinase and regulate cortical cytoskeleton proteins cortactin and vinculin in chick embryonic neurons. *J. Neurosci. Res.* 50:391–401

109. Ignatova EF, Belcheva MM, Bohn LM, Neuman MC, Coscia CJ. 1999. Requirement of receptor internalization for opioid stimulation of mitogen-activated protein kinase: biochemical and immunofluorescence confocal microscopic evidence. *J. Neurosci.* 19:56–63

110. Li JG, Luo LY, Krupnick JG, Benovic JL, Liu-Chen LY. 1999. U50,488-induced internalization of the human κ-opioid receptor involves a β-arrestin- and dynamin-dependent mechanism. κ receptor internalization is not required for mitogen-activating protein kinase activation. *J. Biol. Chem.* 274:12087–94

111. Chuang LF, Killam KF Jr, Chuang RY. 1997. Induction and activation of mitogen-activated protein kinases of human lymphocytes as one of the signaling pathways of the immunomodulatory effects

of morphine sulphate. *J. Biol. Chem.* 272:26815–17

112. Polakiewicz RD, Schieferl SM, Dorner LF, Kansra V, Comb MJ. 1998. A mitogen-activated protein kinase pathway is required for μ-opioid receptor desensitization. *J. Biol. Chem.* 273:12402–6

113. Schultz S, Hollt V. 1998. Opioid withdrawal activates MAP kinase in locus coeruleus neurons in morphine-dependent rats in vivo. *Eur. J. Neurosci.* 10:1196–201

114. Hawes BE, Luttrell LM, van Biesen T, Lefkowitz RJ. 1996. Phosphatidylinositol 3-kinase is an early intermediate in the Gß(-mediated mitogen-activated protein kinase signaling pathway. *J. Biol. Chem.* 271:12133–36

115. Polakiewicz RD, Schieferl SM, Gingras AC, Sonenberg N, Comb MJ. 1998. μ-Opioid receptor activates signaling pathways implicated in cell survival and translational control. *J. Biol. Chem.* 273:23534–41

116. Belcheva MM, Vogel Z, Ignatova E, Avidor-Reiss T, Zippel R, et al. 1998. Opioid modulation of extracellular signal-regulated protein kinase activity is ras-dependent and involves Gβγ subunits. *J. Neurochem.* 70:635–45

117. Nakano K, Osugi T, Kuo CH, Higuchi H, Miki N. 1994. Tyrosine phosphorylation of a 58 kDa protein induced by morphine in SK-N-SH cells. *Biochem. Biophys. Res. Comm.* 200:797–801

118. Mullaney I, Carr IC, Burt AR, Wilson M, Anderson NG, Milligan G. 1997. Agonist-mediated tyrosine phosphorylation of isoforms of the shc adapter protein by the δ opioid receptor. *Cell Signal* 9:423–29

119. Wilson MA, Burt AR, Milligan G, Anderson NG. 1997. Mitogenic signaling by δ opioid receptors expressed in rat-1 fibroblasts involves activation of the p70s6k/p85s6k S6 kinase. *Biochem. J.* 325:217–22

120. Law PY, McGinn TM, Campbell KM, Erickson LE, Loh HH. 1997. Agonist activation of δ-opioid receptor but not μ-opioid receptor potentiates fetal calf serum or tyrosine kinase receptor-mediated cell proliferation in a cell-line specific manner. *Mol. Pharmacol.* 51:152–60

121. Higashita R, Li L, Van Putten V, Yamamura Y, Zarinetchi F, et al. 1997. $G\alpha_{16}$ mimics vasoconstrictor action to induce smooth muscle α-actin in vascular smooth muscle cells through a jun-NH$_2$-terminal kinase-dependent pathway. *J. Biol. Chem.* 272:25845–50

122. Lefkowitz RJ. 1998. G-protein coupled receptors III. New roles for receptor kinases and β-arrestins in receptor signaling and desensitization. *J. Biol. Chem.* 273:18677–80

123. Luttrell LM, Ferguson SSG, Daaka Y, Miller WE, Maudsley S, et al. 1999. β-Arrestin-dependent formation of β2-adrenergic receptor-Src protein kinase complex. *Science* 283:655–61

124. Pei G, Kieffer BL, Lefkowitz RJ, Freedman NJ. 1995. Agonist-dependent phosphorylation of the mouse δ-opioid receptor: involvement of G protein-coupled receptor kinases but not protein kinase C. *Mol. Pharmacol.* 48:173–77

125. Arden JR, Segredo V, Wang A, Lameh J, Sadee W. 1995. Phosphorylation and agonist-specific intracellular trafficking of an epitope-tagged μ-opioid receptor expressed in HEK293 cells. *J. Neurochem.* 65:1636–45

126. Appleyard SM, Patterson TA, Jin W, Chavkin C. 1997. Agonist-induced phosphorylation of the κ-opioid receptor. *J. Neurochem.* 69:2405–12

127. Zhang LY, Yu S, Mackin FF, Weight G, Uhl R, Wang JB. 1996. Differential mu opiate receptor phosphorylation and desensitization induced by agonists and phorbal ester. *J. Biol. Chem.* 271:11449–54

128. El Kouhen R, Maestri-El Kouhen O, Law PY, Loh HH. 1999. The absence of a direct correlation between the loss of

DAMGO inhibition of adenylyl cyclase activity and agonist-induced mu-opioid receptor phosphorylation. *J. Biol. Chem.* 274:9207–15

129. Yu Y, Zhang L, Yin X, Sun H, Uhl GR, Wang JB. 1997. Mu opioid receptor phosphorylation, desensitization and ligand efficacy. *J. Biol. Chem.* 272: 28869–74

130. Zhang J, Ferguson SSG, Barak LS, Bodduluri S, Laporte S, et al. 1998. Role for G protein-coupled receptor kinase in agonist-specific regulation of μ-opioid receptor responsiveness. *Proc. Natl. Acad. Sci. USA* 95:7157–62

131. Chakrabarti S, Law PY, Loh HH. 1998. Distinct differences between morphine- and [δ-Ala²,N-MePhe⁴,Gly-ol⁵]enkephalin-mu-opioid receptor complexes demonstrated by cyclic AMP-dependent protein kinase phosphorylation. *J. Neurochem.* 71:231–39

132. Zhao J, Pei G, Huang YL, Zhong FM, Ma L. 1997. Carboxyl terminus of δ-opioid receptor is required for agonist-dependent receptor phosphorylation. *Biochem. Biophys. Res. Comm.* 238:71–76

133. Murray SR, Evans CJ, von Zastrow M. 1998. Phosphorylation is not required for dynamin-dependent endocytosis of a truncated mutant opioid receptor. *J. Biol. Chem.* 273:24987–91

134. Wang Z, Arden J, Sadee W. 1996. Basal phosphorylation of μ-opioid receptor is agonist modulated and Ca⁺²-dependent. *FEBS Lett.* 387:53–57

135. Koch T, Kroslak T, Mayer P, Raulf E, Hollt V. 1997. Site mutation in the rat μ-opioid receptor demonstrates the involvement of calcium/calmodulin-dependent protein kinase II in agonist-mediated desensitization. *J. Neurochem.* 69:1767–70

136. Pronin AN, Satpaev DK, Slepak VZ, Benovic JL. 1997. Regulation of G protein-coupled receptor kinases by calmodulin and localization of the calmodulin

binding domain. *J. Biol. Chem.* 272: 18273–80

137. Berstein MA, Welch SP. 1998. μ-Opioid receptor down-regulation and cAMP-dependent protein kinase phosphorylation in a mouse model of chronic morphine tolerance. *Mol. Brain Res.* 55:237–42

138. Yang H, Liu D, Vinson GP, Raizada MK. 1997. Involvement of MAP kinase in angiotensin II-induced phosphorylation and intracellular targeting of neuronal AT1 receptors. *J. Neurosci.* 17:1660–69

139. Hasbi A, Polastron J, Allouche S, Stanasila L, Massotte D, Jauzac P. 1998. Desensitization of the δ-opioid receptor correlates with its phosphorylation in SK-N-BE cells: involvement of a G protein-coupled receptor kinase. *J. Neurochem.* 70:2129–38

140. Koover A, Nappey V, Kieffer BL, Chavkin C. 1997. Mu and δ-opioid receptors are differentially desensitized by the coexpression of β-adrenergic receptor kinase 2 and β-arrestin 2 in *Xenopus* oocytes. *J. Biol. Chem.* 272:27605–11

141. Wang C, Zhou D, Cheng Z, Wei Q, Chen J, et al. 1998. The C-truncated δ-opioid receptor underwent agonist-dependent activation and desensitization. *Biochem. Biophys. Res. Comm.* 249:321–24

142. Pak Y, O'Dowd BF, George SR. 1997. Agonist-induced desensitization of the μ-opioid receptor is determined by threonine 394 preceded by acidic amino acids in the COOH-terminal tail. *J. Biol. Chem.* 272:24961–65

143. Fredericks ZL, Picher JA, Lefkowitz RJ. 1996. Identification of the G protein-coupled receptor kinase phosphorylation sites in the human β2-adrenergic receptor. *J. Biol. Chem.* 272:13796–803

144. Zimprich A, Simon T, Hollt V. 1995. Cloning and expression of an isoform of the rat μ-opioid receptor (rMOR1B) which differs in agonist induced desen-

sitization from rMOR1. *FEBS Lett.* 359:142–46

145. Koch T, Schulz S, Schroder H, Wolf R, Raulf E, Hollt V. 1998. Carboxyl-terminal splicing of the rat μ-opioid receptor modulates agonist-mediated internalization and receptor resensitization. *J. Biol. Chem.* 273:13652–57

146. Wolf R, Koch T, Schulz S, Klutzny M, Schroder H, et al. 1999. Replacement of threonine 394 by alanine facilitates internalization and resensitization of the rat μ-opioid receptor. *Mol. Pharmacol.* 55:263–68

147. Pak Y, Kouvelas A, Scheideler MA, Rasmussen J, O'Dowd BF, George SR. 1996. Agonist-induced functional desensitization of the μ-opioid receptor is mediated by loss of membrane receptors rather than uncoupling from G protein. *Mol. Pharmacol.* 50:1214–22

148. Whistler JL, von Zastrow M. 1998. Morphine-activated opioid receptors elude desensitization by β-arrestin. *Proc. Natl. Acad. Sci. USA* 95:9914–19

149. Cheng ZJ, Yu QM, Wu YL, Ma L, Pei G. 1998. Selective interference of β-arrestin 1 with κ- and δ- but not μ-opioid receptor/G protein coupling. *J. Biol. Chem.* 273:24328–33

150. Capeyrou R, Riond J, Corbani M, Lepage JF, Bertin B, Emorine LJ. 1997. Agonist-induced signaling and trafficking of the mu-opioid receptor: role of serine and threonine residues in the third cytoplasmic loop and C-terminal domain. *FEBS Lett.* 415:200–5

151. Chakrabarti S, Law PY, Loh HH. 1995. Neuroblastoma Neuro2A cells stably expressing a cloned μ-opioid receptor: a specific cellular model to study acute and chronic effects of morphine. *Mol. Brain Res.* 30:269–78

152. Koover A, Celver JP, Wu A, Chavkin C. 1998. Agonist induced homologous desensitization of μ-opioid receptors mediated by G protein-coupled receptor kinases is dependent on agonist efficacy. *Mol. Pharmacol.* 54:704–11

153. Koover A, Henry DJ, Chavkin C. 1995. Agonist-induced desensitization of the μ-opioid receptor-coupled potassium channel (GIRK1). *J. Biol. Chem.* 270:589–95

154. Chang KJ, Eckel RW, Blanchard SG. 1982. Opioid peptides induce reduction of enkephalin receptors in cultured neuroblastoma cells. *Nature* 296:446–48

155. Law PY, McGinn TM, Wick MJ, Erickson LJ, Evans CJ, Loh HH. 1994. Analysis of δ-opioid receptor activities stably expressed in CHO cell lines: Function of receptor density? *J. Pharmacol. Exp. Ther.* 271:1689–94

156. Malatynska E, Wang Y, Knapp RJ, Waite S, Dalderon S, et al. 1996. Human δ-opioid receptor: functional studies on stably transfected Chinese hamster ovary cells after acute and chronic treatment with the selective non-peptidic agonist SNC-80. *J. Pharamcol. Exp. Ther.* 278:1083–89

157. Cvejic S, Trapaidze N, Cyr C, Devi LA. 1996. Thr353, located within the COOH-terminal tail of the δ-opiate receptor, is involved in receptor down-regulation. *J. Biol. Chem.* 271:4073–76

158. Law PY, Hom DS, Loh HH. 1984. Down-regulation of opiate receptor in neuroblastoma × glioma NG108–15 hybrid cells: chloroquine promotes accumulation of tritiated enkephalin in the lysosomes. *J. Biol. Chem.* 259:4096–104

159. Keith DE, Murray SR, Zaki PA, Chu PC, Lissin DV, et al. 1996. Morphine activates opioid receptors without causing their rapid internalization. *J. Biol. Chem.* 271:19021–24

160. Trapaidze N, Keith DE, Cvejic S, Evans CJ, Devi LA. 1996. Sequestration of the δ-opioid receptor. Role of the C terminus in agonist-mediated internalization. *J. Biol. Chem.* 271:29279–85

161. Ko JL, Arvidsson U, Williams FG, Law PY, Elde R, Loh HH. 1999. Visualization of time-dependent redistribution of δ-opioid receptors in neuronal cells during

prolonged agonist exposure. *Mol. Brain Res.* 69:171–85

162. Gaudriault GD, Nouel C, Farra D, Beaudet A, Vincent JP. 1997. Receptor-induced internalization of selective peptidic μ- and δ-opioid ligands. *J. Biol. Chem.* 272:2880–88

163. Remmers AE, Clark MJ, Liu XY, Medzihradsky F. 1998. Delta opioid receptor down-regulation is independent of functional G protein yet is dependent on agonist efficacy. *J. Pharmacol. Exp. Ther.* 287:625–32

164. Zadina JE, Harrison LM, Ge LJ, Kastin AJ, Chang SL. 1994. Differential regulation of μ- and δ-opiate receptors by morphine, selective agonists and antagonists and differentiating agents in SHSY5Y human neuroblastoma cells. *J. Pharmacol. Exp. Ther.* 270:1086–96

165. Baumhaker Y, Gafni M, Keren O, Sarne Y. 1993 Selective and interactive down-regulation of μ- and δ-opioid receptors in human neuroblastoma SK-N-SH cells. *Mol. Pharmacol.* 44:461–67

166. Puttfarchen PS, Cox BM. 1989. Morphine-induced desensitization and down-regulation at mu-receptors in 7315C pituitary tumor cells. Life Sci. 45:1937–42

167. Zadina JE, Chang SL, Ge LJ, Kastin AJ. 1993. Mu opiate receptor down-regulation by morphine and up-regulation by naloxone in SHSY5Y human neuroblastoma cells. *J. Pharmacol. Exp. Ther.* 265:254–62

168. Prather PL, Tsai AW, Law PY. 1994. Mu and delta opioid receptor desensitization in undifferentiated human neuroblastoma SHSY5Y cells. *J. Pharmacol. Exp. Ther.* 270:177–84

169. Shapira M, Baumhaker Y, Sarne Y. 1997. Long-term regulation of opioid receptors in neuroblastoma and lymphoma cell lines. *J. Neuroimmunol.* 76:145–52

170. Yabaluri N, Medzihradsky F. 1997. Down-regulation of μ-opioid receptor by full but not partial agonists is indepen-

dent of G protein coupling. *Mol. Pharmacol.* 52:896–902

171. Kato S, Fukuda K, Morikawa H, Shoda T, Mima H, Mori K. 1998. Adaptations to chronic agonist exposure of μ-opioid receptor-expressing Chinese hamster ovary cells. *Eur. J. Pharmacol.* 345:221–28

172. Joseph DB, Bidlack JM. 1995. The κ-opioid receptor expressed on the mouse R1.1 thymoma cell line down-regulates without desensitizing during chronic opioid exposure. *J. Pharmacol. Exp. Ther.* 272:970–76

173. Zhu J, Luo LY, Mao GF, Ashby B, Liu-Chen LY. 1998. Agonist-induced desensitization and down-regulation of the human κ-opioid receptor expressed in Chinese hamster ovary cells. *J. Pharmacol. Exp. Ther.* 285:28–36

174. Segredo V, Burford NT, Lameh J, Sadee W. 1997. A constitutively internalizing and recycling mutant of the μ-opioid receptor. *J. Neurochem.* 68:2395–404

175. Chu P, Murray S, Lissin D, von Zastrow M. 1997. Delta and κ-opioid receptors are differentially regulated by dynamin-dependent endocytosis when activated by the same alkaloid agonist. *J. Biol. Chem.* 272:27124–30

176. Zhang J, Ferguson SSG, Law PY, Barak LS, Caron MG. 1999. Agonist-specific regulation of δ-opioid receptor trafficking by G protein-coupled receptor kinase and β-arrestin. *J. Recept. Signal Transduct. Res.* 19:301–13

177. Burd AL, El-Kouhen R, Erickson LJ, Loh HH, Law PY. 1998. Identification of Serine[356] and Serine[363] as the amino acids involved in etorphine-induced down-regulation of the mu-opioid receptor. *J. Biol. Chem.* 273:34488–95

178. Afify EA, Law PY, Riedl M, Elde R, Loh HH. 1998. Role of carboxyl-terminus of μ- and δ-opioid receptor in agonist-induced desensitization and down-regulation. *Mol. Brain Res.* 54:24–34

179. Law PY, Louie AK, Loh HH. 1985.

Effect of pertussis toxin treatment on the down-regulation of opiate receptors in neuroblastoma × glioma NG108–15 hybrid cells. *J. Biol. Chem.* 260:14818–23

180. ChakrabartiS, Yang W, Law PY, Loh HH. 1997. The μ-opioid receptor down-regulates differently from the δ-opioid receptor: requirement of a high affinity receptor-G-protein complex formation. *Mol. Pharmacol.* 52:105–13

181. Hazum E, Chang KJ, Cuatrecasas P. 1980. Cluster formation of opiate (enkephalin) receptors in neuroblastoma cells: differences between agonists and antagonists and possible relationships to biological functions. *Proc. Natl. Acad. Sci. USA* 77:3038–41

182. Cvejic S, Devi LA. 1997. Dimerization of the δ-opioid receptor: implication for a role in receptor internalization. *J. Biol. Chem.* 272:26959–64

183. Janovich JA, Conn PM. 1996. Gonadotropin releasing hormone agonist provokes homologous receptor microaggregation: an early event in seven-transmembrane receptor mediated signaling. *Endocrinology* 137:3602–5

184. Maggio R, Barbier P, Fornai F, Corsini GU. 1996. Functional role of the third cytoplasmic loop in muscarinic receptor dimerization. *J. Biol. Chem.* 271:31055–60

185. Ng GY, O'Dowd BF, Lee SP, Chung HT, Brann MR, et al. 1996. Dopamine D2 receptor dimers and receptor-blocking peptides. *Biochem. Biophys. Res. Comm.* 227:200–4

186. Kest B, Jenab S, Brodsky M, Elliot K, Inturrisi CE. 1994. Supraspinal δ-opioid receptor mRNA levels are not altered in [δ-Ala2]deltorphin II tolerant mice. *J. Neurosci. Res.* 39:674–79

187. Unterwald EM, Rubenfeld JM, Imai Y, Wang JB, Uhl GR, Kreek MJ. 1995. Chronic opioid antagonist administration upregulates μ-opioid receptor binding without altering μ-opioid receptor

mRNA levels. *Mol. Brain Res.* 33:351–55

188. Buzas B, Rosenberger J. Cox BM. 1996. Mu and delta opioid receptor gene expression after chronic treatment with opioid agonist. *NeuroReport* 7:1505–08

189. Castelli MP, Melis M, Mameli M, Fadda P, Diaz G, Gessa GL. 1997. Chronic morphine and naltrexone fail to modify μ-opioid receptor mRNA level in the rat brain. *Mol. Brain Res.* 45:149–53

190. Ronnekleiv OK, Bosch MA, Cunningham MJ, Wagner EJ, Gandy DK, Kelly MJ. 1996. Down regulation of μ-opioid receptor mRNA in the mediobasal hypothalamus of the female guinea pig following morphine treatment. *Neurosci. Lett.* 216:129–32

191. Quinones-Jena V, Jenab S, Ogawa S, Inturrisi C, Pfaff DW. 1997. Estrogen regulation of μ-opioid receptor mRNA in the forebrain of female rats. *Mol. Brain Res.* 47:134–38

192. Kim DS, Chin H, Klee WA. 1995. Agonist regulation of the expression of the δ-opioid receptor in NG108–15 cells. *FEBS Lett.* 376:11–14

193. Thorlin T, Eriksson PS, Hansson E, Ronnback L. 1997. [D-Pen2,5]enkephalin and glutamate regulate the expression of δ-opioid receptors in rat cortical astrocytes. *Neurosci. Lett.* 232:67–70

194. Charness ME, Hu G, Edwards RH, Querimit LA. 1993. Ethanol increases δ-opioid receptor gene expression in neuronal cell lines. *Mol. Pharmacol.* 44:1119–27

195. Jenab S, Inturrisi CE. 1994. Ethanol and naloxone differentially upregulate δ-opioid receptor gene expression in neuroblastoma hybrid (NG108–15) cells. *Mol. Brain Res.* 27:95–102

196. Jenab S, Inturrisi CE. 1997. Activation of protein kinase A prevents the ethanol-induced up-regulation of δ-opioid receptor mRNA in NG108–15 cells. *Mol. Brain Res.* 47:44–48

197. Shen J, Chan KW, Chen BT, Philippe J,

Sehba F, et al. 1997. The effect of in vivo ethanol consumption on cyclic AMP and δ-opioid receptor in mouse striatum. *Brain Res.* 770:65–71

198. Shah, S, Duttaroy A, Sehba F, Chen B, Philippe J, et al. 1997. The effect of ethanol drinking on opioid analgesia and receptors in mice. *Alcohol* 14:361–66
199. Winkler A, Buzas B, Siems WE, Heder G, Cox BM. 1998. Effect of ethanol drinking on the gene expression of opioid receptors, enkephalinase, and angiotensin-converting enzyme in two inbred mice strains. *Alcohol. Clin. Exp. Res.* 22:1262–71
200. Azaryan AV, Coughlin LJ, Buzas B, Clock BJ, Cox BM. 1996. Effect of chronic cocaine treatment on μ- and δ-opioid receptor mRNA levels in dopaminergically innervated brain regions. *J. Neurochem.* 66:443–48
201. Azaryan AV, Clock BJ, Rosenberger JG, Cox BM. 1998. Transient upregulation of μ-opioid receptor mRNA levels in nucleus accumbens during chronic cocaine administration. *Can. J. Physiol. Pharmacol.* 76:278–83
202. Spangler R, Ho A, Zhou Y, Maggos CE, Yuferouv V, Kreek MJ. 1996. Regulation of κ-opioid receptor mRNA in the rat brain by "binge" pattern cocaine administration and correlation with preprodynorphin mRNA. *Mol. Brain Res.* 38:71–76
203. Azaryan AV, Clock BJ, Cox BM. 1996. Mu opioid receptor mRNA in nucleus accumbens is elevated following dopamine receptor activation. *Neurochem. Res.* 21:1411–15
204. Abood ME, Tao Q. 1995. Characterization of a δ-opioid receptor in rat pheochromocytoma cells. *Pharmacol. Exp. Ther.* 274:1566–73
205. Tryoen-Troth P, Gaveriaux-Ruff C, Maderspach K, Labourdette G. 1998. Regulation of κ-opioid receptor mRNA level by cyclic AMP and growth factors in cul-

tured rat glial cells. *Mol. Brain Res.* 55:141–50
206. Ruzicka BB, Akil H. 1997. The interleukin-1β-mediated regulation of proenkephalin and opioid receptor messenger RNA in primary astrocyte-enriched cultures. *Neuroscience* 79:517–24
207. Ruzicka BB, Thompson RC, Watson SJ, Akil H. 1996. Interleukin-1 β-mediated regulation of μ-opioid receptor mRNA in primary astrocyte-enriched cultures. *J. Neurochem.* 66:425–28
208. Vidal EL, Patel NA, Wu G, Fiala M, Chang SL. 1998. Interleukin-1 induces the expression of μ-opioid receptors in endothelial cells. *Immunopharmacology* 38:261–66
209. Beczkowska IW, Buck J, Inturrisi CE. 1996. Retinoic acid-induced increase in δ-opioid receptor and N-methyl-D-aspartate receptor mRNA levels in neuroblastoma × glioma (NG108–15) cells. *Brain Res. Bull.* 39:193–99
210. Miller B. 1996. Delta opioid receptor expression is induced by concanavalin A in CD cells. *J. Immunol.* 157:5324–28
211. Sharp BM, Shahabi N, McKean D, Li MD, McAllen K. 1997. Detection of basal levels and induction of δ-opioid receptor mRNA in murine splenocytes. *J. Neurochem.* 78:198–202
212. Buzas B, Rosenberger J, Cox BM. 1997. Regulation of δ-opioid receptor mRNA levels by receptor-mediated and direct activation of the adenylyl cyclase-protein kinase A pathway. *J. Neurochem.* 68:610–15
213. Gylys KH, Tran N, Magendzo K, Zaki P, Evans CJ. 1997. cAMP decreases steady-state levels of δ-opioid receptor mRNA in NG108–15 cells. *NeuroReport* 8:2369–72
214. Gies EK, Peters DM, Gelb CR, Knag KM, Peterfreund RA. 1997. Regulation of μ-opioid receptor mRNA levels by activation of protein kinase C in human SHSY5Y neuroblastoma cells. *Anesthesiology* 87:1127–38
215. Buzas B, Rosenberger J, Cox BM. 1998.

Ca^{2+}/calmodulin-dependent transcriptional activation of δ-opioid receptor gene expression induced by membrane depolarization in NG108–15 cells. *J. Neurochem.* 70:105–12

216. Zaki PA, Bilsky EJ, Vanderah TW, Lai J, Evans CJ, Porreca F. 1996. Opioid receptor types and subtypes: the δ receptor as a model. *Annu. Rev. Pharmacol. Toxicol.* 367:379–401

217. Simonin F, Gaveriaux-Ruff C, Befort K, Matthes H, Lannes B, Micheletti G, Mattel MG, Charron G, Block B, Kieffer B. 1995. κ-Opioid receptor in human: cDNA and genomic cloning, chromosomal assignment, functional expression, pharmacology and expression pattern in the central nervous system. *Proc. Natl. Acad. Sci. USA* 92:7006–10

218. Min BH, Augustin LB, Felsheim RF, Fuchs JA, Loh HH. 1994. Genomic structure and analysis of promoter sequence of a mouse μ opioid receptor gene. *Proc. Natl. Acad. Sci. USA* 91:9081–85

219. Kraus J, Horn G, Zimprich A, Simon T, Mayer P, Hollt V. 1995. Molecular cloning and function analysis of the rat mu opioid receptor gene promoter. *Biochem. Biophys. Res. Comm.* 215:591–97

220. Augustine LB, Felsheim RF, Min BH, Fuchs SM, Fuchs JA, Loh HH. 1995. Genomic structure of mouse δ-opioid receptor gene. *Biochem. Biophys. Res. Comm.* 207:111–19

221. Liu HC, Lu S, Augustin LB, Felsheim RF, Chen HC, et al. 1995. Cloning and promoter mapping of mouse κ opioid receptor gene. *Biochem. Biophys. Res. Comm.* 209:639–47

222. Lu S, Loh HH, Wei LN. 1997. Studies of dual promoters of mouse κ-opioid receptor gene. *Mol. Pharmacol.* 52:415–20

223. Ko JL, Minnerath SR, Loh HH. 1997. Dual promoters of mouse μ-opioid receptor gene. *Biochem. Biophys. Res. Comm.* 234:351–57

224. Liu HC, Shen JT, Augustine LB, Ko JL,

Loh HH. 1999. Transcriptional regulation of mouse δ-opioid receptor gene. *J. Biol. Chem.* 274:23617–26

225. Liang YA, Mestek LY, Carr LG. 1995. Cloning and characterization of the promoter region of the mouse mu opioid receptor gene. *Brain Res.* 679:82–88

226. Choe CY, Im HJ, Ko JL, Loh HH. 1998. Mouse μ opioid receptor gene expression: a 34-base pair cis-acting element inhibits transcription of the μ-opioid receptor gene from the distal promoter. *J. Biol. Chem.* 273:34926–32

227. Im HJ, Kang SW, Loh HH. 1999. Opioid receptor gene: cytokine response element and the effect of cytokines. *Brain Res.* 829:174–79

228. Law PY, Loh HH. 1999. Regulation of opioid receptor activities. *J. Pharmacol. Exp. Ther.* 289:607–24

229. Ko JL, Liu HC, Minnerath SR, Loh HH. 1998. Transcriptional regulation of mouse μ-opioid receptor gene. *J. Biol. Chem.* 273:27678–85

230. Matthes HWD, Maldonaldo R, Simonin F, Valverde O, Slowe S, et al. 1996. Loss of morphine induced analgesia, reward effect and withdrawal symptoms in mice lacking the μ opioid receptor gene. *Nature* 383:819–23

231. Sora I, Takahashi N, Funadz M, Ujike H, Revay RS, et al. 1997. Opioid receptor knockout mice define μ receptor roles in endogenous nociceptive responses and morphine-induced analgesia. *Proc. Natl. Acad.Sci. USA* 94:1544–49

231. (a) Sora I, Funada M, Uhl GR. 1997. The m-opioid receptor is necessary for [D-Pen^2, D-Pen^5] enkephalin-induced analgesia. *Eur. J. Pharmacol.* 324:R1–2

232. Tian M, Fan HEB, Lai Z, Zhang S, Aronica S, et al. 1997. Altered hemotopoiesis, behavior and sexual function in μ opioid receptor deficient mice. *J. Exp. Med.* 185:1517–22

233. Loh HH, Liu HC, Cavalli A, Yang W, Chen YF, Wei LN. 1998. μ opioid receptor knockout in mice: effects on

ligand-induced analgesia and morphine lethality. *Mol. Brain Res.* 54:321–26

234. Schuller AGP, King MA, Zheng J, Bolan E, Pan YX, et al. 1999. Retention of heroin and morphine-6β-glucouronide analgesia in a new line of mice lacking exon 1 of MOR-1. *Nature Neurosci.* 2:151–56

235. Simonin F, Valverde O, Smadja C, Slowe S, Kitchen I, et al. 1998. Disruption of the κ-opioid receptor gene in mice enhanced sensitivity to chemical visceral pain, impairs pharmacological actions of the selective κ-agonist U50,488 and attenuates morphine withdrawal. *EMBO J.* 17:886–97

236. Zhu Y, King M, Schuller A, Nitsche JF, Reidl M, et al. 1999. Retention of supraspinal delta-like analgesia and loss of morphine tolerance in delta opioid receptor (DOR-1) knock-out mice. *Neuron* 24:1–10

237. Kitchen I, Slowe SJ, Matthes HW, Kieffer B. 1997. Quantitative autoradiographic mapping of μ-, δ- and κ-opioid receptors in knockout mice lacking the μ-opioid receptor gene. *Brain Res.* 778: 73–88

238. Fuchs PN, Roza C, Sora I, Uhl G, Raja SN. 1999. Characterization of mechanical withdrawal responses and effects of μ- δ- and κ-opioid agonists in normal and μ-opioid receptor knockout mice. *Brain Res.* 821:480–86

239. Kitanaka, N, Sora I, Kinsey S, Zeng Z, Uhl GR. 1998. No heroin or morphine 6β-glucuronide analgesia in μ-opioid receptor knockout mice. *Eur. J. Pharmacol.* 355:R1–R3

240. Jordan BA, Devi LA. 1999. G-protein-coupled receptor heterodimerization modulates receptor function. *Nature* 399:697–700

241. Sora I, Funada M, Uhl GR. 1997. The μ-opioid receptor is necessary for [DPen2,D-Pen5] enkephalin-induced analgesia. *Eur. J. Pharmacol.* 324:R1–R2

242. Rothman RB, Bykov V, Mahboubi A,

Long JB, Jiang Q, et al. 1991. Interaction of β-funaltrexamine with [³H]cyclo-FOXY binding in rat brain: further evidence that β-FNA alkylates the opioid receptor complex. *Synapse* 8:86–99

243. Matthes HWD, Smadja C, Valverde O, Vonesch JL, Foutz AS, et al. 1998. Activity of the δ-opioid receptor is partially reduced, whereas activity of the κ-receptor is maintained in mice lacking the μ-receptor. *J. Neurosci.* 18:7285–95

244. Roy S, Liu HC, Loh HH. 1998. μ-Opioid receptor-knockout mice: the role of μ-opioid receptor in gastrointestinal transit. *Mol. Brain Res.* 56:281–83

245. Gaveriaux-Ruff C, Matthes HW, Peluso J, Kieffer BL. 1998. Abolition of morphine-immunosuppression in mice lacking the μ-opioid receptor gene. *Proc. Natl. Acad. Sci. USA* 95:6326–30

246. Roy S, Barke RA, Loh HH. 1998. Mu-opioid receptor-knockout mice: role of μ-opioid receptor in morphine mediated immune functions. *Mol. Brain Res.* 61:190–94

247. Hepburn MJ, Little PJ, Gingras J, Kuhn CM. 1997. Differential effects of naltrindole on morphine-induced tolerance and physical dependence in rats. *J. Pharmacol. Exp. Ther.* 281:1350–56

248. Kest B, Lee CE, McLenmore GL, Inturrisi CE. 1996. An antisense oligodeoxynucleotide to the delta opioid receptor (DOR-1) inhibits morphine tolerance and acute dependence in mice. *Brain Res. Bull.* 39:185–89

249. Mollereau C, Parmentier M, Mailleux P, Butour JL, Moisand C, et al. 1994. ORL 1, a novel member of opioid receptor family. Cloning, functional expression and localization. *FEBS Lett.* 341:33–38

250. Fukuda K, Kato S, Mori K, Nishi M, Takeshima H, et al. 1994. cDNA cloning and regional distribution of a novel member of the opioid receptor family. *FEBS Lett.* 343:42–46

251. Bunzow JR, Saez C, Mortrud M, Bouvier C, Williams JT, et al. 1994. Molecular

cloning and tissue distribution of a putative member of the rat opioid receptor gene family that is not a mu, delta or kappa opioid receptor type. *FEBS Lett.* 347:284–88

252. Chen Y, Fan Y, Liu J, Mestek A, Tian MT, et al. 1994. Molecular cloning, tissue distribution and chromosomal localization of a novel member of the opioid receptor gene family. *FEBS Lett.* 347:279–83

253. Wang JB, Johnson PS, Imai Y, Persico AM, Ozenberger B, et al. 1994. CDNA cloning an orphan opiate receptor gene family member and its splice variant. *FEBS Lett.* 348:75–79

254. Wick MJ, Minnerath SR, Lin XQ, Elde R, Law PY, Loh H. 1994. Isolation of a novel cDNA encoding a putative membrane receptor with high homology to the cloned mu, delta and kappa opioid receptors. *Mol. Brain Res.* 27:37–44

255. Claude PA, Wotta DR, Zhang XH, Prather PL, McGinn TM, et al. 1996. Mutation of a conserved serine in TM4 of opioid receptors confers full agonistic properties to classical antagonists. *Proc. Natl. Acad. Sci. USA* 93:5715–19

256. Bond C, LaForge KS, Tian M, Melia D, Zhang S, et al. 1998. Single-nucleotide polymorphism in the human mu opioid receptor gene alters β-endorphin binding and activity: possible implications for opiate addiction. *Proc. Natl. Acad. Sci. USA* 95:9608–13

257. Mayer P, Rochlitz H, Rauch E, Rommelspacher H, Hasse HE, et al. 1997. Association between a delta opioid receptor gene polymorphism and heroin dependence in man. *NeuroReport* 8:2547–50

258. Chakrabarti S, Wang L, Tang WJ, Gintzler AR. 1998. Chronic morphine augments adenylyl cyclase phosphorylation: relevence to altered signaling during tolerance/dependence. *Mol. Pharmacol.* 54:949–53

259. Maldonado R, Blendy JA, Tzavara E, Gass P, Roques BP, et al. 1996. Reduction of morphine abstinence in mice with a mutation in the gene encoding CREB. *Science* 273:657–59

260. Truijillo KA, Akil H. 1991. Inhibition of morphine tolerance and dependence by the NMDA receptor antagonist MK-801. *Science* 251:85–87

261. Elliot K, Minami N, Kolesnikov YA, Pasternak GW, Inturrisi CE. 1994. The NMDA receptor antagonists, LY274614 and Mκ-801, and the nitric oxide synthease inhibitor, NG-nitro-L-arginine, attenuate analgesic tolerance to the μ-opioid morphine but not to kappa opioids. *Pain* 56:69–75

262. Pawson, T, Scott JD. 1997. Signaling through scaffold, anchoring and adaptor proteins. *Science* 278:2075–80

263. Tsunoda S, Sierralta J, Sun Y, Bodner R, Suzuki E, et al. 1997. A multivalent PDZ-domain protein assembles signaling complexes in a G protein-coupled cascade. *Nature* 388:243–49

264. Offermann S, Schultz G, Rosenthal W. 1991. Evidence for opioid receptor-mediated activation of G-proteins, G_o and G_{i2} in membranes of neuroblastoma × glioma (NG108–15) hybrid cells. *J. Biol. Chem.* 266:3365–68

Annu. Rev. Pharmacol. Toxicol. 2000. 40:431–58

NICOTINIC RECEPTORS
AT THE AMINO ACID LEVEL

Pierre-Jean Corringer, Nicolas Le Novère, and Jean-Pierre Changeux

Neurobiologie Moléculaire, Unité de recherche associée au Centre National de la Recherche Scientifique D1284 Institut Pasteur, 75724 Paris Cedex 15, France; e-mail: changeux@pasteur.fr

Key Words   nAChR, nicotinic, ion channel, allosteric proteins

■ **Abstract**   nAChRs are pentameric transmembrane proteins into the superfamily of ligand-gated ion channels that includes the $5HT_3$, glycine, $GABA_A$, and $GABA_C$ receptors. Electron microscopy, affinity labeling, and mutagenesis experiments, together with secondary structure predictions and measurements, suggest an all-β folding of the N-terminal extracellular domain, with the connecting loops contributing to the ACh binding pocket and to the subunit interfaces that mediate the allosteric transitions between conformational states. The ion channel consists of two distinct elements symmetrically organized along the fivefold axis of the molecule: a barrel of five M2 helices, and on the cytoplasmic side five loops contributing to the selectivity filter. The allosteric transitions of the protein underlying the physiological ACh-evoked activation and desensitization possibly involve rigid body motion of the extracellular domain of each subunit, linked to a global reorganization of the transmembrane domain responsible for channel gating.

INTRODUCTION

Ligand-gated ion channels mediate intercellular communication by converting the neurotransmitter signal released from the nerve ending into a transmembrane ion flux in the postsynaptic neurone or muscle fiber. According to the classical scheme of fast "wiring" transmission, the neurotransmitter is released in the synaptic cleft at a high concentration (up to 0.3 mM) and brief pulse (approximately 1 ms) (1), whereas in the "volume transmission" or paracrine mode, lower concentrations of the neurotransmitter may more slowly reach a distant target through intercellular space (2). Nicotinic receptors for acetylcholine (nAChRs) may contribute, among the ligand-gated ion channels, to both types of chemical communication in relation to their topological distribution at the pre- and/or post-synaptic levels.

With the use of snake venom α-toxins (3), the identification and purification of the muscle-type electric fish nAChR (4–7) demonstrated that the isolated protein contains all of the structural elements required for chemo-electrical transduction. These physiological properties include the activation response to fast application of ACh in the millisecond timescale resulting in the opening of the ion channel, as well as the slow decrease or even full abolition of the electrical response referred to as desensitization, following a prolonged application of nicotinic agonists and antagonists. A substantial body of biochemical and electron microscopy data subsequently revealed that the nAChR is a heteropentamer, made up of four subunits α1, β1, γ, and δ, pseudosymmetrically arranged with a 2:1:1:1 stoichiometry (6).

The full amino acid sequence of the muscle type, and of several neuronal nAChR subunits have been available for nearly two decades, together with low-resolution three-dimensional (3D) electron microscopy data. Yet most of our knowledge on the functional organization of nAChR derives from affinity labeling and mutagenesis experiments. Crystallographic and nuclear magnetic resonance information of the nAChR molecule are still lacking. At this stage however, the body of available experimental and computational data appears sufficient to define an envelope of structural constraints that justifies the proposal of the general 3D organization of the ACh binding site and of the ion channel at the amino acid level, as plausible anticipations of the experimentally determined 3D structure.

THE nAChR OLIGOMER

The initial cloning (8–10) and sequencing (11–14) of *Torpedo* electric organ nAChR subunits paved the way for the identification of a family of homologous genes encoding nAChR subunits in muscle and brain that belongs to an even larger superfamily of ligand-gated ion channels (15), which includes the 5-HT$_3$ (16), GABA$_A$ (17), GABA$_C$ (18), and glycine receptors (19) in both vertebrate and invertebrate species [amino acid and nucleotide sequences of all the members of the superfamily can be found in Le Novère & Changeux (20)]. The complete sequence of the *Caenorhabditis elegans* genome revealed an unexpected wealth of genes (more than 40) coding for putative subunits in the nicotinic superfamily (21). Many of them are clearly orthologous to known vertebrate subunits. This is the case for ACR7,9,10,11,14,15,16 (Ce21) with α7,8 or ACR6,8,12,13 and UNC38 with α1–6, β1–4, γ, δ, ε. However, according to the sequence analysis, some of the newly discovered genes (for instance DEG3, ACR5, or F18G5.4) do not possess clear orthologs among the known vertebrate nAChR subunits. This would suggest that several new nAChR subunit genes might still be uncovered in the human genome.

The nAChR subunits genes fall into two main classes: The α subunits (α1–9) possess two adjacent cysteines essential for acetylcholine binding (22, 23), whereas the non-α referred to as β, γ, ε, or δ do not (24). Comparative analysis of the available nAChR subunits gene sequences suggests that the first duplication between nAChR subunits is probably older than one and half billion years, whereas the last ones may have occurred around 400 million years ago (such as α7/α8 or β2/β4) (25, 26). The nAChR vertebrate subunits include the following subfamilies, defined on the basis of protein sequence and gene structure (position of the introns in the coding sequence): subfamily I, epithelial α9; subfamily II, neuronal α7,8; subfamily III, neuronal α2–6 and β2–4; and subfamily IV, muscle α1, β1, γ, δ, and ε. The subfamilies III and IV can be further subdivided, on the basis of sequence similarities, into three tribes: tribe III-1, α2,3,4,6; tribe III-2, β2,4; tribe III-3, α5, β3; tribe IV-1, α1; tribe IV-2, γ, δ, ε; and tribe IV-3, β1.

Reconstitution experiments in *Xenopus* oocytes and cultured mammalian cells have shown that for the subunits belonging to each subfamily, the assembly into functional oligomers follows well-defined rules. Members of subfamilies I and II, when expressed alone, are able to form functional homopentamers (27–30). These ancestral type receptors are presumably characterized by a perfect fivefold symmetry. In the case of the recently evolved subfamily III, the coexpression of one member of tribe III-1 and one member of tribe III-2 is required to form an ACh gated ion channel with a currently accepted stoichiometry of 2 α(s) for 3 β(s) (31, 32). Some of these receptors incorporate a third type of subunit from tribe III-3, either α5 (33, 34) or β3 (35). Finally, the assembly of the subunits from the highly evolved muscle subfamily IV appears tightly constrained with a fixed clockwise [α1-γ-α1-δ-β1] order of subunits (6, 36; but see 37).

The more promiscuous assembly of neuronal subunits generates a diversity of receptors, with 24 possible oligomer compositions theoretically generated on the basis of a contribution of one member of tribe III-1 and tribe III-2, plus zero or one member of tribe III-3, and with 14 oligomers actually observed in reconstituted systems. This results in a high diversity in pharmacological specificities, desensitization kinetics, and channel permeabilities, in particular to calcium ions (reviewed in 38), and in diverse cellular and subcellular distributions in the brain (39, 40). The spatiotemporal development of such rich patterns of nAChR gene expression requires complex transcriptional and posttranscriptional regulations, which can hardly be achieved with single promoter species (see 41). As suggested in the case of developmental genes (42, 43), the multiplication of promoters consecutive to gene duplication may allow a fine spatio-temporal control of transcription and thus tentatively explain such large diversity of subunit genes.

TRANSMEMBRANE ORGANIZATION AND SUBUNIT STRUCTURE

At low resolution by electron microscopy, the *Torpedo* receptor appears as an integral elongated transmembrane protein, that protrudes by ~60 and ~20 Å into the synaptic and intracellular compartments, respectively, with an apparent fivefold axis of symmetry perpendicular to the membrane. It creates a central pore, with a diameter of ~25 Å at the synaptic entry, which becomes narrower at the transmembrane level (44) (Figure 1*B*).

Strong experimental evidence supports a commonly accepted transmembrane topology shared by all subunits (reviewed in 45) (Figure 1*A*): (*a*) an amino-terminal domain facing the extracellular environment, glycosylated, and carrying at least one highly conserved cysteine bridge (corresponding to α7 C128–C142); and (*b*) three transmembrane segments (20 amino acids)—M1, M2, and M3—separated by short loops, a large and variable intracellular domain and a fourth

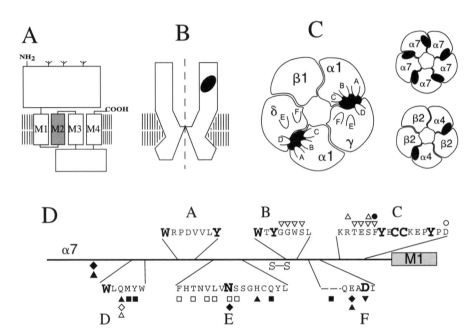

Figure 1 (*A*) The membrane topology of a typical nAChR subunit. (*B*) Schematic drawing of the nAChR in axial section. The ion channel is located along the axis of pseudo-symmetry of the molecule, and the binding site for ACh is shown (*shaded pocket*). (*C*) Schematic drawing of nAChRs in top view, illustrating the quaternary organization of the muscle-type receptor (*left panel*) and of the homooligomeric α7 and heterooligomeric α4β2 receptors (*right panel*). (*Shaded pockets*) The ACh binding sites at the subunit inter-faces, contributed by loops A, B, and C of the "principal component" and loops D, E, and F of the "complementary component." (*D*) Linear representation of the α7 N-terminal domain. (*Bold residues*) Correspond to those affinity labeled on the *Torpedo* receptor (see text). (*Symbols*) Labeled residues homologous to those contributing to the pharmacological diversity in the entire family of nAChR. (*Open symbols*) Neuronal receptors: *triangles* (86), *inverted triangles* (89), *squares* (96), *diamonds* (95), and *circles* (87); (*closed symbols*) muscle-type receptors: *triangles* (92), *inverted triangles* (91), *squares* (67, 93), *diamonds* (68), and *circles* (90).

transmembrane segment M4. The relatively short carboxy-terminal end is then extracellular. A refined prediction of the secondary structure of a typical nAChR subunit (46) has been computed using third-generation algorithms from an alignment of a representative set of 18 nAChR and $5HT_3$ subunit sequences. Incorporation of representative sequences of members of the superfamily carrying an anionic channel (glycine and $GABA_A$ receptors) yields similar predictions, indicating that all subunits from the family share almost identical secondary and tertiary structures. This was anticipated from their sequence similarities and from the observation that a chimera joining the N-terminal domain of the $\alpha7$ nAChR to the transmembrane and cytoplasmic regions of the $5HT_3$ receptor mediates channel activation and desensitization by ACh (47).

Small-scale expression of peptide fragments corresponding to the entire N-terminal extracellular domain of the $\alpha1$ or $\alpha7$ subunits yields soluble proteins (48–51). Whereas the $\alpha1$ fragment appeared to be in a monomeric state, the expression of the $\alpha7$ fragments resulted in a soluble pentameric complex, which displays binding properties resembling those of the native receptor. Thus, the N-terminal domain may spontaneously fold and become stabilized into a native-like conformation, as long as the pentameric organization is preserved. Circular dichroism measurements on the soluble $\alpha1$ extracellular portion reveals the abundance of β-strands (51% β-strand, 12% α-helix) (50). This reasonably agrees with the secondary structure predictions (31.7% β-strand, 13.7% α-helix), depicting two α-helices at the N terminus, followed by a large core of β-strands that extends to the transmembrane segment M1. An all-β portion was also identified by measuring the secondary structure of progressively deleted $GABA_A$ $\alpha1$ subunits (52). Electron microscopy of *Torpedo* receptor at 7.5 Å resolution revealed two cavities located 30 Å above the bilayer surface, which were tentatively assigned to the ACh binding pocket (37), each surrounded by three rods, interpreted as α-helix. On the other hand, at higher resolution (4.6 Å), the pattern of density is more consistent with a seven-stranded β-sheet structure (53), in agreement with the suggested all-β portion.

The ~20–amino acid transmembrane segments M1, M2, M3, and M4 were initially thought to fold into an α-helical structure. Yet, circular dichroism measurements of the M1-M2-M3 portion of the receptor (54), infrared spectroscopy of the *Torpedo* receptor for which the extracellular portion was removed by enzymatic digestion (55), and secondary structure predictions (46) suggest a mixed α/β topology. Extensive mapping of the protein-lipid interfaces using the hydrophobic probes 3-trifluoromethyl-3-(m-iodophenyl) diazirin (TID) (56), 4'-(3-trifluoromethyl-3H-diazin-3-yl)-2'-tributyl stannyl benzyl benzoate (TID-BE) (57), diazofluorene (DAF) (58), cholesterol (59), and promegestone (60) demonstrated a labeling of the M4 as well as of the two third "extracellular" portion of M3, with a pattern of labeling consistent with an α-helix. The "intracellular" one third portion of M1 was also found labeled, but with a pattern inconsistent with either an α-helix or a β-strand. The only non–lipid-exposed segment is M2.

Strong evidence supports its folding in an α-helix and its contribution to the ion channel along the central axis of pseudosymetry of the molecule (see below).

The cytoplasmic domain is predicted to consist of two well-conserved amphipatic helices joined together by a stretch of variable length and sequence devoid of periodic structures (46). Recent electron microscopy images of the cytoplasmic domain reveal that one rod of density protrudes from each subunit, possibly corresponding to one of the predicted α-helices (53).

THE NICOTINIC BINDING SITES

The Nicotinic Binding Sites at Subunit Interface

Concerning both electric organ and muscle nAChR, the following evidence demonstrates the location of the binding site for nicotinic agonists and competitive antagonists at the α1/γ and α1/δ subunit interfaces (Figure 1C).

1. Affinity labeling experiments performed with a series of competitive antagonists of different chemical structures—such as the aryl-cation p-(dimethylamino) benzenediazonium fluoroborate (DDF) (61, 62), the alcaloid d-tubocurarine (dTC) (63), the polypeptide α-bungarotoxin (64) and with the agonist nicotine (65)—show that all probes label primarily the α1 subunits, and to a lesser extent the γ and δ subunits (10%–25% of the α1 subunit labeling).

2. Expression in cell lines of the α1 subunit with either the γ or δ subunits yields an ACh binding pocket with native pharmacology, whereas all other pairwise coexpressions or single expressions of subunit failed to give ACh binding sites (66).

3. The αγ and αδ dimers display marked pharmacological differences, particularly for α-conotoxin MI with a 10,000-fold higher affinity for the α1/δ compared with the α1/γ binding sites of mouse muscle-type receptor (whereas dTC displays a 100-fold preference for the α1/γ site) (67, 68).

The much stronger labeling of α1 compared with that of the γ and δ subunits supports an asymmetric location of the binding site with respect to the interface. We thus proposed to refer to the α1 subunits as carrying the "principal component," and the δ or γ subunits as contributing to the "complementary component" of the nicotinic binding site (69).

The various residues that compose the principal component of the α1 subunit of the *Torpedo* receptor were identified by affinity labeling, proteolysis, and Edman degradation experiments. 4-(N-maleimido) benzyltrimethyl ammonium (22) labels C192 and C193, which form a rather unusual disulfide bridge within, or in close proximity to, the ACh binding site. DDF labels Y93 (loop A), W149 (loop B), and Y190, C192, and C193 (loop C), and in a weak but significant manner W86, Y151, and Y198 (62, 70). These amino acids are also the site of incorporation of the other probes used to date: Y93 is labeled by ACh mustard (71); Y198, C192, and Y190 by nicotine (65); Y190, C192, and Y198 by dTC (63); and Y190 by lophotoxin (72). For the complementary component, the homologous γW55 and δW57 (loop D) were found labeled by nicotine and dTC, whereas the homologous γY111 and δR113 (loop E) were weakly but specifically labeled by dTC (73, 74). In order to identify negatively charged residues contributing to the stabilization of the cationic ligands, a probe 0.9 nm long, grafted onto the reduced C192–C193 disulphide bridge and reacting with aspartates and glutamates, was found to label δD165, δD180, and δE182 (75). Mutation of δD180 (loop F) to asparagine, and of the homologous γD174, but not of δD165 and δE182, was found to decrease the affinity for ACh (76).

Sequence comparison indicates a high conservation of the loop A, B, C, and D motifs in the binding site of neuronal nAChRs. The labeled residues from loops A, B, and C are indeed present in the α2,3,4,6 and α7,8 subunits, and the labeled residue from loop D in the β2,4 and α7,8 subunits. In the homooligomeric α7 receptor, as well as in the α7-V201–5HT$_3$ chimera, which carries the α7 binding site, mutation of the corresponding residues (W54, Y92, W149, and Y188) alters the apparent affinities of binding and activation of ACh, establishing their contribution to the ACh binding site (69, 77). Thus, in this case, the same subunit carries both the principal and the complementary components of binding (Figure 1C). In contrast to this conserved core of amino acids, the labeled residue from loop E appears highly variable, whereas the aspartate of loop F is conserved in all γ-, δ-, ε-, and α7 subunits [where it also contributes to ACh binding (78)], but not in β2,4.

Physical Chemistry of the ACh Binding

The binding site of ACh and nicotinic ligands thus includes a conserved core of aromatic residues, whose electron-rich side chains might provide stabilizing interactions with the cationic ligands. In agreement with this notion, mutations of α1Y93, α1Y190, and α1Y198 affect in the same way the apparent affinities of ACh and tetramethylammonium, which suggests that these tyrosine residues contribute to stabilization of the quaternary ammonium portion of ACh (79). Probing the contribution of these amino acids by incorporation of unnatural amino acids reveals a prominent role of the hydroxyl group and of the aromatic ring of α1Y93 and α1Y198, respectively, whereas the α1Y190 position is found to be too sensitive to structural modifications to be analyzed (80). At position α1W149, the 50% effective concentration (EC$_{50}$) for ACh correlates with the cation-π binding capability of a series of fluorinated tryptophan derivatives (81), which suggests that the indole side chain of W149 makes van der Waals contact (cation-π interactions) with the quaternary ammonium group of ACh. Three lines of evidence further support this notion: (*a*) incorporation of a tyrosine graft with a quaternary ammonium [Tyr-O-(CH$_2$)$_3$-N(CH$_3$)$_3$$^+$] group produces some constitutive activity, thus plausibly mimicking a bound agonist close to W149 (81); (*b*) for the α7 receptor, the ACh apparent affinity is particularly sensitive to mutation at this position, with a 100-fold increase in EC_{50} for W149F compared with a 10-fold increase for Y93F and Y190F (77); and (c) a survey of protein structures indicates that tryptophan presents the most potent cation-π binding site, especially in the case of acetylcholine esterase, within which the quaternary group of ACh makes van der Waals contact with W84 in the X-ray crystallographic structure (82).

Mutation of the homologous γD174 and δD180 to asparagine was also found to decrease the affinities for ACh and tetramethylammonium (76). It is noteworthy that two other aspartates from the principal binding component, α1D152 from loop B (83) and α1D200 from loop C (84), have been shown to decrease the ACh binding affinity when mutated to asparagine. This indicates that aspartates may provide an additional contribution to the stabilization of the ammonium ion, possibly through long-range electrostatic interactions. Finally, mutations such as γY111R and δR113Y, located within the highly variable loop E of the complementary binding component, alter primarily the apparent affinities for dTC and α-conotoxin M1, but not for ACh, indicating the specific contribution of this residue to the binding of these large antagonists (74).

Altogether, these data establish that ACh interacts with a cluster of electron-rich or charged aromatic and acidic amino acid side chains within the nicotinic site, which primarily stabilize the ammonium portion of the molecule.

Mapping the Pharmacological Diversity of nAChR Binding Sites

The pharmacological properties of nAChR vary markedly with subunit composition and species. For instance, the binding affinity of ACh for chick nAChR range from 5 nM (α4β2) to 1 μM (α7). Long- and short-chain α-toxins from snake venoms typically bind with subnanomolar affinities to the muscle-type receptor, whereas only long-chain toxins bind with high affinity to α7 receptor (85). The long-chain κ-bungarotoxin exclusively binds to the α2β2 receptor. α-Conotoxin MII binds specifically to the α3β2 receptor (86).

On the principal side of the site, the construction of α2,3, α7,8, and α4,7 chimeras showed that several segments from the N-terminal domain contribute to the different agonist pharmacologies of α2β2 and α3β2 (87), of α7,8 (88), and of α7 and α4β2 (89). A major role of the C-loop region was found with the 180–208 segment in α7,8 contributing to the relative ACh and DMPP (1,1-dimethyl-4-phenylpiperazinium) affinities, and the 195–215 in α2,3 or 183–191 in α7,4 contributing to the relative ACh and nicotine affinities. In contrast, the 152–155 segment (loop B) in α7,4 chimeras was shown to alter the pharmacology of all agonists, independent of their chemical structure (89). In parallel, some amino acids contributing to toxin binding were found near loop C. A glycosylation at this level was shown to interfere with α-bungarotoxin binding, thus rendering cobra and mongoose resistant to α-toxin (90). Furthermore, mutations at position V188, Y190, P197, and D200 were found to decrease the affinity of the short-chain toxin from *Naja mossambica mossambica* (NmmI) affinity by 60- to 400-fold (91).

On the complementary side of the site, the amino acids involved in the pharmacological diversity were found in most cases located at the level of loops D, E, and F. Mapping the amino acids involved in the different affinities of dTC, α-conotoxin MI, NmmI, and carbamylcholine for the $\alpha1/\gamma$, $\alpha1/\delta$, and $\alpha1/\varepsilon$ binding sites of the mouse muscle-type receptor underlined the contribution of variable residues at position $i + 2$, 3, or 4 from δW55, $i + 4$ or 6 from δY113, and $i - 2$ and $i + 1$ or 2 from δD180. However, two other amino acids outside these loops, δS36 and δK163, were shown to account for some of the differences (67, 68, 92–94). A residue from loop D and several residues from loop E determine, respectively, the different affinities of DHβE/α-conotoxin MII (86, 95) and the different sensitivities of cytisine for $\alpha3\beta2$ and $\alpha3\beta4$ (96).

Altogether, these studies support the notion that variable residues located in the vicinity of the affinity labeled amino acids are the major elements contributing to the pharmacological diversity of the nAChRs. The emerging picture is that the binding site consists of a conserved core of aromatic residues, and that variable amino acids neighboring these positions, as well as several amino acids from the nonconserved loop E and F, confer on each receptor subtype its individual pharmacological properties (Figure 1*D*).

Models of the Extracellular Domain and of the ACh Binding Pocket

In the past few years, two different models of the N-terminal domain appeared in the literature. With a hidden Markov model approach (sequence-sequence comparisons), Tsigelny et al (97) found local resemblance between the nAChR subunits and some members of the cupredoxin superfamily. They hypothesized a common fold and developed a 3D model on this basis. In parallel, Gready et al (98) used a threading approach (sequence-structure comparisons) to find possible templates for the glycine receptor $\alpha1$ subunit. Although they did not find any significant match, they conducted a modeling work based on their highest hit, a SH2–SH3 domain.

Although a unique specific fold is not consistently found by fold recognition approaches, these methods are nevertheless informative. In the analysis we conducted with all the program available, most of the hits belonged to the all-β class of protein. The majority were β-sandwiches generally of the immunoglobulin type, which are consistently aligned with the predicted all-β part of the extracellular moiety of the nAChR subunit. Furthermore, the β-sandwiches of immunoglobulins are flanked at both ends by three loops, analogous to the three loops of the principal and complementary components of the nAChR binding site.

In Figure 2 (see color insert), we propose a plausible model of a typical nAChR N-terminal domain, based on the immunoglobulin structure. The topology cartoon (Figure 2*A*) depicts the arrangement of the predicted nAChR secondary structure elements on the immunoglobulin fold. The A, B, and C components of the binding site would be located on the main β-sheet of the sandwich, whereas the components E and F would be on the side of the smallest sheet. The 60 first amino acids of the nAChR subunit being absent from the model, the D component is not mapped here. The artist's drawings (Figure 2B) tentatively assemble two subunits to account for the formation of the binding site at the interface. The main component of the binding site, on one subunit, would be distal to the lipidic membrane, whereas the complementary component, on the facing subunit, would be proximal to the membrane. Rather than being rod shaped, as often described, the extracellular part of a subunit would be flattened, the interfaces being tilted (in three dimensions) rather than strictly vertical and radial. An actual modeling study will be necessary to verify that the hypothesis described above can account for the large body of experimental data available.

THE ION CHANNEL

The Structural Organization of the Ion Channel

The ion channel was initially chemically identified by photoaffinity labeling with the channel blocker chlorpromazine. Chlorpromazine was found to label, in an agonist-dependent manner, a unique high-affinity site to which contribute all five the subunits of *Torpedo* receptor. The amino acids labeled within the M2 transmembrane segment by chlorpromazine (99–102) by triphenylmethyl phosphonium (103), Meproadifen mustard (104), TID (105), TID-BE (57), DAF (58), and Tetracain (106), as well as by the substituted cysteine accessibility method (SCAM) (23), are consistent with the notion that the ion channel is located along the axis of symmetry of the receptor oligomer, at the fivefold interface of the subunits, each subunit contributing by its M2 segment. The pattern of labeling, i.e. residues homologous to S240, I243/T244, L247/S348, T250/V251, L254, and E258/I259 of the $\alpha 7$ receptor, strongly supports the folding of M2 into an α-helix, in agreement with secondary structure predictions (46). Electron microscopy images of the open conformation of the channel identified five rods bordering the ion channel, attributed to the M2 segment (107). The axis of the rods are ~ 18 and ~ 11.5 Å from the axis of the pore, at the upper and lower faces, respectively, in agreement with a funnel-shaped pore with a minimal diameter of ~ 10 Å. SCAM experiments suggest in addition that the upper part of M1 contributes to the channel (108, 108a), possibly by intercalation between the M2 segment in the upper part.

The reactivity pattern of introduced cysteine side chains with the impermeant methane-thiosulfonate ethyltrimethyl ammonium applied either extra- or intracellularly supports the conclusion that the narrowest portion of the close and open channel is located at the cytoplasmic border of M2 (corresponding to $\alpha 7 K238$ and $\alpha 7 I239$) (109). The diameter of the narrowest portion of the channel in its open conformation was formally estimated to fit a square 6.5 x 6.5 Å wide to accommodate the largest permeant ions (110). Furthermore, the accessibility pattern at this level no longer fits with an α-helix. Residues homologous to α7G236, α7E237, and α7K238 indeed react with the thiosulfonate reagents, a finding consistent with the secondary structure prediction, which proposes this region as an extended loop accessible to solvent.

The ion channel thus appears to be composed of two distinct structural domains: an upper "α-helical component," which delimits both the wide portion of the pore and the pharmacological site for noncompetitive blockers; and a lower "loop component," which contributes to the narrowest portion of the channel (Figure 3) (see also 113–115a).

The Functional Organization of the Ion Channel

The functional contribution of the identified labeled residues to channel block (by QX222) (111), as well as to the intrinsic conductance and ionic selectivity of the pore (112), was further specified by site-directed mutagenesis, pointing to the

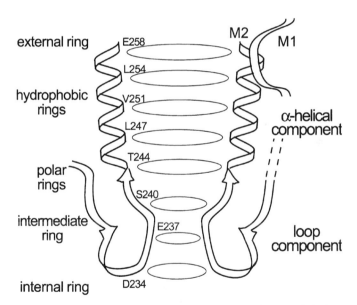

Figure 3   A model for the structural and functional organization of the ion channel. The contribution of two α7 subunits is shown to illustrate the ion channel, which is actually formed by homologous regions from the five subunits of the pentamer. The residues with numbers given are believed to face the lumen of the ion channel, thus forming rings of homologous residues (*circles*). The secondary structure of the M2 segment and M1–M2 loop is tentatively taken from Le Novère et al (46). The data accumulated to date suggest that the upper part of the channel, the α-helical component, acts as a water pore, whereas the lower loop component contributes to the selectivity filter of the ion channel.

contribution of two rings of polar Ser/Thr, three rings of hydrophobic Leu/Val, and three rings of charged Asp/Glu residues, which are highly conserved among the nAChR subunits sequenced to date.

So far, mutations within the loop component were found to alter all aspects of ionic selectivity of the channel:

1. Monovalent cation permeability and selectivity: In the muscle-type receptor, mutations in the rings corresponding to α7S240 and α7E237 progressively decrease the conductance of large cations when the volume of the side chain increases, which suggests that these residues are involved in cation selection according to their size (113–115); furthermore, in the muscle-type receptor, decreasing the net charge of the ring corresponding to α7E237 (and to a lesser extent to α7D234), results in a proportional decrease in potassium unitary conductance, in agreement with their direct or indirect (electrostatic) interaction with cations (116).
2. Divalent cation permeability: Mutation α7E237A abolishes the permeability of the α7 receptor to calcium but preserves that to monovalent cations (117).
3. Charge selectivity: The construction of chimeras between the cationic α7nAChR and the anionic α1GlyR shows that the insertion of a proline residue between positions 234 and 238 converts the selectivity of the E237A/V251T mutant of the α7 receptor from cationic to anionic (118, 119). Scanning mutagenesis indicates that no single residue within this loop is essential for anionic selectivity, stressing a major role of the loop conformation in the selectivity conversion. Yet the E237A mutation is required (but not sufficient) to yield an anionic channel, which suggests that this ring might constitute a negatively charged barrier to chloride ions.

At the level of the α-helical component, decreasing the net charge of the muscle-type ring corresponding to α7E258 results in a proportional decrease in potassium unitary conductance, yet to a lesser extent than in the case of α7E237 (116). At positions α7L247 and V251, introduction of polar or even charged residues is required, along with the proline insertion and the E237A mutation, to yield an anionic channel (118). However, in spite of anion-anion repulsion, mutation V251D also yields an anionic channel, indicating a mechanism not directly related to the nature of the side chain incorporated (119). A similar mechanism may occur in the case of the anionic $GABA_A$ homooligomeric receptor, for which introduction of a positively charged lysine at a position corresponding to α7A257 results in significant cationic permeability (120); also in the case of α7, mutations L254R or T and L255R, T, or G abolish the permeability to calcium (117).

The 10 Å diameter of the α-helical component is consistent with the notion that ions cross the membrane at this level in a fully hydrated state, whereas the narrower diameter of the loop component is expected to accommodate only partially dehydrated ions. The critical role of the loop component in cation discrimination as well as charge selectivity further supports its contribution to the selectivity filter of the channel by specific dehydration of ions. Accordingly, the α-helical component would select on the basis of stabilization of hydrated ions within the membrane, and the several phenotypes observed at this level could be explained in a first attempt on the basis of a structural reorganization of this portion of the channel.

This conception of the nAChR ion channel is reminiscent of that of the tetrameric voltage-gated Na^+, Ca^{2+}, and K^+ channels, composed of similar components, but with an inverted disposition; the loop component (called P-loop) is located on the extracellular side (121), as established by X-ray crystallography in the case of a phylogenetically related bacterial potassium channel (122). Furthermore, the P-loop of the Na^+ and Ca^{2+} channels shows striking similarities with the loop component of nAChR: (*a*) It is made up of two rings of negatively charged residues separated by two amino acids analogous to α7D234/α7E237; and (*b*) mutation of the inner ring of Na^+ channel (DEKA) to the one of the Ca^{2+} channel (EEEE) confers Ca^{2+} permeability (123), which is reminiscent of α7E237A, which abolishes Ca^{2+} permeability (117). One may thus tentatively postulate that similar mechanisms of cation permeation operate in these rather structurally distant receptor channels.

Conjectures About the Three-Dimensional Organization of the Ion Channel

There exists very few resolved transmembrane structures of ionic channels, precluding the use of automated approaches to search possible templates for the nAChR transmembrane part. Synthetic peptides corresponding to the M2 segment of the α1 subunit form ionic pores within the membrane (124). These channels lack the loop component and thus are not likely to mediate ion permeation the same way the native receptor does. Nevertheless, structural model of the helical component was developed from the electron microscopy images (125), and from a minimization method of the channel blockers–M2 helices complexes (126). Also, on the basis of analogy arguments, Ortells et al (127) modeled the entire nAChR transmembrane portion based on the heat-labile enterotoxin B subunits.

Plausible templates are two recently resolved ion channels: the tetrameric potassium channel from *Streptomyces lividans* (1BL8) (122) and the pentameric mechanosensitive receptor from *Mycobacterium tuberculosis* (1MSL) (128) (Figure 2*C*). Both channels are formed by a bundle of inner α-helices arranged in a right-handed cone narrowing at its cytoplasmic side, which may resemble the α-helical component of nAChR formed by M2. However, a hypothetical model of nAChR based on the structure of 1BL8 would require its transformation into a pentamer. In contrast, the pentameric nature of the 1MSL channel fits the nAChR. Furthermore, the outer helices from this receptor contribute to the upper part of the pore, which suggests a possible analogy with the transmembrane segment M1 of nAChR. Using the inner/outer helices as a template for the M2/M1 segments requires a "swap," where the connection between the helices is moved from the upper to the lower side of the channel (for examples of this type of circular permutation, see 129). For the loop component, a plausible template could be generated by inverting the transmembrane organization of the potassium channel, thus locating its P-loop at the cytoplasmic border of the pore. The above proposed templates could guide the design of starting models, which would require further refinement by integrating the structural and functional data accumulated on the nAChR channel.

ALLOSTERIC TRANSITIONS OF THE nAChRS PROBED AT THE AMINO ACID LEVEL

The distance between the ACh binding sites and the ion channel, estimated to be 20–40 Å from fluorescence transfer measurements (130), is such that long-range "allosteric" interactions take place at the level of the nAChR oligomer in the course of the activation and desensitization processes. Agonists binding at topologically distant sites stabilize global conformations of the protein for which the channel is either open (activation) or closed (desensitization), depending on the concentration of the ligand and the kinetics of its application. With *Torpedo* nAChR-rich membranes, rapid mixing experiments following parallel fluorescent agonist binding and ion flux are consistent with a minimal four-state allosteric model, involving discrete B, A, I, and D states, where B is the low-affinity basal state that predominates in the absence of agonist, A is the active open-channel state, and I and D are desensitized states with, respectively, high (micromolar) and very high (nanomolar) dissociation constants (131, 132). Together with the in vivo results of patch clamp recordings (133), these in vitro data are adequately accounted for by an extended allosteric mechanism that involves a cascade of discrete two-state transitions (134–136).

In the case of hemoglobin, often referred to as the prototype of allosteric proteins (137, 138), X-ray structural data have demonstrated that the allosteric transitions that accompany oxygen binding are primarily associated with a reorganization of the quaternary structure with only minor changes in the tertiary structure of the subunits (see 137). In the case of nAChR, the physiologically important sites being located at the subunit interfaces, such global and rigid quaternary reorganizations, are expected to modify "en bloc" the binding site geometry and the state of opening of the ion channel. Consistent with these views, Unwin et al (44) have reported on the basis of the surface-on-views of *Torpedo* nAChR observed by cryoelectron microscopy that before and after equilibration with carbamylcholine, a desensitizing agonist, the whole δ subunit and to a large extent the γ subunit fall away from the pentagonal symmetry, as a consequence of a difference of inclination of 10° tangential to the receptor axis.

Structural Changes Within the N-Terminal Domain

The computed 2D representation of the N-terminal domain and the structural model suggest that this domain consists of a rigid core of β-strands with reduced structural flexibility. Furthermore, a large body of experimental data support the

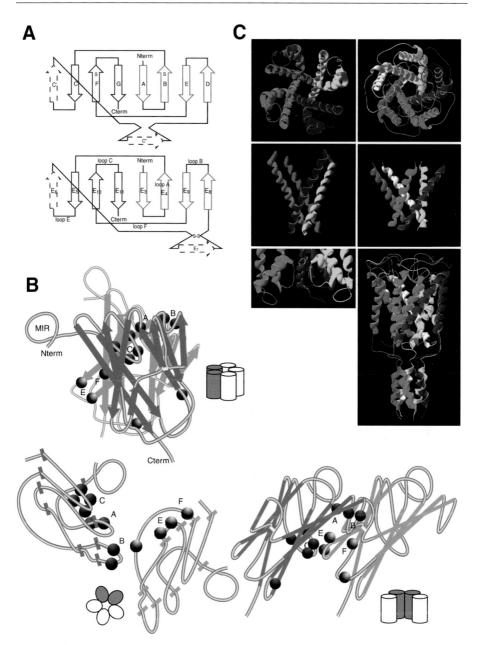

Figure 2 (*A, upper*) Topology cartoon of the immunoglobin (Ig) fold. (*Red strands*) The main sheet of the sandwich; (*blue strands*) the smallest sheet; (*dashed strands*) present only in the variable chains of the IgG. (*A, lower*) Topology cartoon of the proposed nicotinic fold. The strands are named according to Le Novère et al (46). (*B, upper*) Dimer of two subunits (*dark green and light green*) viewed from a line parallel to the membrane and perpendicular to the subunit interface. (*Red balls*) The residues of the main component of the ACh binding

site; (*yellow balls*) the residues of the complementary component. Note the tilt between the subunits in the plane of the interface. (*B, bottom left*) Dimer of subunits viewed from the extracellular side along a line perpendicular to the membrane. Note that the planes of the β-sheets do not contain the axis of symmetry of the receptor. (*B, lower right*) Dimer of subunits viewed from the pore of the receptor. Note the tilt from the vertical, which allows a possible interaction between the two extremities of extracellular domain from adjacent subunits. For sake of clarity, the lateral tilt presented in the *left panel* has been omitted. (*Small drawings*) The position of the represented subunits within the oligomer. (*C, left panels*) *Streptomyces lividans* potassium channel (1BL8). (*Top to bottom*) View from the extracellular side, lateral view of the inner helices, **and** view of the selectivity filter upside-down, as it could be in the nAChR. (*C, right panels*) *Mycobacterium tuberculosis* mechanosensitive channel (1MSL). (*Top to bottom*) View from the extracellular side, lateral view of the inner helices, lateral view of the complete channel. The pictures are screenshots of SWISSPDBVIEWER.

notion that the allosteric transitions mediated by the nAChR molecule are associated with structural modifications of the subunit interfaces in the N-terminal domain: (*a*) Affinity labeling with DDF shows that, in the course of the B-to-D-state transition, the labeling of the loop A and B region increases, whereas that of the γ subunit increases and that of the δ subunit decreases (139). (*b*) Up to now, the mutations of the N-terminal domain that alter the allosteric transitions of the receptor were found at the level of the binding loops of the N-terminal domain that contribute to the subunit interface. For example, single-channel recordings of muscle-type nAChR mutants α1Y198F, εD175N, α1Y93F, and α1Y190F reveal alterations of the gating constants for ACh (140, 141), which may reflect changes of the isomerization constant of the protein between the B and A states. More striking, the mutation of residues 151–155 within loopB of α7, which causes an increase in binding affinity of agonists, alters primarily the isomerization constants leading to the desensitized states (89; see also 142). These mutations also alter the transition leading to the active state because their introduction of these mutations in the α7L247T mutant dramatically increases the fraction of receptor that spontaneously opens (PJ Corringer, JP Changeux & D Bertrand, unpublished observations). (*c*) The allosteric site for nAChR potentiation by Ca^{2+} was identified by scanning mutagenesis on the α7 receptor within the 161–172 segment, which carries loop F of the complementary component of the ACh binding site (78).

Thus, the currently available data are consistent with the view that the N-terminal domain of each subunit would undergo concerted rigid body motion during the allosteric transitions.

Structural Changes Within the Transmembrane Domain

The early observation that the channel blocker chlorpromazine photolabels its M2 site 1000 times faster when the channel is in its open configuration suggests that the α-helical component undergoes a structural reorganization during the activation process (99). Indeed, electron microscopy revealed that when nAChR rich membranes are rapidly mixed with very high concentrations (100 mM) of ACh, the five rods tentatively attributed to the M2 segments bend abruptly near the middle of the membrane and twist around the central axis in the lower part (107). However, SCAM experiments revealed that the residues that are exposed within this region of the pore do not significantly differ in the presence or absence of agonist (143). During desensitization, the labeling by channel blockers known to stabilize the B state [TID (105), TID-BE (57), tetracaine (106), and DAF (58)] shifts in the presence of a desensitizing agonist to a more expanded pattern that includes additional intracellular residues, a finding consistent with a widening of this region of the ionic pathway in the course of desensitization. Still, the same "face" of the helix is labeled both in the presence and in the absence of agonist.

Consistent with an important contribution of the α-helical component in the conformational transitions, mutations within α7 M2 profoundly alter the properties of both activation and desensitization (144). Increasing the polarity of the hydrophobic rings L247, V251, L254, and L255 results in pleiotropic phenotypes, which is well illustrated by the L247T mutation that results in (a) a shift of the ACh dose-response curve to lower concentrations, (b) a dramatic loss of desensitization, (c) the conversion of DHβE from an antagonist to a full agonist, and (d) the occurrence of spontaneous currents blocked by the competitive antagonist α-bungarotoxin (119, 144–147). In the case of the muscle-type nAChR, progressive replacement of homologous leucines leads to progressively larger shifts in the dose-response curves, with symmetrical effects on the α1, β, γ, and δ subunits (148). Congenital myasthenic syndromes were in many cases found to arise from single mutations within M2, generally characterized by prolonged ACh-evoked channel openings, and in some cases spontaneous openings or altered desensitization (149, 150). Autosomal dominant nocturnal frontal lobe epilepsy was also found to arise from mutations S247F and insertion of a leucine (776ins3) within M2 (151, 152) associated, in particular, with an altered agonist apparent affinity and desensitization (153, 154).

For the loop component of the ion channel, SCAM experiments on the α1 of the muscle nAChR indicate that residues corresponding to α7E237, K238, and I239 act as barriers to the permeant methanethiosulfonate ethylammonium when applied either extra- or intracellularly (109). Furthermore, the coapplication of methanethiosulfonate ethylammonium with ACh results in removal of this barrier, and within this region, the insertion of a proline between positions 233 and 238 in the α7 receptor, along with the E237A and V251T mutations, causes an increased ACh EC_{50} and high levels of spontaneous activity (119). These observations suggest that the loop component serves the double function of selectivity filter and physical gate of the channel in the B state. The above mentioned electron microscopy images, which suggest that the gate is located at the middle of the M2 α-helix (107), may thus have to be reinterpreted. Either the two segments making the "kink" do not belong to the same transmembrane segment or the kinked state corresponds to the desensitized rather than to the resting state.

The structural reorganization occurring along the entire length of the pore is, in addition, associated with a global rearrangement of the transmembrane domain.

First, in the M4 segment, mutations α1C418 and β1C447 (155) or γL440 and γM442 of the murine nAChR (156) alter the mean channel open time of ACh-evoked single-channel opening, without alteration of the unitary conductance. These residues belong to the lipid-exposed face of the M4 α-helix (56), supporting a strong link between channel gating and lipid-protein interaction. Along this line, several allosteric effectors of the *Torpedo* receptor were found to act at the lipid-receptor interface, as demonstrated directly by affinity labeling of lipid-exposed residues of M4 by the steroid noncompetitive antagonist promegestone (60). Mutation within M3 of V285I of the human α1 subunit causes a congenital myasthenic syndrome, characterized by single-channel slow opening and fast closing rates in the presence of ACh (157). Labeling experiments support the conclusion that this residue faces the protein interior away from lipids (56). Internal protein motions thus also govern the gating mechanism.

Second, the transmembrane topology of the subunits supports the view that the upper part of M1, as well as the loop linking M2 and M3, may interact with the N-terminal domain, which suggests their possible contribution to the structural coupling between these two domains. In agreement with this idea, the highly conserved successive P and C residues at the middle of M1 were found to be involved in the gating mechanism, because mutation of the *Torpedo* γC230 alters the mean open time of ACh-evoked currents (158), and mutation of the murine receptor at α1P221 to L, A, or G, but not in β1, γ, or δ subunits, appeared nonfunctional electrophysiologically. Introducing at this position α-hydroxy acids corresponding to L, A, or G restores the receptor function, demonstrating that a backbone N-H group interferes with normal gating, probably through hydrogen bonding (159). At the middle of the M2–M3 loop, α7,3 chimeras revealed that mutation of α7D266 resulted in decreased agonist apparent affinities and maximally evoked currents (160). A mutation at this position (α1S269I) is also associated with a myasthenic syndrome, characterized by prolonged ACh-evoked channel openings (161).

In conclusion, many regions of the nAChR are involved in the allosteric transitions. The reorganization of the N-terminal domain is likely to be mainly associated with a change in quaternary structure. The transmembrane domain appear to undergo global conformational changes, associated with local changes at the level of both the α-helical and loop component of the pore, as well as at the lipid-protein interface. Both domains may be allosterically coupled by at least two segments located near the upper side of the membrane.

CONCLUSION

This overview of the nAChR illustrates the advances made in the understanding, at the amino acid level, of mechanisms underlying the chemico-electrical transduction mediated by the protein. In the absence of structural information at atomic resolution, the data presented lead to the proposal of plausible but still hypothetical structural models of the ACh binding sites and of the ion channel, ultimately accounting for their pharmacological and ionic selectivities, respectively. Furthermore, several aspects of the structural changes occurring during signal transduction have been presented involving mainly quaternary reorganizations.

Two mechanisms are currently used to fit nAChR data. On one hand, the Monod-Wyman-Changeux (MWC) theory (162, 163) postulates that the protein spontaneously isomerizes between discrete allosteric states characterized by "all or none" symmetrical changes. On the other hand, the sequential models (164, 165) postulate that the conformational transitions occur only after agonist binding, leading to agonist-induced multiple intermediate states. At this stage, it appears difficult to discriminate unambiguously between these theories. Yet the following observations among others (see 135) support the MWC allosteric model.

1. Mutations altering receptor function and conformational transitions are found widely dispersed throughout the protein structure. In addition, mutations at discrete positions, such as α7L247T within the ion channel, modify the receptor properties in a pleiotropic manner, including the alteration of the apparent affinities of the far distant ACh binding sites. This indicates that global rather than local changes are associated with the transitions.

2. Mutations throughout the structure increase the frequency of spontaneously open states in the absence of ACh, unambiguously establishing that opening of the ion channel does not require, and thus is not induced by, ACh binding and supporting the occurrence of preexisting conformational equilibrium. The MWC theory, adapted to the nAChRs in an extended quantitative model (134), gives a general framework that directly accounts for such extremely pleiotropic phenotypes (166).

The subunit diversity of neuronal nAChRs is such that they may achieve a wide diversity of functions, such as fast wiring (phasic, α7 in CA1 interneurones of the hippocampus) and volume (tonic, α4β2 in CA1 interneurones of the hippocampus) transmission (167), according to both their intrinsic functional properties of activation and desensitization and their subcellular anatomical localization. Understanding these functions will require knowledge of the intimate biochemical and structural organization of these receptors, which has, and continues to, illuminate their physiology.

ACKNOWLEDGMENTS

We thank Stuart Edelstein for critical reading of the manuscript and valuable discussions, and Arthur Karlin and Denis Servent for useful suggestions. This work was supported by research grants from the Association Française contre les Myopathies, the Collège de France, the EEC Biotech and Biomed Programs, the Council for Tobacco Research, and the Reynolds Pharmaceuticals.

Visit the Annual Reviews home page at www.AnnualReviews.org.

LITERATURE CITED

1. Katz B, Miledi R. 1977. Suppression of transmitter release at the neuromuscular junction. *Proc. R. Soc. London Ser. B* 196:465–69

2. Zoli M, Jansson A, Sykova E, Agnati LF, Fuxe K. 1999. Volume transmission in the CNS and its relevance for neuropsy-chopharmacology. *Trends Pharmacol. Sci.* 20:142–50

3. Lee CY, Chang CC. 1966. Modes of actions of purified toxins from elapid venoms on neuromuscular transmission. *Mem. Inst. Butantan Sao Paulo* 33:555–72

4. Changeux JP, Kasai M, Lee CY. 1970. The use of a snake venom toxin to characterize the cholinergic receptor protein. *Proc. Natl. Acad. Sci. USA* 67:1241–47

5. Changeux JP. 1991. Functional architecture and dynamics of the nicotinic acetylcholine receptor: an allosteric ligand-gated ion channel. *Fidia Res. Found. Neurosci. Award Lect.* 4:21–168

6. Karlin A. 1991. Explorations of the nicotinic acetylcholine receptor. *Harvey Lect. Ser.* 85:71–107

7. Lindstrom J. 1996. Neuronal nicotinic acetylcholine receptors. *Ion Channels* 4:377–450

8. Ballivet M, Patrick J, Lee J, Heinemann S. 1982. Molecular cloning of cDNA coding for the gamma subunit of *Torpedo* acetylcholine receptor. *Proc. Natl. Acad. Sci. USA* 79:4466–70

9. Giraudat J, Devillers-Thiery A, Auffray C, Rougeon F, Changeux JP. 1982. Identification of a cDNA clone coding for the acetylcholine binding subunit of *Torpedo marmorata* acetylcholine receptor. *EMBO J.* 1:713–17

10. Sumikawa K, Houghton M, Smith JC, Bell L, Richards BM, Barnard EA. 1982. The molecular cloning and characterisation of cDNA coding for the alpha subunit of the acetylcholine receptor. *Nucleic Acids Res.* 10:5809–22

11. Noda M, Takahashi H, Tanabe T, Toyosato M, Furutani Y, et al. 1982. Primary structure of alpha-subunit precursor of *Torpedo californica* acetylcholine receptor deduced from cDNA sequence. *Nature* 299:793–97

12. Noda M, Takahashi H, Tanabe T, Toyosato M, Kikyotani S, et al. 1983. Primary structures of beta- and delta-subunit precursors of *Torpedo californica* acetylcholine receptor deduced from cDNA sequences. *Nature* 301:251–55

13. Claudio T, Ballivet M, Patrick J, Heinemann S. 1983. Nucleotide and deduced amino acid sequences of *Torpedo Californica* acetylcholine receptor gamma-

subunit. *Proc. Natl. Acad. Sci. USA* 80:1111–15

14. Devillers-Thiery A, Giraudat J, Bentaboulet M, Changeux JP. 1983. Complete mRNA coding sequence of the acetylcholine binding alpha-subunit of *Torpedo marmorata* acetylcholine receptor: a model for the transmembrane organization of the polypeptide chain. *Proc. Natl. Acad. Sci. USA* 80:2067–71

15. Cockcroft VB, Osguthorpe DJ, Barnard EA, Friday AE, Lunt GG. 1992. Ligand-gated ion channels: homology and diversity. *Mol. Neurobiol.* 4:129–69

16. Fletcher S, Barnes NM. 1998. Desperately seeking subunits: Are native 5-HT$_3$ receptors really homomeric complexes? *Trends Pharmacol. Sci.* 19:212–15

17. Macdonald RL, Olsen RW. 1994. GABA$_A$ receptor channels. *Annu. Rev. Neurosci.* 17:569–602

18. Bormann J, Feigenspan A. 1995. GABA$_C$ receptors. *Trends Neurosci.* 18:515–19

19. Bechade C, Sur C, Triller A. 1994. The inhibitory neuronal glycine receptor. *BioEssays* 16:735–44

20. Le Novère N, Changeux JP. 1999. The ligand gated ion channel database. *Nucleic Acids Res.* 27:340–42

21. Mongan NP, Baylis HA, Adcock C, Smith GR, Sansom MS, Sattelle DB. 1998. An extensive and diverse gene family of nicotinic acetylcholine receptor alpha subunits in *Caenorhabditis elegans*. *Recept. Channels* 6:213–28

22. Kao PN, Dwork AJ, Kaldany RRJ, Silver ML, Widemann J, et al. 1984. Identification of the alpha-subunit half-cystine specifically labeled by an affinity reagent for acetylcholine receptor binding site. *J. Biol. Chem.* 259:11662–65

23. Karlin A, Akabas MH. 1995. Toward a structural basis for the function of nicotinic acetylcholine receptors and their cousins. *Neuron* 15:1231–44

24. Sargent PB. 1993. The diversity of neu-

ronal nicotinic acetylcholine receptors. *Annu. Rev. Neurosci.* 16:403–43

25. Le Novère N, Changeux JP. 1995. Molecular evolution of the nicotinic acetylcholine receptor: an example of multigene family in excitable cells. *J. Mol. Evol.* 40:155–72

26. Ortells MO, Lunt GG. 1995. Evolutionary history of the ligand-gated ion-channel superfamily of receptors. *Trends Neurosci.* 18:121–27

27. Couturier S, Bertrand D, Matter JM, Hernandez MC, Bertrand S, et al. 1990. A neuronal nicotinic acetylcholine receptor subunit (alpha 7) is developmentally regulated and forms a homo-oligomeric channel blocked by alpha-BTX. *Neuron* 5:845–56

28. Schoepfer R, Conroy WG, Whiting P, Gore M, Lindstom J. 1990. Brain alpha-bungarotoxin binding protein cDNAs and MAbs reveal subtypes of this branch of the ligand-gated ion channel gene superfamily. *Neuron* 5:35–48

29. Gerzanich V, Anand R, Lindstrom J. 1994. Homomers of alpha 8 and alpha 7 subunits of nicotinic receptors exhibit similar channel but contrasting binding site properties. *Mol. Pharmacol.* 45:212–20

30. Elgoyhen AB, Johnson DS, Boulter J, Vetter DE, Heinemann S. 1994. Alpha 9: an acetylcholine receptor with novel pharmacological properties expressed in rat cochlear hair cells. *Cell* 79:705–15

31. Cooper E, Couturier S, Ballivet M. 1991. Pentameric structure and subunit stoichiometry of a neuronal nicotinic acetylcholine receptor. *Nature* 350:235–38

32. Anand R, Conroy WG, Schoepfer R, Whiting P, Lindstrom J. 1991. Neuronal nicotinic acetylcholine receptors expressed in Xenopus oocytes have a pentameric quaternary structure. *J. Biol. Chem.* 266:11192–98

33. Ramirez-Latorre J, Yu CR, Qu X, Perin F, Karlin A, Role L. 1996. Functional contribution of alpha5 subunit to neu-

ronal acetylcholine receptor channels. *Nature* 380:347–51

34. Wang F, Gerzanich V, Wells G, Anand R, Peng X, et al. 1996. Assembly of human neuronal nicotinic receptor alpha5 subunits with alpha3, beta2, and beta4 subunits. *J. Biol. Chem.* 271:17656–65

35. Groot-Kormelink PJ, Luyten WH, Colquhoun D, Sivilotti LG. 1998. A reporter mutation approach shows incorporation of the "orphan" subunit beta 3 into a functional nicotinic receptor. *J. Biol. Chem.* 273:15317–20

36. Machold J, Weise C, Utkin Y, Tsetlin V, Hucho F. 1995. The handedness of the subunit arrangement of the nicotinic acetylcholine receptor from *Torpedo californica. Eur. J. Biochem.* 234:427–30

37. Unwin N. 1996. Projection structure of the nicotinic acetylcholine receptor: distinct conformations of the alpha subunits. *J. Mol. Biol.* 257:586–96

38. Role LW, Berg DK. 1996. Nicotinic receptors in the development and modulation of CNS synapses. *Neuron* 16:1077–85

39. Wada E, Wada K, Boulter J, Deneris E, Heinemann S, et al. 1989. Distribution of alpha2, alpha3, alpha4, and beta2 neuronal nicotinic receptor subunit mRNAs in the central nervous system: a hybridization histochemical study in the rat. *J. Comp. Neurol.* 284:314–35

40. Le Novère N, Zoli M, Changeux JP. 1996. Neuronal nicotinic receptor alpha6 subunit mRNA is selectively concentrated in catecholaminergic nuclei of the rat brain. *Eur. J. Neurosci.* 8:2428–39

41. Kerszberg M, Changeux JP. 1994. A model for reading morphogenetic gradients: autocatalysis and competition at the gene level. *Proc. Natl. Acad. Sci. USA* 91:5823–27

42. Li X, Noll M. 1994. Evolution of distinct developmental functions of three *Drosophila* genes by acquisition of different cis-regulatory regions. *Nature* 367:83–87

43. Xue L, Noll M. 1996. The functional

conservation of proteins in evolutionary alleles and the dominant role of enhancers in evolution. *EMBO J.* 15:3722–31

44. Unwin N, Toyoshima C, Kubalek E. 1988. Arrangement of the acetylcholine receptor subunits in the resting and desensitized states, determined by cryoelectron microscopy of crystallized *Torpedo* postsynaptic membranes. *J. Cell Biol.* 107:1123–38

45. Hucho F, Tsetlin VI, Machold J. 1996. The emerging three-dimensional structure of a receptor. The nicotinic acetylcholine receptor. *Eur. J. Biochem.* 239:539–57

46. Le Novère N, Corringer PJ, Changeux JP. 1999. Improved secondary structure predictions for a nicotinic receptor subunit. Incorporation of solvent accessibility and experimental data into a 2D representation. *Biophys. J.* 76:2329–45

47. Eiselé JL, Bertrand S, Galzi JL, Devillers-Thiéry A, Changeux JP, Bertrand D. 1993. Chimeric nicotinic-serotoninergic receptor combines distinct ligand binding and channel specificities. *Nature* 366:479–83

48. Schrattenholz A, Pfeiffer S, Pejovic V, Rudolph R, Godovac-Zimmermann J, Maelicke A. 1998. Expression and renaturation of the N-terminal extracellular domain of *Torpedo* nicotinic acetylcholine receptor alpha-subunit. *J. Biol. Chem.* 273:23393–99

49. Wells GB, Anand R, Wang F, Lindstrom J. 1998. Water-soluble nicotinic acetylcholine receptor formed by alpha7 subunit extracellular domains. *J. Biol. Chem.* 273:964–73

50. West AP, Bjorkman PJ, Dougherty DA, Lester HA. 1997. Expression and circular dichroism studies of the extracellular domain of the alpha subunit of the nicotinic acetylcholine receptor. *J. Biol. Chem.* 272:25468–73

51. Alexeev T, Krivoshein A, Shevalier A, Kudelina I, Telyakova O, et al. 1999. Physicochemical and immunological

studies of the N-terminal domain of the *Torpedo* acetylcholine receptor alpha-subunit expressed in *Escherichia coli.* *Eur. J. Biochem.* 259:310–19

52. Xue H, Hang J, Chu R, Xiao Y, Li H, et al. 1999. Delineation of a membrane-proximal beta-rich domain in the GABA$_A$ receptor by progressive deletions. *J. Mol. Biol.* 285:55–61

53. Miyazawa A, Fujiyoshi Y, Stowell M, Unwin N. 1999. Nicotinic acetylcholine receptor at 4.6 Å resolution: transverse tunnels in the channel wall. *J. Mol. Biol.* 288:765–86

54. Corbin J, Methot N, Wang HH, Baenziger JE, Blanton MP. 1998. Secondary structure analysis of individual transmembrane segments of the nicotinic acetylcholine receptor by circular dichroism and Fourier transform infrared spectroscopy. *J. Biol. Chem.* 273:771–77

55. Gorne-Tschelnokow U, Strecker A, Kaduk C, Naumann D, Hucho F. 1994. The transmembrane domains of the nicotinic acetylcholine receptor contain alpha-helical and beta structures. *EMBO J.* 13:338–41

56. Blanton MP, Cohen JB. 1994. Identifying the lipid-protein interface of the *Torpedo* nicotinic acetylcholine receptor: secondary structure implications. *Biochemistry* 33:2859–72

57. Blanton MP, McCardy EA, Huggins A, Parikh D. 1998. Probing the structure of the nicotinic acetylcholine receptor with the hydrophobic photoreactive probes [^{125}I]TID-BE and [^{125}I]TIDPC/16. *Biochemistry* 37:14545–55

58. Blanton MP, Dangott LJ, Raja SK, Lala AK, Cohen JB. 1998. Probing the structure of the nicotinic acetylcholine receptor ion channel with the uncharged photoactivable compound [^{3}H]diazofluorene. *J. Biol. Chem.* 273:8659–68

59. Corbin J, Wang HH, Blanton MP. 1998. Identifying the cholesterol binding domain in the nicotinic acetylcholine

receptor with [^{125}I]azido-cholesterol. *Biochim. Biophys. Acta* 1414:65–74

60. Blanton MP, Xie Y, Dangott LJ, Cohen JB. 1999. The steroid promegestone is a noncompetitive antagonist of the *Torpedo* nicotinic acetylcholine receptor that interacts with the lipid-protein interface. *Mol. Pharmacol.* 55:269–78

61. Langenbuch-Cachat J, Bon C, Goeldner M, Hirth C, Changeux JP. 1988. Photoaffinity labeling by aryldiazonium derivatives of *Torpedo marmorata* acetylcholine receptor. *Biochemistry* 27:2337–45

62. Dennis M, Giraudat J, Kotzyba-Hibert F, Goeldner M, Hirth C, et al. 1988. Amino acids of the *Torpedo marmorata* acetylcholine receptor subunit labeled by a photoaffinity ligand for the acetylcholine binding site. *Biochemistry* 27:2346–57

63. Pedersen SE, Cohen JB. 1990. d-Tubocurarine binding sites are located at the alpha-gamma and alpha-delta subunit interfaces of the nicotinic acetylcholine receptor. *Proc. Natl. Acad. Sci. USA* 87:2785–89

64. Oswald RE, Changeux JP. 1982. Cross-linking of alpha-bungarotoxin to the acetylcholine receptor from *Torpedo marmorata* by ultraviolet light irradiation. *FEBS Lett.* 139:225–29

65. Middleton RE, Cohen JB. 1991. Mapping of the acetylcholine binding site of the nicotinic acetylcholine receptor: [^{3}H]nicotine as an agonist photoaffinity label. *Biochemistry* 30:6987–97

66. Blount P, Merlie JP. 1989. Molecular basis of the two nonequivalent ligand binding sites of the muscle nicotinic receptor. *Neuron* 3:349–57

67. Sine SM. 1993. Molecular dissection of subunit interfaces in the acetylcholine receptor: identification of residues that determine curare selectivity. *Proc. Natl. Acad. Sci. USA* 90:9436–40

68. Sine SM, Kreienkamp HJ, Bren N, Maeda R, Taylor P. 1995. Molecular dissection of subunit interfaces in the ace-

tylcholine receptor: identification of determinants of alpha-conotoxin M1 selectivity. *Neuron* 15:205–11

69. Corringer PJ, Galzi JL, Eiselé JL, Bertrand S, Changeux JP, Bertrand D. 1995. Identification of a new component of the agonist binding site of the nicotinic alpha 7 homooligomeric receptor. *J. Biol. Chem.* 270:11749–52

70. Galzi JL, Revah F, Black D, Goeldner M, Hirth C, Changeux JP. 1990. Identification of a novel amino acid alpha-Tyr 93 within the active site of the acetylcholine receptor by photoaffinity labeling: additional evidence for a three-loop model of the acetylcholine binding site. *J. Biol. Chem.* 265:10430–37

71. Cohen JB, Sharp SD, Liu WS. 1991. Structure of the agonist-binding site of the nicotinic acetylcholine receptor. *J. Biol. Chem.* 266:23354–64

72. Abramson SN, Li Y, Culver P, Taylor P. 1989. An analog of lophotoxin reacts covalently with Tyr 190 in the alpha-subunit of the nicotinic acetylcholine receptor. *J. Biol. Chem.* 264:12666–72

73. Chiara DC, Middleton RE, Cohen JB. 1998. Identification of tryptophan 55 as the primary site of [^{3}H]nicotine photoincorporation in the gamma-subunit of the *Torpedo* nicotinic acetylcholine receptor. *FEBS Lett.* 423:223–26

74. Chiara DC, Xie Y, Cohen JB. 1999. Structure of the agonist-binding sites of the *Torpedo* nicotinic acetylcholine receptor: affinity-labeling and mutational analyses identify gamma Tyr-111/delta Arg-113 as antagonist affinity determinants. *Biochemistry* 38:6689–98

75. Czajkowski C, Karlin A. 1995. Structure of the nicotinic receptor acetylcholine-binding site. Identification of acidic residues in the delta subunit within 0.9 nm of the 5 alpha subunit-binding. *J. Biol. Chem.* 270:3160–64

76. Martin M, Czajkowski C, Karlin A. 1996. The contributions of aspartyl residues in the acetylcholine receptor gamma

and delta subunits to the binding of agonists and competitive antagonists. *J. Biol. Chem.* 271:13497–503

77. Galzi JL, Bertrand D, Devillers-Thiéry A, Revah F, Bertrand S, Changeux JP. 1991. Functional significance of aromatic amino acids from three peptide loops of the alpha 7 neuronal nicotinic receptor site investigated by site-directed mutagenesis. *FEBS Lett.* 294:198–202

78. Galzi JL, Bertrand S, Corringer PJ, Changeux JP, Bertrand D. 1996. Identification of calcium binding sites that regulate potentiation of a neuronal nicotinic acetylcholine receptor. *EMBO J.* 15: 5824–32

79. Sine SM, Quiram P, Papanikolaou F, Kreienkamp HJ, Taylor P. 1994. Conserved tyrosines in the alpha subunit of the nicotinic acetylcholine receptor stabilize quaternary ammonium groups of agonists and curariform antagonists. *J. Biol. Chem.* 269:8808–16

80. Nowak MW, Kearney PC, Sampson JR, Saks ME, Labarca CG, et al. 1995. Nicotinic receptor binding site probed with unnatural amino acid incorporation in intact cells. *Science* 268:439–42

81. Zhong W, Gallivan JP, Zhang Y, Li L, Lester HA, Dougherty DA. 1998. From ab initio quantum mechanics to molecular neurobiology: a cation-π binding site in the nicotinic receptor. *Proc. Natl. Acad. Sci. USA* 95:12088–93

82. Sussman J, Harel M, Frolow F, Oefner C, Goldman A, et al. 1991. Atomic structure of acetylcholinesterase from *Torpedo californica:* a prototypic acetylcholine-binding protein. *Science* 253: 872–79

83. Sugiyama N, Boyd AE, Taylor P. 1996. Anionic residue in the alpha-subunit of the nicotinic acetylcholine receptor contributing to subunit assembly and ligand binding. *J. Biol. Chem.* 271:26575–81

84. O'Leary ME, White MM. 1992. Mutational analysis of ligand-induced activation of the *Torpedo* acetylcholine receptor. *J. Biol. Chem.* 267:8360–65

85. Servent D, Winckler-Dietrich V, Hu HY, Kessler P, Drevet P, et al. 1997. Only snake curaremimetic toxins with a fifth disulfide bond have high affinity for the neuronal alpha7 nicotinic receptor. *J. Biol. Chem.* 272:24279–86

86. Harvey SC, McIntosh JM, Cartier GE, Maddox FN, Luetje CW. 1997. Determinants of specificity for alpha-conotoxin MII on alpha3beta2 neuronal nicotinic receptors. *Mol. Pharmacol.* 51:336–42

87. Luetje CW, Piattoni M, Patrick J. 1993. Mapping of ligand binding sites of neuronal nicotinic acetylcholine receptors using chimeric alpha subunits. *Mol. Pharmacol.* 44:657–66

88. Anand R, Nelson ME, Gerzanich V, Wells GB, Lindstrom J. 1998. Determinants of channel gating located in the N-terminal extracellular domain of nicotinic alpha7 receptor. *J. Pharmacol. Exp. Ther.* 287:469–79

89. Corringer PJ, Bertrand S, Bohler S, Edelstein SJ, Changeux JP, Bertrand D. 1998. Critical elements determining diversity in agonist binding and desensitization of neuronal nicotinic acetylcholine receptors. *J. Neurosci.* 18:648–57

90. Kreienkamp HJ, Sine SM, Maeda RK, Taylor P. 1994. Glycosylation sites selectively interfere with alpha-toxin binding to the nicotinic acetylcholine receptor. *J. Biol. Chem.* 269:8108–14

91. Ackermann EJ, Taylor P. 1997. Nonidentity of the alpha-neurotoxin binding sites on the nicotinic acetylcholine receptor revealed by modification in alpha-neurotoxin and receptor structures. *Biochemistry* 36:12836–44

92. Prince RJ, Sine SM. 1996. Molecular dissection of subunit interfaces in the acetylcholine receptor. Identification of residues that determine agonist selectivity. *J. Biol. Chem.* 271:25770–77

93. Bren N, Sine SM. 1997. Identification of

residues in the adult nicotinic acetylcholine receptor that confer selectivity for curariform antagonists. *J. Biol. Chem.* 272:30793–98

94. Osaka H, Malany S, Kanter JR, Sine SM, Taylor P. 1999. Subunit interface selectivity of the alpha-neurotoxins for the nicotinic acetylcholine receptor. *J. Biol. Chem.* 274:9581–86

95. Harvey SC, Luetje CW. 1996. Determinants of competitive antagonist sensitivity on neuronal nicotinic receptor beta subunits. *J. Neurosci.* 16:3798–806

96. Figl A, Cohen BN, Quick MW, Davidson N, Lester HA. 1992. Regions of beta 4.beta 2 subunit chimeras that contribute to the agonist selectivity of neuronal nicotinic receptors. *FEBS Lett.* 308:245–48

97. Tsigelny I, Sugiyama N, Sine SM, Taylor P. 1997. A model of the nicotinic receptor extracellular domain based on sequence identity and residue location. *Biophys. J.* 73:52–66

98. Gready JE, Ranganathan S, Schofield PR, Matsuo Y, Nishikawa K. 1997. Predicted structure of the extracellular region of ligand-gated ion-channel receptors shows SH2-like and SH3-like domains forming the ligand-binding site. *Protein Sci.* 6:983–98

99. Heidmann T, Changeux JP. 1984. Time-resolved photolabeling by the noncompetitive blocker chlorpromazine of the acetylcholine receptor in its transiently open and closed ion channel conformations. *Proc. Natl. Acad. Sci. USA* 81:1897–901

100. Giraudat J, Dennis M, Heidmann T, Chang JY, Changeux JP. 1986. Structure of the high-affinity site for noncompetitive blockers of the acetylcholine receptor: serine-262 of the delta subunit is labeled by [³H]chlorpromazine. *Proc. Natl. Acad. Sci. USA* 83:2719–23

101. Giraudat J, Galzi JL, Revah F, Changeux JP, Haumont PY, Lederer F. 1989. The noncompetitive blocker chlorpromazine labels segment MII but not segment MI

102. Revah F, Galzi JL, Giraudat J, Haumont PY, Lederer F, Changeux JP. 1990. The noncompetitive blocker [³H]chlorpromazine labels three amino acids of the acetylcholine receptor gamma subunit: implications for the alpha-helical organization of the M2 segments and the structure of the ion channel. *Proc. Natl. Acad. Sci. USA* 87:4675–79

103. Hucho F, Oberthür W, Lottspeich F. 1986. The ion channel of the nicotinic acetylcholine receptor is formed by the homologous helices MII of the receptor subunits. *FEBS Lett.* 205:137–42

104. Pedersen SE, Sharp SD, Liu WS, Cohen JB. 1992. Structure of the noncompetitive antagonist-binding site of the *Torpedo* nicotinic acetylcholine receptor. [³H]meproadifen mustard reacts selectively with alpha-subunit Glu-262. *J. Biol. Chem.* 267:10489–99

105. White BH, Cohen JB. 1992. Agonist-induced changes in the structure of the acetylcholine receptor M2 regions revealed by photoincorporation of an uncharged nicotinic noncompetitive antagonist. *J. Biol. Chem.* 267:15770–83

106. Middleton RE, Strand NP, Cohen JB. 1999. Photoaffinity labeling the *Torpedo* nicotinic acetylcholine receptor with [³H]tetracaine, a nondesensitizing noncompetitive antagonist. *Mol. Pharmacol.* 56:290–99

107. Unwin N. 1995. Acetylcholine receptor channel imaged in the open state. *Nature* 373:37–43

108. Akabas MH, Karlin A. 1995. Identification of acetylcholine receptor channel-lining residues in the M1 segment of the alpha-subunit. *Biochemistry* 34:12496–500

108. (a) Zhang H, Karlin A. 1997. Identification of acetylcholine receptor channel-lining residues in the M1 segment of the β subunit. *Biochemistry* 36:15856–64

109. Wilson GG, Karlin A. 1998. The location

of the gate in the acetylcholine receptor. *Neuron* 20:1269–81

110. Hille B. 1992. *Ion Channels of Excitable Membranes.* Sunderland, MA: Sinauer

111. Charnet P, Labarca C, Leonard RJ, Vogelaar NJ, Czyzyk L, et al. 1990. An open-channel blocker interacts with adjacent turns of alpha-helices in the nicotinic acetylcholine receptor. *Neuron* 2:87–95

112. Imoto K, Methfessel C, Sakmann B, Mishina M, Mori Y, et al. 1986. Location of a delta-subunit region determining ion transport through the acetylcholine receptor channel. *Nature* 324:670–74

113. Villarroel A, Sakmann B. 1992. Threonine in the selectivity filter of the acetylcholine receptor channel. *Biophys. J.* 62:196–205

114. Wang F, Imoto K. 1992. Pore size and negative charge as structural determinants of permeability in the *Torpedo* nicotinic acetylcholine receptor channel. *Proc. R. Soc. London Ser. B* 250:11–17

115. Cohen BN, Labarca C, Czyzyk L, Davidson N, Lester HA. 1992. Tris + /Na + permeability ratios of nicotinic acetylcholine receptors are reduced by mutations near the intracellular end of the M2 region. *J. Gen. Physiol.* 99:545–72

115. (a) Dani JA. 1989. Open channel structure and ion binding sites of the nicotinic acetylcholine receptor channel. *J. Neurosci.* 9:884–92

116. Imoto K, Busch C, Sakmann B, Mishina M, Konno T, et al. 1988. Rings of negatively charged amino acids determine the acetylcholine receptor channel conductance. *Nature* 335:645–48

117. Bertrand D, Galzi JL, Devillers-Thiéry A, Bertrand S, Changeux JP. 1993. Mutations at two distinct sites within the channel domain M2 alter calcium permeability of neuronal alpha7 nicotinic receptor. *Proc. Natl. Acad. Sci. USA* 90:6971–75

118. Galzi JL, Devillers-Thiéry A, Hussy N, Bertrand S, Changeux JP, Bertrand D. 1992. Mutations in the ion channel domain of a neuronal nicotinic receptor convert ion selectivity from cationic to anionic. *Nature* 359:500–5

119. Corringer PJ, Bertrand S, Galzi JL, Devillers-Thiéry A, Changeux JP, Bertrand D. 1999. Mutational analysis of the charge selectivity filter of the alpha7 nicotinic acetylcholine receptor. *Neuron* 22:831–43

120. Wang CT, Zhang HG, Rocheleau TA, ffrench-Constant RH, Jackson MB. 1999. Cation permeability and cation-anion interactions in a mutant GABA-gated chloride channel from *Drosophila*. *Biophys. J.* 77:691–700

121. Armstrong CM, Hille B. 1998. Voltage-gated ion channels and electrical excitability. *Neuron* 20:371–80

122. Doyle DA, Cabral JM, Pfuetzner RA, Kuo A, Gulbis JM, et al. 1998. The structure of the potassium channel: molecular basis of K + conduction and selectivity. *Science* 280:69–77

123. Heinemann SH, Terlau H, Stuhmer W, Imoto K, Numa S. 1992. Calcium channel characteristics conferred on the sodium channel by single mutations. *Nature* 356:441–43

124. Opella SJ, Marassi FM, Gesell JJ, Valente AP, Kim Y, et al. 1999. Structures of the M2 channel-lining segments from nicotinic acetylcholine and NMDA receptors by NMR spectroscopy. *Nat. Struct. Biol.* 6:374–79

125. Adcock C, Smith GR, Sansom MS.P. 1998. Electrostatics and the ion selectivity of ligand gated channels. *Biophys. J.* 75:1211–22

126. Tikhonov DB, Zhorov BS. 1998. Kinked-helices model of the nicotinic acetylcholine receptor ion channel and its complexes with blockers: simulation by the Monte Carlo minimization method. *Biophys. J.* 74:242–55

127. Ortells MO, Barrantes GE, Wood C, Lunt GG, Barrantes FJ. 1997. Molecular modeling of the nicotinic acetylcholine recep-

tor transmembrane region in the open state. *Protein Eng.* 10:511–17

128. Chang G, Spencer RH, Lee AT, Barclay MT, Rees DC. 1998. Structure of the MscL homolog from *Mycobacterium tuberculosis:* a gated mechanosensitive ion channel. *Science* 282:2220–26

129. Lindqvist Y, Schneider G. 1997. Circular permutations of natural protein sequences: structural evidence. *Curr. Opin. Struct. Biol.* 7:422–27

130. Herz JM, Johnson DA, Taylor P. 1989. Distance between the agonist and non-competitive inhibitor sites on the nicotinic acetylcholine receptor. *J. Biol. Chem.* 264:12439–48

131. Heidmann T, Changeux JP. 1980. Interaction of a fluorescent agonist with the membrane-bound acetylcholine receptor from *Torpedo marmorata* in the millisecond time range: resolution of an "intermediate" conformational transition and evidence for positive cooperative effects. *Biochem. Biophys. Res. Commun.* 97:889–96

132. Neubig RR, Cohen JB. 1980. Permeability control by cholinergic receptors in *Torpedo* post-synaptic membranes: agonist dose response relations measured at second and millisecond times. *Biochemistry* 19:2770–79

133. Colquhoun D, Sakmann B. 1985. Fast events in single-channel currents activated by acetylcholine and its analogues at the frog muscle endplate. *J. Physiol.* 369:501–7

134. Edelstein SJ, Schaad O, Henry E, Bertrand D, Changeux JP. 1996. A kinetic mechanism for nicotinic acetylcholine receptor based on multiple allosteric transitions. *Biol. Cybern.* 75:361–79

135. Changeux JP, Edelstein SJ. 1998. Allosteric receptors after 30 years. *Neuron* 21:959–80

136. Colquhoun D, Sakmann B. 1998. From muscle endplate to brain synapses: a short history of synapses and agonist-activated ion channels. *Neuron* 20:381–87

137. Perutz MF. 1989. Mechanisms of cooperativity and allosteric regulation in proteins. *Quart. Rev. Biophys.* 22:139–236

138. Brunori M. 1999. Hemoglobin is an honorary enzyme. *Trends Biochem. Sci.* 24:158–61

139. Galzi JL, Revah F, Bouet F, Ménez A, Goeldner M, et al. 1991. Allosteric transitions of the acetylcholine receptor probed at the amino acid level with a photolabile cholinergic ligand. *Proc. Natl. Acad. Sci. USA* 88:5051–55

140. Chen J, Zhang Y, Akk G, Sine S, Auerbach A. 1995. Activation kinetics of recombinant mouse nicotinic acetylcholine receptors: mutations of alpha-subunit tyrosine 190 affect both binding and gating. *Biophys. J.* 69:849–59

141. Akk G, Zhou M, Auerbach A. 1999. A mutational analysis of the acetylcholine receptor channel transmitter binding site. *Biophys. J.* 76:207–18

142. Sine SM, Ohno K, Bouzat C, Auerbach A, Milone M, et al. 1995. Mutation of the acetylcholine receptor alpha subunit causes a slow-channel myasthenic syndrome by enhancing agonist binding affinity. *Neuron* 15:229–39

143. Akabas MH, Kaufmann C, Archdeacon P, Karlin A. 1994. Identification of acetylcholine receptor channel-lining residues in the entire M2 segment of the alpha subunit. *Neuron* 13:919–27

144. Revah F, Bertrand D, Galzi JL, Devillers-Thiéry A, Mulle C, et al. 1991. Mutations in the channel domain alter desensitization of a neuronal nicotinic receptor. *Nature* 353:846–49

145. Bertrand D, Devillers-Thiéry A, Revah F, Galzi JL, Hussy N, et al. 1992. Unconventional pharmacology of a neuronal nicotinic receptor mutated in the channel domain. *Proc. Natl. Acad. Sci. USA* 89:1261–65

146. Devillers-Thiéry A, Galzi JL, Bertrand S, Changeux JP, Bertrand D. 1992. Strati-

fied organization of the nicotinic acetyl-choline receptor channel. *NeuroReport* 3:1001–4

147. Bertrand S, Devillers-Thiéry A, Palma E, Buisson B, Edelstein SJ, et al. 1997. Paradoxical allosteric effects of competitive inhibitors on neuronal alpha7 nicotinic receptor mutants. *NeuroReport* 8:3591–96

148. Labarca C, Nowak MW, Zhang H, Tang L, Deshpande P, Lester HA. 1995. Channel gating governed symmetrically by conserved leucine residues in the M2 domain of nicotinic receptors. *Nature* 376:514–16

149. Engel AG, Ohno K, Sine SM. 1999. Congenital myasthenic syndromes: recent advances. *Arch. Neurol.* 56:163–67

150. Léna C, Changeux JP. 1997. Pathological mutations of nicotinic receptors and nicotine-based therapies for brain disorders. *Curr. Opin. Neurobiol.* 7:674–82

151. Steinlein OK, Mulley JC, Propping P, Wallace RH, Phillips HA, et al. 1995. A missense mutation in the neuronal nicotinic acetylcholine receptor alpha 4 subunit is associated with autosomal dominant nocturnal frontal lobe epilepsy. *Nat. Genet.* 11:201–3

152. Steinlein OK, Magnusson A, Stoodt J, Bertrand S, Weiland S, et al. 1997. An insertion mutation of the CHRNA4 gene in a family with autosomal dominant nocturnal frontal lobe epilepsy. *Hum. Mol. Genet.* 6:943–47

153. Bertrand S, Weiland S, Berkovic SF, Steinlein OK, Bertrand D. 1998. Properties of neuronal nicotinic acetylcholine receptor mutants from humans suffering from autosomal dominant nocturnal frontal lobe epilepsy. *Br. J. Pharmacol.* 125:751–60

154. Kuryatov A, Gerzanich V, Nelson M, Olale F, Lindstrom J. 1997. Mutation causing autosomal dominant nocturnal frontal lobe epilepsy alters Ca2+ permeability, conductance, and gating of

human alpha4beta2 nicotinic acetylcholine receptors. *J. Neurosci.* 17:9035–47

155. Lee YH, Li L, Lasalde J, Rojas L, McNamee M, et al. 1994. Mutations in the M4 domain of *Torpedo californica* acetylcholine receptor dramatically alter ion channel function. *Biophys. J.* 66:646–53

156. Bouzat C, Bren N, Sine SM. 1994. Structural basis of the different gating kinetics of fetal and adult acetylcholine receptors. *Neuron* 13:1395–402

157. Wang HL, Milone M, Ohno K, Shen XM, Tsujino A, et al. 1999. Acetylcholine receptor M3 domain: stereochemical and volume contributions to channel gating. *Nat. Neurosci.* 2:226–33

158. Lo DC, Pinkham JL, Stevens CF. 1991. Role of a key cysteine residue in the gating of the acetylcholine receptor. *Neuron* 6:31–40

159. England PM, Zhang Y, Dougherty DA, Lester HA. 1999. Backbone mutations in transmembrane domains of a ligand-gated ion channel: implications for the mechanism of gating. *Cell* 96:89–98

160. Campos-Caro A, Sala S, Ballesta JJ, Vicente-Agullo F, Criado M, Sala F. 1996. A single residue in the M2-M3 loop is a major determinant of coupling between binding and gating in neuronal nicotinic receptors. *Proc. Natl. Acad. Sci. USA* 93:6118–23

161. Croxen R, Newland C, Beeson D, Oosterhuis H, Chauplannaz G, et al. 1997. Mutations in different functional domains of the human muscle acetylcholine receptor alpha subunit in patients with the slow-channel congenital myasthenic syndrome. *Hum. Mol. Genet.* 6:767–74

162. Monod J, Wyman J, Changeux JP. 1965. On the nature of allosteric transitions: a plausible model. *J. Mol. Biol.* 12:88–118

163. Karlin A. 1967. On the application of "a plausible model" of allosteric proteins to the receptor for acetylcholine. *J. Theoret. Biol.* 16:306–20

164. Del Castillo J, Katz B. 1957. Interaction at endplate receptors between different choline derivatives. *Proc. R. Soc. London Ser. B* 146:369–81

165. Koshland D, Nemethy G, Filmer D. 1966. Comparison of experimental binding data and theoretical models in proteins containing subunits. *Biochemistry* 5:365–85

166. Galzi JL, Edelstein SJ, Changeux JP. 1996. The multiple phenotypes of allosteric receptor mutants. *Proc. Natl. Acad. Sci. USA* 93:1853–58

167. Alkondon M, Pereira EF, Eisenberg HM, Albuquerque EX. 1999. Choline and selective antagonists identify two subtypes of nicotinic acetylcholine receptors that modulate GABA release from CA1 interneurons in rat hippocampal slices. *J. Neurosci.* 19:2693–705

Annu. Rev. Pharmacol. Toxicol. 2000. 40:459–89

THE ROLE OF RHO IN G PROTEIN-COUPLED RECEPTOR SIGNAL TRANSDUCTION

Valerie P. Sah, Tammy M. Seasholtz, Sarah A. Sagi, and Joan Heller Brown

Department of Pharmacology, University of California, San Diego, California 92093–0636; e-mail: vtansah@ucsd.edu, tseasholtz@ucsd.edu, ssagi@ucsd.edu, and jhbrown@ucsd.edu

Key Words   RhoA, small G proteins, heterotrimeric G proteins, RhoGEF, $G_{12/13}$

■ **Abstract**   Low molecular weight G proteins of the Rho subfamily are regulators of actin cytoskeletal organization. In contrast to the heterotrimeric G proteins, the small GTPases are not directly activated through ligand binding to G protein–coupled receptors (GPCRs). However, a subset of GPCRs, including those for lysophosphatidic acid and thrombin, induce stress fibers, focal adhesions, and cell rounding through Rho-dependent pathways. C3 exoenzyme has been a useful tool for demonstrating Rho involvement in these and other responses, including Ca^{2+} sensitization of smooth muscle contraction, cell migration, transformation, and serum response element–mediated gene expression. Most of the GPCRs that induce Rho-dependent responses can activate G_q, but this is not a sufficient signal. Recent data demonstrate that $G\alpha_{12/13}$ can induce Rho-dependent responses. Furthermore, $G\alpha_{12/13}$ can bind and activate Rho-specific guanine nucleotide exchange factors, providing a mechanism by which GPCRs that couple to $G\alpha_{12/13}$ could activate Rho and its downstream responses.

INTRODUCTION

Low molecular weight G proteins are well recognized as mediators of cell growth and actin cytoskeletal rearrangement in mammalian cells. The discovery that extracellular stimuli regulate these proteins suggested their role in signal transduction pathways. Studies in the early 1990s focused on the Ras family proteins and delineated the steps leading to Ras and mitogen-activated protein (MAP) kinase activation by receptor tyrosine kinases. G protein–coupled receptors (GPCRs) were also demonstrated to activate Ras and MAP kinase cascades, albeit with relatively low efficacy compared with receptor tyrosine kinases. Although interest in small G proteins of the Rho family was limited, a role for Rho in signal transduction had also been discovered in the early 1990s. This was demonstrated not through the effects of tyrosine kinase growth factors, but rather through the remarkable effects of the GPCR agonists lysophosphatidic acid (LPA), thrombin, bombesin, and endothelin on cell morphology and tyrosine phosphorylation. The

0362–1642/00/0415–0459$14.00

concept that Rho proteins are mediators of responses to certain GPCRs has now become well recognized and is the subject of this and a previous review (1).

PROPERTIES AND REGULATORS OF RHO FAMILY PROTEINS

Rho Family Proteins

The first Rho family protein was identified as a Ras homolog in the sea snail *Aplysia* (2). Currently at least 14 distinct Rho family proteins ranging from 20–25 kDa have been identified. These can be broadly divided into subfamilies (Rac, Cdc42, Rnd, and Rho) based on amino acid sequence identities and cellular functions (reviewed in 3, 4). The members of the Rho subfamily, RhoA, RhoB, and RhoC, share >85% homology. Differences in their lipid modification have been proposed to influence their interaction with regulators and their subcellular localization (5). RhoA is the best-characterized member of the Rho family of low molecular weight GTPases. Most studies examining cellular responses to Rho have utilized transiently expressed or microinjected RhoA protein or cDNA expression plasmid. On the other hand, studies implicating Rho in cellular responses through the use of inhibitors such as C3 exoenzyme, dominant negative Rho, guanine nucleotide dissociation inhibitors (GDIs), or mutant guanine nucleotide exchange factors (GEFs) do not target specific Rho subfamily members (RhoA vs RhoB vs RhoC). Thus, although it is assumed that it is RhoA that regulates the pathways discussed in this review, the more general terminology Rho is used.

Studies investigating the involvement of Rho in various cellular responses have been facilitated by the generation of mutant proteins that interfere with or enhance Rho function. G proteins cycle between an inactive GDP-bound state and an active GTP-bound state. Studies of Ras identified several critical amino acids that modulate the GTP-bound state. Analogous mutations were made in RhoA. Mutation of Ser[19] to Asn[19] results in a protein with increased affinity for GEFs. Hence, by competing for required activators, these proteins serve as dominant negative inhibitors of endogenous Rho activation. Dominant negative Rho proteins have been widely used to block Rho-dependent responses (see, for example, 6–8) but have been noted to be unstable (P Chardin, personal communication). Conversely, mutation of Gly[14] to Val[14] or of Gln[63] to Leu[63] on RhoA renders the protein GTPase deficient and thus constitutively GTP-bound and active.

RhoGAPs, GEFs, and GDIs

In vivo, the activation of Rho is regulated by GTPase activating proteins (GAPs), GEFs, and GDIs and can be modulated by bacterial toxins. GAPs regulate the inactivation of small G proteins by accelerating their intrinsic GTPase activity.

Protein tyrosine phosphatase PTPL1-associated RhoGAP (PARG1) has been shown to have GAP activity for Rho family GTPases, with a preference for Rho (10). Other Rho-specific GAPs include Graf (11, 12), p190RhoGAP (13), and p122RhoGAP (15). Graf and p190RhoGAP have been demonstrated to localize to the actin cytoskeleton, providing a possible mechanism for rapid termination of Rho-mediated cytoskeletal rearrangements. Graf is ubiquitously expressed and can be phosphorylated by MAP kinase (11). The p190RhoGAP is tyrosine phosphorylated in response to activation of c-Src, resulting in enhanced RhoGAP activity and actin disorganization (13, 14). The p122RhoGAP, when transiently transfected or microinjected into Swiss 3T3 cells, inhibits LPA-stimulated, Rho-dependent stress fiber formation (15). The concept that the activity and localization of GAPs may be regulated makes them potential targets in the control of responses to GPCRs.

RhoGEFs catalyze the exchange of GDP for GTP and thereby activate Rho. The proteins in this family contain a number of well-characterized domains. The dbl homology (DH) domain, named for Dbl the first identified Rho family GEF (16), and an adjacent pleckstrin homology (PH) domain are common to all Rho GEFs. The DH domain possesses the nucleotide exchange activity, and the PH domain contributes to this as well as to the cellular localization of the GEF. Microinjection or expression of RhoGEFs has been shown to induce changes in cell shape, gene expression, DNA synthesis, and cell transformation (17–20). Conversely, mutant forms of RhoGEFs lacking DH domains have been used as inhibitors of GPCR responses requiring Rho function (17–19).

Many of the RhoGEFs were first identified as oncogenes in DNA isolated from malignant cells. Dbl stimulates guanine nucleotide exchange on both Cdc42 and RhoA (16). Other Rho-specific GEFs isolated as oncogenes include Lbc (20), Lfc (21), and Lsc (22). RIP2 is a putative RhoGEF isolated as a Rho-interacting protein (RIP) using the yeast two-hybrid system (23). In addition to DH and PH domains, RIP2 contains a leucine-rich motif and a zinc-finger–like motif similar to those present in Lfc. These domains could contribute to protein or DNA binding. The p115RhoGEF (24) also contains regulatory sites in addition to DH and PH domains. This GEF has an N-terminal domain similar to that found in regulators of G protein signaling (RGS) proteins and has been shown to catalyze GTPase-stimulated inactivation of $G\alpha_{12/13}$ proteins (25). Another GEF was named PDZ-RhoGEF based on inclusion of an N-terminal PDZ domain (17). It is the lsc homology (LH) domain that is of greater potential interest for GPCR signaling, however, because this domain (which shows limited sequence similarity to RGS14) is required for binding of PDZ-RhoGEF to $G\alpha_{12}$ and $G\alpha_{13}$. The RGS and related LH domains in RhoGEFs may provide negative feedback at the level of $G\alpha$ subunits for GPCR-mediated responses. Another group of RhoGEFs, including Trio (26) and Duet (27), possess serine/threonine kinase activity. Thus, RhoGEFs may regulate responses other than the activation of small G proteins.

GDIs bind Rho family GTPases, targeting the major fraction of Rho to the cytosol in unstimulated cells (for reviews, see 28, 29). Binding of Rho to

RhoGDIs inhibits guanine nucleotide exchange and activation of the Rho GTPases. The ubiquitously expressed RhoGDI as well as GDI/D4, expressed only in hematopoietic cells, inhibit nucleotide exchange on all the Rho family proteins (RhoA, Rac and Cdc42). On the other hand, the homologous protein RhoGDIγ, which is preferentially expressed in brain and pancreas, only binds Rho and Cdc42 (29a). The RhoGDIs have been shown to inhibit various Rho-dependent functions, such as cell spreading and stress fiber formation in baby hamster kidney cells (29a), exocytosis in mast cells (30), and activation of phospholipase D (PLD) in response to GTPγS in plasma membranes from rat liver (31). Although GDIs show little relative specificity for particular Rho family members, they possess several protein domains subject to modification by serine-threonine kinases, which suggests their potential for regulation (for a review, see 29).

Bacterial Toxins

A number of bacterial toxins that inactivate Rho have been identified (reviewed in 32). The clostridial cytotoxins *Clostridium difficile* toxin A and toxin B inactivate all Rho family proteins by glucosylating the nucleotide binding site. Another family of Rho-inactivating enzymes consists of ADP-ribosyltransferases, including the *Clostridium botulinum* C3 exoenzyme, the *Clostridium limosum* transferase, and the *Staphylococcus aureus* transferase epidermal differentiation inhibitor. These toxins show greater specificity than those of the *C. difficile* family for Rho subfamily proteins (RhoA, RhoB, and RhoC). Although Rac was originally identified as a substrate for C3 exoenzyme (33), it has been demonstrated that C3-catalyzed ribosylation of RhoA is at least 100–400 times more efficient than that of Rac or Cdc42 (34). Thus, C3 can specifically target the Rho subfamily although they do not distinguish between RhoA, RhoB, or RhoC.

C3 exoenzyme irreversibly ADP-ribosylates Rho at Asn[41] located in the effector region. Mutation of this residue to Ile[41] prevents ribosylation by C3 (35). The exact mechanism by which ADP-ribosylation confers loss of Rho function and inhibition of Rho-mediated responses is unclear. One hypothesis is that ribosylation renders Rho unstable. Indeed, several studies have noted a substantial loss of Rho protein following C3 treatment (36, 37, 37a). Another possibility is that ribosylation alters RhoA localization. This is supported by a recent study demonstrating that GTPγS treatment increases RhoA localization in caveolar membranes, and that C3 pretreatment leads to a loss of RhoA from this compartment (38). Likewise, localization of RhoA in caveolae has been associated with cytoskeletal reorganization in astrocytes stimulated with endothelin-1 (38a).

The purified C3 exoenzyme possesses no cell surface binding or translocation components, thus various modes of achieving C3 expression and Rho blockade in intact cells have been devised. One strategy is to express the C3 cDNA by plasmid transfection (39) or Sindbis viral infection (37). Alternatively, purified recombinant C3 exoenzyme has been introduced into the cells by scrape-loading

(36), permeabilization (40), osmotic shock (41), or electroporation (42). A hybrid toxin consisting of the cell-binding and translocation subunit of the diphtheria toxin fused to C3 exoenzyme has also been used (43). The most common approaches have been either microinjection or prolonged incubation of cells with purified C3, which results in passive uptake (see, for example, 34, 35, 77, 83).

Measurement of Rho Activation

There is a substantial body of work utilizing tools such as C3 exoenzyme and dominant negative Rho to support the involvement of Rho in GPCR-mediated responses. In contrast, relatively few studies have directly examined the ability of GPCRs to activate Rho. As previously mentioned, the major cellular fraction of Rho is cytosolic, and upon stimulation by either guanine nucleotide or GPCR agonist, the amount of Rho associated with the membrane fraction is increased while cytosolic Rho is decreased. This phenomenon has been exploited in order to measure activation of Rho in response to LPA or endothelin in Swiss 3T3 fibroblasts (44), thrombin in astrocytoma and vascular smooth muscle cells (45, 46), and angiotensin II in cardiac myocytes (47). Increases in membrane-associated Rho have also been detected in response to GTPγS or GTP plus phenylephrine in permeabilized blood vessels (48), and decreases in cytosolic Rho have been described following addition of carbachol to permeabilized GTPγS-stimulated HEK cells (49).

Activation of Rho based on increased GTP binding has been more difficult to demonstrate, but a few groups have reported increased binding of radiolabeled guanine nucleotides to Rho following GPCR stimulation. Formylmethionylleu-cylphenylalanine (fMLP) increased both [^{32}P]GTP- and [^{32}P]GDP-bound Rho in leukocytes (50, 51). [^{35}S]GTPγS binding to Rho was increased in response to fMLP in leukocytes and in response to thrombin in rat aortic smooth muscle cells (46, 51). α_2-Adrenergic receptor stimulation increased [^{32}P]GTP binding to Rho and decreased [^{32}P]GDP-Rho binding in preadipocytes (52). Expression of various constitutively activated Gα subunits of heterotrimeric G proteins in COS-7 cells has also been shown to increase Rho-[^{32}P]GTP binding (53).

Recent studies have used Rho binding proteins in pull-down assays to measure Rho activation (54, 55). This method is based on the enhanced ability of activated (GTP bound vs GDP bound) Rho to bind the Rho binding domain (RBD) of Rho effectors. GST-fusion proteins of the RBDs of Rho kinase (54) and rhotekin (55) have been generated and used to affinity precipitate activated Rho. Using this assay, stimulation of COS-7 or Swiss 3T3 cells with LPA was shown to increase the amount of activated Rho (54, 55). Expression of activated $G\alpha_{12}$ or $G\alpha_{13}$ in COS-7 cells also resulted in increased Rho-RBD binding (54). The development of these apparently more sensitive Rho-RBD assays should expedite the elucidation of the molecular mechanisms involved in Rho activation in response to GPCR stimulation.

RHO-MEDIATED CELLULAR RESPONSES

Effectors of Rho

A large number of Rho-binding proteins have been identified by gel overlay, yeast two-hybrid screening, and related approaches (reviewed in 56, 57). Among the many Rho effectors identified, the serine/threonine-directed Rho kinases (Rho kinase/ROKα/ROCK-II and p160ROCK/ROCKβ, hereafter generically referred to as Rho kinase) are the best characterized (58–61).

Dominant negative mutants of Rho kinase have been utilized to demonstrate a requirement for Rho kinase in various cellular responses (see, for example, 58, 62–64, 98). Studies assessing the involvement of Rho kinase in cellular responses have been facilitated by the development of a selective inhibitor, Y27632 (65). Y27632 acts as a competitive inhibitor of ATP binding and has been shown to be ~200 times more selective for inhibiting Rho kinase than protein kinase C (PKC), cAMP-dependent protein kinase, and myosin light chain (MLC) kinase (65). In addition, effector mutants of RhoA that are unable to interact with Rho kinase have been generated (66, 67). Experiments using the aforementioned tools confirm a requirement for Rho kinase in the regulation of stress fibers, focal adhesions and cell transformation.

Much less is known about the specific functions of another group of Rho effectors that are PKC–related serine/threonine kinases (PKN/PRK1 and PRK2) (68–70). PKN has been demonstrated to be phosphorylated in a C3-sensitive manner on stimulation of Swiss 3T3 cells with LPA (69). PRK2 has been shown to cooperate with RhoA to induce serum response factor (SRF)-dependent transcriptional activation (70). However, studies with RhoA effector domain mutants indicate that RhoA-mediated stress fiber formation, SRF activation, and transformation can occur in the absence of RhoA-PKN interactions (66). Other Rho effectors include citron kinase, which regulates cytokinesis (71), p140mDia, which regulates actin reorganization (72), and rhophilin and rhotekin (68, 73), the functions of which remain unknown.

Cytoskeletal Responses

Pioneering work by several independent laboratories in the early 1990s established a direct role for Rho in the regulation of the actin cytoskeleton. Elegant microinjection experiments (34, 35) demonstrated that a constitutively active RhoA mutant stimulated actin stress fiber formation and focal adhesion complex assembly in serum-starved Swiss 3T3 cells, whereas inactivation of Rho prevented these serum-induced cytoskeletal responses. The factor in serum that was responsible for these cytoskeletal effects was later identified as LPA (34), an agonist that is now known to act through a GPCR (74). Other GPCR agonists, including endothelin and bombesin, were subsequently shown to elicit stress fiber formation and focal adhesion complex assembly in a Rho-dependent manner (75,

76). A distinct but related Rho-dependent cytoskeletal response characterized by process retraction and cell rounding is observed in neuronal and astroglial cells stimulated by GPCR agonists such as LPA and thrombin (77–79).

Studies by Rozengurt and coworkers (80–82) demonstrated that stimulation of GPCRs also led to rapid tyrosine phosphorylation of the cytoskeleton-associated proteins, p125 focal adhesion kinase (FAK) and paxillin, and to their clustering at focal adhesions. Agonist- or GTPγS-induced tyrosine phosphorylation of these proteins was not dependent on PKC activation or Ca^{2+} mobilization but was inhibited by C3 exoenzyme (75, 80–84), implicating Rho as a mediator of these responses. It is interesting to note that cytochalasin D, which disrupts the actin filament network, prevented tyrosine phosphorylation of FAK and paxillin in response to GPCR activation. This finding suggests that the response is dependent on the integrity of the actin cytoskeleton (80–82). Tyrosine phosphorylation of FAK and paxillin results in the creation of binding sites for other proteins, e.g. Src family kinases and phosphatidylinositol 3-kinase (PI(3)K), facilitating their recruitment to focal adhesion complexes for structural or signaling functions (85, 86). However, it is not yet clear how the phosphorylation of FAK and paxillin and recruitment of structural and signaling molecules to focal adhesion plaques contribute to downstream Rho-dependent responses.

The basis for the involvement of the actin cytoskeleton in focal adhesion formation and associated tyrosine phosphorylation is suggested by the work of Chrzanowska-Wodnicka & Burridge (87). They demonstrated that stimulation of fibroblasts with LPA increased MLC phosphorylation with a time course preceding that for the detection of tyrosine phosphorylation, stress fibers, and focal adhesions. Pharmacological inhibition of MLC kinase activity with KT5926 prevented the formation of stress fibers and focal adhesions (87), which suggests a role for contractile responses mediated through MLC phosphorylation.

Recent studies have shown that Rho and Rho kinase regulate MLC phosphorylation. Rho kinase phosphorylates the myosin-binding subunit of MLC phosphatase, rendering the phosphatase inactive and thus preventing MLC dephosphorylation (88, 89). In addition, Rho kinase has been reported to directly phosphorylate MLC in vitro (89). Together, these events result in an accumulation of phosphorylated MLC that promotes actin-myosin interaction. Considerable evidence indicates that Rho kinase mediates LPA-, thrombin-, and RhoA-induced actin stress fibers, focal adhesion complexes, endothelial cell contractility, and cell rounding through its effect on MLC phosphorylation (63, 78, 90–93). Thrombin-induced cell rounding and MLC phosphorylation in 1321N1 astrocytoma cells are C3-sensitive and prevented by Y27632 (19, 78). In N1E-115 cells, expression of activated Rho kinase was shown to promote MLC phosphorylation and neurite retraction, and dominant negative Rho kinase blocked both of these responses. In addition, a mutant MLC (T18D, S19D) that mimics the phosphorylated state of myosin also induced neurite retraction (91).

Although numerous studies suggest an association between MLC phosphorylation and cytoskeletal reorganization (42, 78, 87, 90–93), some caution in interpretation is warranted. The MLC kinase inhibitor KT5926 was recently shown to inhibit PKC (42). Additionally, KT5926 completely inhibits astrocytoma cell rounding at concentrations that only partially blocked MLC phosphorylation (78). These observations suggest some dissociation between MLC phosphorylation and the cytoskeletal response. Other mechanisms by which Rho and Rho kinase could mediate actin cytoskeletal responses must therefore be considered. LPA has been demonstrated to phosphorylate ezrin/radixin/moesin (ERM) proteins in a Rho-dependent manner (94). Furthermore, phosphorylation of ERM proteins is regulated by Rho kinase and the myosin-binding subunit of myosin phosphatase (94, 95). ERM phosphorylation regulates the ability of these proteins to cross-link the plasma membrane and actin filaments. Additionally, Maekawa et al recently identified LIM kinase as a Rho kinase target involved in stress fiber formation in HeLa cells (96). These investigators reported that LIM kinase is phosphorylated and activated by Rho kinase, resulting in phosphorylation of cofilin, an actin depolymerizing protein. Phosphorylation of cofilin has been demonstrated to suppress its activity, thus contributing to actin cytoskeletal reorganization. Although neither LIM kinase nor ERM proteins has been demonstrated to be involved in GPCR signaling to the cytoskeleton, investigations into the role of these proteins are likely to be forthcoming.

Stress fiber formation in fibroblasts has also been suggested to occur via activation of the ubiquitously expressed Na^+-H^+ exchanger NHE1 (97), which regulates intracellular pH homeostasis and is associated with cellular growth responses. Barber's laboratory demonstrated that the induction of stress fibers by LPA and activated RhoA was abolished in NHE1-deficient cells and also by treatment with ethylisopropylamiloride, a pharmacological inhibitor of NHE1 (97). LPA-stimulated phosphorylation and activation of NHE1 in vivo was inhibited by a catalytically inactive Rho kinase or pretreatment of the cells with Y27632, which suggests that Rho kinase mediates LPA- and RhoA-induced NHE1 activity (98).

Phospholipid Metabolism

A number of phospholipid metabolizing enzymes appear to be regulated through Rho-dependent pathways. PI(3)K is an enzyme known to signal responses from receptor tyrosine kinases and to regulate the actin cytoskeleton (reviewed in 99). GPCRs including the thrombin receptor in platelets and the LPA receptor in Swiss 3T3 cells have been shown to activate PI(3)K, and studies using C3 exoenzyme indicate that this requires Rho function (83, 100). The isoform of PI(3)K regulated by Rho in platelets is the p85/p110 heterodimer. In contrast, the p110 catalytic subunit, PI(3)Kγ, which is regulated by GPCRs and controlled through Gβγ subunits, is not Rho-dependent (101). The products of PI(3)K, $PI(3,4)P_2$, and $PI(3,4,5)P_3$ function in the regulation of downstream effectors such as Akt/PKB (99), thus alterations in PI(3)K activity could contribute to Rho-mediated apoptosis (see below).

Phosphatidylinositol-4-phosphate 5-kinase (PIP5K), another Rho-activated phosphoinositide kinase, has been shown to interact with both GTP- and GDP-bound recombinant Rho (102). GTP-bound Rho and GTPγS increase PIP5K activity, and this is inhibited by C3 exoenzyme (103). PIP5K catalyzes the resynthesis of $PI(4,5)P_2$, the substrate for phospholipase C (PLC). Because cellular $PI(4,5)P_2$ levels are limited, $PI(4,5)P_2$ resynthesis is required to prevent depletion of hormonally regulated stores of this lipid. Accordingly, C3 treatment was shown to attenuate Ca^{2+} mobilization by PLC-coupled receptors (103). Similar conclusions were reached in studies examining $PI(4,5)P_2$ levels and inositol phosphate formation in N1E-115 cells (104). In these cells, inositol phosphate formation induced by bradykinin and LPA was inhibited by pretreatment with C3 exoenzyme and *C. difficile* toxin B. This was associated with a marked reduction in total cellular $PI(4,5)P_2$ levels in the absence of diminished PLC catalytic activity (104). Thus Rho-dependent pathways can regulate the supply of $PI(4,5)P_2$ needed to sustain Ca^{2+} mobilization and presumably PKC signaling by PLC-coupled receptors.

Changes in $PI(4,5)P_2$ levels could also contribute to control of the actin cytoskeleton. $PI(4,5)P_2$ associates with actin binding proteins such as profilin and gelsolin, uncaps the barbed ends of actin filaments, and promotes actin polymerization. Microinjection of $PI(4,5)P_2$ antibodies inhibits assembly of stress fibers and focal adhesions (105). Conversely, when PIP5K was microinjected into COS-7 cells, actin polymerization was induced (106). The delta isoform of PLC is also regulated by $PI(4,5)P_2$, and both Rho and p122RhoGAP have been suggested to directly modulate $PLC\delta_1$ activity (15, 107).

Stimulation of the LPA, endothelin, m_3 muscarinic, bradykinin, sphingosine 1-phosphate, and α_2-adrenergic GPCRs leads to Rho-dependent PLD activation (36, 37, 40, 108, 109). A GTPase-deficient $G\alpha_{13}$ mutant also stimulated PLD activity in a C3-sensitive manner (110). The Rho-dependent stimulation of PLD by the m_3 mAChR was inhibited by Rho kinase mutants and a Rho kinase inhibitor, HA-1077, which suggests that this response is mediated through Rho kinase-dependent phosphorylation (111). How Rho functions in the regulation of PLD activity is still unclear. Although Rho may regulate PLD indirectly via its effect on synthesis of the PLD cofactor $PI(4,5)P_2$, several studies demonstrate a direct interaction between Rho and PLD (112, 113).

Smooth Muscle Contraction

The traditional Ca^{2+}-dependent biochemical pathway responsible for vascular smooth muscle contraction has been well characterized. Heterotrimeric G protein-linked contractile agonists that couple to G_q and/or G_i increase intracellular Ca^{2+}, and subsequently Ca^{2+}-bound calmodulin activates MLC kinase. Increases in the phosphorylation state of MLC stimulate the actinomyosin ATPase, resulting in cross bridge cycling and contraction. A mechanism for Rho involvement in GPCR stimulation of vascular contraction has been more recently elucidated. Initial studies revealed that in permeabilized blood vessels, where Ca^{2+} concentrations can be maintained constant, nonhydrolyzable GTP analogs or GTP plus agonists elicit a contractile response (114, 115). This led to the hypothesis that a G protein(s) is involved in Ca^{2+} sensitization, i.e. contraction in the absence of increases in intracellular Ca^{2+}. The observation that C3 exoenzyme blocked agonist and guanine nucleotide-induced contraction of permeabilized vessels (116, 117) and the associated increase in MLC phosphorylation (118) led to the conclusion that Rho is responsible for Ca^{2+} sensitization. Consistent with this theory, a study by the Somlyo laboratory showed that redistribution of Rho to the plasma membrane correlated with Ca^{2+} sensitization (48).

The mechanism for this Rho-dependent response has been elucidated. As described previously, activation of Rho kinase leads to accumulation of phosphorylated MLC (88). Addition of the catalytic subunit of Rho kinase to permeabilized vessels results in contraction (120) whereas Y27632 inhibits contraction induced by phenylephrine or GTPγS (65). These data provide evidence that Rho kinase is the effector that mediates Ca^{2+} sensitization. Recently, Rho kinase-mediated Ca^{2+} sensitization has been implicated in the pathophysiology of hypertension. Narumiya's laboratory has shown that acute administration of Y27632 reduces blood pressure in three forms of experimental hypertension (65). This observation along with the previously observed increase in serotonin-stimulated Ca^{2+} sensitization in permeabilized vessels from hypertensive rats suggests that Ca^{2+} sensitization may be enhanced in hypertension (121). Studies performed in our laboratory reveal a role for Rho and Rho kinase as mediators of thrombin-stimulated vascular smooth muscle cell DNA synthesis and migration (46), two responses thought to be enhanced in experimental hypertension and possibly involved in the pathophysiology of atherosclerosis, restenosis, and graft rejection.

Cell Migration and Tumor Cell Invasion

Cell migration is required for physiological processes such as embryonic development, wound healing, and inflammation as well as for pathophysiological responses such as atherosclerosis and metastasis of cancer cells. Recently, Rho has been established as a critical mediator of cell migration in response to a host of interventions, including stimulation of GPCRs. Migration of J82 carcinoma cells is stimulated by LPA and thrombin but not by bradykinin, bombesin, and histamine, other G_q-coupled agonists (122). Responses to both LPA and thrombin were inhibited by C3 exoenzyme. We reported that migration of vascular smooth muscle cells was likewise induced by thrombin, but not phenylephrine, in a C3-sensitive manner (46). Using Y27632, we suggested the involvement of Rho kinase in GPCR-stimulated vascular smooth muscle cell migration. Consistent with these observations, Kaibuchi's laboratory showed that microinjection of dominant negative Rho kinase inhibited migration of NRK49F cells in a wound healing assay (123). Y27632 was also shown to inhibit chemotactic peptide-(fNLPNTL) stimulated migration of human neutrophils (124).

Phosphorylation of cytoskeletal-associated proteins such as FAK, paxillin, MLC, and α-adducin have been associated with cell migration, and phosphorylated forms of both α-adducin and MLC have been observed at the leading edge of migrating cells (123, 125). Consistent with involvement of myosin phosphorylation in cell migration, microinjection of an antibody to MLC phosphorylated at Ser[19] (the site of phosphorylation by Rho kinase and MLCK) inhibited fNLPNTL-stimulated migration of human neutrophils (124). It was further demonstrated that Rho kinase can phosphorylate α-adducin and that a mutant form of α-adducin, which cannot be phosphorylated, was able to inhibit migration of NRK49F cells (123). Therefore, Rho kinase-mediated phosphorylation of α-adducin and MLC appears to be important in regulating cell migration.

Studies investigating biochemical pathways involved in cancer cell invasion, a critical event in malignant metastasis, have also indicated a role for GPCRs and Rho. Early studies of cell invasion revealed that rat MM1 hepatoma cells could penetrate a cell monolayer in the presence of serum in vitro. It was later found that the response to serum could be fully reproduced by LPA (126). Studies using C3 exoenzyme have implicated Rho as a necessary signal transducer of LPA-stimulated cell invasion (127). In addition, expression of activated RhoA enhanced LPA-mediated MM1 cell invasion, consistent with a potential positive feedback loop involved in Rho activation (128).

MAP Kinase Activation and Gene Transcription

On activation by extracellular stimuli, the MAP kinase family of serine/threonine kinases phosphorylate transcription factors, increasing their transcriptional activity and thereby regulating gene expression. Receptor tyrosine kinases and GPCRs that activate the small G proteins Ras or Rac initiate kinase cascades leading to MAP kinase activation. The ability of Rho family proteins to activate MAP kinase cascades has also been examined. Rho alone is not sufficient to activate extracellular signal-regulated kinase (ERK) (129, 130, 130a), although it can cooperate with and enhance other stimulatory signals that lead to ERK activation (130, 131). In addition, whereas activated forms of Rac and Cdc42 are potent stimulators of c-Jun N-terminal kinase (JNK) and p38, RhoA is ineffective in the same assays (129, 130, 130a, 132, 133). Furthermore, although dominant interfering mutants of Rac and Cdc42 attenuated JNK activation, dominant negative RhoA had no effect (129, 132). A paper by Teramoto et al (134), however, reported that constitutively active RhoA, -B, or -C stimulated JNK in 293T cells (134). Paradoxically, it has also been noted that C3 stimulates JNK and p38 in Rat-1 cells, possibly due to stress activation of these kinases (37a). Although some cell type–specific effects of Rho on MAP kinases may exist, these kinases do not appear to be the primary downstream targets of Rho activation.

A role for Rho in transcriptional regulation was first demonstrated by Hill et al (39). Their work established that activated RhoA stimulates gene expression through the c-fos serum response element (SRE). SRE sites are regulated by serum response factor (SRF) acting in conjunction with ternary complex factor. Hill et al showed that RhoA stimulated the transcriptional activity of several mutants of the c-fos SRE including one (SRE.L) that has a high affinity-binding site for SRF but does not bind ternary complex factor. A variety of GPCRs stimulate transcription from the SRE.L, and these responses are largely inhibited by C3 exoenzyme or dominant negative RhoA (6, 8, 39).

Constitutively active mutants of the Rho effectors, Rho kinase and PRK2 have been shown to weakly activate SRE-mediated gene expression (66, 70, 135). Studies utilizing mutant constructs of activated RhoA identified three residues in the effector loop that are vital for activating SRF-mediated gene expression (136). However, the loss of SRF activation could not be correlated with the loss of binding of Rho to any known effector (66). It is interesting to note that these effector loop mutants were able to dissociate the ability of RhoA to induce SRF and to induce stress fibers, indicating that different effectors (or different combinations of effectors) mediate these two responses (66). Y27632 failed to block c-fos SRE activation, further indicating that SRF activation is not dependent on Rho kinase activity (137).

Nuclear factor (NF) κB plays a key role in immune function, inflammation, and lymphoid differentiation. GPCR agonists such as bradykinin and LPA have been demonstrated to regulate NFκB transcriptional activation (138–140). Activation of an NFκB reporter gene by bradykinin was inhibited by dominant negative RhoA or C3 exoenzyme and mimicked by constitutively active RhoA (9). A possible mechanism by which RhoA mediates NFκB activation is by enhancing the phosphorylation of IκBα, which leads to IκBα degradation and the subsequent nuclear translocation of NFκB. Montaner et al (141) found that a nonphosphorylatable mutant of IκBα prevented NFκB activation by Rho. Of particular note, the ability of Rho and Rho-specific GEFs to stimulate the SRE.L was also inhibited, which suggests that NFκB- and SRE-mediated gene expression might be interdependent.

Some recent reports have shown an involvement of Rho in AP-1–mediated transcription. Chang et al (142) reported that activated RhoA potentiated phorbol ester-induced AP-1–mediated gene expression in T cells, which suggests that RhoA- and PKC-mediated pathways interact. This was suggested to occur through the binding of RhoA to PKCα, because expression of the N terminus of PKCα prevented this effect of Rho (142). Studies from our lab also suggest the involvement of Rho in thrombin-induced AP-1 activation (SA Sagi, S Schubbert & JH Brown, unpublished observations). Expression of N19RhoA inhibited thrombin-induced AP-1–luciferase expression in 1321N1 astrocytoma cells, whereas activated RhoA or a RhoGEF (Lbc) mimicked the effect of thrombin. Although the full extent of Rho involvement in AP-1–mediated gene transcription is unknown, further investigation is warranted.

Cell Growth and Survival Responses

GPCR-induced signals can stimulate proliferative cell growth. Indeed, activation of a number of these serpentine receptors has been shown to display mitogenic effects and to have transforming potential (reviewed in 143, 144). Aberrant cell growth has also been observed with mutationally activated mutants of various G protein α subunits, including those of $G\alpha_i$, $G\alpha_q$, $G\alpha_{12}$, and $G\alpha_{13}$ (reviewed in 143). A role for Rho in regulating cell proliferation was first suggested by studies in which it was demonstrated that C3-mediated inhibition of Rho caused fibroblasts to arrest in the G_1 phase of the cell cycle (145). Inhibition of protein geranylgeranylation also results in G_0/G_1 cell cycle arrest. This arrest has been attributed to blockade of Rho function, because newly synthesized RhoA is geranylgeranylated and translocates to the membrane fraction during G_1-S progression in growth-stimulated cells (146, 147). Consistent with the observed involvement of Rho in cell cycle progression, the incorporation of the thymidine analog, bromodeoxyuridine, into nascent DNA (an indicator of G_1-S progression) was stimulated by microinjection of GTPase-deficient RhoA into quiescent fibroblasts (130a). The finding that Rho is required for serum- and Ras-induced DNA synthesis may be explained by the ability of activated Rho to stimulate the degradation of cyclin-dependent kinase inhibitors, thereby permitting G_1-S progression and DNA synthesis (147a). DNA synthesis induced by thrombin and endothelin-1 has been reported to be C3 sensitive, which suggests a role for Rho in GPCR-stimulated cell proliferation (46, 78, 148a).

Although RhoA alone displays weak transforming ability, it can strongly cooperate with the Ras-Raf pathway in focus formation (7, 148). When constitutively activated mutants of RhoA and Ras were coexpressed, a synergistic enhancement in transforming activity was observed, and a dominant negative RhoA mutant reduced oncogenic Ras-induced transformation (7, 148). Similarly, we observed that although expression of activated RhoA alone was insufficient to induce DNA synthesis, it acted synergistically with activated Ras (46). The involvement of Rho kinase in cellular transformation has been implicated through studies utilizing Y27632 and Rho effector domain mutants (66, 136, 137).

The muscle cells of the heart are terminally differentiated at birth. In response to growth-promoting signals, these cells undergo hypertrophy, a phenomenon whereby cell size is increased without increased cell number. Cardiomyocyte hypertrophy is characterized by the induction of a specific subset of genes, including that of c-fos, atrial natriuretic factor, MLC 2, and skeletal α-actin and by the organization of sarcomeric proteins into contractile units. In cultured neonatal rat cardiomyocytes, these hypertrophic responses are elicited through stimulation of receptors coupled to G_q, including the α_1-adrenergic, endothelin, prostaglandin $F_{2\alpha}$, and angiotensin II receptors. Work from our laboratory and that of others has shown that GPCR agonist-induced hypertrophic gene expression and actin myofibrillar organization are RhoA-dependent events (47, 62, 129, 149–151). Additional data suggest that RhoA is a downstream mediator of $G\alpha_q$ signaling in a pathway that acts synergistically with that activated by Ras (129, 150). Rho kinase was implicated as a mediator of hypertrophy, because inhibitory mutants of Rho kinase and Y27632 were able to attenuate the hypertrophic responses triggered by constitutively active RhoA and endothelin (62, 151).

To study the role of RhoA in regulating cardiac function in vivo, transgenic mice with cardiac-specific expression of wild-type or activated forms of RhoA were generated. It is surprising to note that these mice did not manifest cardiac hypertrophy but instead had greatly reduced survival rates due to the development of severe bradycardia, conduction system disturbances, and left ventricular contractile dysfunction (152). RhoA has been demonstrated to associate with and suppress the activity of a delayed rectifier K^+ channel Kv1.2 (153). It was suggested, therefore, that the phenotype seen in the transgenic mice could result from effects of RhoA on K^+ channel function, either directly or through changes in the actin cytoskeleton.

GPCR agonists not only elicit growth responses, they can also activate cell death. Constitutively active mutants of G protein α subunits, including those of the $G_{q/11}$ and $G_{12/13}$ families, have been shown to trigger programmed cell death (apoptosis) when heterologously expressed in COS-7 cells or cardiomyocytes (154–156). Although constitutively activated $G\alpha_q$ was shown to induce apoptosis through a PKC-dependent mechanism, $G\alpha_{13}$ did so via a RhoA-dependent pathway (154). In cardiomyocytes, a low level of $G\alpha_q$ promoted cell growth whereas excessive activation induced apoptosis (156). Similarly, in neuronal and astroglial cells, the GPCR agonist thrombin is neuroprotective at moderate concentrations (157), but at higher concentrations, it induces apoptosis (45). The ability of thrombin to protect from hypoglycemia and induce apoptosis was attenuated by C3 exoenzyme treatment, suggesting that Rho can participate in both cell protection and cell death (45, 158).

Several mechanisms through which GPCRs regulate cell survival and apoptosis have been proposed. For example, it has been shown that m_1 and m_2 muscarinic receptor stimulation can lead to phosphorylation and activation of a serine/threonine protein kinase Akt/PKB (159). Akt/PKB is regulated through PI(3)K and synthesis of PI(3,4)P$_2$ and PI(3,4,5)P$_3$ (99). Thus, it is possible that GPCRs utilize Rho to regulate this cell survival pathway. Rho activation has also been reported to regulate dynamic membrane blebbing (a process that may be mediated by MLC phosphorylation) during the final stages of apoptotic cell death (160). The Rho effector PKN is another possible mediator of apoptosis, because it is proteolytically cleaved by caspases to generate a constitutively activated kinase fragment (161). However, there is as yet no direct evidence implicating specific signaling molecules or pathways downstream of Rho in the apoptotic signaling cascade.

Other Responses

In addition to the numerous Rho-dependent cellular processes described above, Rho function has also been implicated in the regulation of endocytosis, exocytosis, glucose transport, and ion channels. Internalization of m_1 and m_2 mAChRs, via clathrin-coated pit-dependent and -independent mechanisms, respectively, was inhibited by overexpression of wild-type RhoA, although Rho did not appear to be an endogenous mediator of mAChR sequestration (162). It had previously been noted that activated RhoA inhibits clathrin-coated vesicular endocytosis (163) and that Rho is a mediator of the effects of $G\beta\gamma$ on clathrin-dependent endocytosis (164). In chromaffin cells, mastoparan-mediated activation of G_o inhibits Ca^{2+}-induced disassembly of the actin network and accompanying exocytotic catecholamine secretion (165). These effects of mastoparan are inhibited by C3 exoenzyme, which suggests that the regulatory effect of G_o on exocytosis requires Rho, possibly via its effects on the actin cytoskeleton.

Glucose transport is an early cellular response to growth factors and is essential for cell proliferation. Several reports suggest a role for Rho in regulating glucose transport (166, 167). For instance, LPA-stimulated deoxyglucose uptake was shown to be inhibited by C3 exoenzyme (166). Furthermore, GTPγS-induced GLUT4 translocation and glucose transport were inhibited by C3 exoenzyme and dominant negative forms of RhoA and PKN (167). Thus, RhoA-dependent pathways appear to be required for the regulation of glucose transport.

A role for Rho in regulating ion channel function has been demonstrated by Cachero et al (153). These investigators initially showed that stimulation of the m_1 mAChR resulted in a tyrosine kinase-dependent suppression of the basal K^+ current generated by the delayed rectifier, Kv1.2 ($I_{Kv1.2}$). A yeast two-hybrid screen identified RhoA as a Kv1.2-interacting protein. Overexpression of RhoA was shown to mimic the effects of carbachol on $I_{Kv1.2}$, and this appeared to be dependent on the physical interaction between RhoA and Kv1.2. In addition, C3 exoenzyme blocked the carbachol-mediated tyrosine kinase-dependent suppression of Kv1.2 (153), demonstrating a role for RhoA in the modulation of GPCR-mediated Kv1.2 activity. These provocative data suggest the possibility that additional ion channels will be found to be regulated through Rho-dependent mechanisms.

MECHANISMS OF RHO ACTIVATION

Pertussis Toxin Sensitivity

Most of the GPCR agonists that regulate actin cytoskeletal responses, smooth muscle contraction, gene transcription, and cell growth through Rho-dependent pathways can couple to more than a single class of heterotrimeric G proteins. For example LPA and thrombin elicit cellular responses through both pertussis toxin–sensitive and –insensitive G proteins (74, 168, 169, 176). GPCR agonist-induced stress fiber formation, focal adhesion complex assembly, and cell rounding are generally pertussis toxin–insensitive (76, 78, 170–171a). Comparison of the effects of microinjected activated $G\alpha$ subunits demonstrated negligible cytoskeletal effects of $G\alpha_i$ relative to those of the pertussis toxin–insensitive G proteins $G_{q/11}$ and $G_{12/13}$ (172, 173). Furthermore, expression of activated $G\alpha_i$ in COS-7 cells produced no increase in the level of activated Rho (54). These observations indicate that $G_{i/o}$ proteins are not sufficient or necessary for GPCR-mediated activation of Rho or Rho-dependent cytoskeletal responses.

There are exceptions to this pattern, however. For example, stimulation of heterologously expressed α_2-adrenergic receptors in preadipocytes led to Rho-mediated changes in cell morphology and increases in FAK phosphorylation. These responses were shown to be sensitive to pertussis toxin but not to $G\beta\gamma$ sequestration by the βARK1 C-terminal domain and therefore appeared to be mediated through the $G\alpha_{i/o}$ subunit (52). Increases in membrane association of and $[^{32}P]GTP$ binding to Rho were also observed in response to α_2-adrenergic receptor stimulation in this system. In addition, LPA-mediated increases in membrane-associated Rho in Swiss 3T3 fibroblasts and migration of J82 carcinoma cells were pertussis toxin–sensitive (44, 122). Paradoxically, $\beta\gamma$ subunits isolated from $G_{i/o}$ were shown to bind to Rho and inhibit Rho-GTPγS binding, which suggests the opposite, i.e. a possible inhibitory effect of $G_{i/o}$ proteins on Rho (174).

Regulation by $G_{q/11}$

Most of the GPCR agonists shown to activate Rho are coupled to G_q-mediated pathways. In spite of this, considerable evidence suggests that G_q-mediated signaling pathways are not sufficient as regulators of Rho-mediated cytoskeletal and other responses. First, it is clear that not all receptors that couple to G_q and activate PLC are able to elicit Rho-dependent cytoskeletal responses, cell migration, or DNA synthesis (46, 78, 79, 122, 175, 176). For example, cell rounding is elicited by thrombin but not by carbachol in 1321N1 and N1E115 cells (78, 175), and by LPA but not bradykinin in PC12 cells (79). Second, G_q/PLC-generated second messenger pathways (Ca^{2+}, PKC) are not sufficient (76, 79) or required for cytoskeletal responses to GPCR agonists such as thrombin and LPA (78, 171a, 175). In addition, recent studies used platelets and fibroblast cell lines derived from wild-type and $G\alpha_q/G\alpha_{11}$-deficient mice to unequivocally demonstrate that activation of several receptors that can couple to $G_{q/11}$ (including those for thrombin, LPA, thromboxane A_2, and endothelin) induce shape changes even in the absence of $G\alpha_q$ and $G\alpha_{11}$ (92, 176). Consistent with this, $G\alpha_q$ antibodies only weakly inhibit the Rho-dependent effects of LPA and thrombin on the cytoskeleton (19, 53).

On the other hand, a signaling pathway dependent on Ca^{2+} and PKC leads to neurite retraction in response to expression of constitutively activated $G\alpha_q$ in PC12 cells (173). Furthermore, heterologously expressed m_1 muscarinic and metabotropic glutamate receptors induce Rho-dependent stress fiber formation in mouse fibroblasts, and this response is abolished in fibroblasts from $G\alpha_{q/11}$-deficient mice (176). This finding implies that coupling of $G_{q/11}$ to at least some GPCRs is required for the cytoskeletal response (176). Rho-dependent regulation of the SRE.L by GPCR agonists, as described above, can also be induced by expression of activated $G\alpha_q$ and through heterologously expressed m_1 mAChRs or α_1-adrenergic receptors in wild-type but not G_q-deficient cells (8, 18). Thus, heterologously expressed G_q-coupled receptors or GTPase-deficient $G\alpha_q$ can activate signaling pathways that contribute to Rho activation or its ability to elicit downstream responses, although the contribution of these pathways to endogenous signaling is not clear.

Regulation by $G_{12/13}$

Recent evidence indicates that activation of Rho and its downstream effectors is primarily mediated through G proteins of the $G_{12/13}$ family. $G_{12/13}$ proteins, isolated as oncogenes and cloned by homology to other G proteins, have been unique in their failure to regulate known $G\alpha$ effectors such as adenylyl cyclase or phospholipases (reviewed in 177). The ability of activated $G\alpha_{12/13}$ subunits to induce stress fiber formation was first demonstrated by Buhl et al in studies using 3T3 fibroblasts (172). Constitutively active forms of $G\alpha_{12}$ and $G\alpha_{13}$ have subsequently been shown to induce stress fiber and focal adhesion formation, as well as tyrosine phosphorylation of FAK and paxillin, in a Rho-dependent manner (53, 180). Both $G\alpha_{12}$ and $G\alpha_{13}$ also induce neurite retraction and cell rounding when expressed in PC12, N1E-115, or 1321N1 cells (19, 54, 173). In addition, activated $G\alpha_{12}$ and $G\alpha_{13}$ cause transcriptional activation of the SRE.L reporter in a Rho-dependent manner (6, 8, 17, 18, 181).

The ability of these constitutively active G protein α subunits to induce the aforementioned responses suggests, but does not prove, their involvement in agonist-mediated responses. This question has been addressed by microinjection of G protein C-terminal antibodies, which block receptor–G protein coupling. Experiments carried out in several laboratories demonstrate that thrombin and LPA effects on the cytoskeleton can be blocked by antibodies to $G\alpha_{12}$ and $G\alpha_{13}$ (19, 53). Both of these receptors have been shown by GTP-labeling studies to couple to $G\alpha_{12}$ and $G\alpha_{13}$ (178, 179). Specificity in receptor coupling to $G\alpha_{12}$ vs $G\alpha_{13}$ was suggested by the microinjection experiments (19, 53) and confirmed by the use of inhibitory mutants of $G\alpha_{12}$ and $G\alpha_{13}$ and by the use of $G\alpha_{13}$-deficient fibroblasts (176). The results of these studies suggest that the LPA receptor functions primarily through G_{13} and the thrombin receptor primarily acts through G_{12}.

Involvement of Tyrosine Kinases

It is interesting to note that the pathways by which G_{12} and G_{13} signal to Rho also appear distinct. Early studies had suggested that a tyrphostin A25–sensitive tyrosine kinase functioned upstream of Rho in agonist-induced cytoskeletal pathways (182). In a recent report, tyrphostin A25 was shown to inhibit $G\alpha_{13}$-induced morphological changes in PC12 cells (173), as well as LPA- and $G\alpha_{13}$-induced stress fibers and focal adhesion assembly in 3T3 cells (53), but failed to block the effects of $G\alpha_{12}$ in the same systems. In addition, tyrphostin AG1478, an epidermal growth factor (EGF) receptor-specific tyrosine kinase inhibitor, blocked cytoskeletal responses induced by $G\alpha_{13}$ and LPA but not those induced by thrombin or $G\alpha_{12}$ (53, 176). Thus, tyrosine kinases and the EGF receptor have been implicated in the $G\alpha_{13}$ but not $G\alpha_{12}$ pathways.

Two groups have now independently shown that expression of activated forms of either $G\alpha_{12}$ or $G\alpha_{13}$ in COS-7 cells increases Rho activation, as measured by increases in [^{32}P]GTP-binding to Rho (53) and increases in Rho binding to the GST-RBD of Rho kinase (54). Results of these studies also suggest that the EGF receptor tyrosine kinase is upstream of Rho, i.e. involved in the pathway by which $G\alpha_{13}$ leads to Rho-GTP loading (53). Tyrosine kinase involvement in LPA-mediated Rho activation was further substantiated by a study demonstrating inhibition of LPA-stimulated Rho-RBD binding by pretreatment with either genistein or tyrphostin 47 (54).

The EGF receptor is not the only tyrosine kinase that affects Rho activation. Nonreceptor tyrosine kinases of the Tec/Bmx family may be involved in $G\alpha_{12/13}$-induced Rho and SRE.L activation (181). Transfection of Tec into COS-7 cells was shown to increase membrane-associated Rho indicative of Rho activation. This family of tyrosine kinases was also suggested to function in response to $G\alpha_{12/13}$, because synergistic activation of the SRE.L was observed when activated $G\alpha_{13}$ and Tec or Bmx were coexpressed, and because constitutively active $G\alpha_{13}$ was shown to increase the tyrosine phosphorylation and activation of Tec. In addition, thrombin-induced SRE.L activation in $G_{q/11}$-deficient cells was shown to be inhibited by a kinase-dead mutant of Tec (181). Other recent evidence suggests that calpeptin may prevent Rho activation through inhibition not only of calpeptin, but also of membrane-associated tyrosine phosphatase activity (183, 184). Thus, it appears likely that tyrosine phosphorylation of an as-yet-unidentified signaling molecule(s) plays a key role in the control of Rho activation.

Involvement of RhoGEFs

The most exciting development concerning mechanisms by which GPCRs and $G\alpha_{12/13}$ activate Rho is the discovery that $G\alpha_{12/13}$ family proteins can interact directly with and activate RhoGEFs. Two papers describe this novel and important regulatory pathway (25, 185). The authors observed that the p115RhoGEF contained an RGS-like domain at its N terminus and demonstrated that this domain was required for binding to $G\alpha_{12}$ and $G\alpha_{13}$. Significantly, they showed that p115RhoGEF, like other RGS proteins and Gα protein effectors, served as a GAP for both $G\alpha_{12}$ and $G\alpha_{13}$. The finding of most fundamental importance, however, was that $G\alpha_{13}$ stimulated p115RhoGEF activity, providing a direct mechanism by which the $G\alpha_{13}$ protein could induce Rho activation. It is also of interest that although p115RhoGEF bound to and acted as a GAP for $G\alpha_{12}$, its activity as a GEF was not activated by $G\alpha_{12}$. This is consistent with work cited above that suggests that $G\alpha_{12}$ and $G\alpha_{13}$ activate Rho through different mechanisms. Mao et al (18) used the SRE.L reporter gene in transient transfection assays to demonstrate that $G\alpha_{13}$ synergizes with p115RhoGEF and thus presumably acts through p115RhoGEF to activate SRE.L. They further demonstrated that a mutant p115RhoGEF lacking the DH domain served as a dominant negative inhibitor of

LPA and thrombin effects on the SRE.L. These data are significant in that they implicate this or similar RhoGEFs in Rho-mediated agonist-induced gene transcription. The PDZ-RhoGEF, analyzed by Fukuhara et al (17), was also shown to bind to both $G\alpha_{12}$ and $G\alpha_{13}$. A mutant PDZ-RhoGEF with the DH and PH domains deleted blocked both $G\alpha_{12/13}$-and LPA-mediated activation of the SRE.L. Recent work from our laboratory demonstrated that $G\alpha_{12/13}$ mediate the effects of thrombin on the cytoskeleton in 1321N1 cells and that inactive forms of either p115RhoGEF or Lbc inhibit cell rounding induced by either $G\alpha_{12}$ or thrombin (19).

Although much of the work above indicates that $G\alpha_{12/13}$ can interact directly with RhoGEFs, it is likely that second messenger pathways and kinase cascades also regulate Rho activity. For instance, activation of phospholipase A_2 by Rac was shown to increase arachidonic acid and, subsequently, activation of the SRE.L reporter gene (186). This was blocked by dominant negative RhoA or a C3 expression plasmid, indicating a potential role for PLA_2 signaling in Rho activation. Activation of PI(3)K in response to serum also leads to Rho-mediated c-fos SRE activation (187). RhoGAPs can be phosphorylated by protein kinases such as Src and MAP kinase (11, 13, 14), and GDIs contain sequences for phosphorylation by casein kinase II, PKC, and cGMP-dependent protein kinase (29). Phosphorylation of RhoGEFs has not to our knowledge been described, but the RacGEF Tiam has been shown to be phosphorylated by PKC in response to LPA (187a). There is also evidence that cAMP and cAMP-dependent protein kinase can affect Rho activation. Agonist-stimulated [^{35}S]GTPγS binding to Rho was shown to be inhibited by 8-bromo-cAMP (51). In addition, cAMP-dependent protein kinase phosphorylates Rho; this has been demonstrated to be associated with increases in cytosolic Rho (188) and to inhibit the ability of Rho to alter cell morphology and bind Rho kinase (189). Thus phosphorylation of Rho or its regulators (GAPs, GDIs, or GEFs) is likely to provide additional mechanisms by which GPCRs can modulate Rho signaling pathways.

Visit the Annual Reviews home page at www.AnnualReviews.org.

LITERATURE CITED

1. Seasholtz TM, Majumdar M, Brown JH. 1999. Rho as a mediator of G protein-coupled receptor signaling. *Mol. Pharmacol.* 55:949–56

2. Madaule P, Axel R. 1985. A novel *ras*-related gene family. *Cell* 41:31–40

3. Zohn IM, Campbell SL, Khosravi-Far R, Rossman KL, Der CJ. 1998. Rho family proteins and Ras transformation: the RHOad less traveled gets congested. *Oncogene* 17:1415–38

4. Aspenstrom P. 1999. The Rho GTPases have multiple effects on the actin cytoskeleton. *Exp. Cell. Res.* 246:20–25

5. Hori Y, Kikuchi A, Isomura M, Katayama M, Miura Y, et al. 1991. Post-translational modifications of the C-terminal region of the *rho* protein are important for its interaction with membranes and the stimulatory and inhibitory GDP/GTP exchange proteins. *Oncogene* 6:515–22

6. Fromm C, Coso OA, Montaner S, Xu N, Gutkind JS. 1997. The small GTP-binding protein Rho links G protein-coupled

receptors and $G\alpha_{12}$ to the serum response element and to cellular transformation. *Proc. Natl. Acad. Sci. USA* 91:10098–103

7. Khosravi-Far R, Solski PA, Clark GJ, Kinch MS, Der CJ. 1995. Activation of Rac1, RhoA, and mitogen-activated protein kinases is required for Ras transformation. *Mol. Cell. Biol.* 15:6443–53

8. Mao J, Yuan H, Xie W, Simon MI, Wu D. 1998. Specific involvement of G proteins in regulation of serum response factor-mediated gene transcription by different receptors. *J. Biol. Chem.* 273:27118–23

9. Perona R, Montaner S, Saniger L, Sánchez-Pérez I, Bravo R, Lacal JC. 1997. Activation of the nuclear factor-κB by Rho, CDC42, and Rac-1 proteins. *Genes Dev.* 11:463–75

10. Saras J, Franzen P, Aspenstrom P, Hellman U, Gonez LJ, Heldin C-H. 1997. A novel GTPase-activating protein for Rho interacts with a PDZ domain of the protein tyrosine-phosphatase PTPL1. *J. Biol. Chem.* 272:24333–38

11. Taylor JM, Hildebrand JD, Mack CP, Cox ME, Parsons JT. 1998. Characterization of Graf, the GTPase-activating protein for Rho associated with focal adhesion kinase. Phosphorylation and possible regulation by mitogen-activated protein kinase. *J. Biol. Chem.* 273:8063–70

12. Taylor JM, Macklem M, Parsons JT. 1999. Cytoskeletal changes induced by Graf, The GTPase regulator associated with focal adhesion kinase, are mediated by Rho. *J. Cell Sci.* 112:231–42

13. Roof RW, Haskell MD, Dukes BD, Sherman N, Kinter M, Parsons SJ. 1998. Phosphotyrosine (p-Tyr)-dependent and -independent mechanisms of p190 RhoGAP-p120 RasGAP interaction: Tyr 1105 of p190, a substrate for c-Src, is the sole p-Tyr mediator of complex formation. *Mol. Cell. Biol.* 18:7052–63

14. Chang J-H, Gill S, Settleman J, Parsons SJ. 1995. c-Src regulates the simultaneous rearrangement of actin cytoskeleton, p190RhoGAP, and p120RasGAP following epidermal growth factor stimulation. *J. Cell Biol.* 130:355–68

15. Sekimata M, Kabuyama Y, Emori Y, Homma Y. 1999. Morphological changes and detachment of adherent cells induced by p122, a GTPase-activating protein for Rho. *J. Biol. Chem.* 274:17757–62

16. Hart MJ, Eva A, Zangrilli D, Aaronson SA, Evans T, et al. 1994. Cellular transformation and guanine nucleotide exchange activity are catalyzed by a common domain on the dbl oncogene product. *J. Biol. Chem.* 269:62–65

17. Fukuhara S, Murga C, Zohar M, Igishi T, Gutkind JS. 1999. A novel PDZ domain containing guanine nucleotide exchange factor links heterotrimeric G proteins to Rho. *J. Biol. Chem.* 274:5868–79

18. Mao J, Yuan H, Wu D. 1998. Guanine nucleotide exchange factor GEF115 specifically mediates activation of Rho and serum response factor by the G protein α subunit $G\alpha13$. *Proc. Natl. Acad. Sci. USA* 95:12973–76

19. Majumdar M, Seasholtz TM, Buckmaster C, Toksoz D, Brown JH. 1999. A Rho exchange factor mediates thrombin and $G\alpha_{12}$-induced cytoskeletal responses. *J. Biol. Chem.* 274:26815–21

20. Zheng Y, Olson MF, Hall A, Cerione RA, Toksoz D. 1995. Direct involvement of the small GTP-binding protein Rho in lbc oncogene function. *J. Biol. Chem.* 270:9031–34

21. Whitehead I, Kirk H, Tognon C, Trigo-Gonzalez G, Kay R. 1995. Expression cloning of lfc, a novel oncogene with structural similarities to guanine nucleotide exchange factors and to the regulatory region of protein kinase C. *J. Biol. Chem.* 270:18388–95

22. Whitehead IP, Khosravi-Far R, Kirk H, Trigo-Gonzalez G, Der CJ, Kay R. 1996. Expression cloning of lsc, a novel onco-

gene with structural similarities to the Dbl family of guanine nucleotide exchange factors. *J. Biol. Chem.* 271:18643–50

23. Gebbink MFBG, Kranenburg O, Poland M, van Horck FPG, Houssa B, Moolenaar WH. 1997. Identification of a novel, putative Rho-specific GDP/GTP exchange factor and a RhoA-binding protein: control of neuronal morphology. *J. Cell Biol.* 137:1603–13

24. Hart MJ, Sharma S, elMasry N, Qiu R-G, McCabe P, et al. 1996. Identification of a novel guanine nucleotide exchange factor for the Rho GTPase. *J. Biol. Chem.* 271:25452–58

25. Kozasa T, Jiang X, Hart MJ, Sternweis PM, Singer WD, et al. 1998. p115 RhoGEF, a GTPase activating protein for $G\alpha_{12}$ and $G\alpha_{13}$. *Science* 280:2109–11

26. Bellanger J-M, Lazaro J-B, Diriong S, Fernandez A, Lamb N, Debant A. 1998. The two guanine nucleotide exchange factor domains of Trio link the Rac1 and the RhoA pathways *in vivo*. *Oncogene* 16:147–52

27. Kawai T, Sanjo H, Akira S. 1999. Duet is a novel serine/threonine kinase with Dbl-homology (DH) and pleckstrin-homology (PH) domains. *Gene* 227:249–55

28. Sasaki T, Takai Y. 1998. The Rho small G protein family—Rho GDI system as a temporal and spatial determinant for cytoskeletal control. *Biochem. Biophys. Res. Commun.* 245:641–45

29. Olofsson B. 1999. Rho guanine dissociation inhibitors: pivotal molecules in cellular signalling. *Cell. Signal.* 11:545–54

29. (a) Adra CN, Manor D, Ko JL, Zhu S, Horiuchi T, et al. 1997. RhoGDIγ: a GDP-dissociation inhibitor for Rho proteins with preferential expression in brain and pancreas. *Proc. Natl. Acad. Sci. USA* 94:4279–84

30. Mariot P, O'Sullivan AJ, Brown AM, Tatham PER. 1996. Rho guanine nucleotide dissociation inhibitor protein (RhoGDI) inhibits exocytosis in mast cells. *EMBO J.* 15:6476–82

31. Malcolm KC, Ross AH, Qiu R-G, Symons M, Exton JH. 1994. Activation of rat liver phospholipase D by the small GTP-binding protein RhoA. *J. Biol. Chem.* 269:25951–54

32. Schmidt G, Aktories K. 1998. Bacterial cytotoxins target Rho GTPases. *Naturwissenschaften* 85:253–61

33. Didsbury J, Weber RF, Bokoch GM, Evans T, Snyderman R. 1989. *rac,* a novel *ras*-related family of proteins that are botulinum toxin substrates. *J. Biol. Chem.* 264:16378–82

34. Ridley AJ, Hall A. 1992. The small GTP-binding protein rho regulates the assembly of focal adhesions and actin stress fibers in response to growth factors. *Cell* 70:389–99

35. Paterson HF, Self AJ, Garrett MD, Just I, Aktories K, Hall A. 1990. Microinjection of recombinant $p21^{rho}$ induces rapid changes in cell morphology. *J. Cell Biol.* 111:1001–7

36. Malcolm KC, Elliott CM, Exton JH. 1996. Evidence for Rho-mediated agonist stimulation of phospholipase D in Rat1 fibroblasts. Effects of *Clostridium botulinum* C3 exoenzyme. *J. Biol. Chem.* 271:13135–39

37. Meacci E, Vasta V, Moorman JP, Bobak DA, Bruni P, et al. 1999. Effects of Rho and ADP-ribosylation factor GTPases on phospholipase D activity in intact human adenocarcinoma A549 cells. *J. Biol. Chem.* 274:18605–12

37. (a) Beltman J, Erickson JR, Martin GA, Lyons JF, Cook SJ. 1999. C3 toxin activates the stress signaling pathways, JNK and p38, but antagonizes the activation of AP-1 in Rat-1 cells. *J. Biol. Chem.* 274:3772–80

38. Michaely PA, Mineo C, Ying Y-S, Anderson RGW. 1999. Polarized distribution of endogenous Rac1 and RhoA at the cell surface. *J. Biol. Chem.* 274:21430–36

38. (a) Teixeira A, Chaverot N, Schröder C, Strosberg AD, Couraud PO, Cazaubon, S. 1999. Requirement of caveolae microdomains in extracellular signal-regulated kinase and focal adhesion kinase activation induced by endothelin-1 in primary astrocytes. *J. Neurochem.* 72:120–28

39. Hill CS, Wynne J, Treisman R. 1995. The Rho family GTPases RhoA, Rac1, and CDC42Hs regulate transcriptional activation by SRF. *Cell* 81:1159–70

40. Schmidt M, Rumenapp U, Bienek C, Keller J, von Eichel-Streiber C, Jakobs KH. 1996. Inhibition of receptor signaling to phospholipase D by *Clostridium difficile* toxin B: role of Rho proteins. *J. Biol. Chem.* 271:2422–26

41. Rubin EJ, Gill DM, Boquet P, Popoff MR. 1988. Functional modification of a 21-kilodalton G protein when ADP-ribosylated by exoenzyme C3 of *Clostridium botulinum*. *Mol. Cell. Biol.* 8:418–26

42. Strassheim D, May LG, Varker KA, Puhl HL, Phelps SH, et al. 1999. M₃ muscarinic acetylcholine receptors regulate cytoplasmic myosin by a process involving RhoA and requiring conventional protein kinase C isoforms. *J. Biol. Chem.* 274:18675–85

43. Aullo P, Giry M, Olsnes S, Popoff MR, Kocks C, Boquet P. 1993. A chimeric toxin to study the role of the 21 kDa GTP binding protein Rho in the control of actin microfilament assembly. *EMBO J.* 12:921–31

44. Fleming IN, Elliot CM, Exton JH. 1996. Differential translocation of Rho family GTPases by lysophosphatidic acid, endothelin-1, and platelet-derived growth factor. *J. Biol. Chem.* 271:33067–73

45. Donovan FM, Pike CJ, Cotman CW, Cunningham DD. 1997. Thrombin induces apoptosis in cultured neurons and astrocytes via a pathway requiring tyrosine kinase and RhoA activities. *J. Neurosci.* 17:5316–26

46. Seasholtz TM, Majumdar M, Kaplan DD, Brown JH. 1999. Rho and Rho kinase mediate thrombin-stimulated vascular smooth muscle cell DNA synthesis and migration. *Circ. Res.* 84:1186–93

47. Aoki H, Izumo S, Sadoshima J. 1998. Angiotensin II activates RhoA in cardiac myocytes: a critical role of RhoA in angiotensin II-induced premyofibril formation. *Circ. Res.* 82:666–76

48. Gong MC, Fujihara H, Somlyo AV, Somlyo AP. 1997. Translocation of *rhoA* associated with Ca²⁺ sensitization of smooth muscle. *J. Biol. Chem.* 272:10704–9

49. Keller J, Schmidt M, Hussein B, Rumenapp U, Jakobs KH. 1997. Muscarinic receptor-stimulated cytosol-membrane translocation of RhoA. *FEBS Lett.* 403:299–302

50. Laudanna C, Campbell JJ, Butcher EC. 1996. Role of Rho in chemoattractant-activated leukocyte adhesion through integrins. *Science* 271:981–83

51. Laudanna C, Campbell JJ, Butcher EC. 1997. Elevation of intracellular cAMP inhibits RhoA activation and integrin-dependent leukocyte adhesion induced by chemoattractants. *J. Biol. Chem.* 272:24141–44

52. Betuing S, Daviaud D, Pages C, Bonnard E, Valet P, et al. 1998. Gβγ-independent coupling of α₂-adrenergic receptor to p21^rhoA in preadipocytes. *J. Biol. Chem.* 273:15804–10

53. Gohla A, Harhammer R, Schultz G. 1998. The G-protein G₁₃ but not G₁₂ mediates signaling from lysophosphatidic acid receptor via epidermal growth factor receptor to Rho. *J. Biol. Chem.* 273:4653–59

54. Kranenburg O, Poland M, van Horck FPG, Drechsel D, Hall A, Moolenaar WH. 1999. Activation of RhoA by lysophosphatidic acid and Gα₁₂/₁₃ subunits in neuronal cells: induction of neurite retraction. *Mol. Biol. Cell* 10:1851–57

55. Ren X-D, Kiosses WB, Schwartz MA. 1999. Regulation of the small GTP-bind-

ing protein Rho by cell adhesion and the cytoskeleton. *EMBO J.* 18:578–85

56. Van Aelst L, D'Souza-Schorey C. 1997. Rho GTPases and signaling networks. *Genes Dev.* 11:2295–322

57. Aspenstrom P. 1999. Effectors for the Rho GTPases. *Curr. Opin. Cell Biol.* 11:95–102

58. Leung T, Chen X-Q, Manser E, Lim L. 1996. The p160 RhoA-binding kinase ROKα is a member of a kinase family and is involved in the reorganization of the cytoskeleton. *Mol. Cell. Biol.* 16: 5313–27

59. Ishizaki T, Maekawa M, Fujisawa K, Okawa K, Iwamatsu A, et al. 1996. The small GTP-binding protein Rho binds to and activates a 160 kDa Ser/Thr protein kinase homologous to myotonic dystrophy kinase. *EMBO J.* 15:1885–93

60. Matsui T, Amano M, Yamamoto T, Chihara K, Nakafuku M, et al. 1996. Rho-associated kinase, a novel serine/threonine kinase, as a putative target for small GTP binding protein Rho. *EMBO J.* 15:2208–16

61. Nakagawa O, Fujisawa K, Ishizaki T, Saito Y, Nakao K, Narumiya S. 1996. ROCK-I and ROCK-II, two isoforms of Rho-associated coiled-coil forming protein serine/threonine kinase in mice. *FEBS Lett.* 392:189–93

62. Hoshijima M, Sah VP, Wang Y, Chien KR, Brown JH. 1998. The low molecular weight GTPase Rho regulates myofibril formation and organization in neonatal rat ventricular myocytes: involvement of Rho kinase. *J. Biol. Chem.* 273:7725–30

63. Amano M, Chihara K, Kimura K, Fukata Y, Nakamura N, et al. 1997. Formation of actin stress fibers and focal adhesions enhanced by Rho-kinase. *Science* 275:1308–11

64. Ishizaki T, Naito M, Fujisawa K, Maekawa M, Watanabe N, et al. 1997. p160[ROCK], a Rho-associated coiled-coil forming protein kinase, works down-

stream of Rho and induces focal adhesions. *FEBS Lett.* 404:118–24

65. Uehata M, Ishizaki T, Satoh H, Ono T, Kawahara T, et al. 1997. Calcium sensitization of smooth muscle mediated by a Rho-associated protein kinase in hypertension. *Nature* 389:990–94

66. Sahai E, Alberts AS, Treisman R. 1998. RhoA effector mutants reveal distinct effector pathways for cytoskeletal reorganization, SRF activation and transformation. *EMBO J.* 17:1350–61

67. Fujisawa K, Madaule P, Ishizaki T, Watanabe G, Bito H, et al. 1998. Different regions of Rho determine Rho-selective binding of different classes of Rho target molecules. *J. Biol. Chem.* 273:18943–49

68. Watanabe G, Saito Y, Madaule P, Ishizaki T, Fujisawa K, et al. 1996. Protein kinase N (PKN) and PKN-related protein rhophilin as targets of small GTPase Rho. *Science* 271:645–48

69. Amano M, Mukai H, Ono Y, Chihara K, Matsui T, et al. 1996. Identification of a putative target for Rho as the serine-threonine kinase protein kinase N. *Science* 271:648–50

70. Quilliam LA, Lambert QT, Mickelson-Young LA, Westwick JK, Sparks AB, et al. 1996. Isolation of a NCK-associated kinase, PRK2, an SH3-binding protein and potential effector of Rho protein signaling. *J. Biol. Chem.* 271:28772–76

71. Madaule P, Eda M, Watanabe N, Fujisawa K, Matsuoka T, et al. 1998. Role of citron kinase as a target of the small GTPase Rho in cytokinesis. *Nature* 394:491–94

72. Watanabe N, Madaule P, Reid T, Ishizaki T, Watanabe G, et al. 1997. p140mDia, a mammalian homolog of *Drosophila* diaphanous, is a target protein for Rho small GTPase and is a ligand for profilin. *EMBO J.* 16:3044–56

73. Reid T, Furuyashiki T, Ishizaki T, Watanabe G, Watanabe N, et al. 1996. Rho-tekin, a new putative target for Rho

bearing homology to a serine/threonine kinase, PKN, and rhophilin in the Rho-binding domain. *J. Biol. Chem.* 271: 13556–60

74. Fukushima N, Kimura Y, Chun J. 1998. A single receptor encoded by vzg-1/lpA1/edg-2 couples to G proteins and mediates multiple cellular responses to lysophosphatidic acid. *Proc. Natl. Acad. Sci. USA* 95:6151–56

75. Rankin S, Morii N, Narumiya S, Rozengurt E. 1994. Botulinum C3 exo-enzyme blocks the tyrosine phosphory-lation of p125^{FAK} and paxillin induced by bombesin and endothelin. *FEBS Lett.* 354:315–19

76. Ridley AJ, Hall A. 1994. Signal trans-duction pathways regulating Rho-medi-ated stress fibre formation: requirement for a tyrosine kinase. *EMBO J.* 13:2600–10

77. Jalink K, van Corven EJ, Hengeveld T, Morii N, Narumiya S, Moolenaar WH. 1994. Inhibition of lysophosphatidate- and thrombin-induced neurite retraction and neuronal cell rounding by ADP ribo-sylation of the small GTP-binding pro-tein Rho. *J. Cell Biol.* 126:801–10

78. Majumdar M, Seasholtz TM, Goldstein D, de Lanerolle P, Brown JH. 1998. Requirement for Rho-mediated myosin light chain phosphorylation in thrombin-stimulated cell rounding and its dissoci-ation from mitogenesis. *J. Biol. Chem.* 273:10099–106

79. Tigyi G, Fischer DJ, Sebok A, Yang C, Dyer DL, Miledi R. 1996. Lysophospha-tidic acid-induced neurite retraction in PC12 cells: control by phosphoinositide-Ca^{2+} signaling and Rho. *J. Neurochem.* 66:537–48

80. Zachary I, Sinnett-Smith J, Turner CE, Rozengurt E. 1993. Bombesin, vasopres-sin, and endothelin rapidly stimulate tyrosine phosphorylation of the focal adhesion-associated protein paxillin in Swiss 3T3 cells. *J. Biol. Chem.* 268: 22060–65

81. Sinnett-Smith J, Zachary I, Valverde AM, Rozengurt E. 1993. Bombesin stimulation of p125 focal adhesion kinase tyrosine phosphorylation: role of protein kinase C, Ca^{2+} mobilization, and the actin cytoskeleton. *J. Biol. Chem.* 268:14261–68

82. Seufferlein T, Rozengurt E. 1994. Lyso-phosphatidic acid stimulates tyrosine phosphorylation of focal adhesion kinase, paxillin, and p130. Signaling pathways and cross-talk with platelet-derived growth factor. *J. Biol. Chem.* 269:9345–51

83. Kumagai N, Morii N, Fujisawa K, Nemoto Y, Narumiya S. 1993. ADP-ribosylation of rho p21 inhibits lyso-phosphatidic acid-induced protein tyrosine phosphorylation and phosphati-dylinositol 3-kinase activation in cul-tured swiss 3T3 cells. *J. Biol. Chem.* 268:24535–38

84. Seckl MJ, Morii N, Narumiya S, Roz-engurt E. 1995. Guanosine 5'-3-*O*-(thio)triphosphate stimulates tyrosine phosphorylation of p125^{FAK} and paxillin in permeabilized Swiss 3T3 cells. *J. Biol. Chem.* 270:6984–90

85. Schaller MD, Hildebrand JD, Shannon JD, Fox JW, Vines RR, Parsons JT. 1994. Autophosphorylation of the focal adhe-sion kinase, pp125FAK, directs SH2-dependent binding of pp60src. *Mol. Cell. Biol.* 14:1680–88

86. Chen H-C, Appeddu PA, Isoda H, Guan J-L. 1996. Phosphorylation of tyrosine 397 in focal adhesion kinase is required for binding phosphatidylinositol 3-kinase. *J. Biol. Chem.* 271:26329–34

87. Chrzanowska-Wodnicka M, Burridge K. 1996. Rho-stimulated contractility drives the formation of stress fibers and focal adhesions. *J. Cell Biol.* 133:1403–15

88. Kimura K, Ito M, Amano M, Chihara K, Fukata Y, et al. 1996. Regulation of myo-sin phosphatase by Rho and Rho-asso-ciated kinase (Rho-kinase). *Science* 273:245–48

89. Amano M, Ito M, Kimura K, Fukata Y, Chihara K, et al. 1996. Phosphorylation and activation of myosin by Rho-associated kinase (Rho-kinase). *J. Biol. Chem.* 271:20246–49

90. Essler M, Amano M, Kruse H-J, Kaibuchi K, Weber PC, Aepfelbacher M. 1998. Thrombin inactivates myosin light chain phosphatase via Rho and its target Rho kinase in human endothelial cells. *J. Biol. Chem.* 273:21867–74

91. Amano M, Chihara K, Nakamura N, Fukata Y, Yano T, et al. 1998. Myosin II activation promotes neurite retraction during the action of Rho and Rho-kinase. *Genes Cells* 3:177–88

92. Klages B, Brandt U, Simon MI, Schultz G, Offermanns S. 1999. Activation of G_{12}/G_{13} results in shape change and Rho/Rho kinase-mediated myosin light chain phosphorylation in mouse platelets. *J. Cell Biol.* 144:745–54

93. Hirose M, Ishizaki T, Watanabe N, Uehata M, Kranenburg O, et al. 1998. Molecular dissection of the Rho-associated protein kinase (p160ROCK)-regulated neurite remodeling in neuroblastoma N1E-115 cells. *J. Cell Biol.* 141:1625–36

94. Matsui T, Maeda M, Doi Y, Yonemura S, Amano M, et al. 1998. Rho-kinase phosphorylates COOH-terminal threonines of ezrin/radixin/moesin (ERM) proteins and regulates their head-to-tail association. *J. Cell Biol.* 140:647–57

95. Fukata Y, Kimura K, Oshiro N, Saya H, Matsuura Y, Kaibuchi K. 1998. Association of the myosin-binding subunit of myosin phosphatase and moesin: dual regulation of moesin phosphorylation by Rho-associated kinase and myosin phosphatase. *J. Cell Biol.* 141:409–18

96. Maekawa M, Ishizaki T, Boku S, Watanabe N, Fujita A, et al. 1999. Signaling from Rho to the actin cytoskeleton through protein kinases ROCK and LIM-kinase. *Science* 285:895–98

97. Vexler ZS, Symons M, Barber DL. 1996. Activation of Na^+-H^+ exchange is necessary for RhoA-induced stress fiber formation. *J. Biol. Chem.* 271:22281–84

98. Tominaga T, Ishizaki T, Narumiya S, Barber DL. 1998. p160ROCK mediates RhoA activation of Na^+-H^+ exchange. *EMBO J.* 17:4712–22

99. Toker A, Cantley LC. 1997. Signalling through the lipid products of phosphoinositide-3-OH kinase. *Nature* 387:673–76

100. Zhang J, King W, Dillon S, Hall A, Feig L, Rittenhouse SE. 1993. Activation of platelet phosphatidylinositide 3-kinase requires the small GTP-binding protein rho. *J. Biol. Chem.* 268:22251–54

101. Zhang J, Zhang J, Benovic JL, Sugai M, Wetzker R, Gout I, Rittenhouse SE. 1995. Sequestration of a G-protein βγ subunit or ADP-ribosylation of Rho can inhibit thrombin-induced activation of platelet phosphoinositide 3-kinases. *J. Biol. Chem.* 270:6589–94

102. Ren X-D, Bokoch GM, Traynor-Kaplan A, Jenkins GH, Anderson RA, Schwartz MA. 1996. Physical association of the small GTPase Rho with a 68-kDa phosphatidylinositol 4-phosphate 5-kinase in Swiss 3T3 cells. *Mol. Biol. Cell* 7:435–42

103. Chong LD, Traynor-Kaplan A, Bokoch GM, Schwartz MA. 1994. The small GTP-binding protein Rho regulates a phosphatidylinositol 4-phosphate 5-kinase in mammalian cells. *Cell* 79:507–13

104. Zhang C, Schmidt M, von Eichel-Streiber C, Jakobs KH. 1996. Inhibition by toxin B of inositol phosphate formation induced by G protein-coupled and tyrosine kinase receptors in N1E-115 neuroblastoma cells: involvement of Rho proteins. *Mol. Pharmacol.* 50:864–69

105. Gilmore AP, Burridge K. 1996. Regulation of vinculin binding to talin and actin by phosphatidylinositol-4-5-bisphosphate. *Nature* 381:531–35

106. Shibasaki Y, Ishihara H, Kizuki N, Asano

T, Oka Y, Yazaki Y. 1997. Massive actin polymerization induced by phosphatidylinositol-4-phosphate 5-kinase *in vivo. J. Biol. Chem.* 272:7578–81

107. Homma Y, Emori Y. 1995. A dual functional signal mediator showing RhoGAP and phospholipase C-δ stimulating activities. *EMBO J.* 14:286–91

108. Jinsi-Parimoo A, Deth RC. 1997. Reconstitution of α_{2D}-adrenergic receptor coupling to phospholipase D in PC12 cell lysate. *J. Biol. Chem.* 272:14556–61

109. Exton JH. 1997. New developments in phospholipase D. *J. Biol. Chem.* 272:15579–82

110. Plonk SG, Park S-K, Exton JH. 1998. The α-subunit of the heterotrimeric G protein G_{13} activates a phospholipase D isozyme by a pathway requiring Rho family GTPases. *J. Biol. Chem.* 273:4823–26

111. Schmidt M, Voss M, Oude Weernink PA, Wetzel J, Amano M, et al. 1999. A role for Rho-kinase in Rho-controlled phospholipase D stimulation by the m_3 muscarinic acetylcholine receptor. *J. Biol. Chem.* 274:14648–54

112. Yamazaki M, Zhang Y, Watanabe H, Yokozeki T, Ohno S, et al. 1999. Interaction of the small G protein RhoA with the C terminus of human phospholipase D1. *J. Biol. Chem.* 274:6035–38

113. Bae CD, Min DS, Fleming IN, Exton JH. 1998. Determination of interaction sites on the small G protein RhoA for phospholipase D. *J. Biol. Chem.* 273:11596–604

114. Nishimura J, Kolber M, van Breemen C. 1988. Norepinephrine and GTP-γ-S increase myofilament Ca^{2+} sensitivity in α-toxin permeabilized arterial smooth muscle. *Biochem. Biophys. Res. Commun.* 157:677–83

115. Kitazawa T, Kobayashi S, Horiuti K, Somlyo AV, Somlyo AP. 1989. Receptor-coupled, permeabilized smooth muscle. Role of the phosphatidylinositol cascade, G-proteins, and modulation of the contractile response to Ca^{2+}. *J. Biol. Chem.* 264:5339–42

116. Kokubu N, Satoh M, Takayanagi I. 1995. Involvement of botulinum C3-sensitive GTP-binding proteins in α_1-adrenoceptor subtypes mediating Ca^{2+}-sensitization. *Eur. J. Pharmacol.* 290:19–27

117. Hirata K-I, Kikuchi A, Sasaki T, Kuroda S, Kaibuchi K, et al. 1992. Involvement of *rho* p21 in the GTP-enhanced calcium ion sensitivity of smooth muscle contraction. *J. Biol. Chem.* 267:8719–22

118. Noda M, Yasuda-Fukazawa C, Moriishi K, Kato T, Okuda T, et al. 1995. Involvement of *rho* in GTPγS-induced enhancement of phosphorylation of 20 kDa myosin light chain in vascular smooth muscle cells: inhibition of phosphatase activity. *FEBS Lett.* 367:246–50

119. Deleted in proof

120. Kureishi Y, Kobayashi S, Amano M, Kimura K, Kanaide M, et al. 1997. Rho-associated kinase directly induces smooth muscle contraction through myosin light chain phosphorylation. *J. Biol. Chem.* 272:12257–60

121. Satoh S, Kreutz R, Wilm C, Ganten D, Pfitzer G. 1994. Augmented agonist-induced Ca^{2+} sensitization of coronary artery contraction in genetically hypertensive rats. Evidence for altered signal transduction in the coronary smooth muscle cells. *J. Clin. Invest.* 94:1397–403

122. Lummen G, Virchow S, Rumenapp U, Schmidt M, Wieland T, et al. 1997. Identification of G protein-coupled receptors potently stimulating migration of human transitional-cell carcinoma cells. *Naunyn-Schmiedebergs Arch. Pharmacol.* 356:769–76

123. Fukata Y, Oshiro N, Kinoshita N, Kawano Y, Matsuoka Y, et al. 1999. Phosphorylation of adducin by Rho-kinase plays a crucial role in cell motility. *J. Cell Biol.* 145:347–61

124. Niggli V. 1999. Rho-kinase in human neutrophils: a role in signalling for myo-

sin light chain phosphorylation and cell migration. *FEBS Lett.* 445:69–72

125. Yano Y, Saito Y, Narumiya S, Sumpio BE. 1996. Involvement of rho p21 in cyclic strain-induced tyrosine phosphorylation of focal adhesion kinase (pp125FAK), morphological changes and migration of endothelial cells. *Biochem. Biophys. Res. Commun.* 224: 508–15

126. Imamura F, Horai T, Mukai M, Shinkai K, Sawada M, Akedo H. 1993. Induction of in vitro tumor cell invasion of cellular monolayers by lysophosphatidic acid or phospholipase D. *Biochem. Biophys. Res. Commun.* 193:497–503

127. Imamura F, Shinkai K, Mukai M, Yoshioka K, Komagome R, et al. 1996. Rho-mediated protein tyrosine phosphorylation in lysophosphatidic-acid-induced tumor-cell invasion. *Int. J. Cancer* 65:627–32

128. Yoshioka K, Matsumura F, Akedo H, Itoh K. 1998. Small GTP-binding protein Rho stimulates the actomyosin system, leading to invasion of tumor cells. *J. Biol. Chem.* 273:5146–54

129. Sah VP, Hoshijima M, Chien KR, Brown JH. 1996. Rho is required for $G\alpha_q$ and α_1-adrenergic receptor signaling in cardiomyocytes: dissociation of Ras and Rho pathways. *J. Biol. Chem.* 271: 31185–90

130. Frost JA, Xu S, Hutchison MR, Marcus S, Cobb MH. 1996. Actions of Rho family small G proteins and p21-activated protein kinases on mitogen-activated protein kinase family members. *Mol. Cell. Biol.* 16:3707–13

130. (a) Olson MF, Ashworth A, Hall A. 1995. An essential role for Rho, Rac, and Cdc42 GTPases in cell cycle progression through G_1. *Science* 269:1270–72

131. Kumagai N, Morii N, Ishizaki T, Watanabe N, Fujisawa K, et al. 1995. Lysophosphatidic acid-induced activation of protein Ser/Thr kinases in cultured rat 3Y1 fibroblasts. Possible involvement in

rho p21-mediated signalling. *FEBS Lett.* 366:11–16

132. Coso OA, Chiariello M, Yu J-C, Teramoto H, Crespo P, et al. 1995. The small GTP-binding proteins Rac1 and Cdc42 regulate the activity of the JNK/SAPK signaling pathway. *Cell* 81:1137–46

133. Minden A, Lin A, Claret F-X, Abo A, Karin M. 1995. Selective activation of the JNK signaling cascade and c-Jun transcriptional activity by the small GTPases Rac and Cdc42Hs. *Cell* 81:1147–57

134. Teramoto H, Crespo P, Coso OA, Igishi T, Xu N, Gutkind JS. 1996. The small GTP-binding protein Rho activates c-Jun N-terminal kinases/stress-activated protein kinases in human kidney 293T cells: evidence for a Pak-independent signaling pathway. *J. Biol. Chem.* 271:25731–34

135. Chihara K, Amano M, Nakamura N, Yano T, Shibata M, et al. 1997. Cytoskeletal rearrangements and transcriptional activation of c-*fos* serum response element by Rho-kinase. *J. Biol. Chem.* 272:25121–27

136. Zohar M, Teramoto H, Katz B-Z, Yamada KM, Gutkind JS. 1998. Effector domain mutants of Rho dissociate cytoskeletal changes from nuclear signaling and cellular transformation. *Oncogene* 17:991–98

137. Sahai E, Ishizaki T, Narumiya S, Treisman R. 1999. Transformation mediated by RhoA requires activity of ROCK kinases. *Curr. Biol.* 9:136–45

138. Pan ZK, Zuraw BL, Lung C-C, Prossnitz ER, Browning DD, Ye RD. 1996. Bradykinin stimulates NF-κB activation and interleukin 1β gene expression in cultured human fibroblasts. *J. Clin. Invest.* 98:2042–49

139. Pan ZK, Ye RD, Christiansen SC, Jagels MA, Bokoch GM, Zuraw BL. 1998. Role of the Rho GTPase in bradykinin-stimulated nuclear factor-κB activation and IL-1β gene expression in cultured

human epithelial cells. *J. Immunol.* 160:3038–45

140. Shahrestanifar M, Fan X, Manning DR. 1999. Lysophosphatidic acid activates NF-κB in fibroblasts. *J. Biol. Chem.* 274:3828–33

141. Montaner S, Perona R, Saniger L, Lacal JC. 1998. Multiple signalling pathways lead to the activation of the nuclear factor κB by the Rho family of GTPases. *J. Biol. Chem.* 273:12779–85

142. Chang J-H, Pratt JC, Sawasdikosol S, Kapeller R, Burakoff SJ. 1998. The small GTP-binding protein Rho potentiates AP-1 transcription in T cells. *Mol. Cell Biol.* 18:4986–93

143. Dhanasekaran N, Heasley LE, Johnson GL. 1995. G protein-coupled receptor systems involved in cell growth and oncogenesis. *Endocrine Rev.* 16:259–70

144. Gutkind JS. 1998. Cell growth control by G protein-coupled receptors: from signal transduction to signal integration. *Oncogene* 17:1331–42

145. Yamamoto M, Marui N, Sakai T, Morii N, Kozaki S, et al. 1993. ADP-ribosylation of the *rhoA* gene product by botulinum C3 exoenzyme causes Swiss 3T3 cells to accumulate in the G1 phase of the cell cycle. *Oncogene* 8:1449–55

146. Noguchi Y, Nakamura S, Yasuda T, Kitagawa M, Kohn LD, et al. 1998. Newly synthesized Rho A, not Ras, is isoprenylated and translocated to membranes coincident with progression of the G_1 to S phase of growth-stimulated rat FRTL-5 cells. *J. Biol. Chem.* 273:3649–53

147. Adnane J, Bizouarn FA, Qian Y, Hamilton AD, Sebti SM. 1998. p21*WAF1/CIP1* is upregulated by the geranylgeranyltransferase I inhibitor GGTI-298 through a transforming growth factor β- and Sp1-responsive element: involvement of the small GTPase RhoA. *Mol. Cell. Biol.* 18:6962–70

147. (a) Olson MF, Paterson HF, Marshal CJ. 1998. Signals from Ras and Rho

GTPases interact to regulate expression of p21[Waf1/Cip1]. *Nature* 394:295–99

148. Qiu R-G, Chen J, McCormick F, Symons M. 1995. A role for Rho in Ras transformation. *Proc. Natl. Acad. Sci. USA* 92:11781–85

148. (a) Cazaubon S, Chaverot N, Romero IA, Girault J-A, Adamson P, et al. 1997. Growth factor activity of endothelin-1 in primary astrocytes mediated by adhesion-dependent and -independent pathways. *J. Neurosci.* 17:6203–12

149. Thorburn J, Xu S, Thorburn A. 1997. MAP kinase- and Rho-dependent signals interact to regulate gene expression but not actin morphology in cardiac muscle cells. *EMBO J.* 16:1888–900

150. Hines WA, Thorburn A. 1998. Ras and Rho are required for Gαq-induced hypertrophic gene expression in neonatal rat cardiac myocytes. *J. Mol. Cell. Cardiol.* 30:485–94

151. Kuwahara K, Saito Y, Nakagawa O, Kishimoto I, Harada M, et al. 1999. The effects of the selective ROCK inhibitor, Y27632, on ET-1-induced hypertrophic response in neonatal rat cardiomyocytes—possible involvement of Rho/ROCK pathway in cardiac muscle cell hypertrophy. *FEBS Lett.* 452:314–18

152. Sah VP, Minamisawa S, Tam SP, Wu TH, Dorn GW, et al. 1999. Cardiac-specific overexpression of RhoA results in sinus and atrioventricular nodal dysfunction and contractile failure. *J. Clin. Invest.* 103:1627–34

153. Cachero TG, Morielli AD, Peralta EG. 1998. The small GTP-binding protein RhoA regulates a delayed rectifier potassium channel. *Cell* 93:1077–85

154. Althoefer H, Eversole-Cire P, Simon MI. 1997. Constitutively active Gαq and Gα13 trigger apoptosis through different pathways. *J. Biol. Chem.* 272:24380–86

155. Berestetskaya YV, Faure MP, Ichijo H, Voyno-Yasenetskaya TA. 1998. Regulation of apoptosis by α-subunits of G12 and G13 proteins via apoptosis signal-

regulating kinase-1. *J. Biol. Chem.* 273:27816–23

156. Adams JW, Sakata Y, Davis MG, Sah VP, Wang Y, et al. 1998. Enhanced $G\alpha_q$ signaling: a common pathway mediates cardiac hypertrophy and apoptotic heart failure. *Proc. Natl. Acad. Sci. USA* 95:10140–45

157. Vaughan PJ, Pike CJ, Cotman CW, Cunningham DD. 1995. Thrombin receptor activation protects neurons and astrocytes from cell death produced by environmental insults. *J. Neurosci.* 15:5389–401

158. Donovan FM, Cunningham DD. 1998. Signaling pathways involved in thrombin-induced cell protection. *J. Biol. Chem.* 273:12746–52

159. Murga C, Laguinge L, Wetzker R, Cuadrado A, Gutkind JS. 1998. Activation of Akt/protein kinase B by G protein-coupled receptors. A role for α and $\beta\gamma$ subunits of heterotrimeric G proteins acting through phosphatidylinositol-3-OH kinaseγ. *J. Biol. Chem.* 273:19080–85

160. Mills JC, Stone NL, Erhardt J, Pittman RN. 1998. Apoptotic membrane blebbing is regulated by myosin light chain phosphorylation. *J. Cell Biol.* 140:627–36

161. Takahashi M, Mukai H, Toshimori M, Miyamoto M, Ono Y. 1998. Proteolytic activation of PKN by caspase-3 or related protease during apoptosis. *Proc. Natl. Acad. Sci. USA* 95:11566–71

162. Vogler O, Krummenerl P, Schmidt M, Jakobs KH, van Koppen CJ. 1999. RhoA-sensitive trafficking of muscarinic acetylcholine receptors. *J. Pharmacol. Exp. Ther.* 288:36–42

163. Lamaze C, Chuang T-H, Terlecky LJ, Bokoch GM, Schmid SL. 1996. Regulation of receptor-mediated endocytosis by Rho and Rac. *Nature* 382:177–79

164. Lin HC, Duncan JA, Kozasa T, Gilman AG. 1998. Sequestration of the G protein $\beta\gamma$ subunit complex inhibits receptor-mediated endocytosis. *Proc. Natl. Acad. Sci. USA* 95:5057–60

165. Gasman S, Chasserot-Golaz S, Popoff MR, Aunis D, Bader M-F. 1997. Trimeric G proteins control exocytosis in chromaffin cells. G_o regulates the peripheral actin network and catecholamine secretion by a mechanism involving the small GTP-binding protein Rho. *J. Biol. Chem.* 272:20564–71

166. Thomson FJ, Jess TJ, Moyes C, Plevin R, Gould GW. 1997. Characterization of the intracellular signalling pathways that underlie growth-factor-stimulated glucose transport in *Xenopus* oocytes: evidence for *ras-* and *rho-* dependent pathways of phosphatidylinositol 3-kinase activation. *Biochem. J.* 325:637–43

167. Standaert M, Bandyopadhyay G, Galloway L, Ono Y, Mukai H, Farese R. 1998. Comparative effects of GTPγS and insulin on the activation of Rho, phosphatidylinositol 3-kinase, and protein kinase N in rat adipocytes. Relationship to glucose transport. *J. Biol. Chem.* 273:7470–77

168. van Corven EJ, Groenink A, Jalink K, Eichholtz T, Moolenaar WH. 1989. Lysophosphatidate-induced cell proliferation: identification and dissection of signaling pathways mediated by G proteins. *Cell* 59:45–54

169. Trejo JA, Connolly AJ, Coughlin SR. 1996. The cloned thrombin receptor is necessary and sufficient for activation of mitogen-activated protein kinase and mitogenesis in mouse lung fibroblasts. *J. Biol. Chem.* 271:21536–41

170. Jalink K, Eichholtz T, Postma FR, van Corven EJ, Moolenaar WH. 1993. Lysophosphatidic acid induces neuronal shape changes via a novel, receptor-mediated signaling pathway: similarity to thrombin action. *Cell Growth Diff.* 4:247–55

171. Tigyi G, Fischer DJ, Sebök A, Marshall F, Dyer DL, Miledi R. 1996. Lysophos-

phatidic acid-induced neurite retraction in PC12 cells: neurite-protective effects of cyclic AMP signaling. *J. Neurochem.* 66:549–58

171. (a) Vouret-Craviari V, Boquet P, Pouysségur J, Van Obberghen-Schilling E. 1998. Regulation of the actin cytoskeleton by thrombin in human endothelial cells: role of Rho proteins in endothelial barrier function. *Mol. Biol. Cell* 9:2639–53

172. Buhl AM, Johnson NL, Dhanasekaran N, Johnson GL. 1995. $G\alpha_{12}$ and $G\alpha_{13}$ stimulate Rho-dependent stress fiber formation and focal adhesion assembly. *J. Biol. Chem.* 270:24631–34

173. Katoh H, Aoki J, Yamaguchi Y, Kitano Y, Ichikawa A, Negishi M. 1998. Constitutively active $G\alpha_{12}$, $G\alpha_{13}$, and $G\alpha_q$ induce Rho-dependent neurite retraction through different signaling pathways. *J. Biol. Chem.* 273:28700–7

174. Harhammer R, Gohla A, Schultz G. 1996. Interaction of G protein $G\beta\gamma$ dimers with small GTP-binding proteins of the Rho family. *FEBS Lett.* 399:211–14

175. Jalink K, Moolenaar WH. 1992. Thrombin receptor activation causes rapid neural cell rounding and neurite retraction independent of classic second messengers. *J. Cell Biol.* 118:411–19

176. Gohla A, Offermanns S, Wilkie TM, Schultz G. 1999. Differential involvement of $G\alpha_{12}$ and $G\alpha_{13}$ in receptor-mediated stress fiber formation. *J. Biol. Chem.* 274:17901–7

177. Dhanasekaran N, Dermott JM. 1996. Signaling by the G_{12} class of G proteins. *Cell. Signal.* 8:235–45

178. Offermanns S, Laugwitz K-L, Spicher K, Schultz G. 1994. G proteins of the G_{12} family are activated via thromboxane A_2 and thrombin receptors in human platelets. *Proc. Natl. Acad. Sci. USA* 91:504–8

179. Barr AJ, Brass LF, Manning DR. 1997. Reconstitution of receptors and GTP-binding regulatory proteins (G proteins) in Sf9 cells. A direct evaluation of selectivity in receptor-G protein coupling. *J. Biol. Chem.* 272:2223–29

180. Needham LK, Rozengurt E. 1998. $G\alpha_{12}$ and $G\alpha_{13}$ stimulate Rho-dependent tyrosine phosphorylation of focal adhesion kinase, paxillin, and p130 Crk-associated substrate. *J. Biol. Chem.* 273:14626–32

181. Mao J, Xie W, Yuan H, Simon MI, Mano H, Wu D. 1998. Tec/BMX non-receptor tyrosine kinases are involved in regulation of Rho and serum response factor by $G\alpha 12/13$. *EMBO J.* 17:5638–46

182. Nobes CD, Hawkins P, Stephens L, Hall A. 1995. Activation of the small GTP-binding proteins rho and rac by growth factor receptors. *J. Cell Sci.* 108:225–33

183. Schoenwaelder SM, Burridge K. 1999. Evidence for a calpeptin-sensitive protein-tyrosine phosphatase upstream of the small GTPase Rho. A novel role for the calpain inhibitor calpeptin in the inhibition of protein-tyrosine phosphatases. *J. Biol. Chem.* 274:14359–67

184. Kulkarni S, Saido TC, Suzuki K, Fox JE. 1999. Calpain mediates integrin-induced signaling at a point upstream of Rho family members. *J. Biol. Chem.* 274:21265–75

185. Hart MJ, Jiang X, Kozasa T, Roscoe W, Singer WD, et al. 1998. Direct stimulation of the guanine nucleotide exchange activity of p115 RhoGEF by $G\alpha_{13}$. *Science* 280:2112–14

186. Kim B-C, Lim C-J, Kim J-H. 1997. Arachidonic acid, a principal product of Rac-activated phospholipase A_2, stimulates c-fos serum response element via Rho-dependent mechanism. *FEBS Lett.* 415:325–28

187. Wang Y, Falasca M, Schlessinger J, Malstrom S, Tsichlis P, et al. 1998. Activation of the c-fos serum response element by phosphatidyl inositol 3-kinase and rho pathways in HeLa cells. *Cell Growth Diff.* 9:513–22

187. (a) Fleming IN, Elliott CM, Collard JG,

Exton JH. 1997. Lysophosphatidic acid induces threonine phosphorylation of Tiam1 in Swiss 3T3 fibroblasts via activation of protein kinase C. *J. Biol. Chem.* 272:33105–10

188. Lang P, Gesbert F, Delespine-Carmagnat M, Stancou R, Pouchelet M, Bertoglio J. 1996. Protein kinase A phosphorylation of RhoA mediates the morphological and functional effects of cyclic AMP in cytotoxic lymphocytes. *EMBO J.* 15:510–19

189. Dong J-M, Leung T, Manser E, Lim L. 1998. cAMP-induced morphological changes are counteracted by the activated RhoA small GTPase and the Rho kinase ROKα. *J. Biol. Chem.* 273:22554–62

Annu. Rev. Pharmacol. Toxicol. 2000. 40:491–518

CENTRAL ROLE OF PEROXISOME PROLIFERATOR–ACTIVATED RECEPTORS IN THE ACTIONS OF PEROXISOME PROLIFERATORS

J. Christopher Corton, Steven P. Anderson[1], and Anja Stauber

Chemical Industry Institute of Toxicology, 6 Davis Drive, Research Triangle Park, North Carolina 27709–2137; e-mail: corton@ciit.org, stauber@ciit.org

Key Words   hepatocarcinogenesis, inflammation, growth suppression

■ **Abstract**   Peroxisome proliferators (PPs) are a large class of structurally dissimilar chemicals that have diverse effects in rodents and humans. Most, if not all, of the diverse effects of PPs are mediated by three members of the nuclear receptor superfamily called peroxisome proliferator-activated receptors (PPARs). In this review, we define the molecular mechanisms of PPs, including PPAR binding specificity, alteration of gene expression through binding to DNA response elements, and cross talk with other signaling pathways. We discuss the roles of PPARs in growth promotion in rodent hepatocarcinogenesis and potential therapeutic effects, including suppression of cancer growth and inflammation.

INTRODUCTION

Peroxisomes are subcellular organelles that are found in most animal cells and that perform diverse metabolic functions, including H_2O_2-derived respiration, β-oxidation of fatty acids, and cholesterol metabolism (1). Peroxisome proliferators (PPs) are a large class of structurally dissimilar industrial and pharmaceutical chemicals that were originally identified as inducers of both the size and the number of peroxisomes in rat and mouse livers or hepatocytes in vitro after exposure. Rodent exposure to PPs leads to a stereotypical orchestration of adaptations consisting of hepatocellular hypertrophy and hyperplasia, and to transcriptional induction of fatty acid–metabolizing enzymes regulated in parallel with peroxisome proliferation (1). Chronic exposure to many PPs causes an increased incidence of liver tumors in male and female mice and rats (2).

---

[1]Present Address: Strategic Toxicologic Sciences, Glaxo Wellcome Research and Development, 5 Moore Drive, Research Triangle Park, NC 27709

0362–1642/00/0415–0491$14.00   **491**

Recent research points toward a pivotal role for a subset of nuclear receptor superfamily members, called peroxisome proliferator–activated receptors (PPARs), in mediating many, or all, of the adaptive consequences of PP exposure (3). PPs may activate PPARs by binding directly to the receptor, or possibly by perturbing lipid metabolism to generate PPAR ligands. Upon activation, PPAR regulates the expression of genes involved in lipid metabolism and peroxisome proliferation, as well as genes involved in cell growth. Other factors, both positive and negative, influence the ability of PPARs to modulate gene expression.

In this review, we describe the molecular mode of action of PPAR transcription factors, including ligand binding, interaction with specific DNA response elements, transcriptional activation, and cross talk with other signaling pathways. We discuss the evidence that suggests that PPARs play a central role in mediating rodent hepatocarcinogenesis. Lastly, we discuss evidence that has recently emerged on the potential therapeutic actions of PPs, including suppression of cancer cell growth and inflammation. Readers are referred to a number of excellent reviews focusing more specifically on the role of PPARs in hyperlipidemia (4), type II diabetes (5), adipocyte differentiation (6), and atherosclerosis (7, 8).

STRUCTURE AND FUNCTION OF PPAR ISOFORMS

The rapid and coordinate induction of liver cell hyperplasia, peroxisome proliferation, and increases in lipid-metabolizing enzymes by PPs gave an early indication that a receptor-mediated mechanism was involved (9). A member of the nuclear receptor superfamily that was transcriptionally activated by PPs was cloned from mouse liver in 1990 and was named the peroxisome proliferator–activated receptor (PPAR) (10). Like other members of the vertebrate steroid-nuclear receptor superfamily, PPARs exist in distinct isoforms encoded by separate genes. There are three known PPAR isoforms: PPARα, PPARδ (also known as NUC1 and PPARβ), and PPARγ (11).

Similar to other nuclear receptors, PPAR proteins exhibit a generic organization consisting of a number of functional domains: A/B, C, D, and E/F (reviewed in 12). The A/B region encodes a ligand-independent transcriptional activation domain (activation function-1) that is active in some cell types. The C domain encodes the highly conserved DNA binding domain consisting of two zinc finger DNA binding motifs. This domain targets the receptor to specific DNA sequences in responsive genes called peroxisome proliferator response elements (PPREs). The ligand binding domain (LBD), or E domain of PPARs, is responsible for ligand-binding and converting PPARs to an active form that binds DNA and modulates gene expression. In addition, the E region is also important in dimerization, nuclear localization, and association with modulators of transcription, such as coactivators and corepressors, through interaction with a transactivation domain [activation function-2 (AF-2)] located within the C-terminal α-helix. PPARs lack a C-terminal extension (the F domain) found in other nuclear receptors that may modulate transactivation. The D region encodes a flexible hinge region, thought to allow independent movement of the LBD relative to the DNA binding domain.

PPAR isoforms perform different physiological functions, based on their divergent patterns of tissue-specific expression, different ligand-binding specificities, and divergent physiological consequences when activated (Table 1). PPARα regulates fatty acid metabolism and is highly expressed in liver, kidney, and intestine. PPARα also down-regulates inflammatory responses (13, 14). PPARβ/δ is ubiquitously expressed, but its physiological function is yet to be fully defined. By using a specific agonist, PPARβ/δ has been shown to be involved in embryo implantation and decidualization in the mouse (15). PPARγ exists in two distinct isoforms, designated PPARγ1 and PPARγ2, that have different tissue distributions and functions. Expression of these isoforms, differing only in their N-terminal 30 amino acids (γ2 has 30 extra amino acids), is driven from the same gene by alternative promoter usage and splicing (16). PPARγ1 is found in liver and to a lesser extent in other organs, including adipose tissue. PPARγ2 is expressed exclusively in adipose tissue and is a potent regulator of adipocyte differentiation. When PPARγ2 is expressed in fibroblasts, adipocyte genes are activated, leading to conversion of fibroblasts to adipocytes (reviewed in 6, 17). Activation of PPARγ inhibits angiogenesis (18) and inflammatory processes, which are involved in a number of disease states (5). Thiazolidinedione drug activation of PPARγ induces the antidiabetic effects of this important class of compounds (5).

Recent evidence demonstrates that PPARs modulate gene expression in a manner similar to that of other nuclear receptors (Figure 1). Many important clues to the mechanism of PPAR activation have come from resolving the crystal structures of the LBDs of the human PPARγ (19, 20) and human PPARβ/δ (21) determined both with and without ligands. The PPAR ligand binding pocket, encompassing ~ 1300 Å^3, is unusual in that it is two to three times larger than pockets in other nuclear receptors (22). This difference in size allows these receptors to accommodate a host of structurally diverse chemicals (see below). In the absence of ligand activation, PPAR AF-2 helix is positioned away from the ligand binding pocket (19, 20). Ligand binding induces a conformational change in the

TABLE 1   Properties of rodent isoforms of the peroxisome proliferator-activated receptor

Isoform	Tissue distribution[a]					Physiological role
	Liver	Kidney	Intestine	Spleen	Fat	
α	+ + + +	+ +	+ + + +	+	−	Lipid metabolism, regulation of inflammation
β/δ	+ +	+ +	+ + +	+ +	−	Embryo implantation
γ	−	+/−	+ +	+ + +	+ + + +	Adipocyte differentiation, regulation of inflammation

[a]Tissue distribution is based on in situ hybridization of rat tissue (90).

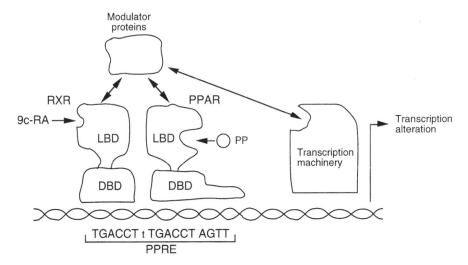

Figure 1   Modulation of gene transcription by a peroxisome proliferator–activated receptor (PPAR). Ligand binding of the peroxisome proliferator (PP) leads to PPAR activation and heterodimerization with the retinoid X receptor (RXR), the receptor for 9-*cis*-retinoic acid (9c-RA). The PPAR-RXR heterodimer, through their DNA-binding domains (DBD), binds to the consensus sequence 5'-TGACCT T TGACCT AGTT-3' (or variant), with PPAR occupying the 3' position. Interactions between the PPAR-RXR heterodimer, modulator proteins, and the transcription machinery affect transcription initiation and mRNA abundance. LBD, ligand-binding domain; PPRE, peroxisome proliferator response element.

LBD, resulting in the AF-2 helix swinging shut behind the ligand, in what has been termed the mouse trap model (19). Critical interactions between the acidic group on the ligand and specific amino acids on the AF-2 helix are required for ligand binding and associated transcriptional activation. The pivotal role of AF-2 helix amino acids in the transactivation function of PPARs and other nuclear receptors had been previously demonstrated (reviewed in 23). The ligand-induced conformation of the LBD, including the AF-2 helix across the opening of the ligand binding pocket, creates the proper orientation for binding to a coactivator protein called the steroid receptor coactivator-1 (SRC-1). A number of proteins, including coactivators, encode one or more short α-helices, called nuclear receptor boxes, which are important in nuclear receptor interaction and transcriptional activation. A nuclear receptor box from SRC-1 associates with the PPARδ LBD between a glutamic acid on the AF-2 helix and a lysine on helix 3. This arrangement of the nuclear receptor box helix held between PPAR LBD amino acids has been called the charged clamp (19). In addition to interaction with transcriptional modulators, PP binding to PPARs leads to dimerization with the retinoid X receptor (RXR), the receptor for 9-*cis* retinoic acid. The PPAR-RXR heterodimer binds to the consensus sequence 5'-TGACCT T TGACCT AGTT-3' (or variant), with PPARs occupying the 3' position. Interaction between the PPAR-RXR heterodimer and other factors that modulate the PP-induced activation, such as coactivators, the transcription machinery, or both, leads to either increases or decreases in transcription of target genes that contain PPREs. Transcription may also be modulated by phosphorylation of the A/B domains of PPARα (24) and -γ (25) through a mitogen-activated protein kinase-dependent pathway (23).

PPAR LIGANDS

Exogenous Ligands

PPs are unique, compared with the structurally restricted ligands that interact with other nuclear receptors, in that they are structurally diverse. PPs do have similar structural requirements for interacting with and activating PPARs in vitro and for eliciting biological effects in humans or animals. Most PPs are amphipathic molecules containing a hydrophobic backbone (aliphatic or aromatic) linked to an acidic function. This acidic function is essential for ligand activity and typically consists of a carboxyl group present in the parent compound or a group that may be converted metabolically to a carboxyl group. PPs resemble endogenous lipid activators of PPARs that also require an acidic function linked to an aliphatic backbone for activity.

Several PPs have been shown to bind to PPARs and to act as exogenous PPAR activators in cell transactivation assays (Table 2). These include hypolipidemic drugs such as clofibrate and gemfibrozil and the experimental drug WY-14,643 (26, 27), leukotriene D4 receptor antagonists (28–30), and industrial compounds (10, 31). Several of these PPs have been shown to preferentially activate the PPARα isoform, which suggests that some PPs may be PPARα-selective ligands (26, 27). There is a good correlation between the ability of a PP to bind to and/or activate PPARα and the potency of the PP as an inducer of hepatocarcinogenesis. For example, one of the strongest inducers of hepatocarcinogenesis is WY-14,643, which binds strongly to PPARα and activates PPARα to high levels. In contrast, bezafibrate is a relatively weak hepatocarcinogen and binds and activates PPARα weakly (32). Taken together, these studies strongly suggest that many hepatocarcinogenic PPs are ligands of the PPARα isoform, and they support the hypothesis that PPARα is the major cellular target of hepatocarcinogenic PPs in the liver.

Antidiabetic thiazolidinediones enhance adipocyte differentiation, a process shown to be mediated by PPARγ (6). One such compound, BRL49653, specifically binds and activates PPARγ in transactivation assays (27, 33). Other thiazolidinedione and non-thiazolidinedione chemicals have more recently been identified as PPARγ-specific ligands. The non-thiazolidinedione L-764406 binds to PPARγ with high affinity, forms a covalent linkage with Cys^{313} in helix 3 of

TABLE 2 Chemical activators of peroxisome proliferator-activated receptors (PPARs)[a]

Peroxisome proliferator compounds	PPAR		
	α	β/δ	γ
Hypolipidemic drugs			
WY-14,643[b]	$+++$[c]	$+$	$++$
Clofibrate[a]	$++$[c]	$-$	$+$
Ciprofibrate[b]	$++$[c]	$-$	$+$
Gemfibrozil[a]	$++$[c]	$-$	$+$
Nafenopin[b]	$++$[c]	ND	ND
GW2331	$+++$[c]	$+/-$	$++$[c]
Bezafibrate[b]	$+$[c]	$+++$[c]	$-$
Miscellaneous peroxisome proliferators			
Phthalate ester			
Monoethylhexyl phthalate[b,d]	$+++$	$+$	$++$
Organic Solvent			
Trichloroacetic acid[a]	$+$	ND	ND
Synthetic arachidonic acid			
ETYA	$+++$[c]	$-$	$+/-$
Leukotriene B4 antagonists			
MK-571	$++$	ND	ND
LY-171883	$++$[c]	ND	ND
Antidiabetic thiazolidinediones			
BRL-49653	$-$	$-$	$+++$[c]
Pioglitazone	$-$	$-$	$++$[c]
Ciglitazone	$-$	$-$	$++$[c]
Englitazone	$-$	$-$	$+$[c]
KRP-297	$++$[c]	$-$	$++$[c]
MCC-555	ND	ND	$++$
Nonsteroidal ant-inflammatory drugs			
Indomethacin	$+$	$-$	$+++$[c]
Ibuprofen	$+$	$-$	$+$[c]
Fenoprofen	$++$	$-$	$+$[c]
Piroxicam	$-$	$-$	$+$
GW2433	$-$	$+++$	$-$
GW0072	$-$	$-$	$+$
L-764406	$-$	$-$	$+++$
L-165041	$-$	$+++$	$+$

[a] $+$, Activator of this isoform in a transactivation assay; $-$, not an activator of this isoform in a transactivation assay; $+/-$, conflicting reports in the literature about this compound being an activator in a transactivation assay; ND, not determined for this compound.
[b] This compound has been shown to cause hepatocarcinogenesis in rats and mice (see Reference 3).
[c] This compound has been determined to be a ligand for the PPAR isoform.
[d] This compound is believed to be the proximate carcinogen of di(2-ethylhexyl)phthalate (see text and Reference 3).

the LBD, and acts as a partial agonist (25% of highest activity obtained with a thiazolidinedione) in transactivation of PPARγ and induction of the adipogenic gene program (34). Another non-thiazolidinedione has been identified that is similar to classical receptor antagonists. GW0072 binds to PPARγ with high affinity and is a weak agonist, but it potently inhibits the ability of a thiazolidinedione to activate PPARγ and the associated adipocyte differentiation program (35). Interference of thiazolidinedione activation by GW0072 occurs through a unique mode of binding. The bound receptor adopts a conformation similar to the unliganded apo-receptor in which the carboxylic acid of GW0072 is oriented away from the AF-2 helix, preventing the charged clamp to be stabilized through direct interactions with the ligand. GW0072 may be the prototype of ligands with unique biological activities mechanistically distinct from conventional agonists and antagonists. A number of other non-thiazolidinedione chemicals have been identified that interact with both PPARγ and PPARδ (36).

Several nonsteroidal anti-inflammatory drugs (NSAIDS), such as indomethacin and ibuprofen, that are cyclooxygenase (COX) inhibitors have been shown to activate and bind PPARγ and promote adipocyte differentiation at concentrations incrementally higher than those required to inhibit COX (37). Certain NSAIDS also activate PPARα (37).

Endogenous Ligands

A summary of the large number of endogenous PPAR ligands is shown in Table 3. Diverse fatty acids bind and activate all three PPAR isoforms to varying degrees (28, 38–40). The ligand binding pocket accommodates a diverse array of saturated, monounsaturated, and polyunsaturated fatty acids. Fatty acids with chain lengths under 16 and over 22 carbons activate the PPARs weakly, if at all. PPARα is the most promiscuous of the PPAR family members, exhibiting strong binding affinity for both saturated and unsaturated fatty acids. Although more selective, PPARδ will also bind diverse fatty acids, but with a lower affinity than PPARα. PPARγ is the most selective receptor because it binds primarily to polyunsaturated fatty acids (21).

An intriguing observation, which potentially implicates PPAR activation with a number of diverse functions, including tumor promotion and anti-inflammatory effects, is the recent demonstration that several leukotriene and prostaglandin (PG) eicosanoid metabolites bind and activate PPARs (28, 33, 40, 41). PGs play an important role in cancer development and progression (reviewed in 42). Decreased levels of PGs, perhaps a result of increased catabolism (43), are seen in rats and rat hepatocyte cultures treated with PPs (44). PG can increase the transcription of genes encoding enzymes involved in their own catalysis through fatty acid β- and ω-oxidation pathways, which suggests that PPARs are involved in an autoregulatory loop in lipid homeostasis (10). The inflammatory mediator leukotriene B_4 (LTB4) binds and activates PPARα, and this reportedly decreased the duration of the inflammatory response by increasing LTB4 degradation (13).

TABLE 3 Endogenous activators of peroxisome proliferator-activated receptors[a]

Activator	α	β/δ	γ
Saturated fatty acids			
Palmitic (16:0)	+ + +[b]	+ +	−
Stearic (18:0)	+ + +	+ +	−
Monounsaturated fatty acids			
Palmitoleic (16:1)	+ + +[b]	+	+ +[b]
Oleic (18:1)	+ + +[b]	+ +	+ +
Elaidic (20:1)	+ +	−	+
Polyunsaturated fatty acids			
Linoleic (18:2, n-6)	+ + +[b]	+ +	+
α-Linoleic (18:3, n-3)	+ + +	+	+ +
γ-Linoleic (18:3, n-6)	+ + +	+ + +	+ +
Dihomo-γ-linoleic (20:3, n-6)	+ + +	+ +	+ + +
Arachidonic (20:4, n-3)	+ + +[b]	+ +[b]	+ + +
Eicosapentaenoic (22:5, n-3)	+ + +[b]	+ +	+ + +
Docosahexaenoic (22:6, n-3)	+ +[b]	+ +	+/−
Eicosanoids			
PGA1	+	+ +	+
PGA2	+	+	+
PGD1	+ +	+	+ +
PGD2	+ +	+	+ +
PGJ2	+	+/−	+ + +
15-Deoxy-$\Delta^{12,14}$-Prostaglandin J_2	+	+/−	+ + +[b]
8(S)-HETE	+ + +[b]	−	−
8-HEPE	+ +[b]	−	−
LTB4	+/−	ND	ND
9-HODE	ND	ND	+ + +[b]
13-HODE	ND	ND	+ + +[b]

[a] +, Activator of this isoform in a transactivation assay; −, not an activator of this isoform in a transactivation assy; +/−, conflicting reports in the literature about this compound being an activator in a transactivation assay; ND, not determined for this compound. LT, leukotriene; PG, prostaglandins; HETE, hydroxyeicosatetraenoic acid; HEPE, hydroxyeicosapentaenoic acid; HODE, hydroxyoctadecadiemoic acid.
[b] This compound has been determined to be a ligand for the peroxisome proliferator-activated receptor isoform.

The identification of eicosanoid metabolites as PPAR ligands should clarify the metabolic and regulatory roles of PPAR-dependent pathways in hepatocarcinogenesis and suppression of inflammation.

Lastly, oxidized low-density lipoproteins thought to play a central role in the pathogenesis of atherosclerosis are partly composed of 9-hydroxyoctadecadienoic acid (HODE) and 13-HODE, which bind and activate PPARγ and regulate some of the events important in foam cell formation (45, 46).

PEROXISOME PROLIFERATOR RESPONSE ELEMENTS

PP binding induces a conformational change in PPARs that enables binding to specific DNA sequences upstream of the transcription initiation site called peroxisome proliferator response elements (PPREs). In most cases this leads to transcriptional activation of the target gene. The first PPRE sequences were identified by promoter analysis of the PP-responsive gene, acyl-coenzyme A oxidase (ACO) (47, 48). Through similar analysis of the promoters of several other PP-responsive genes, a PPRE sequence motif was defined as two direct TG(A/T)CCT repeats, known as half-sites, separated by a single nucleotide and thus called a direct repeat one (DR1). PPREs located at variable distances upstream of the transcription initiation site have been identified in other genes known to be activated by PPs, including genes encoding peroxisomal, microsomal, mitochondrial, nuclear, and cytosolic or extracellular proteins (reviewed in 3). Comparison of PPRE sequences with the DNA-binding motifs of other nuclear receptors, including the thyroid hormone receptor (TR), the retinoic acid receptor (RAR), retinoid X receptor (RXR), and vitamin D_3 receptor (VDR), revealed that these receptors all recognize the same half-site sequence motifs (TGACCT). Like PPARs, these receptors bind to direct repeats as heterodimers with a common partner, RXR. The relative spacing and orientation of the half-site motifs determine which nuclear receptor-RXR heterodimer binds to the response element. The RXR heterodimers with RAR, TR, VDR, RAR, and PPAR recognize direct repeats separated by five, four, three, two, or one nucleotide, respectively. In addition to the DR1 sequence, PPAR-RXR heterodimers have also been shown to bind to and activate at a direct repeat element separated by two nucleotides in the promoter of the human rev-erb α gene (49) and at estrogen response elements (50).

A number of studies point to the importance of the sequences flanking the PPREs for maintaining the optimal conformation of the PPAR-RXR heterodimer on the PPREs. In rabbit cytochrome P450 4A6 PPREs, six nucleotides adjacent to the DR1 element are necessary for both optimal receptor binding and receptor gene activation (51). Likewise, in human ACO PPREs, the flanking sequences protect the PPAR/RXR heterodimer from protease digestion (52). Although these extended sequences are not essential for PPAR/RXR binding to the PPREs, they may allow the optimal positioning of the PPAR-RXR heterodimer for interactions with the transcriptional machinery, resulting in either activation or repression. In addition, these flanking sequences may provide an extra level of specificity to different nuclear receptors that recognize the DR1 element (53).

Not all of the PPREs in responsive genes act to mediate increases in transcription. A growing number of genes including transthyretin, some apolipoprotein genes, transferrin, and hepatocyte nuclear factor-4 possess DR1-like motifs but are negatively regulated by PPs through PPARs (reviewed in 3). As discussed below, PPARs may negatively regulate some genes through DR1-like elements by competing for binding to the DR1 with other nuclear receptors that constitutively activate expression.

CONVERGENCE OF PEROXISOME PROLIFERATOR AND NUCLEAR RECEPTOR SIGNALING

Several studies have demonstrated cross talk between the PPAR signaling pathway and other nuclear receptor pathways. This convergence and interaction of different pathways can occur at multiple levels, including competition between PPARs and other nuclear receptors for (a) a common heterodimerization partner or (b) binding to the same DNA response element (Figure 2). Cross talk between PPs and other signaling pathways could explain some of the diverse biological effects of PP exposure.

One type of cross talk results from the heterodimerization of PPARs and RXR. Transactivation assays have demonstrated that PPAR-RXR heterodimers interacting at a PPRE can respond to either PPs or the RXR ligand, 9-*cis*-retinoic acid, by activation of the reporter gene. In the presence of both activators, synergistic activation of reporter gene expression occurs (54). In the absence of RXRs, PPARs cannot bind to the PPREs and activate transcription (54–56). A number of retinoids have been shown to activate the PPAR-RXR heterodimer through binding RXRs (57–59). In intact animals or cell cultures, exposure to these retinoids results in peroxisome proliferation and increases in β-oxidation enzymes

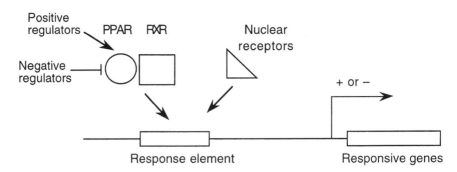

Figure 2 Mechanisms of cross talk with peroxisome proliferator–activated receptors (PPARs). Two general mechanisms of cross talk with PPAR exist. A large number of proteins interact with PPARs and may modulate the ability of PPARs to interact with a retinoid X receptor (RXR), bind a peroxisome proliferator response element, and increase transcription initiation. In addition, PPARs compete with other nuclear receptors for response element binding. The outcome is influenced by availability of the competing receptors and also by relative binding affinities for a particular response element.

(59). It is interesting to note that activation of the PPAR-RXR heterodimers through RXRs is not equivalent to activation through PPARs, as some retinoids elicit a unique set of responses not shared with PPs (59). These studies demonstrate how certain retinoids can act as PPs indirectly, through activation of the heterodimer via the back door (RXRs).

The fact that the RXR is a heterodimerization partner shared by PPARs and other nuclear receptors provides a level of cross talk through competition of available RXRs. The consequence of this competition is well-defined for PPARs and TRs. In transactivation assays, overexpression of PPARs in the presence of limiting amounts of RXRs prevents TR-RXR heterodimers from forming, resulting in inhibition of the expression of TR-regulated genes. On the other hand, an excess of TR prevents PPAR-RXR heterodimerization, resulting in repression of PPAR-regulated genes (60–63). Competition between PPARs and other nuclear receptors for RXR binding is also possible but has not been reported.

Modulation of PPAR activation by PPAR-binding proteins may also occur by either direct competition with RXRs for PPAR binding or by interaction with PPAR-RXR heterodimers on the PPREs. The large number of proteins now known to interact with PPARs is shown in Table 4. They belong to a number of predictable categories of proteins, including nuclear receptors, coactivators, and corepressors. A number of proteins have been isolated that heterodimerize with PPARs, preventing PPARs from interacting with RXRs and activating at PPRE-containing genes. These proteins include (*a*) a member of the nuclear receptor family that lacks a DNA-binding domain called SHP (64), (*b*) the nuclear receptor LXRα (65), and (*c*) deoxyuridine triphosphatase (66). The product of the nuclear oncogene *c-jun* was also shown to inhibit the ability of PPARs to activate a PPRE-linked gene, possibly through a direct interaction (67). Conversely, PPARs were able to inhibit the ability of Jun protein to activate transcription of the glutathione S-transferase–placental gene (67). The relevance of these interactions for repression of PPAR activation in mammals is not known. It is possible that these PPAR-containing heterodimers have new DNA binding targets and transcriptional properties.

Like many other nuclear receptors, PPARs are also regulated by factors referred to as coactivators and corepressors. Coactivators or corepressors act as bridging proteins between nuclear receptors and the transcriptional machinery and enhance or decrease transcriptional activation, respectively. A number of PPAR-interactive proteins have been isolated that enhance PPAR-mediated activation of reporter genes in vitro. These coactivators include p300/CBP (68), tuberous sclerosis 2 (69), PPAR binding protein (70), PGC-1 (71), PGC-2 (72), Ara70 (73), and the steroid receptor coactivator-1 (SRC-1) (74, 75). SRC-1 makes an insignificant contribution to PPARα activation in the liver because PPARα-dependent activation of PP-inducible liver genes was not altered in a mouse strain lacking a functional SRC-1 gene (76). Given the large number of coactivators that can interact with PPARs, it is likely that coactivators carry out functionally redundant roles with PPARs and other transcription factors. Although not a coac-

TABLE 4   Peroxisome proliferator-activated receptor (PPAR)-interactive proteins[a]

Protein	Interacts with PPAR			Functional consequence of interaction
	α	β/δ	γ	
Nuclear receptors				
RXR	+	+	+	Increased activation
LXRα	+	ND	ND	Inhibition of PPAR-RXR
SHP	+	ND	ND	Unknown
Coactivators				
SRC-1/TIF2	+	ND	+	
P300/CBP	ND	ND	+	
PBP	+	ND	+	
PGC-1	ND	ND	+	
PGC-2	−	−	+	
ARA70	ND	ND	+	
TSC2	ND[b]	ND	ND	
Corepressors				
N-CoR/RIP13	+	ND	+/−	Inhibition of activation
SMRT/TRAC	+	ND	+	
RIP140	+	ND	+	
Miscellaneous proteins				
c-Jun	+	ND	ND	Inhibition of activation
dUTPase	+	+	+	Prevents PPAR-RXR heterodimerization
HMG-CoA synthase	+	ND	ND	Increased activation
NRBF-1	+	ND	ND	Unknown

[a] +, Physical interaction with indicated PPAR isoform; −, no interaction; +/−, conflicting reports in the literature about interaction; ND, not determined for this isoform. RXR, retinoid X receptor; HMG, 3-hydroxy-3-methylglutaryl.
[b] Increased transactivation of designated isoform.

tivator, the 3-hydroxy-3-methylglutaryl–coenzyme A synthase protein may positively regulate its own gene by interacting with PPARα (77).

Two corepressors for RARs and TRs have been characterized that interact with unliganded receptors to keep them in a repressed state. These corepressors are termed nuclear receptor corepressor or RXR–interacting protein 13 (N-COR/RIP13) and silencing mediator for retinoid and thyroid hormone receptors or TR-associating cofactor (SMRT/TRAC). By using the two-hybrid system, interactions were detected between N-COR/RIP13 or SMRT/TRAC and PPARα (78, 79), and N-COR/RIP13 was shown to suppress PPARα-RXR transcription at a PPRE in a human kidney cell line (80). PPARγ was shown to interact with both N-COR/RIP13 and SMRT/TRAC in solution (81), although interaction between PPARγ and N-COR/RIP13 in yeast was not detected. In contrast to PPARα, these corepressors lacked the ability to interact with PPARγ-RXR heterodimers bound to the PPRE or to repress transcription (81). Although originally identified as a coactivator, RIP140 was found to down-regulate PPARα coactivation mediated by SRC-1 possibly by competition with SRC-1 for binding to the PPARα AF-2 domain (82, 83).

In addition to competition for common heterodimerization partners, a second form of cross talk between PPARs and other nuclear receptor pathways involves competition for DNA binding at common response elements. Competition for response element binding by multiple nuclear receptor complexes can have reciprocal effects on gene expression. On the one hand, competing nuclear receptor complexes could interfere with PPAR-RXR binding to a PPRE. On the other hand, PPAR-RXR can bind to other DNA response elements and interfere with signaling by other nuclear receptors. Several nuclear receptors other than PPARs can bind to PPRE-like DR1 elements, resulting in either transcriptional repression or activation. TRα homodimers bind to PPREs, resulting in thyroid hormone-independent activation of acyl-coenzyme A oxidase (61, 63). Heterodimers of RAR-RXR have also been shown to activate at a PPRE (84). COUP-TFI (85) and COUP-TFII (also called ARP-1) (86) block PPAR action by binding PPREs when cotransfected into cell lines. Heterodimers of TR-RXR (87) and homodimers of another nuclear receptor, TAK1 (88), also inhibit PP signaling in this manner.

There are two well-characterized examples where PPAR-RXR heterodimers bind to response elements recognized by other nuclear receptors and interfere with nuclear receptor signaling. First, PPAR-RXR heterodimers were shown to compete with hepatocyte nuclear factor-4 (HNF-4) homodimers for binding to DR1 elements, resulting in decreases in transcription of apolipoprotein cIII and transferrin genes (89, 90). HNF-4 binding and activation is necessary for constitutive expression of some liver-specific genes, and binding of PPAR-RXR to these HNF-4–dependent DR1 elements blocks gene expression by an unknown mechanism. It is possible that the sequences flanking the DR1 (discussed above) necessary for correctly orienting the PPAR-RXR heterodimers on the PPREs for optimal activation are lacking in these DR1 elements. Additionally, the antagonism is believed to be partially due to PPAR-RXR down-regulation of the HNF-4 gene itself, by decreasing HNF-4 autoactivation through a DR1 in the HNF-4 promoter region (90), although down-regulation of HNF-4 gene by fibrates was not observed in another study (91). Because there are many liver-specific genes whose expression appears to be dependent on HNF-4, suppression by PPAR activation could dramatically alter liver-specific functions.

In the second example, PPAR-RXR heterodimers were shown to compete with the estrogen receptor (ER) homodimer for binding to estrogen response elements (50). By using a reporter gene construct with an artificial promoter consisting of an estrogen response element linked to a basal promoter, PPAR-RXR expression was shown to activate gene expression. On a more natural promoter that contained an estrogen response element from an ER-dependent gene, PPAR-RXR heterodimers prevented ER from activating reporter gene expression (50). The ability of PPAR-RXR to prevent ER-mediated gene expression may account for estrogen insensitivity in cells that express both ERs and PPARs (92).

PEROXISOME PROLIFERATOR-INDUCED HEPATOCARCINOGENESIS

PPs belong to a class of carcinogens whose mode of action does not involve direct damage to the DNA. Assays measuring covalent DNA binding of DNA adducts and short-term tests of mutagenicity have been uniformly negative when PPs were used (reviewed in 93). In addition, two of the most potent PPs, Wy-14,643 and ciprofibrate, were negative in classic initiation assays (94, 95). Therefore, to understand how PPs induce hepatic tumors in rodents, alternative mechanisms of action must be considered.

PPARα plays a central role in the hepatocarcinogenesis by PPs. Ligand binding studies with PPs of different affinities show a good correlation between PPARα binding or activation and its potency as a hepatocarcinogen (discussed above). An important step toward understanding the role of PPARα in PP-induced hepatocarcinogenesis came from the development of a mouse strain in which the PPARα gene was functionally inactivated by targeted disruption of the ligand-binding domain (96). Short-term treatment of PPARα-null mice with hypolipidemic PPs (96) or the phthalate ester plasticizers di-n-butyl phthalate and diethylhexylphthalate (31) failed to induce classical short-term responses associated with PP exposure, including peroxisome proliferation and transcriptional activation of peroxisomal β-oxidation and microsomal ω-oxidation genes. In this mouse model, in the liver, a large number of genes with diverse functions have also been shown to depend on a functional PPARα for constitutive and altered regulation by PPs (summarized in 97).

To determine if PPARα was necessary for PPs to induce liver cancer, wild-type and PPARα-null mice were fed for 11 months a diet containing 0.1% Wy-14,643. There was a 100% incidence of hepatic neoplasms in the treated wild-type mice (98). In contrast, none of the PPARα-null mice developed liver tumors. The mechanism through which PPARα mediates the carcinogenic effects remains to be elucidated. However, it is clear that this receptor plays a necessary role in both peroxisome proliferation and cell proliferation in the liver, both of which have been linked to the observed increases in hepatocellular tumors.

Two hypotheses have been proposed to account for PP-induced hepatocarcinogenesis in rodents (Figure 3). The oxidative stress hypothesis proposes that the carcinogenicity of PPs is initiated by oxidative damage due to excessive production of peroxisomal hydrogen peroxide (93). The alternative hypothesis centers around imbalances in hepatocyte growth control resulting from increases in cell proliferation and suppression of apoptosis (99, 100).

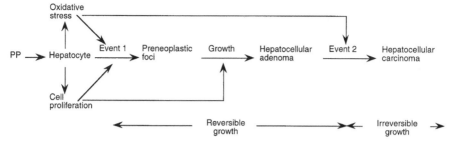

Figure 3 Cancer model for peroxisome proliferators (PPs). The different stages of PP-induced conversion of normal hepatocytes to hepatocellular carcinomas are shown. Two critical events (Event 1 and Event 2) are thought to occur that convert a normal hepatocyte to a hepatocellular carcinoma. Hepatocytes exposed to PPs have increases in oxidative stress and cell proliferation, which can enhance the probability of Event 1, converting a normal hepatocyte to an altered hepatocyte. Event 1 could arise through a mutagenic or an epigenetic process. In the presence of PPs, a subpopulation of altered cells exhibit increased cell proliferation and progress to become preneoplastic basophilic foci and, ultimately, hepatocellular adenomas. Cessation of exposure results in involution of these lesions through an increased rate of apoptosis. A mutational event (Event 2) likely drives conversion of adenomas to carcinomas because carcinomas persist after compound withdrawal.

The oxidative stress hypothesis is based on early observations that chronic exposure to PPs results in a sustained increase in oxidative stress in target rodent hepatocytes because of an imbalance between the production and degradation of hydrogen peroxide or other reactive oxygen species (101). PP treatment induces peroxisomal ACO and urate oxidase (93), and as a consequence of substrate oxidation, hydrogen peroxide is produced as a by-product. Under homeostatic conditions, hydrogen peroxide is neutralized by catalase; however, in this hypothesis, the excess hydrogen peroxide generated during PP exposure is not neutralized by a concomitant increase in catalase levels. The excess hydrogen peroxide may then diffuse through the peroxisomal membrane and attack DNA directly or via other reactive oxygen species (e.g. hydroxyl radical). 8-Hydroxydeoxyguanosine (8-OH-dG) is a frequently used marker of DNA damage produced by oxygen radicals. PPs increase 8-OH-dG levels in livers of treated rodents, but there is no clear link between the observed increase and carcinogenesis (102). The oxidative stress hypothesis predicts a central role for ACO in generating the PP-induced hydrogen peroxide. Mice that lack functional ACO exhibit PP-independent increases in the expression of genes normally regulated by PPARα (103). Furthermore, these mice have increased incidence of liver tumors (104). Based on these results, ACO has an insignificant role in PP-induced oxidative stress and was hypothesized to negatively regulate the levels of endogenous PPARα activators that have carcinogenic activity. Likely candidates include ω_6-unsaturated fatty acids and PGs that (*a*) activate PPARα, (*b*) are metabolized by the fatty acid β-oxidation system, and (c) have growth-promoting effects (reviewed in 105). Therefore, although peroxisome proliferation and the accompanying increases in reactive oxygen species may play a role in the carcinogenicity of PPs, it is clear that oxidative damage alone is not sufficient for the hepatocarcinogenicity.

Carcinogenesis is a multistep process that can be conceptually divided into three stages: initiation, promotion, and progression (106). Initiation of a cell involves two steps: mutational events that irreversibly damage DNA, and fixation of these lesions through rounds of cell division. Initiated cells must undergo further genetic alterations before acquiring a malignant phenotype (106, 107). Cell proliferation induced by PPs has been extensively characterized and likely plays a central role in the hepatocarcinogenesis (Figure 3). PPARα is necessary for PP-mediated hepatocyte proliferation. Within 48 h of treatment, cell proliferation is increased in the livers of PP-treated rodents (108). Increases in cell proliferation in the liver of wild-type mice treated with Wy-14,643 in the diet for 1 or 5 weeks is abolished in PPARα-null mice (98). Although the mechanism of cell proliferation is unclear, recent work suggests that sustained PPARα-dependent alterations in cell cycle regulatory proteins play a role in PP-induced hepatocarcinogenesis (109). The early increase in cell replication induced by PPs could increase the frequency of spontaneous mutations (93), and these spontaneous mutations and those induced by exogenous sources could be fixed by further rounds of cell division or clonal expansion. With chronic Wy-14,643 treatment, cell proliferation in the liver is sustained; however, with weaker PPs [e.g. di(2-ethylhexyl)phthalate or nafenopin], cell proliferation in the liver returns to control levels (110, 111). In general, the magnitude of the sustained increase in cell proliferation during chronic PP treatment has been a good predictor of eventual tumor yield in rodents, but not when the level of exposure or potency of the PPs is low (100, 108, 110–112).

Elimination of initiated cells via apoptosis is one defense mechanism against neoplastic transformation. In addition to increasing hepatocellular proliferation, PPs decrease apoptosis in normal and initiated cell populations, and this likely contributes to the hepatocarcinogenic effects of PPs. Nafenopin and Wy-14,643 inhibit transforming growth factor-β1–induced apoptosis in vitro (113), and this suppressive effect of nafenopin could be ablated with increasing concentrations of a dominant negative PPARα (114). These data suggest that PPs may interfere with the mito-inhibitory and apoptotic effects of this cytokine through a PPARα-dependent mechanism (114).

PPs are commonly classified as tumor promoters. PPs can promote the clonal expansion of anchorage-independent hepatocytes in vitro (115, 116), which suggests that these compounds perturb the balance of mitosis and apoptosis, leading to the net outgrowth of initiated clones. PPs selectively stimulate growth of initiated cells exhibiting a phenotype different from cells composing either spontaneous tumors or tumors induced by other nongenotoxic chemicals (117). PP-induced foci are predominantly basophilic and do not express proteins such as glutathione S-transferase–placental form or γ-glutamyl transpeptidase, which are normally associated with foci and tumors induced by other nongenotoxic carcinogens or DNA-damaging agents (118). Cell proliferation within PP-induced basophilic foci and adenomas is increased during PP exposure (94, 119, 120). Apoptosis is also increased in these foci and adenomas, but the lesions continue to grow because of an imbalance favoring cell replication over cell death (120a). Progression from initiated cell to hepatic carcinomas is dependent on the continued presence of the PPs. Five weeks after withdrawal of nafenopin there was a 20% reduction in the number of hepatocytes in the noninvolved tissue and 85% reduction of cells in foci, adenomas, and carcinomas (120). The data indicate that continual activation of PPARα is necessary for the growth and maintenance of initiated cells in foci, adenomas, and carcinomas in the liver of PP-treated rodents.

Although rodents are sensitive to the hepatocarcinogenic effects of PPs, there is little evidence that humans are at increased risk of liver cancer, even after chronic exposure. The hypolipidemic agents gemfibrozil and clofibrate have been clinically used for 15 and 30 years, respectively, and epidemiological studies do not reveal a statistically significant increase in cancer up to 8 years after initiation of therapy (93). Human liver contains a functionally active PPARα; however, the human PPARα is expressed to only about 10% of that in mouse liver, and extracts from human liver contain little PPARα that can bind to a PPRE (121). These dramatic differences in PPARα expression and activity may account for the absence of indicators of PP exposure in human liver, including increases in peroxisome proliferation and cell proliferation (93). Because the rodent hepatocarcinogenesis following PP exposure is mediated via PPARα, the current evidence suggests that humans exposed to these compounds are not at increased risk for developing liver tumors.

SUPPRESSION OF TUMOR GROWTH BY PEROXISOME PROLIFERATORS

Emerging evidence indicates that PPs have the ability to suppress the growth of different types of human cancer. Early indications that PPs can suppress growth of tumors came from traditional studies of the growth promotion effects of PPs in the livers of rats. Although PPs promote the growth of basophilic lesions (discussed above), there was a paradoxical suppression of both γ-glutamyl transpeptidase-positive and ATPase-deficient foci (122, 123), indicating that PPs through PPARs may inhibit growth in these lesions.

A large number of studies have demonstrated growth inhibition properties of PPARα and PPARγ ligands on human tumor cell lines. A large number of tumor types appear to be sensitive to PPs, including cells from prostate cancer (124), monocytic leukemia (125), ovarian carcinoma (126), hepatoma (127), liposarcoma (128), and breast cancer (129–131). Growth inhibition of these cell lines occurred through a number of distinct mechanisms, including increases in necrosis (124), apoptosis (127, 129), and growth arrest (125, 126). In addition, increases in differentiation to a cell type expressing markers of adipocyte phenotype also occurred in liposarcoma (128) and breast cancer (131) cell lines. Increases in PPAR expression do not seem to be required for growth inhibition, as PPARα was not altered in hepatoma cells (127) and PPARγ was unchanged in monocytic leukemia (125) and prostate cancer (137) cells. In all cases examined, however, PPARs were expressed to varying degrees in the target tissues (124, 127, 129, 131).

PPAR ligands have potent anticancer activity in vivo. In studies using immunodeficient mice injected with human prostate (124) or human breast (129) cancer cells, treatment of mice with the PPARγ ligand troglitazone decreased tumor volume and weight. It is interesting to note that treatment with a combination of troglitazone and all-*trans*-retinoic acid was more potent at inhibition of tumor growth in these two studies. Treatment with dehydroepiandrosterone, a primary steroid precursor and a PP, decreased the number of ethylnitrosourea-induced rat mammary tumors (130). Lastly, the intermediate-to-high-grade liposarcomas in patients treated with a thiazolidinedione exhibited extensive lipid accumulation and up-regulation of genes involved in terminal adipocyte differentiation, as well as down-regulation of a marker of cell proliferation (128). In summary, many different types of cancer may respond favorably to PP therapy, providing a rational basis for anticancer medicines that work through PPAR family members.

There is conflicting evidence of the effects of PP treatment on colon cancer cell growth. Similar to the therapeutic effects of PPs, discussed above, treatment of human colon cancer cell lines with troglitazone resulted in decreases in cell replication, in G1 cell-cycle arrest, and in increases in expression of markers of enterocyte cell differentiation (120a). Consistent with the therapeutic effects of PPs, mutations in PPARγ were found in human colon cancers that resulted in a decreased ability of PPARγ to be activated by ligands (133). These data indicate that a functional PPARγ is required for normal growth properties of human colon cells. In contrast, treatment of *Min* mice predisposed to intestinal neoplasia with the PPARγ ligands troglitazone or BRL-49,653 resulted in increases in the number of colon tumors but not small-intestine tumors (134, 135). Increases in the protein β-catenin, which has been linked to colon cancer, were observed in the colon in these mice after BRL-49,653 treatment, pointing to a reprogramming of gene expression important in tumorigenesis (135). Thus, the promise of using thiazolidinediones to treat colon cancer is overshadowed by the possibility that these compounds may actually increase susceptibility of colon cancer in certain human subpopulations. Further work on the significance of findings in the *Min* mice is needed.

PPARS AND INFLAMMATION

There is increasing evidence that PPARs are capable of inhibiting inflammatory responses in certain cell types. This effect may be mediated by at least two mechanisms. First, proinflammatory lipid metabolites may serve as ligands for PPARs, thereby activating PPAR-responsive enzymes responsible for their clearance. This has been demonstrated for PPARα-mediated catabolism of LTB4 (13), and PPARγ-induced 12/15-lipoxygenase catabolism of linoleic acid and arachidonic acid (136) to PPARγ ligands. It is interesting to note that interleukin (IL)-4 up-regulates both 12/15-lipoxygenase and PPARγ, which suggests a new paradigm for the regulation of nuclear receptor function by cytokines. Second, PPARs may influence cytokine induction by other transcription factors with roles in mediating inflammation, such as signal tranducers and activators of transcription, NF-κB, and activator protein-1. This mechanism appears to be operative via PPARγ, as well as PPARα. For example, activation of PPARγ inhibits transcription of inducible nitric oxide synthase, gelatinase B, and scavenger receptor A in activated macrophages (137), and alpha tumor necrosis factor, IL-1β, and IL-6 in monocytes (138), by a mechanism that occurs in the absence of PPARγ-DNA interaction. In a similar fashion, activation of PPARα in activated aortic smooth muscle cells leads to decreased expression of IL-6 and cyclooxygenase 2 (COX-2) (14). Possible explanations for these effects include PPAR titration of essential transcriptional cofactors, such as CBP/p300 and SRC-1 (138, 14), used by other transcription factors, or perhaps by direct inactivation by PPAR-transcription factor interaction.

A direct role for PPARα in down-regulating inflammatory responses in vivo is now well established. Treatment of wild-type but not PPARα-null mice with diverse PPs resulted in down-regulation of a number of acute-phase response genes normally induced in the liver after a localized inflammatory stimulus (139, 140). In PPARα-null mice, acute-phase response genes are expressed at higher levels than in wild-type mice (139, 140), LTB4- and arachidonic acid-induced ear swelling is prolonged (13), and there are higher levels of age-associated NF-κB activity and regulated genes, including IL-6, IL-12, COX-2, and tumor necrosis factor alpha (TNFα) (141, 142). Similar responses may occur in humans because patients receiving therapeutic doses of hypolipidemic drugs have decreased acute-phase proteins and cytokine levels in serum (14). These data indicate that the PPAR family members may be attractive candidates for therapeutic intervention in chronic inflammatory diseases often associated with aging.

FUTURE DIRECTIONS

In the decade since the first PPAR was cloned, a substantial body of research has revealed that PPARs exist in three isoforms with distinct, sometimes overlapping, roles in regulating fatty acid metabolism, glucose homeostasis, cell growth and differentiation, and inflammation. Although much has been accomplished, many important questions remain. A large number of both endogenous and exogenous PPAR ligands have been identified. It is likely that additional natural ligands, and the conditions under which they are produced, will be uncovered. Considerable effort has already been directed toward understanding the complex interactions between PPARs, other nuclear receptors, and receptor cofactors. Forthcoming research will address how the architecture of these complexes determines tissue-specific patterns of gene expression. This, in turn, should facilitate identification of additional genes that are both directly and indirectly regulated by the different PPARs. Clinically, PPs are already emerging as important mediators in the progression of certain chronic human diseases. Thus, it will be important to explore how these receptors can be manipulated therapeutically to delay disease progression or alleviate symptoms. Finally, given that several PPs are potent rodent carcinogens, another significant challenge will be to gain a more complete understanding of how accurately rodent cells predict human responses. If they are not good surrogates, it will be important to understand why. Answers to these questions will greatly enhance our ability to more accurately estimate the true relative risk of adverse health effects in humans receiving chronic therapeutic or environmental exposure to various PPs. Looking toward the future, research on the mechanisms of PPAR activation promises to continue to yield exciting and biomedically beneficial information.

ACKNOWLEDGMENTS

We thank Dr. Greg Kedderis for reviewing the manuscript, Kathy Claypoole for preparation of the manuscript, and Stan Piestrak for artwork. We apologize to our colleagues whose work we were not able to cite because of space limitations.

Visit the Annual Reviews home page at www.AnnualReviews.org.

LITERATURE CITED

1. Lock EA, Mitchell AM, Elcombe CR. 1989. Biochemical mechanisms of induction of hepatic peroxisome proliferation. *Annu. Rev. Pharmacol. Toxicol.* 29:145–63
2. Reddy JK, Azarnoff DL. 1980. Hypolipidemic hepatic peroxisome proliferators form a novel class of chemical carcinogens. *Nature* 283:397–98
3. Lapinskas PJ, Corton JC. 1998. Molecular mechanisms of hepatocarcinogenic peroxisome proliferators. In *Molecular Biology of the Toxic Response,* ed. A Puga, KB Wallace, pp. 219–53. Philadelphia, PA: Taylor & Francis
4. Staels B, Dallongeville J, Auwerx J, Schoonjans K, Leithersdort E, Fruchart JC. 1998. Mechanism of action of fibrates on lipid and lipoprotein metabolism. *Circulation* 98:2088–93
5. Kliewer SA, Willson TM. 1998. The nuclear receptor PPARgamma-bigger than fat. *Curr. Opin. Genet. Dev.* 5:576–81
6. Spiegelman BM, Flier, JS. 1996. Adipogenesis and obesity: rounding out the big picture. *Cell* 87:337–89
7. Spiegelman BM. 1998. PPARgamma in monocytes: less pain, any gain? *Cell* 93:153–55
8. Wolf G. 1999. The role of oxidized low-density lipoprotein in the activation of peroxisome proliferator-activated receptor gamma: implications for atherosclerosis. *Nutr. Rev.* 57:88–91
9. Reddy JK, Rao MS. 1986. Peroxisome proliferators and cancer: mechanisms and implications. *Trends Pharmacol. Sci.* 7:438–43
10. Issemann I, Green S. 1990. Activation of

a member of the steroid hormone receptor superfamily by peroxisome proliferators. *Nature* 347:645–50

11. Lemberger T, Desvergne B, Wahli W. 1996. Peroxisome proliferator-activated receptors: a nuclear receptor signaling pathway in lipid physiology. *Annu. Rev. Cell Dev. Biol.* 12:335–63

12. Mangelsdorf DJ, Thummel C, Beato M, Herrlich P, Schutz G, et al. 1995. The nuclear receptor superfamily: the second decade. *Cell* 83:835–39

13. Devchand PR, Keller H, Peters JM, Vazquez M, Gonzalez FJ, et al. 1996. The PPARα-leukotriene B$_4$ pathway to inflammation control. *Nature* 384:39–43

14. Staels B, Wolfgang K, Habib A, Merval R, Lebret M, et al. 1998. Activation of human aortic smooth-muscle cells is inhibited by PPARα but not PPARγ activators. *Nature* 393:790–93

15. Lm H, Gupta RA, Ma W-g, Paria BC, Moller DE, et al. 1999. Cyclo-oxygenase-2-derived prostacyclin mediates embryo implantation in the mouse via PPARδ. *Genes Dev.* 13:561–74

16. Zhu Y, Qi C, Korenberg JR, Chen XN, Noya D, et al. 1995. Structural organization of mouse peroxisome proliferator-activated receptor gamma (mPPAR) gamma gene: alternative promoter use and different splicing yield two mPPAR gamma isoforms. *Proc. Natl. Acad. Sci. USA* 92:7921–25

17. MacDougald OA, Lane MD. 1995. Transcriptional regulation of gene expression during adipocyte differentiation. *Annu. Rev. Biochem.* 64:345–73

18. Xin X, Yang S, Kowalski J, Gerritsen ME. 1999. Peroxisome proliferator-activated receptor γ ligands are potent inhibitors of angiogenesis in vitro and in vivo. *J. Biol. Chem.* 274:9116–21

19. Nolte RT, Wisely GB, Westin S, Cobb JE, Lambert MH, et al. 1998. Ligand binding and co-activator assembly of the peroxisome proliferator-activated receptor-gamma. *Nature* 395:137–43

20. Uppenberg J, Svensson C, Jaki M, Bertilsson G, Jendeberg L, et al. 1998. Crystal structure of the ligand binding domain of the human nuclear receptor PPAR-gamma. *J. Biol. Chem.* 273:31108–12

21. Xu HE, Lambert MH, Montana VG, Parks DJ, et al. 1999. Molecular recognition of fatty acids by peroxisome proliferator-activated receptors. *Mol. Cell* 3:397–403

22. Moras D, Gronemeyer H. 1998. The nuclear receptor ligand-binding domain: structure and function. *Curr. Opin Cell Biol.* 3:384–91

23. Sorensen HN, Treuter E, Gustafsson JA. 1998. Regulation of peroxisome proliferator-activated receptors. *Vitam. Horm.* 54:121–66

24. Juge-Aubry CE, Hammar E, Siegrist-Kaiser C, Pernin A, Takeshita A, et al. 1999. Regulation of the transcriptional activity of the peroxisome proliferator-activated receptor alpha by phosphorylation of a ligand-independent transactivating domain. *J. Biol. Chem.* 274:10505–10

25. Hu E, Kim JB, Sarraf P, Spiegelman BM. 1996. Inhibition of adipogenesis through MAP kinase-mediated phosphorylation of PPARgamma. *Science* 274:2100–3

26. Kliewer SA, Forman BM, Blumberg B, Ong ES, Borgmeyer U, et al. 1994. Differential expression and activation of a family of murine peroxisome proliferator-activated receptors. *Proc. Natl. Acad. Sci. USA* 91:7355–559

27. Lehmann JM, Moore LB, Smith-Oliver TA, Wilkson WO, Willson TM, et al. 1995. An antidiabetic thiazolidinedione is a high affinity ligand for peroxisome proliferator-activated receptor γ (PPARγ). *J. Biol. Chem.* 270:12953–56

28. Forman BM, Chen J, Evans RM. 1997. Hypolipidemic drugs, polyunsaturated fatty acids, and eicosanoids are ligands for peroxisome proliferator-activated receptors α and δ. *Proc. Natl. Acad. Sci. USA* 94:4312–17

29. Dowell P, Peterson VJ, Zabriskie TM, Leid M. 1997. Ligand-induced peroxisome proliferator-activated receptor α conformational change. *J. Biol. Chem.* 272:2013–20

30. Kliewer SA, Lenhard JM, Wilson TM, Patel I, Morris DC, et al. 1995. A prostaglandin J$_2$ metabolite binds peroxisome proliferator-activated receptor γ and promotes adipocyte differentiation. *Cell* 83:813–19

31. Lapinskas PJ, Corton JC. 1997. Phthalate ester plasticizers differentially activate the peroxisome proliferator-activated receptors. *Fundam. Appl. Toxicol.* 36:144

32. Krey G, Braissant O, L'Horset F, Kalkhoven E, Perroud M, et al. 1997. Fatty acids, eicosanoids, and hypolipidemic agents identified as ligands of peroxisome proliferator-activated receptors by coactivator-dependent receptor ligand assay. *Mol. Endocrinol.* 11:779–91

33. Kliewer SA, Lenhard JM, Wilson TM, Patel I, Morris DC, et al. 1995. A prostaglandin J$_2$ metabolite binds peroxisome proliferator-activated receptor γ and promotes adipocyte differentiation. *Cell* 83:813–19

34. Elbrecht A, Chen Y, Adams A, Berger J, Griffin P, et al. 1999. L-764406 is a partial agonist of human peroxisome proliferator-activated receptor gamma. The role of Cys313 in ligand binding. *J. Biol. Chem.* 274:7913–22

35. Oberfield JL, Collins JL, Holmes CP, Goreham DM, Cooper JP, et al. 1999. A peroxisome proliferator-activated receptor gamma ligand inhibits adipocyte differentiation. *Proc. Natl. Acad. Sci. USA* 96:6102–6

36. Berger J, Leibowitz MD, Doebber TW, Elbrecht A, Zhang B, et al. 1999. Novel peroxisome proliferator-activated receptor (PPAR) gamma and PPAR delta ligands produce distinct biological effects. *J. Biol. Chem.* 274:6718–25

37. Lehmann JM, Lenhard JM, Oliver BB, Ringold GM, Kliewer SA. 1997. Peroxisome proliferator-activated receptors α and γ are activated by indomethacin and other non-steroidal anti-inflammatory drugs. *J. Biol. Chem.* 272:3406–10

38. Gottlicher M, Widmark E, Li Q, Gustafsson J-Å. 1992. Fatty acids activate a chimera of the clofibric acid-activated receptor and the glucocorticoid receptor. *Proc. Natl. Acad. Sci. USA* 89:4653–57

39. Krey G, Keller H, Mahfoudi A, Medin J, Ozato K, et al. 1993. Xenopus peroxisome proliferator activated receptors: genomic organization, response element recognition, heterodimer formation with retinoid X receptor and activation by fatty acids. *J. Steroid Biochem.* 47:65–73

40. Kliewer SA, Sundseth SS, Jones SA, Brown PJ, Wisely GB, et al. 1997. Fatty acids and eicosanoids regulate gene expression through direct interactions with peroxisome proliferator-activated receptors α and γ. *Proc. Natl. Acad. Sci. USA* 94:4318–23

41. Yu K, Bayona W, Kallen CB, Hardings HP, Ravera CP, et al. 1995. Differential activation of peroxisome proliferator-activated receptors by eicosanoids. *J. Biol. Chem.* 270:23975–83

42. Karmali RA. 1986. Eicosanoids and cancer. *Prog. Clin. Biol. Res.* 222:687–97

43. Diczfalusy UG, Alexson SEH. 1992. Role of peroxisomes in the degradation of prostaglandins. In *New Developments in Fatty Acid Oxidation,* ed. PM Coates, K Tanaka, pp. 253–61. New York: Wiley-Liss

44. Leug LK, Glauert HP. 1996. Reduction of the concentrations of prostaglandins E2 and F2α, and thromboxane B2 in cultured rat treated with the peroxisome proliferator ciprofibrate. *Toxicol. Lett.* 85:143–49

45. Nagy L, Tontonoz P, Alvarex JG, Chen H, Evans RM. 1998. Oxidized LDL regulates macrophage gene expression through ligand activation of PPAR-gamma. *Cell* 93:229–40

46. Tontonoz P, Nagy L, Alvarez JG, Thom-azy VA, Evans RM. 1998. PPARgamma promotes monocyte/macrophage differ-entiation and uptake of oxidized LDL. *Cell* 93:241–52

47. Tugwood JD, Aldridge TC, Lambe KG, Macdonald N, Woodyatt NJ. 1996. Per-oxisome proliferator-activated receptors: structures and function. *Ann. NY Acad. Sci.* 27:252–65

48. Osumi T, Osada S, Tsukamoto T. 1996. Analysis of peroxisome proliferator-responsive enhancer of the rat acyl-CoA oxidase gene. *Ann. NY Acad. Sci.* 804:202–13

49. Gervois P, Chopin-Delannoy S, Fadel A, Dubois G, Kosykh V, et al. 1999. Fibrates increase human REV-ERB alpha expres-sion in liver via a novel peroxisome pro-liferator-activated receptor response element. *Mol. Endocrinol.* 3:400–9

50. Nunez SB, Medin JA, Braissant O, Kemp L, Wahli W, et al. 1997. Retinoid X receptor and peroxisome proliferator-activated receptor activate an estrogen responsive gene independent of the estro-gen receptor. *Mol. Cell. Endocrinol.* 127:27–40

51. Palmer CAN, Hsu M-H, Griffin KJ, Johnson EF. 1995. Novel sequence deter-minants in peroxisome proliferator sig-naling. *J. Biol. Chem.* 270:16114–21

52. Varanasi U, Chu R, Huang Q, Castellon R, Yeldandi AV, et al. 1996. Identifica-tion of a peroxisome proliferator-respon-sive element upstream of the human peroxisomal fatty acyl coenzyme A oxi-dase gene. *J. Biol. Chem.* 271:2147–55

53. Johnson EF, Palmer CNA, Griffin KJ, Hsu M-H. 1996. Role of the peroxisome proliferator-activated receptor in cyto-chrome P450 4A gene regulation. *FASEB J.* 10:1241–48

54. Kliewer SA, Umeson K, Noonan DJ, Heyman RA, Evans RM. 1992. Conver-gence of 9-cis retinoic acid and peroxi-some proliferator signaling pathways

through heterodimer of formation of their receptors. *Nature* 358:771–74

55. Gearing KL, Gottlicher M, Teboul M, Widmark E, Gustafsson J-Å. 1993. Inter-action of the peroxisome-proliferator-activated receptor and retinoid X receptor. *Proc. Natl. Acad. Sci. USA* 90:1440–44

56. Keller H, Dreyer C, Medin J, Mahfoudi A, Ozato K, et al. 1993. Fatty acids and retinoids control lipid metabolism through activation of peroxisome proli-ferator-activated receptor-retinoid X receptor heterodimers. *Proc. Natl. Acad. Sci. USA* 90:2160–64

57. Mukherjee R, Davies PJ, Crombie DL, Bischoff ED, Cesario RM, et al. 1997. Sensitization of diabetic and obese mice to insulin by retinoid X receptor agonists. *Nature* 386:407–10

58. Canan Koch SS, Dardashti LJ, Cesario RM, Croston GE, Boehm MF, et al. 1999. Synthesis of retinoid X receptor-specific ligands that are potent inducers of adipogenesis in 3T3-L1 cells. *J. Med. Chem.* 42:742–50

59. Standeven AM, Escobar M, Beard RL, Yuan YD, Chandraratna RA. 1997. Mito-genic effect of retinoid X receptor ago-nists in rat liver. *Biochem. Pharmacol.* 54:517–24

60. Juge-Aubry CE, Gorla-Bajszczak A, Per-nin A, Lemberger T, Wahli W, et al. 1995. Peroxisome proliferator-activated receptor mediates cross-talk with thyroid hormone receptor by competition for retinoid X receptor. Possible role of a leucine zipper-like heptad repeat. *J. Biol. Chem.* 270:18117–22

61. Chu R, Madison LD, Lin Y, Kopp P, Rao MS, et al. 1995. Thyroid hormone (T_3) inhibits ciprofibrate-induced transcrip-tion of genes encoding β-oxidation enzymes: cross talk between peroxisome proliferator and T_3 signaling pathways. *Proc. Natl. Acad. Sci. USA* 92:11593–97

62. Jow L, Mukherjee R. 1995. The human peroxisome proliferator-activated recep-

tor (PPAR) subtype NUC1 represses the activation of hPPAR alpha and thyroid hormone receptors. *J. Biol. Chem.* 270:3836–40

63. Hunter J, Kassam A, Winrow CJ, Rachubinski RA, Capone JP. 1996. Crosstalk between the thyroid hormone and peroxisome proliferator-activated receptors in regulating proliferator-response genes. *Mol. Cell. Endocrinol.* 116:213–21

64. Masuda N, Yasumo H, Tamura T, Hashiguchi N, Furusawa T, et al. 1997. An orphan nuclear receptor lacking a zinc-finger DNA-binding domain: interaction with several nuclear receptor. *Biochim. Biophys. Acta* 1350:27–32

65. Miyata KS, McCaw SE, Patel HV, Rachubinski RA, Capone JP. 1996. The orphan nuclear hormone receptor LXR alpha interacts with the peroxisome proliferator-activated receptor and inhibits peroxisome proliferator signaling. *J. Biol. Chem.* 271:9189–92

66. Chu R, Lin Y, Rao MS, Reddy JK. 1996. Cloning and identification of rat deoxyuridine triphosphatase as an inhibitor of peroxisome proliferator-activated receptor α. *J. Biol. Chem.* 271:27670–76

67. Sakai M, Matsushima-Hibiya Y, Nishizawa M, Nishi S. 1995. Suppression of rat glutathione transferase P expression by peroxisome proliferators: interaction between jun and peroxisome proliferator-activated receptor alpha. *Cancer Res.* 55:5370–76

68. Dowell P, Ishmael JE, Avram D, Peterson VJ, Nevrivy DJ, Leid M. 1997. p300 functions as a coactivator for the peroxisome proliferator-activated receptor alpha. *J. Biol. Chem.* 272:33435–43

69. Henry KW, Yuan X, Koszewski NJ, Onda H, Kwiatkowski DJ, et al. 1998. Tuberous sclerosis gene 2 product modulates transcription mediated by steroid hormone receptor family members. *J. Biol. Chem.* 273:20535–39

70. Zhu Y, Qi C, Jain S, Sambasiv RM, Reddy JK. 1997. Isolation and character-

ization of PBP, a protein that interacts with peroxisome proliferator-activated receptor. *J. Biol. Chem.* 272:25500–6

71. Puigserver P, Wu Z, Park CW, Graves R, Wright M, Spiegelman BM. 1998. A cold-inducible coactivator of nuclear receptors linked to adaptive thermogenesis. *Cell* 92:829–39

72. Castillo G, Brun RP, Rosenfield JK, Hauser S, Park CW, et al. 1999. An adipogenic cofactor bound by the differentiation domain of PPARγ. *EMBO J.* 13:3676–87

73. Heinlein CA, Ting HJ, Yeh S, Chang C. 1999. Identification of ARA70 as a ligand-enhanced coactivator for the peroxisome proliferator-activated receptor γ. *J. Biol. Chem.* 23:16147–52

74. Zhu Y, Qi C, Calandra C, Rao MS, Reddy JK. 1996. Cloning and identification of mouse steroid receptor coactivator-1 (MSRC-1), as a coactivator of peroxisome proliferator-activated receptor gamma. *Gene Exp.* 6:185–95

75. DiRenzo J, Söderström M, Kurokawa R, Ogliastro M-H, Ricote M, et al. 1997. Peroxisome proliferator-activated receptors and retinoic acid receptors differentially control the interactions of retinoid X receptor heterodimers with ligands, coactivators, and corepressors. *Mol. Cell. Biol.* 17:2166–76

76. Qi C, Zhu Y, Pan J, Yeldandi AV, Rao MS, et al. 1999. Mouse steroid receptor coactivator-1 is not essential for peroxisome proliferator-activated receptor alpha-regulated gene expression. *Proc. Natl. Acad. Sci. USA* 96:1585–90

77. Meertens LM, Miyata KS, Cechetto JD, Rachubinski RA, Capone JP. 1998. A mitochondrial ketogenic enzyme regulates its gene expression by association with the nuclear hormone receptor PPARα. *EMBO J.* 23:6972–78

78. Sande S, Privalsky M. 1996. Identification of TRACs (T₃ receptor-associating cofactors), a family of cofactors that associate with, and modulate the activity

of, nuclear hormone receptors. *Mol. Endocrinol.* 10:813–25

79. Seol W, Mahon MJ, Lee Y-K, Moore DD. 1996. Two receptor interacting domains in the nuclear hormone receptor corepressor RIP13/N-CoR. *Mol. Endocrinol.* 10:1646–55

80. Dowell P, Ishmael JE, Avram D, Peterson VJ, Nevrivy DJ, et al. 1999. Identification of nuclear receptor corepressor as a peroxisome proliferator-activated receptor alpha interacting protein. *J. Biol. Chem.* 274:15901–7

81. Zamir I, Zhang J, Lazar MA. 1997. Stoichiometric and steric principles governing repression by nuclear hormone receptors. *Genes Dev.* 11:835–46

82. Treuter E, Albrektsen T, Johansson L, Leers J, Gustafsson JA. 1998. A regulatory role for RIP140 in nuclear receptor activation. *Mol. Endocrinol.* 12:864–81

83. Miyata KS, McCaw SE, Meertens LM, Patel HV, Rachubinski RA, et al. 1998. Receptor-interacting protein 140 interacts with, and inhibits transactivation by, peroxisome proliferator-activated receptor alpha and liver-X-receptor alpha. *Mol. Cell. Endocrinol.* 146:69–76

84. Jansen JH, Mahfoudi A, Rambaud S, Lavau C, Wahli W, Dejean A. 1995. Multimeric complexes of the PML-retinoic acid receptor α fusion protein in acute promyelocytic leukemia cells and interference with retinoid and peroxisome-proliferator signaling pathways. *Proc. Natl. Acad. Sci. USA* 92:7401–5

85. Miyata KS, Zhang B, Marcus SL, Capone JP, Rachubinski RA. 1993. Chicken ovalbumin upstream promoter transcription factor (COUP-TF) binds to a peroxisome proliferator-responsive element and antagonizes peroxisome proliferator-mediating signaling. *J. Biol. Chem.* 268:19169–72

86. Marcus SL, Capone JP, Rachubinski RA. 1996. Identification of COUP-TFII as a peroxisome proliferator response element binding factor using genetic selec-

tion in yeast: COUP-TFII activates transcription in yeast but antagonizes PPAR signaling in mammalian cells. *Mol. Cell. Endocrinol.* 120:31–39

87. Miyamoto T, Kaneko A, Kakizawa T, Yajima H, Kamijo K, et al. 1997. Inhibition of peroxisome proliferator signaling pathways by thyroid hormone receptor. *J. Biol. Chem.* 272:7752–58

88. Yan ZH, Karam WG, Staudinger JL, Medvedev A, Ghanayem BI, et al. 1999. Regulation of peroxisome proliferator-activated receptor alpha-induced transactivation by the nuclear orphan receptor TAK1/TR4. *J. Biol. Chem.* 273:10948–57

89. Hertz R, Bishara-Shieban J, Bar-Tana J. 1995. Mode of action of peroxisome proliferators as hypolipidemic drugs: suppression of apolipoprotein C-III. *J. Biol. Chem.* 270:13470–75

90. Hertz R, Seckback M, Zaki MM, Bar-Tana J. 1996. Transcriptional suppression of the transferrin gene by hypolipidemic peroxisome proliferators. *J. Biol. Chem.* 271:218–24

91. Vu-Dac N, Chopin-Delannoy S, Gervois P, Bonnelye E, Martin G, et al. 1998. The nuclear receptors peroxisome proliferator-activated receptor α and rev-erbα mediate the species-specific regulation of apolipoprotein A-1 expression by fibrates. *J. Biol. Chem.* 273:25713–20

92. Shyamala G, Schneider W, Schott D. 1990. Developmental regulation of murine mammary progesterone receptor expression. *Endocrinology* 126:2882–89

93. Ashby J, Brady A, Elcombe CR, Elliott BM, Ishnmael J, et al. 1994. Mechanistically-based human hazard assessment of peroxisome proliferator-induced hepatocarcinogenesis. *Hum. Exp. Toxicol.* 13:S1–117

94. Cattley RC, Marsman DS, Popp JA. 1989. Failure of the peroxisome proliferator WY-14,643 to initiate growth-selectable foci in rat liver. *Toxicology* 56:1–7

95. Glauert HP, Clark TD. 1989. Lack of ini-

tiating activity of the peroxisome proliferator clofibrate in two-stage hepatocarcinogenesis. *Cancer Lett.* 44:95–100

96. Lee SS, Pineau T, Drago J, Lee EJ, Owens JW, et al. 1995. Targeted disruption of the alpha isoform of the peroxisome proliferators. *Mol. Cell. Biol.* 15:3012–22

97. Gonzalez FJ, Peters JM, Cattley RC. 1998. Mechanism of action of the nongenotoxic peroxisome proliferators: role of the peroxisome proliferator-activated receptor α. *J. Natl. Cancer Inst.* 90:1702–9

98. Peters JM, Cattley RC, Gonzalez FJ. 1997. Role of PPARα in the mechanism of action of the nongenotoxic carcinogen and peroxisome proliferator Wy-14,643. *Carcinogenesis* 18:2029–33

99. Bursch W, Lauer LB, Timmermann-Troseiner, Barthel G, Schuppler J, et al. 1984. Controlled death (apoptosis) of normal and putative preneoplastic cells in rat liver following withdrawal of tumor promoters. *Carcinogenesis* 5:453–58

100. Marsman DS, Goldsworthy TL, Popp JA. 1992. Contrasting hepatocyte peroxisome proliferation, lipofuscin accumulation and cell turnover for the hepatocarcinogens Wy-14,643 and clofibric acid. *Carcinogenesis* 13:1011–17

101. Reddy JK, Rao MS. 1986. Peroxisome proliferators and cancer: mechanisms and implications. *Trends. Pharmacol. Sci.* 7:438–43

102. Sausen PJ, Lee DC, Rose ML, Cattley RC. 1995. Elevated 8-hydroxydeoxyguanosine in hepatic DNA of rats following exposure to peroxisome proliferators: relationship to mitochondrial alterations. *Carcinogenesis* 16:1795–801

103. Fan C-Y, Pan J, Chu R, Lee D, Kluckman KD, et al. 1996. Hepatocellular and hepatic peroxisome alterations in mice with a disrupted peroxisomal fatty acyl-coenzyme A oxidase gene. *J. Biol. Chem.* 271:24698–710

104. Fan C-Y, Pan J, Usuda N, Yeldandi AV, Rao MS, et al. 1998. Steatohepatitis, spontaneous peroxisome proliferation and liver tumors in mice lacking peroxisomal fatty acyl-CoA oxidase: implications for peroxisome proliferator-activated receptor alpha natural ligand metabolism. *J. Biol. Chem.* 273:15639–45

105. Masters C. 1996. Omega-3 fatty acids and the peroxisome. *Mol. Cell. Biochem.* 165:83–93

106. Farber E, Sarma DSR. 1987. Hepatocarcinogenesis: a dynamic cellular perspective. *Lab. Invest.* 56:4–22

107. Barrett JC. 1993. Mechanisms of multistep carcinogenesis and carcinogen risk assessment. *Env. Health Perspect.* 100:9–20

108. Marsman DS, Cattley RC, Conway JG, Popp JA. 1988. Relationship of hepatic peroxisome proliferation and replicative DNA synthesis to the hepatocarcinogenicity of the peroxisome proliferators di(2-ethylhexyl)phthalate and [4-chloro-6-(2,3-xylidino)-2-pyrimidinylthio]acetic acid (Wy-14,643) in rats. *Cancer Res.* 48:6739–44

109. Peters JM, Aoyama T, Cattley RC, Nobumitsu U, Hashimoto T, et al. 1998. Role of peroxisome proliferator-activated receptor α in altered cell cycle regulation in mouse liver. *Carcinogenesis* 19:1989–94

110. Eacho PI, Lanier TL, Brodhecker CA. 1991. Hepatocellular DNA synthesis in rats given peroxisome proliferating agents: comparison of Wy-14,643 to clofibric acid, nafenopin and LY171883. *Carcinogenesis* 12:1557–61

111. Barrass NC, Price RJ, Lake BG, Orton TC. 1993. Comparison of the acute and mitogenic effects of the peroxisome proliferator methylclofenapate and clofibric acid in rat liver. *Carcinogenesis* 14:1451–56

112. Tanaka K, Smith PF, Stromberg PC, Eydelloth RS, Herold EG, et al. 1992.

Studies of early hepatocellular proliferation and peroxisomal proliferation in Sprague-Dawley rats treated with tumorigenic doses of clofibrate. *Toxicol. Appl. Pharmacol.* 116:71–77

113. Bayly AC, Roberts RA, Dive C. 1994. Suppression of liver cell apoptosis in vitro by the non-genotoxic hepatocarcinogen and peroxisome proliferator nafenopin. *J. Cell Biol.* 125:197–203

114. Roberts RA, James NH, Woodyatt NJ, Nacdonald N, Tugwood JD. 1998. Evidence for the suppression of apoptosis by the peroxisome proliferator activated receptor alpha (PPARα). *Carcinogenesis* 19:43–48

115. James NH, Roberts RA. 1994. The peroxisome proliferator class of non-genotoxic hepatocarcinogens synergize with epidermal growth factor to promote clonal expansion of initiated rat hepatocytes. *Carcinogenesis* 15:2687–94

116. James NH, Ashby S, Roberts RA. 1995. Enhanced hepatocyte colony growth in soft agar after in vivo treatment with a genotoxic carcinogen: a potential assay for hepatocarcinogens? *Cancer Lett.* 93:121–28

117. Rao MS, Tatematsu M, Subbarao V, Ito N, Reddy JK. 1986. Analysis of peroxisome proliferator-induced preneoplastic and neoplastic lesions of rat liver for placental form of glutathione S-transferase γ-glutamyltranspeptidase. *Cancer Res.* 46:5287–90

118. Rao MS, Nenali MR, Usuda N, Scarpelli DG, Makino T, et al. 1988. Lack of expression of glutathione-s-transferase p, gamma-glutamyl transpeptidase and alpha-fetoprotein messenger RNAs in liver tumors induced by peroxisome proliferators. *Cancer* 48:4919–25

119. Grasl-Kraupp B, Huber W, Just W, Gibson G, Schulte-Hermann R. 1993. Enhancement of peroxisomal enzymes, cytochrome P-450 and DNA synthesis in putative preneoplastic foci of rat liver

treated with the peroxisome proliferator nafenopin. *Carcinogenesis* 14:1007–12

120. Grasl-Kraupp B, Ruttkay-Nedecky B, Mullauer L, Taper H, Huber W, et al. 1997. Inherent increase of apoptosis in liver tumors: implications for carcinogenesis and tumor regression. *Hepatology* 25:906–12

120. (a) Kitamura S, Miyazaki Y, Shinomura Y, Kondo S, Kanayama S, et al. 1999. Peroxisome proliferator-activated receptor gamma induces growth arrest and differentiation markers of human colon cancer cells. *Jpn. J. Cancer Res.* 90:75–85

121. Palmer CN, Hsu MH, Griffin KJ, Raucy JL, Johnson EF. 1998. Peroxisome proliferator activated receptor-alpha expression in human liver. *Mol. Pharmacol.* 53:14–22

122. DeAngelo AB, Queral AE, Garrett CT. 1985. Concentration-dependent inhibition of development of GGT positive foci in rat liver by the environmental contaminant di(2-ethylhexyl) phthalate. *Environ. Health Perspect.* 60:381–85

123. Cattley RC, Popp JA. 1989. Differences between the promoting activities of the peroxisome proliferator WY-14,643 and phenobarbital in rat liver. *Cancer Res.* 49:3246–51

124. Kubota T, Koshizuka K, Williamson EA, Hiroya A, Said JW, et al. 1998. Ligand for peroxisome proliferator-activated receptor γ (troglitazone) has potent antitumor effect against human prostate cancer both *in vitro* and *in vivo*. *Cancer Res.* 58:3344–52

125. Zhu L, Gong B, Bisgaier CL, Aviram M, Newton RS. 1998. Induction of PPAR-gamma1 expression in human THP-1 monocytic leukemia cells by 9-cis-retinoic acid is associated with cellular growth suppression. *Biochem. Biophys. Res. Commun.* 251:842–48

126. Ferrandina G, Melichar B, Loercher A, Verschraegen CF, Kudelka AP, et al. 1997. Growth inhibitory effects of

sodium phenylacetate (NSC 3039) on ovarian carcinoma cells *in vitro. Cancer Res.* 57:4309–15

127. Canuto RA, Muzio G, Bonelli G, Maggiora M, Autelli R, et al. 1998. Peroxisome proliferators induce apoptosis in hepatoma cells. *Cancer Detect. Prev.* 22:357–66

128. Demetri GD, Fletcher CDM, Mueller E, Sarraf P, Naujoks R, et al. 1999. Induction of solid tumor differentiation by the peroxisome proliferator-activated receptor-γ ligand troglitazone in patients with liposarcoma. *Proc. Natl. Acad. Sci. USA* 96:3951–56

129. Elstner E, Muller C, Koshizuka K, Williamson EA, Park D, et al. 1998. Ligands for peroxisome proliferator-activated receptor γ and retinoic acid receptor inhibit growth and induce apoptosis of human breast cancer cell *in vitro* and in BNX mice. *Proc. Natl. Acad. Sci. USA* 95:8806–11

130. Lubet RA, Gordon GB, Prough RA, Lei XD, You M, et al. 1998. Modulation of methylnitrosourea-induced breast cancer in Sprague Dawley rats by dehydroepiandrosterone: dose-dependent inhibition, effects of limited exposure, effects on peroxisomal enzymes, and lack of effects on levels of Ha-Ras mutations. *Cancer Res.* 58:921–26

131. Mueller E, Sarraf P, Tontonoz P, Evans RM, Martin KJ, et al. 1998. Terminal differentiation of human breast cancer through PPAR gamma. *Mol. Cell* 1:465–70

132. Deleted in proof

133. Sarraf P, Mueller E, Smith WM, Wright HM, Kum JB, et al. 1999. Loss-of-function mutations in PPARγ associated with human colon cancer. *Mol. Cell* 3:799–804

134. Saez E, Tontonoz P, Nelson MC, Alvarez JGA, U TM, et al. 1998. Activators of the nuclear receptor PPARγ enhance colon polyp formation. *Nat. Med.* 4:1058–61

135. Lefebvre AM, Chen I, Desreumaux P, Najib J, Fruchart JC, et al. 1998. Activation of the peroxisome proliferator-activated receptor γ promotes the development of colon tumors in C57BL/6J-APC^{min}/+ mice. *Nat. Med.* 4:1053–57

136. Huang JT, Welch JS, Ricote M, Binder CJ, Willson TM, et al. 1999. Interleukin-4-dependent production of PPAR-gamma ligands in macrophages by 12/156-lipoxygenase. *Nature* 400:378–82

137. Ricote M, Li AC, Willson TM, Kelly CJ, Glass CK. 1998. The peroxisome proliferator-activated receptor-γ is a negative regulator of macrophage activation. *Nature* 391:79–82

138. Jiang C, Ting AT, Seed B. 1998. PPAR-γ agonists inhibit production of monocyte inflammatory cytokines. *Nature* 391:82–86

139. Corton JC, Fan LQ, Brown S, Anderson SP, Bocos C, et al. 1998. Down-regulation of cytochrome P450 2C family members and positive acute-phase response gene expression by peroxisome proliferator chemicals. *Mol. Pharmacol.* 54:463–73

140. Anderson SP, Cattley RC, Corton JC. 1999. Upregulation of acute-phase protein gene expression in peroxisome proliferator-induced hepatocellular adenomas in the rat. *Mol. Carcinog.* 26: 226–38

141. Spencer NF, Poynter ME, Im SY, Daynes RA. 1997. Constitutive activation of NF-kappa B in an animal model of aging. *Int. Immunol.* 9:1581–88

142. Poynter ME, Daynes RA. 1998. Peroxisome proliferator-activated receptor alpha activation modulates cellular redox status, represses nuclear factor-kappa B signaling, and reduces inflammatory cytokine production in aging. *J. Biol. Chem.* 273:32833–41

Annu. Rev. Pharmacol. Toxicol. 2000. 40:519–61

THE PAS SUPERFAMILY: Sensors of Environmental and Developmental Signals

Yi-Zhong Gu, John B. Hogenesch, and Christopher A. Bradfield

McArdle Laboratory for Cancer Research, University of Wisconsin School of Medicine, Madison, Wisconsin 53706; e-mail: ygu@oncology.wisc.edu, johnh@scripps.edu, bradfield@oncology.wisc.edu

Key Words PAS domains, LOV domains, dioxin, hypoxia, circadian rhythm, signaling

■ **Abstract** Over the past decade, PAS domains have been identified in dozens of signal transduction molecules and various forms have been found in animals, plants, and prokaryotes. In this review, we summarize this rapidly expanding research area by providing a detailed description of three signal transduction pathways that utilize PAS protein heterodimers to drive their transcriptional output. It is hoped that these model pathways can provide a framework for use in understanding the biology of the less well-understood members of this emerging superfamily, as well as of those to be characterized in the days to come. We use this review to develop the idea that most eukaryotic PAS proteins can be classified by functional similarities, as well as by predicted phylogenetic relationships. We focus on the α-class proteins, which often act as sensors of environmental signals, and the β-class proteins, which typically act as broad-spectrum partners that target these heterodimers to their genomic targets.

INTRODUCTION

A major thesis of this review is that the PAS domain is a signature of proteins that play roles in the detection of and adaptation to environmental change. For all eukaryotic PAS proteins to be included under this rubric, we must put forth a fairly broad definition of environment. Put another way, we accept the idea that through evolution, mechanisms of environmental adaptation have also been put to use in a number of developmentally important processes. Results from *Hif*, *Arnt*, and *Ahr* null alleles support this idea and demonstrate that in many cases, environmental stresses and developmental signals may be functionally similar. Although this relationship may not turn out to be absolute, we have found it useful to view the developing embryo as an organism adapting to the environmental challenges imposed by multicellularity.

0362–1642/00/0415–0519$14.00

To make the above points, we first provide a description of three of the most well-understood PAS-dependent pathways found in higher eukaryotes. Given historical precedent and our own scientific interests, we will begin with a discussion of the aryl hydrocarbon (Ah) receptor (AHR) pathway that allows animals to adapt to environments contaminated with planar aromatic compounds. We follow this with the description of signal transduction pathways that allow organisms to adapt to changes in atmospheric and cellular oxygen [the hypoxia inducible factor (HIF) system], as well as the pathway that entrains an animal's activity to its illuminated environment (the circadian response pathway). Finally, we provide support for the environmental sensor thesis by describing more recent observations that demonstrate that rudimentary PAS domains are found in a number of light and oxygen sensors of prokaryotes and plants. For additional viewpoints on these various pathways, the reader is also referred to a number of excellent reviews (1–4).

BACKGROUND

The PAS domain is found in a rapidly growing number of proteins. The term PAS comes from the first letter of each of the three founding members of the family: PER, ARNT, and SIM (Figure 1). The PER protein, the product of the *Drosophila* (d) *Period* (*per*) gene, was discovered as a result of its involvement in the regulation of circadian rhythms (5, 6). ARNT, the AHR nuclear translocator, was originally identified as a protein that was essential for normal signal transduction by the AHR (7). SIM, the product of the *Drosophila Single-minded* locus, was

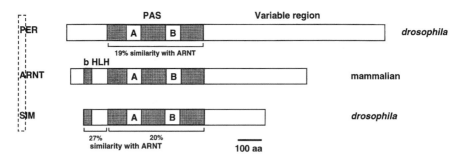

Figure 1 The founding PAS family members. Domain structures of the founding PAS proteins PER, ARNT, and SIM are shown. The name PAS stems from the first letters of PER, ARNT, and SIM (*boxed*). The basic region (b), helix-loop-helix (HLH), PAS, and C-terminal variable domains are labeled on *top*. The A and B repeat regions are shown within the PAS domain as *white boxes*. The percentage amino acid similarities of SIM and PER, as compared with ARNT, are labeled *beneath* their respective domains. See text for details.

identified through its role as a regulator of midline cell lineage (8, 9). The PAS domain is best described as a region of homology to these three founding members. It typically encompasses 250–300 amino acids and contains a pair of highly degenerate 50 amino acid subdomains termed the A and B repeats (7–9).

In higher eukaryotes, the PAS domain functions as a surface for both homotypic interactions with other PAS proteins and heterotypic interactions with cellular chaperones, such as the 90-kDa heat shock protein (Hsp90) (10, 11). In the case of the AHR, the PAS domain can also function as a binding surface for small-molecule ligands, such as the environmental contaminant 2,3,7,8-tetrachlorodibenzo-p-dioxin (dioxin) (12–14). Most of the PAS proteins that have been cloned to date also contain basic-helix-loop-helix (bHLH) motifs immediately N-terminal to their PAS domain. The HLH domains participate in homotypic dimerization between two bHLH-PAS proteins, and they position the basic regions to allow specific contacts within the major groove of target regulatory elements found in DNA (15, 16). Consistent with their activities as signal transduction molecules, most PAS proteins have transcriptionally active domains within their C-terminal ends. It is interesting to note that despite the relative conservation of the bHLH and PAS domains and their apparent functional similarities, most PAS proteins show little sequence homology in their C-terminal sequences.

THE AH RECEPTOR PATHWAY

One way in which vertebrates adapt to adverse chemical environments is by up-regulating batteries of xenobiotic metabolizing enzymes (XMEs), thus decreasing the biological half-life of the insulting chemical. It has long been observed that a number of XMEs are up-regulated upon exposure to their substrates (17–19). The most well-understood example is the induction of the microsomal cytochrome P450–dependent monooxygenases, such as CYP1A1 and CYP1A2, that occurs in response to exposure to planar aromatic hydrocarbons (PAHs) or dioxins (1, 20, 21). Compounds like benzo(a)pyrene and 3-methylcholanthrene are examples of a large number of highly toxic PAHs that are widely distributed in the environment. These compounds are byproducts of industrial processes, can be produced naturally, and are most commonly generated from the incomplete combustion of organic material (22). Prior exposure to many PAHs will decrease the biological half-life of structurally related compounds upon subsequent exposures. This adaptive response is a direct result of the up-regulation of XMEs.

A protein known as the AHR mediates the adaptive response to PAHs. This receptor was identified using both genetic and pharmacological approaches. Early on it was observed that the inductive response to PAHs was polymorphic among strains of mice. For example, it was observed that some murine strains were highly responsive to PAH induction of XMEs whereas others were relatively nonresponsive (23). Crosses, backcrosses, and intercrosses of these mouse lines demonstrated that the difference in response was mediated by a single autosomal locus, termed *Ah* (for aryl hydrocarbon responsiveness) (24, 25). Segregation with the responsive and nonresponsive alleles is still an important method by which a role for the *Ah* locus is proven. It was later learned that halogenated aromatic compounds such as dioxin were much more potent agonists of this signal transduction system than were the PAHs (26). This greater potency was predicted to be related to their greater binding affinity for an *Ah*-encoded receptor, AHR (26). The increased binding affinity of halogenated agonists provided direction for the synthesis of high-affinity radioligands and supported a pharmacological approach to the study of this receptor (27–32).

The development of radioligands, purified receptor preparations, and AHR-specific antibodies provided initial insights into the mechanism of PAH/dioxin signal transduction. Reversible radiolabeled ligands allowed the biochemical demonstration of a saturable, high-affinity receptor present in the target cells (33, 34). Competitive binding studies allowed the correlation of congener binding affinity to biological response (27, 35, 36). Structure-activity relationships are still a central aspect of any proof that the AHR mediates a given biological response (37, 38). Radiolabeled ligands were also used to demonstrate that agonist exposure induced a change in the oligomeric state of AHR (10, 39–41). This change was coincident with a receptor species that gained a higher affinity for the nuclear compartment and specific sequences of the target DNA (30, 39, 42, 43). More recent saturation binding isotherms with[125]I-labeled congeners demonstrated that the AHR had a remarkably high binding affinity for halogenated agonists (e.g. the K_D of dioxin is approximately 1×10^{-12} M) (31). Related studies with these ligands demonstrated that the nonresponsive *Ah* alleles (*Ah^d*) encoded a receptor with a 2- to 10-fold lower binding affinity for agonists compared with AHRs encoded by responsive alleles (e.g. *Ah^{b-1}* and *Ah^{b-2}*) (14, 44–49). The development of the photoaffinity label, [^{125}I]2-azido-3-iodo-7,8-dibromodibenzo-p-dioxin provided the tool that led to the biochemical purification of the AHR and the generation of the first receptor-specific antibodies (31, 50, 51). These reagents also revealed the fact that size of the AHR can differ dramatically between species and strains of mice (51–53).

Protein sequence information from the purified protein lead to the molecular cloning of the receptor's cDNA and revealed that it was a member of the PAS superfamily (Figure 2) (12, 54). It is interesting to note that the ARNT protein was cloned about a year before the AHR (Figure 2). Its cDNA was cloned as the result of a genetic screen designed to identify gene products that played roles in AHR signal transduction in mouse hepatoma cells (7). In one class of signaling mutants identified in this screen, the AHR was present and bound ligand normally but did not attain an increased affinity for the nuclear compartment. A human gene fragment encoding the ARNT protein rescued this loss-of-function mutation. Further experiments demonstrated that the ARNT protein was required to direct the ligand-activated AHR to enhancer elements upstream of genomic targets similar to those found upstream of the *Cyp1a1* gene (7, 55). The realization that the

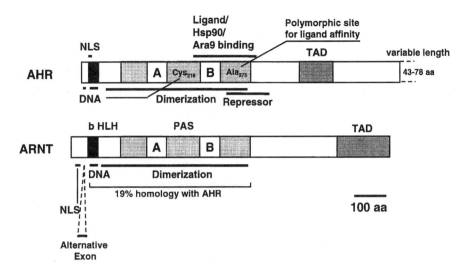

Figure 2 The molecular structures of Ah receptor (AHR) and ARNT. The basic region (b), helix-loop-helix (HLH), PAS, and transactivation (TAD) domains are labeled. The regions that have been shown to play a role in nuclear translocation (NLS), DNA binding (DNA), PAS protein dimerization, ligand/Hsp90/Ara9 binding, TAD, and repression of AHR activity are marked with *thick lines* and labeled. For AHR, Cys_{216} is marked for its role in DNA binding (264). Ala_{375} is marked for its importance for high-affinity ligand binding (14). The C-terminal end variable length represents the length of different AHR alleles (ahr^{b-1}, ahr^{b-2}, ahr^{b-3}, and ahr^d) in various mouse strains (14). For ARNT, the location of the alternative exon, the amino acid sequences that are involved in nuclear translocation (NLS), DNA binding, PAS protein dimerization, TAD, and its percentage similarity with AHR are marked. See text for details.

AHR and ARNT were structurally related bHLH-PAS proteins shed light on the model of AHR signal transduction and provided the first example of a bHLH-PAS heterodimer.

The current model of the adaptive response pathway to PAHs is the result of research from a number of laboratories (Figure 3). A widely held model is that the unliganded AHR is maintained in a complex with a dimer of HSP90 and additional cellular chaperones such as ARA9 (also known as AIP1 or XAP2) and p23 (56–59). The interaction of an HSP90 dimer with the AHR is essential and is believed to help fold the C-terminal half of the PAS domain in a conformation that can bind ligand (60–63). Our understanding of the roles of ARA9 or p23 is more nascent. Although the ARA9-AHR interaction was originally identified in two-hybrid screens, copurification and coimmunoprecipitation experiments have confirmed the biological relevance of this association (57, 58, 64). Recent evidence suggests that the ARA9 protein enhances signal transduction in mammalian cells by increasing the functional receptor number in the cytosolic compartment (65, 66). Presumably, the ARA9 protein acts by stabilizing the AHR-chaperone

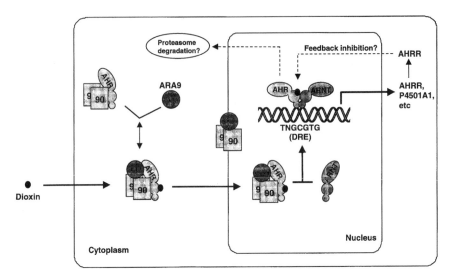

Figure 3 Model of dioxin signaling pathways. The Ah receptor (AHR) normally resides in cytoplasm with a dimer of Hsp90 holding it in a ligand binding form. ARA9 also stabilizes the ligand binding form of AHR and increases the number of functional receptors through this stabilization. On activation by its ligand, AHR translocates from cytoplasm into the nucleus and exchanges its chaperones for ARNT. The AHR-ARNT heterodimer then binds to the dioxin responsive element (DRE) with the core sequence of TNGCGTG and activates transcription of downstream target genes. Among the activated target genes, the cytochrome p450 isozymes are involved in the adaptive response, and the AHR repressor (AHRR) may form a feedback inhibition loop by competing for the binding of ARNT with AHR and by actively repressing transcription from DRE-driven promoters. AHR may finally be degraded through a proteasome pathway. See text for details.

complex. An argument against an absolute requirement for ARA9 comes from the observation that AHR functions normally in the yeast *Saccharomyces cerevisiae,* an organism that has no clear structural homologues of ARA9 (67). Recent data also suggest that the AHR is associated with the same p23 protein that is associated with the glucocorticoid receptor-HSP90 complex (59). Although this physical association is intriguing, it has not been proven that p23 has functional significance in the AHR signal transduction pathway.

The unliganded AHR complex appears to be primarily cytosolic, although in some cell types it may also be nuclear (43, 68, 69). The ligand-induced translocation from the cytosolic to nuclear compartments is associated with a reduction in the size of the receptor's oligomeric state that appears to result from a shedding of cellular chaperones and/or their exchange for the nuclear ARNT protein (39, 41, 70, 71). The nuclear localization sequences for both AHR and ARNT have recently been identified (Figure 2) (68, 72). Within the nucleus, the AHR-ARNT heterodimer is formed and becomes competent to bind specific dioxin response elements (DREs) and drive transcription from adjacent target promoters (13, 42, 71, 73–78). Molecular analysis, coupled with the identification of consensus DREs from known target genes, has defined the core DRE as TNGCGTG (73, 75, 79–82). Evidence generated in vitro indicates that the AHR binds to the TNGC half site, whereas ARNT binds to the GTG half site (79, 80). The target genes of this adaptive response include a battery of XMEs such as CYP1A1, CYP1B1, CYP1A2, the glutathione S transferase Ya subunit and quinone oxidoreductase (1). The protein sequences required to drive transcription appear to reside in the C-terminal halves of both the AHR and ARNT (83–86). Some laboratories have proposed that these two proteins contribute differently to transcriptional activation (87, 88). For a recent review on AHR-mediated gene transcription, see Whitlock (1).

In addition to the induction of XMEs, exposure of most vertebrates to halo-genated aromatic hydrocarbons, like dioxin, can lead to epithelial changes, por-phyria, liver damage, thymic involution, cancer, teratogenicity, a severe wasting syndrome, and death (89, 90). Application of the pharmacological and genetic proofs outlined above indicates that the AHR is directly involved in mediating many, if not all, of these toxic endpoints. Although it should be emphasized that there is no proof that alterations in gene transcription lie at the root of receptor-mediated toxicity, there is an understandable expectation that the toxic pathway will in some way be a reflection of the adaptive pathway as defined in Figure 3. Although this may ultimately be proven true, it is important to emphasize that the pharmacological and genetic proofs for AHR involvement do not necessarily implicate the ARNT protein or DRE-mediated gene expression in any toxic mech-anism. Thus, although the mechanism of XME induction is well characterized, the molecular mechanism underlying most aspects of the AHR-mediated toxic response is currently unknown.

Other than a role for the AHR, little is understood about the mechanisms that underlie most of dioxin's toxic effects. Two important exceptions are that tumor necrosis factor α has been implicated in dioxin-induced hyperinflammation, and there is recent evidence to indicate that thymic involution may be the result of dioxin signaling in bone marrow stromal cells (91–94). In a search to explain this broad spectrum of toxic effects, links have been proposed between the AHR and the regulation of genes involved in epithelial cell growth and differentiation (95, 96) as well as in dioxin-induced alterations in the levels of various cytokines (91, 97–99). Potential mechanisms for toxicity include the existence of low-affinity DRE sites upstream of genes involved in the above processes, the potential for the AHR to signal through nontranscriptional pathways, and the possibility that the AHR competes for and sequesters ARNT or other limiting factors from par-allel cellular pathways (see cross talk below) (90, 100–102). In our view, each of these potential mechanisms is plausible, yet none has particularly compelling experimental support.

Recent data suggest that other PAS proteins may be involved in dioxin sig-naling. A novel PAS protein, an AHR repressor (AHRR), containing only one of the conserved 50 amino acid PAS repeats, was found to inhibit AHR signal transduction (103). This repression appears to be the result of two events. First, when expressed, the AHRR is a constitutively active protein that competes with AHR for ARNT dimerization and DRE binding. Second, the AHRR protein has activity as a transcriptional repressor and may directly inhibit gene expression from DRE-linked promoters. It has been suggested that AHRR may be a part of a negative feedback loop to down-regulate or attenuate an activated AHR pathway. The feedback inhibition idea is based upon the observations that the AHRR promoter is driven by a functional DRE and that the level of the AHRR mRNA is up-regulated by agonists of the AHR (103). It is interesting to note that the AHRR is now one of two mechanisms by which the AHR signal can be down-regulated. It has also been demonstrated that the ligand-activated AHR is rapidly proteolyzed, leading to a decreased receptor number immediately following agonist exposure of many cell types (104–106). This agonist-dependent degradation may provide an additional mechanism to attenuate this response and to protect cells from the consequences of prolonged exposure to high concentrations of agonists.

A close structural homologue of the ARNT molecule (ARNT2) has also been described (107, 108). The ARNT2 protein has been proposed to play a role in PAH/dioxin signal transduction by acting as an alternate partner for the AHR (107). This assertion is based upon the observations that ARNT2 dimerizes with the AHR in vitro and that the resultant complex is capable of driving transcription from a DRE-linked promoter in a heterologous expression system. Developmental profiling suggests that if ARNT2 is active in AHR signal transduction, it may only be playing a role in a small subset of cells. Side-by-side analysis of the AHR, ARNT, and ARNT2 expression in the developing mouse embryo has been performed by in situ hybridization (109, 110). These results suggest that although the AHR and ARNT are coexpressed in a variety of cell types, ARNT2 is expressed in the central nervous system, primarily in areas where the AHR expression is low (107, 109, 110). This result suggests that at most cellular locations, ARNT is the more common partner of the AHR in vivo and that ARNT2 has other important biological roles (see below). Another ARNT homologue, MOP3 (member of PAS 3) [also called BMAL1 (brain and muscle ARNT-like protein 1)] (111–113) is coexpressed with the AHR in a number of cell types (111–113). Yet, initial studies indicate that the dimerization affinity between MOP3 and AHR may be too low to have consequences in vivo (111, 114). Thus, ARNT may be the most prominent bHLH-PAS partner of the AHR that has been cloned to date, with the roles of ARNT2 and MOP3 in this pathway still to be understood.

It is hard to imagine that the AHR and ARNT evolved solely as a defense against PAHs or related environmental toxicants. If this idea is correct, then the characterization of functional AHRs and ARNTs in marine, aquatic, avian, and mammalian species is an indication that there has been significant evolutionary pressure for conservation of this adaptive system due to a common chemical stress (7, 12, 115–117). A second explanation for the conservation of this system is that the AHR-ARNT dimer has a physiological purpose in addition to its role in xenobiotic adaptation. Evidence to support an important physiological role has come from gene targeting experiments in mice, where the AHR has been shown to have an important role in mouse development. Mouse strains deficient in the AHR protein have recently been developed by three independent laboratories (118–121). Although there are some phenotypic differences, these mouse lines commonly show defects in liver development, decreased animal weights, and poor fecundity (118, 119). As predicted, AHR null mice fail to show up-regulation of XMEs in response to agonists or the classical toxic endpoints on exposure to dioxins (119, 122, 123). Taken together, these data suggest that the developing organism has a developmental requirement for this adaptive pathway, possibly due to some unavoidable or endogenous toxicant, and/or that the receptor system plays other roles in addition to its known adaptive functions.

HYPOXIA RESPONSE PATHWAY

Hypoxia can stimulate a variety of systemic, local, and cellular responses (124). In mammalian systems, the systemic response includes the transcriptional up-regulation of the gene encoding the peptide hormone erythropoietin (EPO). This cytokine increases the red blood cell count by stimulating erythropoiesis, thus increasing the efficiency of O_2 transport throughout the body (125). A second aspect of the systemic response to low oxygen tension is the increase in respiration rate that occurs through dopaminergic input to the carotid body. The up-regulation of dopamine is due to the hypoxia-induced transcriptional activation of tyrosine hydroxylase, the rate-limiting enzyme of catecholamine synthesis (126). Local areas of hypoxia can arise during embryogenesis, wound healing, and tumor growth. In these processes, hypoxic tissues up-regulate the transcription of genes encoding various angiogenic factors, such as vascular endothelial growth factor (VEGF), platelet-derived growth factor (PDGF), and fibroblast growth factor (FGF) (127–129), as well as vasodilators produced by enzymes, such as inducible nitric oxide synthase and heme oxygenase-1 (130, 131). The up-regulation of these factors results in an increased vascular bed density, vascular permeability, and oxygen availability to the starved tissues. At the cellular level, hypoxia can limit oxidative metabolism and thus decrease energy production. To adapt to a low-oxygen environment, many cell-types convert to glycolysis for energy. This cellular response is mounted through the transcriptional activation of genes encoding glycolytic enzymes such as aldolase A, phosphoglycerate kinase 1, lactate dehydrogenase A, and phosphofructokinase L and glucose transporters such as GLUT-1 (132–135).

The connection between oxygen homeostasis and PAS proteins was revealed through studies designed to understand the regulation of hypoxia-induced genes, such as *Epo*. Early on, the up-regulation of EPO production by hypoxia was shown to be due in large part to increased transcription of the *Epo* gene (136, 137). This regulation was shown to be mediated by a hypoxia-inducible factor

(HIF1), which bound to a hypoxia responsive element (HRE) found in a region of the *Epo* gene that corresponded to the 3' untranslated portion of its mRNA (136, 138, 139). Purification of the HIF1 protein from induced HeLa cells revealed that this transcription factor was composed of two subunits, HIF1α and HIF1β (140, 141). Amino acid sequence analysis demonstrated that HIF1β was identical to the ARNT protein previously shown to be required for AHR signal transduction (140, 141). Protein sequencing and cDNA cloning experiments also demonstrated that the HIF1α subunit was a novel member of the PAS superfamily. The characterization of the HIF1α-ARNT dimer provided the second example of a bHLH-PAS heterodimer that played an important role in sensing and adapting to environmental change.

The observation that HIF1 was a heterodimer of two bHLH-PAS proteins suggested that the mechanism underlying the hypoxia response would share certain features with that of PAH/dioxin signal transduction pathway (Figure 4). In this regard, the core sequences found in the HRE and the DRE share a number of similarities. Based upon functionally active HREs identified in known target genes, the core consensus sequence for the binding of HIF1α-ARNT dimer has been defined as either 5'-TACGTG-3' or 5'-RCGTG-3' (133, 142). Methylation interference assays support this core element and indicate contact between the HIF1 dimer and all four guanine residues found in both strands of the *Epo* HRE, i.e. 5'-TA*CGTGC*T-3' (143). This result is consistent with the consensus data and indicates that contacts between HIF1α and its response element extend beyond the minimal core sequence. The length of the core sequence and the idea that recognition extends beyond the core element is similar to that seen for the AHR-ARNT heterodimer (79, 80, 144, 145). Based upon these similarities, one can predict that the ARNT protein maintains the same half-site specificity within the HRE as it does within the DRE (i.e. the 3' GTG half-site). This prediction is based upon the observations that the AHR has been definitively shown to bind to the 5' TNGC half-site and ARNT to the 3'GTG half-site of the core DRE sequence, TNGCGTG (79, 80). It follows that the HIF1α subunit would bind to the 5' TAC half-site of the HRE whereas ARNT would bind to the 3' GTG. This latter prediction has not been formally tested.

The mechanism by which HIF1α transduces the hypoxia signal is an area of active investigation. Early studies of hypoxia-driven gene expression by pO_2, iron chelators, and divalent metal ions provided evidence that a heme protein was involved in this process (125). Experiments using antibodies against HIF1α indicated that the levels of the HIF1α protein rise dramatically in response to hypoxia, desferoxamine, or $CoCl_2$, whereas levels of the ARNT protein are relatively nonresponsive to these treatments (100, 140, 146). This observation is consistent with the idea that HIF1α functions directly in the hypoxia sensor pathway and that ARNT is a constitutively active factor required for the hypoxia signal to reach its nuclear targets. Thus, it seems fair to describe HIF1α as a sensor and ARNT as a broad-spectrum partner. In keeping with the terminology of the hypoxia field,

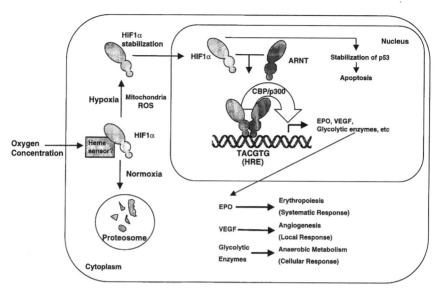

Figure 4   Model of hypoxia signaling pathways. Under normoxic conditions, HIF1α protein is degraded through the ubiquitin-proteasome pathway. When a cell is exposed to a hypoxic environment, the HIF1α protein is stabilized. A heme protein and/or the generation of mitochondrially generated reactive oxygen species (ROS) may be necessary for hypoxia induction of HIF1α protein levels. HIF1α protein is translocated from cytoplasm to nucleus, where it dimerizes with ARNT. The HIF1α-ARNT heterodimer then binds to the hypoxia responsive element (HRE) and activates the transcription of downstream target genes. The transcription coactivator CBP/p300 is involved in this transcription activation event. The target genes include erythropoietin (EPO), vascular endothelial growth factor (VEGF), and a series of glycolytic enzymes involved in the systematic, local, and cellular hypoxic responses. HIF1α also is involved in the stabilization of p53 protein and may play a role in the hypoxia-induced apoptosis. See text for details.

as well as of that proposed at the outset of this review, we propose to classify these proteins as α and β class, respectively.

The primary mechanism by which hypoxia regulates HIF1α appears to reside mainly at the level of the protein. In the majority of published reports, the levels of HIF1α protein rise in response to hypoxia, $CoCl_2$, etc, whereas its mRNA level remains stable (146–149). Moreover, it has been observed that under normoxic conditions, the HIF1α protein undergoes rapid degradation via the ubiquitin-proteasome pathway, whereas under hypoxic conditions the protein is relatively stable (138, 143, 150–152). The mechanism by which the HIF1α protein's stability is achieved is poorly understood, although a dependence on the ARNT protein has been proposed (147). Metabolic inhibitors, such as cycloheximide, actinomycin D, and 2-aminopurine, have been used to demonstrate a requirement for cellular translation, transcription, and protein phosphorylation in the hypoxia response (138, 143, 153). Furthermore, results from a number of laboratories have indicated that HIF1α activation is dependent on the red-ox state of the cell (148, 150, 154). Recently, it has been shown that hypoxia- but not Co^{2+}-induced HIF1α activation requires the production of reactive oxygen species (ROS) that is dependent on the mitochondria. This observation suggests that hypoxia and Co^{2+} induction of HIF1α may employ different pathways (154). Taken in sum, these results suggest an extremely complicated regulatory mechanism for the stabilization of the HIF1α protein. To add to this complexity, results from a number of labs have indicated that under certain circumstances, the level of HIF1α mRNA can also be up-regulated (143, 155, 156). Although this has not been a widely reproduced finding, it should not be discounted and may be an indication that alternative methods of regulation are at play. In this regard, recent reports have demonstrated that IFN-β, but not IFN-α or IFN-γ, can up-regulate HIF1α mRNA by about sevenfold in a human fibrosarcoma cell line (157).

The bHLH and PAS domains of HIF1α and ARNT domains confer both DNA binding and dimerization specificity, as would be predicted based upon data from the AHR and ARNT studies (158). Using GAL4 chimeras and a GAL-UAS–driven reporter system, two hypoxia responsive domains (HRDs) have been mapped to the C-terminal half of HIF1α (134, 159, 160). The exact boundaries and identifiers for these domains vary between labs. For simplicity, we use the definitions of Jiang et al (160). That is, HRD1 lies between residues 531 and 575 and HRD2 lies between residues 786 and 826 of the human HIF1α protein (160). It is interesting to note that these two HRDs appear to influence HIF1α activity by different mechanisms. The HRD1 domain responds to low O_2 tension by stabilizing the HIF1α protein (159, 160), whereas HRD2 appears to act as a hypoxia-activated transcriptionally active domain (134, 159, 160). The transactivational activity of HIF1α is found to be potentiated by the general coactivator CBP/p300 (161, 162).

Just as in the AHR system, screens of expressed sequence tag (EST) databases have added to the number of PAS proteins at play in the hypoxia pathway. In addition to HIF1α, two α-class homologues have the capacity to sense low-oxygen tension, HIF2α (also called EPAS1 or MOP2) and HIF3α (107, 111, 112, 163–166). HIF2α was identified by a number of laboratories and is highly homologous to HIF1α in the bHLH-PAS domains (111, 164–166). In addition, HIF2α contains structural and functional similarity to the HRD1 and HRD2 domains found in HIF1α (167, 168). In contrast to the widespread expression of HIF1α, HIF2α is expressed mainly in endothelial cells and in certain nonendothelial tissues such as the olfactory epithelium and the adrenal gland (109, 165). HIF3α is a newly identified hypoxia-inducible factor that shares considerable sequence homology with HIF1α and HIF2α in the basic region, the HLH and PAS domain. It dimerizes with ARNT, and this complex activates transcription of reporter genes driven by HRE elements in a heterologous expression system (163). Less is known about the expression of the 3α homologue, although preliminary evidence from our laboratory suggests high-level expression in the developing trachea and olfactory epithelium (Y-Z Gu, SM Moran & CA Bradfield, unpublished observation). It is interesting to note that both sequence analysis and functional analysis suggest that HIF3α contains an HRD1 domain but does not harbor a domain equivalent to HRD2 (163).

The ARNT2 and MOP3 homologues of ARNT (described above) may also play roles as β-class partners of the α-class HIF sensor subunits. The ARNT2 protein shares 81% identity with ARNT in the bHLH-PAS domains (57% overall sequence identity) and thus was predicted to be a second partner of AHR (107, 108). In DNA binding assays, the ARNT2 protein is able to substitute for ARNT, directing HIF1α, HIF2α, and HIF3α to HREs (JB Hogenesch, Y-Z Gu & CA Bradfield, unpublished results). Coupled with these in vitro results and the overlapping developmental profiles of ARNT2 and the α-class HIF proteins, it seems highly likely that these proteins are biologically relevant partners in vivo (109). The third ARNT homologue MOP3 was originally cloned in EST screens for novel PAS-encoding cDNAs (111–113). It has homology with the ARNT protein in both its bHLH and PAS domains (66% and 40% identity, respectively). Although MOP3 and HIF1α are coexpressed in a number of tissues, MOP3 is a fairly weak dimerization partner of the α-class HIFs (109, 114). Thus, it is unclear if MOP3 plays a significant role in hypoxia signal transduction.

To understand the biological roles of these PAS proteins in hypoxia signaling, a number of gene inactivation models have been exploited. Murine strains lacking the ARNT protein were the first to be developed (169, 170). These mice displayed embryonic lethality between 9.5 and 10.5 days of gestation. Although some controversy remains as to whether the yolk sac circulation was affected, both ARNT knockout mouse strains display major blocks in developmental angiogenesis, which suggests that this failure is the primary cause of embryonic lethality (169, 170). The phenotype of the ARNT null mice provided important genetic support for the idea that hypoxia is an important signal in normal development. Null alleles at loci encoding either of the other putative β-class partners, i.e. ARNT2 or MOP3, have not been reported.

In keeping with the idea that hypoxia is an important signal for normal development, mice homozygous for disruption at the *Hif1α* locus (*Hif1α-/-*) display embryonic lethality at day 11 of gestation with neural tube defects, cardiovascular malformation, and lack of cephalic vascularization (171, 172). In addition, these mice display a lack of the classic hypoxia responses, such as the up-regulation of VEGF, glycolytic enzymes, and glucose transporters (171–173). This phenotype is similar to the ARNT null mice discussed earlier and is consistent with the role of HIF1 heterodimer in the hypoxia-driven transcriptional activation of a number of genes involved in developmental angiogenesis, such as VEGF, FGF, and PDGF. Like many null alleles, the phenotype of *Hif2α* null mice provided a surprising result. The *Hif2α-/-* embryos die at day 12.5 of gestation because of pronounced bradycardia related to substantially decreased catecholamine levels (174). This phenotype is consistent with the high level of expression of HIF2α in the organ of Zuckerkandl (OZ), the principal source of catecholamine production (174).

Because of the early death of HIF2α homozygous embryo, it is unclear whether HIF2α plays a role in hypoxia responses in later stages of life or whether this protein plays a role in angiogenesis, as might have been predicted based upon its expression in the vascular endothelium. Conditional knockout of this gene may shed more light on such physiological functions.

The above discussion should also highlight the fact that hypoxia signal transduction is a complex pathway and that this pathway is likely to take multiple forms in different cell types and under different physiological conditions. Moreover, attempts to model this biology must explain how a similar response can be elicited from low O_2 tension, ferric ions, cobalt, and oxidative stress. In addition, it must explain how some responses to hypoxia can be evoked at moderately low levels (8% O_2) (175, 176), whereas other responses require more extreme hypoxia (close to 1% O_2) (177). It must also take into account the apparent redundancy of both the α- and β-class partners (e.g. HIF1α, HIF2α, HIF3α, ARNT, and ARNT2), as well as the multiple levels of control that appear to be exerted over this system (i.e. evidence for the importance of translation, transcription, phosphorylation, ROS, heme, and protein stability).

This complexity leads us to apply Occam's razor and state the simplest possibility, that the α-class HIFs are in fact the heme sensors themselves or that they directly interact with an upstream PAS-containing heme sensor. If we use the similarity to the AHR system (above), as well as the prokaryotic systems (below), we might also predict that the PAS domain is the region of the α-class HIFs or the upstream protein that senses oxygen through a bound heme group. One version of this model would be that the α-class HIF senses the oxygen environment as it comes off of the ribosome. This oxygen sensing could occur through the integration of a heme moiety or through a PAS-PAS interaction with an upstream heme-containing PAS protein. Under low oxygen, the α-class HIF conformation could be such that it avoids the ubiquitination, whereas in normoxia, the folded state leads the protein down a rapid degradative pathway. Such a model is based more upon our belief that the AHR is a prototype of signaling through PAS proteins rather than an exception.

Experiments from a number of laboratories have demonstrated the importance of heterodimerization of the α- and β-class subunits in the regulation of the systematic, local, and cellular responses to hypoxia (2, 127, 132, 133, 136, 139). Despite the importance of heterodimerization, recent evidence also suggests that HIFs may signal through heterologous interactions with non-PAS containing proteins. In this regard, HIF1α has also been shown to be involved in the stabilization of p53 protein and may play a role in hypoxia-induced apoptosis (178) (Figure 4). This stabilization appears to be directly related to protein-protein interactions between HIF1α and p53 protein. Such a mechanism of protein stabilization may be a common activity of HIF1α. More recent evidence has suggested that the interaction between HIF1α and the VHL protein, the product of the von Hippel-Lindau (VHL) tumor suppressor gene, is necessary for the oxygen-dependent degradation of HIF α subunits (179). Such a relationship may explain the highly

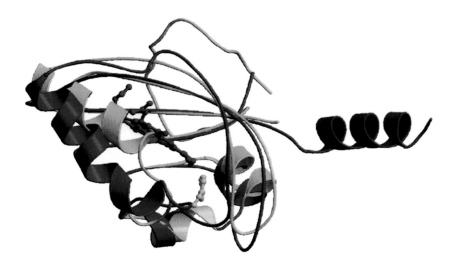

Figure 8 Structure of model prokaryotic PAS domains. Superimposed tertiary structure of FixL (*red*) and PYP (*yellow*) and their respective cofactors, heme and hydroxycinnamate (Credit: Weimin Gong and Michael K. Chan, Ohio State University) (259).

vascularized tumors of VHL patients because α-class HIF subunits would be constitutively up-regulated in the absence of the VHL protein (180).

THE CIRCADIAN RESPONSE PATHWAY

Biological clocks help entrain an organism's activity to changes in daily and seasonal environment. In keeping with our thesis that PAS is a signature of proteins involved in environmental adaptation, we view diurnal changes in light and temperature as some of the most fundamental environmental variables that challenge terrestrial species. To meet this environmental challenge, circadian rhythms of various biological activities are maintained through both an internal clock and responsiveness to environmental cues that keep that clock in tune (3).

Nowhere is the PAS domain more prominent and nowhere are the PAS proteins more structurally diverse than in pathways regulating circadian rhythmicity. Vertebrates and invertebrates employ orthologues of a number of PAS proteins, including PER, CLOCK, and MOP3, to control this important biological process (3). Even simple eukaryotes, such as the slime mold *Neurospora crassa*, control circadian rhythmicity through the gene products of the *white collar* loci. The WHITE COLLAR (WC) proteins, WC-1 and WC-2, display a single PAS repeat motif instead of containing the signature A and B domains found in the PAS domains of *Drosophila* and mammals (8, 181). WC proteins have been shown to be required for transcriptional activation of *Neurospora* circadian responsive gene *FRQ* and are essential for maintaining circadian rhythms (181). Like the PAS domains of their mammalian counterparts, the PAS domains of the WC proteins appear to serve as dimerization surfaces. This is demonstrated by the fact that these domains mediate the formation of WC homodimers and heterodimers, as well as the formation of WC-heterodimers with mammalian PAS proteins such as the AHR (182, 183).

The first PAS factor ever to be characterized was the product of the *Drosophila period* (*per*) locus, a regulator of the circadian rhythms of locomotor activity (5, 6, 8). Proof for the involvement of this locus in rhythmicity was provided through genetic screens for mutants with an aberrant circadian free-running time (184, 185). The three original mutant alleles at this locus were designated *per$_s$* (*short*), *per$_l$* (*long*), and *per$_0$* (*null*). The *per* locus encodes a 1218–amino acid protein generated from eight exons (8). When SIM and ARNT were later cloned, the consensus PAS domain emerged from sequence comparisons (186). Compared with the wild type, the *per$_s$* mutants shorten whereas the *per$_l$* mutants lengthen the free-running locomotor rhythms. The *per$_0$* mutants are arrhythmic under free-running conditions. It is interesting to note that the *per$_l$* mutation (valine 243 to aspartic acid) resides within the PAS domain whereas the other two mutations reside immediately C-terminal to the PAS domain (i.e. *per$_s$* mutation, serine 589 to asparagine; *per$_0$* mutation, glutamine 464 to stop). A second observation that supports a role for this locus in rhythmicity is that the PER protein and mRNA levels oscillate in a circadian manner (187, 188). Not only does the PER protein level display a rhythm, its localization into the nucleus also appears to be regulated in a similar fashion (189–191).

A number of early observations provided important insights into how the PER protein might work at a molecular level. The cloning of the dSIM and the mammalian ARNT and AHR cDNAs revealed that the dPER protein was a unique member of this superfamily in that it did not harbor a bHLH domain. It was also shown that the PAS domain of PER could act as a dimerization surface to support interactions with other PAS domain-containing proteins, such as SIM and ARNT (192). Coupling these observations to the evidence that constitutive overexpression of PER inhibited the cycling of its own mRNA (193) led to the suspicion that PER was a dominant negative inhibitor of its own transcription (possibly acting by inhibiting another bHLH-PAS pair) (114). Such a model had precedence from a similar mechanism in the myoD field (194). This model has now gained support from experiments in both mice and flies (see below) (195–198).

The fact that PAS proteins were found to play important roles in the circadian rhythm pathways of organisms as diverse as arthropods and mammals has allowed investigators to apply what is learned from one model system to another. This convergence of ideas has led to a rapid advancement in the field and the development of a model that describes the core working of the circadian clock in a wide variety of species. The first mammalian gene shown to play a central role in maintenance of rhythmicity was encoded by the murine *Clock* locus (199). Because there was precedence for autosomal dominant and semidominant mutations in *Drosophila* and *Neurospora* (6, 181), a genetic screen was employed to identify mutations in mice that would alter their normal free-running period of 24 h (199). In an ethylnitrosourea (ENU) mutagenesis screen of mice, a mutant locus, called *Clock,* was identified that displayed a free-running period of slightly longer than 25 h. Mice homozygous for the *Clock* mutant allele had an even longer period, and this period degraded more quickly while in free-running conditions (200). The positional cloning of the murine *Clock* gene was undertaken by a number of parallel approaches and was aided by the identification of exons encoding a bHLH-PAS domain within the target genomic region (199). Complementation with the corresponding bacterial artificial chromosome confirmed the biological importance of the PAS gene product (201). The ENU-induced mutation in *Clock* was found to generate the deletion of a single exon encoding a region within the C terminus of the CLOCK protein (199). Corresponding regions in other bHLH-PAS members have been shown to harbor transactivation activity (83, 86, 160, 167).

Following the cloning of murine *Clock,* three mammalian homologues of *Drosophila* PER were identified by genomic sequencing, searches of ESTs, and degenerate polymerase chain reaction (202–205). Like their *Drosophila* homologue, mRNA levels of the mammalian PERs responded to light and phase shifted in a circadian manner in the suprachiasmatic nucleus, the site of the master circadian oscillator in mammals. Another observation that allowed the decoding of the circadian clock pathway was the demonstration that a 69-bp region upstream of the *Drosophila per* promoter was sufficient to drive in vivo cycling of synthetic reporter genes in flies (206). Further analysis revealed that an element harboring an E-box core sequence, *CACGTG*AGC (the E-box is underlined), was necessary for the robust amplitude of this cycling (206). These results coupled with the observation that β-class PAS proteins such as ARNT recognize the 5'GTG of an E-box prompted the idea that this element was bound by an α- and β-class bHLH-PAS heterodimer. These observations were also consistent with the idea that the PER protein acted as an inhibitor of a CLOCK-bHLH-PAS heterodimer in both *Drosophila* and mammals.

The characterization of this E-box–bound heterodimer came in a flurry of papers shortly after the cloning of CLOCK. It is interesting to note that the partner of CLOCK was identified as the putative β-class bHLH-PAS protein, known as MOP3/BMAL1, that was pulled out in earlier EST screens (111, 112). Using yeast two-hybrid screens, it was determined that a partnership was formed between the mammalian MOP3 and CLOCK proteins in vivo (114, 195, 207). In parallel experiments, *Drosophila* homologues of these proteins were identified as the result of screens for circadian rhythm mutants (208, 209). Mutations in the *Drosophila cycle* and *clock* loci were shown to result in a significant decrease in the expression of both PER and TIM, and both mutations resulted in arrhythmia as homozygous alleles (208, 209). Sequence analysis of the gene products of these loci indicated that they were orthologues of the mammalian MOP3 and CLOCK, respectively. These experiments provided both the biochemical and genetic proofs that MOP3 (CYCLE) and CLOCK were components of the circadian clock in various species and that the mammalian and *Drosophila* circadian pathways would be functionally similar.

Proof that the MOP3-CLOCK heterodimer bound the circadian response element came from three lines of evidence. First, our own lab was aided by the fact that a CLOCK homologue, MOP4/NPAS2, was identified from earlier EST screens like those that revealed MOP3 (111, 210). The observation that the CLOCK and MOP4 proteins share 84% and 73% identity in their bHLH and PAS domains, respectively, indicated that MOP3-MOP4 interactions provided a model system for MOP3-CLOCK interactions. In a randomized screen for the response element recognized by the human MOP3-MOP4 heterodimer, the sequence *CACGTG*ACC was identified and named the M34 responsive element (M34RE) (114). Heterologous expression experiments demonstrated that MOP3-MOP4 and MOP3-CLOCK combinations were capable of driving transcription from this M34 element (114). It is important to note that this sequence differs at only a single nucleotide (*CACGTG*AGC) from the circadian enhancer found upstream of the *Drosophila per* gene (206). In addition, this sequence appears three times in the structural gene of the hPER3 gene. Second, in parallel experiments, other laboratories had also demonstrated that a similar circadian element was harbored in the mammalian PER1 promoter, and that the CLOCK-MOP3 heterodimer was capable of driving transcription of synthetic promoters harboring this element (207). Third, concurrent experiments from *Drosophila* also supported this model. These experiments demonstrated that the *Drosophila* CLOCK activates *per* transcription through the previously described 69-bp 5' flanking sequence containing the E-box element (195). It was also shown that PER and TIM could inhibit CLOCK/CYCLE-induced transcription of their own messages (195), which supports the feedback inhibition hypothesis for PER and provides a role for two additional bHLH-PAS protein in circadian rhythms of flies, mice, and humans.

The circadian rhythm pathway also depends on a number of heterotypic interactions between bHLH-PAS proteins and non-PAS proteins. The *Drosophila* protein timeless (TIM) was the first such non-PAS protein to be identified (190, 191). The cyclic expression of TIM appears to dictate the timing of PER protein accumulation and nuclear localization, and it is hypothesized that PER and TIM translocate to the nucleus as a complex (191, 211, 212). In addition, both the TIM message and protein levels have been found to cycle in a circadian manner (211, 213). The recently cloned *Drosophila* gene *double-time* (DBT) encodes a protein closely related to human casein kinase Iε and fine-tunes the length of circadian rhythm by promoting PER phosphorylation and subsequent degradation (214, 215). In *double-time* mutants, the PER protein accumulates in the nucleus in a noncircadian fashion, leading to abnormal locomotor rhythms.

Besides TIM and DBT, other heterotypic non-PAS interactors are involved in circadian regulation. Although the PER protein oscillates and phase shifts in response to light, PER may not be the first molecule that senses light. In fact, evidences suggest that there is an upstream mediator of the light-sensing process. Recently, the *Drosophila* cryptochrome (CRY) and mouse CRY1 and CRY2 cDNAs were cloned and were found to be members of the plant blue-light photoreceptor and photolyase family (216, 217). Mutational analysis proved that these proteins were essential for maintenance of circadian rhythms (216, 218–220). Both the *Drosophila* CRY and mammalian CRYs are shown to interact with the core components of the circadian clock, PER and TIM (196, 221). The functional consequences of this interaction are the relief of the repression by PER and TIM in flies, thereby allowing for light input into the circadian clock (196, 221).

The research of the past few years has led to a plausible mechanism for cellular mRNA oscillations (Figure 5): Two bHLH-PAS transcription factors, CLOCK and MOP3, form a heterodimer and bind to response element sequences termed M34RE (or a circadian responsive E-box). These elements are present in the enhancer/promoter regions of circadian-regulated genes such as *per.* As a result, The MOP3-CLOCK heterodimer positively regulates the levels of circadian responsive gene products (191). In return, PER and TIM negatively regulate the CLOCK/MOP3 complex, either by binding to one member of the complex and disrupting its function or by indirectly influencing the signaling of the MOP3/CLOCK complex through interactions with the basal transcriptional machinery (195–198). These mechanisms are in agreement with the observation of feedback

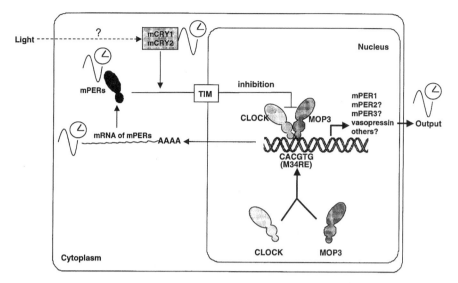

Figure 5   Model of the mammalian circadian response pathways. The mammalian and fruit fly circadian response pathways may be slightly different; thus, the model of the mammalian pathway is shown here. The expression of PERs and CRYs are circadian regulated (*clock icon*). CLOCK and MOP3 form a heterodimer. The heterodimer binds to the responsive element M34RE (the MOP3 and MOP4 responsive element) containing the core sequence of CACGTG and activates the transcription of downstream target genes such as mPER1 and vasopressin. It is not known whether or how CRYs respond to light, but mCRYs interact with mPERs and help in translocating mPERs from cytoplasm into nucleus. PER, TIM, and CRY can block the CLOCK-MOP3–dependent transcriptional activation and, therefore, complete the feedback inhibition loop of PER. See text for details.

inhibition by PER and TIM. Because these genes negatively regulate their own transcription, and because there is a delay between their translation and functional interference in the CLOCK-MOP3/CYCLE complex, an oscillation occurs and is maintained (Figure 5).

PAS PROTEINS IN OTHER RESPONSE PATHWAYS

Our choice to focus on AHR, hypoxia, and circadian biology was the result of our interest in emphasizing pathways where bHLH-PAS heterodimers played important roles. A number of excellent reviews are recommended to learn more about these pathways (4, 222–224).

Among the important signal transduction molecules not discussed here is one of the founding members of this superfamily, the product of the *single-minded* locus (SIM) (225). This protein is a regulator of midline development in flies. The recent cloning of two mammalian SIM homologues has also been reported

(SIM1 and SIM2) (226–230). Although it has not been clearly shown that either of the mammalian SIMs is a bona fide orthologue of the *Drosophila* SIM, gene-targeting experiments have demonstrated that homozygous *Sim1* mutant mice die shortly after birth. The death is due to developmental defect of the hypothalamic-pituitary axis marked by a lack of secretory neurons (231).

The product of the *Drosophila trachealess* locus (TRH) is another interesting bHLH-PAS protein that is essential for the development of tracheal pits in *Drosophila* (232, 233). Given the role hypoxia has as a developmental signal in the development of vascular tubes (234), it is tempting to speculate that trachealogenesis may also respond directly to low oxygen and that TRH is a sensor in that pathway (232, 233). It is interesting to note that in vitro experiments indicate that the mammalian SIMs dimerize with ARNT and that both the dSIM and dTRH appear to dimerize with TANGO, the putative *Drosophila* orthologue of ARNT (235, 236). Using our simplified classification scheme, this would lead us to predict that TRH and the SIMs are sensors of some input signal (α-class PAS proteins). Another *Drosophila* PAS protein that has been identified is Similar (dSIMA) (237). dSIMA contains both bHLH and PAS domains and is inducible by hypoxia, cobaltous ions, and desferrioxamine in transient transfection experiments (238), which suggests that dSIMA functions as a hypoxia sensor in *Drosophila* and that the hypoxia signaling pathway is also conserved between flies and humans.

Not all proteins fit neatly under the title of sensor or broad-spectrum partner or have been shown to participate in heterodimeric interactions to bind DNA. Most notably, three bHLH-PAS proteins have been shown to act as coactivators for members of the nuclear receptor superfamily (239). This surprising result came from a number of two-hybrid screens using steroid receptors as the baits. The cDNA identified in these screens were a unique γ-class of PAS proteins, commonly referred to as coactivators (240–244) (Figure 6). These coactivators mediate the interaction of the nuclear receptors and the transcriptional activator/integrators such as CBP/p300 and are required for the full transcriptional activity of the nuclear receptors (241, 242, 245). It is interesting to note that it appears that neither the bHLH nor PAS domains of these proteins are required for coactivator activity (246). This suggests that this class of proteins may have more than one cellular role and that bHLH-PAS partners of this class of proteins may also exist.

SENSORS, PARTNERS, AND COACTIVATORS

An examination of the bHLH-PAS superfamily suggests that these proteins can be classified based upon functional similarities (sensors, partners, and coactivators) or evolutionary relatedness (α, β, and γ class) (Figure 6). In most cases, these two methods of classification overlap. Our understanding of the above signaling pathways provides evidence that many PAS proteins can act as either sensors of an input signal or as general partners required for the dimers to interact with their nuclear targets. With respect to sensors, we have reviewed the considerable evidence that proteins such as the AHR, HIF1α, HIF2α, and HIF3α are directly sensing environmental signals. In the case of the AHR, direct binding of a ligand is the mechanism at play, whereas in the case of the HIFα subunits, they appear to be either directly sensing oxygen or being influenced by an oxygen-sensing protein. Similarly, the function of the ARNT, ARNT2, and MOP3 proteins appears to act as partners that target the multiple sensor PAS proteins to their cognate enhancer elements. The ARNT protein is the best characterized in vivo and clearly serves as a partner for both the AHR and some or all of the HIFαs. As mentioned above, the putative *Drosophila* orthologue of ARNT, the TANGO protein, has also shown to be a partner of SIM and TRH (235). The dimerization profile of ARNT2 strongly suggests its in vivo function will be similar to ARNT and that ARNT2 is a broad-spectrum partner for many of the same sensor proteins as ARNT (albeit in neuronal tissue). The published data also provide support for the classification of MOP3 as a general partner based upon the observation that it can dimerize with CLOCK and MOP4, and to a lesser degree with the HIFα subunits. To date, all biologically relevant PAS heterodimers are composed of one α-class and one β-class partner. The γ-class coactivators participate in transcriptional activation of steroid receptors, and they form a special subgroup of this superfamily, with the functions of their PAS domains unknown. To date, coactivators have not been shown to form heterodimers with other bHLH-PAS proteins. This class of transcriptional coactivators (γ-class) has received less attention from this chapter but has been the focus of a number of recent reviews (239, 247).

An amino acid sequence comparison of the PAS domains can also be used to classify members of this superfamily. This phylogenetic analysis suggests that proteins classified as general partners are more closely related to each other than to other members of this superfamily (Figure 6). This can also be said for the γ-class coactivators and for the larger number of proteins that fall under the rubric of sensor (α-class). By extension, the above classifications allow us to make some predictions about many of the less well-understood PAS proteins. Based upon the above pairing rules and phylogenetic comparisons, we would place CLOCK, MOP4, and SIM in the α-sensor class. Calling these proteins sensors is a bit premature; nevertheless, it is provocative to think of the CLOCK protein as sensing photic input and playing a role in adjusting circadian rhythms to the environmental surroundings. Perhaps this sensing of environmental input comes from direct interactions with the PER protein that is also in this sensing pathway.

CROSS TALK BETWEEN PAS PROTEIN–MEDIATED SIGNALING PATHWAYS

The fact that bHLH-PAS proteins could be involved in more than one cellular pathway leads to the possibility that signaling through one pathway could influence the responsiveness of another (90). Such a situation could arise when parallel

540

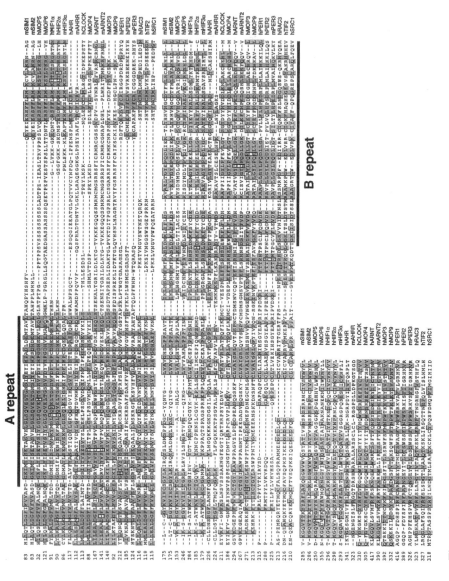

Figure 6a See Figure 6b for this caption.

B

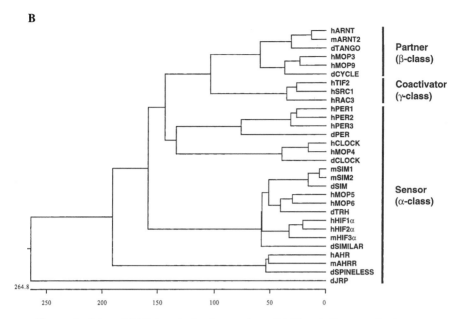

Figure 6   Selected PAS domain family members. (*A*) Clustal alignment for the sequences corresponding to the PAS domains of mammalian family members (265). Besides the published sequences, two newly identified PAS proteins in our lab, hMOP6 and hMOP9, are also included (RS Thomas, JB Hogenesch & CA Bradfield, unpublished observation). The consensus residues are *shaded.* The alignment conditions were as follows. Multiple: gap penalty, 10; gap length penalty, 10. Pairwise: ktuple, 1; gap penalty, 3. Species prefix h represents human and m represents mouse. (*Thick lines*) The PAS A and B repeats. For hARNT, the A repeat starts at ETGR and ends at REQL and the B repeat starts at EGIF and ends at QQVV. See text for details. (*B*). A phylogenetic tree constructed using clustal alignment. The *axis below* denotes sequence distance. JRP is the drosophila juvenile hormone-resistance protein (266). The PAS proteins are classified into sensors (α-class), partners (β-class), and coactivators (γ-class), as indicated on the *right*. Species prefix h represents human, m represents mouse, and d represents drosophila. See text for details.

pathways within the same cell share a limiting common partner, such as ARNT. In support of this idea, it has been shown that AHR and HIF1α compete for the binding of ARNT in vitro and that under certain conditions parallel signaling can be inhibitory (100, 146, 248). Although the simplest explanation of these data is that ARNT is a limiting factor, these experiments do not formally exclude other explanations, such as the possibility that other shared and limiting factors are important. In this regard, the significance of limiting heterologous factors is suggested by the recent demonstration of interference between the dioxin and the progesterone signaling pathway (249). Adding to the potential complexity of the cross-talk concept is the observation that certain responsive genes may be protected from such an event. For example, it has been shown that although there is interference between the dioxin and the hypoxia pathways in vitro and in cell culture, the human *Epo* gene was protected from this interference in hepatoma cells. This protection appears to be due to the fact that the Epo promoter is influenced by both the classical HREs in its 3' regions, as well as a number of degenerate DREs immediately upstream of its promoter (100). Thus, for an EPO response, an additive effect of dioxin and hypoxia was observed instead of an inhibition, as might be predicted by the cross-talk model (100). It will be interesting to see whether this is a common mechanism of regulation for other hypoxia inducible genes.

THE PAS PROTEINS AS ENVIRONMENTAL SENSORS IN PROKARYOTES AND PLANTS

Any discussion of the mammalian PAS superfamily would be incomplete without mention of its more distant relatives in prokaryotes and plants. Although prokaryotes harbor no consensus bHLH proteins, they do express proteins that contain local homology to PAS domains (Figure 7) (250, 251). Members of this group of proteins are involved in oxygen regulation (FixL), sporulation (KinA), nitrogen fixation (NtrB), and negative phototropism [photoactive yellow protein (PYP)] (Figure 7) (252–254). Like their eukaryotic PAS relatives, these proteins often transduce signals in response to environmental change. Unlike their eukaryotic relatives, these prokaryotic proteins often harbor histidine kinase activity and transduce their signals via phosphorylation cascades that lead to activation of transcription factors (255).

The PYP protein, a bacterial blue-light photosensor that contains a rudimentary PAS repeat, was the first PAS-like molecule from which the three-dimensional structure was obtained (257, 258). This solution provided the first look into the structure of a simple PAS repeat (254). The idea that such prokaryotic domains were models of PAS was followed by the crystalization of the heme binding domain of the oxygen sensor FixL (259). The examination of these models shows that the structure of PAS repeat is highly conserved evolutionarily [Figure 8 (see

Figure 7 Alignment of selected prokaryotic and eucaryotic minimal PAS domains. (*Top*). A clustal alignment for mammalian PAS protein hARNT, hMOP3, hHIF1α, mCLOCK, and mAHR and bacterial PAS protein PYP and FixL. The consensus residues are *boxed*. The alignment conditions are as follows. Multiple: gap penalty, 10; gap length penalty, 20. Pairwise: ktuple, 1; gap penalty, 3. (*Bottom*). A phylogenetic tree was constructed based upon results from the above clustal alignment. The *axis below* denotes sequence distance. (*Thick line*) The PAS B repeat. For hARNT, the B repeat starts at EGIF and ends at QQVV. See text for details.

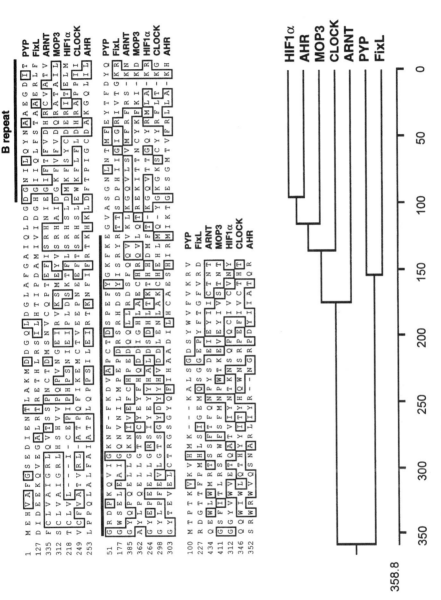

Figure 7 Figure caption on bottom of facing page.

color insert)] and indicates the functional importance of this structure as an interface for an environmental sensor. The cocrystalization of the chromophore 4-hydroxycinnamic acid with PYP (258) and heme bound with FixL (259) provided additional evidence that PAS domains can be directly involved in sensing environmental change. This observation is also consistent with the idea that this sensing process requires a bound low-molecular-weight ligand and that these prokaryotic domains are the forerunners of the AHR dioxin binding domain.

Structural homology with the PAS domain has also been identified in several photoreceptors in plants. In *Arabidopsis,* these proteins include NPH1, phytochromes from PhyA to PhyE, and the phytochrome interacting factor PIF3 (223, 224). The blue-light photoreceptor NPH1 is required for directional growth toward light (phototropism) (260). This protein has two repeats of approximately 110 amino acids, referred to as light, oxygen, voltage (LOV) sensor domains (261). The LOV domains share sequence homology to the PAS domains and have been shown to function as the binding sites for the chromophore flavin mononucleotide (261). Five types of phytochromes (from PhyA to PhyE) have been identified. They respond mainly to light at the red/far-red region of the spectrum and are involved in many aspects of plant development (224). These phytochromes contain two repeats homologous to the typical PAS domain and a histidine kinase–like domain at their C terminus (224). In keeping with the importance of homotypic interactions in PAS protein function, a yeast two-hybrid screen using the C-terminal region of PhyB as the bait lead to the identification of PIF3. This protein was shown to harbor the bHLH-PAS domain and to participate in the signaling pathways of both PhyA and PhyB (262). The presence of both bHLH and PAS domains as well as their involvement in PhyA and PhyB signaling suggest that PIF3 is a transcription factor (262).

SUMMARY

With the help of the rapidly expanding EST database and the fast pace of PAS protein research, more than 20 mammalian PAS cDNAs have been cloned to date, with related proteins being found in flies, plants, and prokaryotes (Figure 6). Many of these proteins function in heterodimeric pairs and can be classified as either sensors or broad-spectrum partners. The sensors, such as the AHR, the HIFαs, and possibly even CLOCK or PER, detect changes in the environment and regulate an adaptive response. The partners, such as the ARNTs and MOP3, dimerize with a broad spectrum of sensors and are essential for the transcriptional output of a number of these biologically important pathways. The sensors often act by directly detecting environmental change (AHR ligand binding) or by transducing a signal from an upstream sensor (HIF1α from low O_2 tension or PER from light). The mechanism by which the signal transduction occurs in response to environmental cues are diverse and can involve ligand binding (AHR), protein stability (HIF1α), or subcellular localization (PER). Finally, cross talk between different bHLH-PAS pathways may be an important mechanism by which these proteins can signal through or attenuate parallel pathways.

Describing these models of signal transduction was performed as part of our interest in predicting how novel PAS proteins function and how their pathways mediate environmental adaptation in adults and developing embryos. Although we have focused on heterodimers of bHLH-PAS proteins with transcriptional outputs, it is not clear if this will prove to be the most common mechanism by which these proteins act. In this regard, bHLH-PAS coactivators have been shown to directly interact with and modify the transcriptional responses of nuclear receptors (241–245). Although these PAS proteins have bHLH and PAS domains, they have not yet been shown to heterodimerize with other bHLH-PAS proteins, nor have they been shown to directly contact specific DNA response elements (239). Thus, their participation in bHLH-PAS heterodimers might be predicted but has not been demonstrated. In addition, individual PAS proteins have recently emerged that are being shown to have a function apart from the nuclear compartment. An important example of this is the recent identification and crystalization of a PAS domain within the HERG K^+ channel (263). The PAS domain at the N terminus of this channel molecule may participate in regulating the rate of channel deactivation (263).

It is now easy to predict that the PAS domain will be found in one of the largest families of signal transduction molecules encoded by the mammalian genome, rivaling the size of the nuclear receptor superfamily. The elucidation of dioxin, hypoxia, and circadian signal transduction pathways has provided valuable information about this superfamily and has allowed us to make a number of generalizations about PAS protein function. The more recent realizations that rudimentary PAS domains are found in prokaryotic light and oxygen sensors, as well as in plant photoreceptors, adds strength to our assertion that these proteins represent a primary mechanism by which organisms adapt to environmental change. The idea that normal development would utilize many of these same pathways should not be a surprise and should serve as a reminder that ontogeny of complex organisms can also be viewed as a cellular struggle to adapt to environmental change.

ACKNOWLEDGMENTS

This work was supported by The National Institutes of Health (grants R01-ES05703, T32-CA09681, and P30-CA07175) and a fellowship from The Burroughs Wellcome Fund.

Visit the Annual Reviews home page at www.AnnualReviews.org.

LITERATURE CITED

1. Whitlock JP Jr. 1999. Induction of cytochrome P4501A1. *Annu. Rev. Pharmacol. Toxicol.* 39:103–25
2. Semenza GL. 1998. Hypoxia-inducible factor 1: master regulator of O_2 homeostasis. *Curr. Opin. Genet. Dev.* 8:588–94
3. Dunlap JC. 1999. Molecular bases for circadian clocks. *Cell* 96:271–90
4. Crews ST. 1998. Control of cell lineage-specific development and transcription by bHLH-PAS proteins. *Genes Dev.* 12:607–20
5. Reddy P, Jacquier AC, Abovich N, Petersen G, Rosbash M. 1986. The period clock locus of *D. melanogaster* codes for a proteoglycan. *Cell* 46:53–61
6. Citri Y, Colot HV, Jacquier AC, Yu Q, Hall JC, et al. 1987. A family of unusually spliced biologically active transcripts encoded by a Drosophila clock gene. *Nature* 326:42–44
7. Hoffman EC, Reyes H, Chu FF, Sander F, Conley LH, et al. 1991. Cloning of a factor required for activity of the Ah (dioxin) receptor. *Science* 252:954–58
8. Jackson FR, Bargiello TA, Yun SH, Young MW. 1986. Product of per locus of Drosophila shares homology with proteoglycans. *Nature* 320:185–88
9. Nambu JR, Lewis JO, Wharton KA Jr, Crews ST. 1991. The Drosophila single-minded gene encodes a helix-loop-helix protein that acts as a master regulator of CNS midline development. *Cell* 67:1157–67
10. Denis M, Cuthill S, Wikstrom AC, Poellinger L, Gustafsson JA. 1988. Association of the dioxin receptor with the Mr 90,000 heat shock protein: a structural kinship with the glucocorticoid receptor. *Biochem. Biophys. Res. Commun.* 155:801–7
11. Perdew GH. 1988. Association of the Ah receptor with the 90-kDa heat shock protein. *J. Biol. Chem.* 263:13802–5
12. Burbach KM, Poland A, Bradfield CA. 1992. Cloning of the Ah receptor cDNA reveals a distinctive ligand-activated transcription factor. *Proc. Natl. Acad. Sci. USA* 89:8185–89
13. Dolwick KM, Swanson HI, Bradfield CA. 1993. *In vitro* analysis of Ah receptor domains involved in ligand-activated DNA recognition. *Proc. Natl. Acad. Sci. USA* 90:8566–70
14. Poland A, Palen D, Glover E. 1994. Analysis of the four alleles of the murine aryl hydrocarbon receptor. *Mol. Pharmacol.* 46:915–21
15. Murre C, Bain G, van Dijk MA, Engel I, Furnari BA, et al. 1994. Structure and function of helix-loop-helix proteins. *Biochim. Biophys. Acta* 1218:129–35
16. Kadesch T. 1993. Consequences of heteromeric interactions among helix-loop-helix proteins. *Cell Growth Differ.* 4:49–55
17. Conney AH, Miller EC, Miller JA. 1956. The metabolism of methylated aminoazo dyes. V. Evidence for induction of enzyme synthesis in the rat by 3-methylcholanthrene. *Cancer Res.* 16:450–59
18. Conney AH, Gillette JR, Inscoe JK, Trams ER, Posner HS. 1959. Induced synthesis of liver microsomal enzymes which metabolize foreign compounds. *Science* 130:1478–79
19. Remmer H, Merker HJ. 1963. Drug-induced changes in the liver endoplasmic reticulum: association with drug-metabolizing enzymes. *Science* 142:1657–58
20. Quattrochi LC, Vu T, Tukey RH. 1994. The human CYP1A2 gene and induction by 3-methylcholanthrene. *J. Biol. Chem.* 269:6949–54
21. Li W, Harper PA, Tang BK, Okey AB. 1998. Regulation of cytochrome P450 enzymes by aryl hydrocarbon receptor in human cells: CYP1A2 expression in the LS180 colon carcinoma cell line after

treatment with 2,3,7,8-tetrachlorodi-benzo-p-dioxin or 3-methylcholanthrene. *Biochem. Pharmacol.* 56:599–612

22. Skene SA, Dewhurst IC, Greenberg M. 1989. Polychlorinated dibenzo-*p*-dioxins and polychlorinated dibenzofurans: the risks to human health. A review. *Hum. Toxicol.* 8:173–203

23. Nebert DW, Gelboin HV. 1969. The *in vivo* and *in vitro* induction of aryl hydrocarbon hydroxylase in mammalian cells of different species, tissues, strains, and development and hormonal states. *Arch. Biochem. Biophys.* 134:76–89

24. Gielen JE, Goujon FM, Nebert DW. 1972. Genetic regulation of aryl hydrocarbon hydroxylase induction. *J. Biol. Chem.* 247:1125–37

25. Nebert DW, Goujon FM, Gielen JE. 1972. Aryl hydrocarbon hydroxylase induction by polycyclic hydrocarbons: simple autosomal dominant trait in the mouse. *Nat. New Biol.* 236:107

26. Poland AP, Glover E, Robinson JR, Nebert DW. 1974. Genetic expression of aryl hydrocarbon hydroxylase activity. Induction of monooxygenase activities and cytochrome P_1-450 formation by 2,3,7,8-tetrachlorodibenzo-p-dioxin in mice genetically "nonresponsive" to other aromatic hydrocarbons. *J. Biol. Chem.* 249:5599–606

27. Poland A, Glover E. 1979. An estimate of the maximum *in vivo* covalent binding of 2,3,7,8-tetrachlorodibenzo-*p*-dioxin to rat liver protein, ribosomal RNA, and DNA. *Cancer Res.* 39:3341–44

28. Poland A, Greenlee WF, Kende AS. 1979. Studies on the mechanism of action of the chlorinated dibenzo-p-dioxins and related compounds. *Ann. NY Acad. Sci.* 320:214–30

29. Poellinger L, Kurl RN, Lund J, Gillner M, Carlstedt-Duke J, et al. 1982. High-affinity binding of 2,3,7,8-tetrachlorodi-benzo-p-dioxin in cell nuclei from rat liver. *Biochim. Biophys. Acta* 714:516–23

30. Poland A, Glover E, Ebetino FH, Kende AS. 1986. Photoaffinity labeling of the Ah receptor. *J. Biol. Chem.* 261:6352–65

31. Bradfield CA, Kende AS, Poland A. 1988. Kinetic and equilibrium studies of Ah receptor-ligand binding: use of [^{125}I] 2-iodo-7,8-dibromodibenzo-p-dioxin. *Mol. Pharmacol.* 34:229–37

32. Poland A, Teitelbaum P, Glover E. 1989. [^{125}I]2-iodo-3,7,8-trichlorodibenzo-p-dioxin-binding species in mouse liver induced by agonists for the Ah receptor: characterization and identification. *Mol. Pharmacol.* 36:113–20

33. Gasiewicz TA, Ness WC, Rucci G. 1984. Ontogeny of the cytosolic receptor for 2,3,7,8-tetrachlorodibenzo-p-dioxin in rat liver, lung, and thymus. *Biochem. Biophys. Res. Commun.* 118:183–90

34. Poland A, Glover E, Kende AS. 1976. Stereospecific, high affinity binding of 2,3,7,8-tetrachlorodibenzo-*p*-dioxin by hepatic cytosol. *J. Biol. Chem.* 251: 4936–46

35. Goldstein JA. 1979. The structure-activity relationship of halogenated biphenyls as enzyme inducers. *Ann. NY Acad. Sci.* 320:164–71

36. Poland A, Greenlee WF, Kende AS. 1979. Studies on the mechanism of action of the chlorinated dibenzo-p-dioxins and related compounds. *Ann. NY Acad. Sci.* 320:214–30

37. Kende AS, Ebetino FH, Drendel WB, Sundaralingam M, Glover E, Poland A. 1985. Structure-activity relationship of bispyridyloxybenzene for induction of mouse hepatic aminopyrine N-demethylase activity. Chemical, biological, and X-ray crystallographic studies. *Mol. Pharmacol.* 28:445–53

38. Denomme MA, Homonoko K, Fujita T, Sawyer T, Safe S. 1985. Effects of substituents on the cytosolic receptor-binding avidities and aryl hydrocarbon

hydroxylase induction potencies of 7-substituted 2,3-dichlorodibenzo-p-dioxins. A quantitative structure-activity relationship analysis. *Mol. Pharmacol.* 27:656–61

39. Wilhelmsson A, Cuthill S, Denis M, Wikstrom AC, Gustafsson JA, Poellinger L. 1990. The specific DNA binding activity of the dioxin receptor is modulated by the 90 kd heat shock protein. *EMBO J.* 9:69–76

40. Prokipcak RD, Denison MS, Okey AB. 1990. Nuclear Ah receptor from mouse hepatoma cells: effect of partial proteolysis on relative molecular mass and DNA-binding properties. *Arch. Biochem. Biophys.* 283:476–83

41. Gasiewicz TA, Elferink CJ, Henry EC. 1991. Characterization of multiple forms of the Ah receptor: recognition of a dioxin-responsive enhancer involves heteromer formation. *Biochemistry* 30: 2909–16

42. Tukey RH, Hannah RR, Negishi M, Nebert DW, Eisen HJ. 1982. The Ah locus: correlation of intranuclear appearance of inducer-receptor complex with induction of cytochrome P_1-450 mRNA. *Cell* 31:275–84

43. Pollenz RS, Sattler CA, Poland A. 1994. The aryl hydrocarbon receptor and aryl hydrocarbon receptor nuclear translocator protein show distinct subcellular localizations in Hepa 1c1c7 cells by immunofluorescence microscopy. *Mol. Pharmacol.* 45:428–38

44. Thomas PE, Kouri RE, Hutton JJ. 1972. The genetics of aryl hydrocarbon hydroxylase induction in mice: a single gene difference between C57BL/6J and DBA/2J. *Biochem. Genet.* 6:157–68

45. Thomas PE, Hutton JJ. 1973. Genetics of aryl hydrocarbon hydroxylase induction in mice: additive inheritance in crosses between C3H/HeJ and DBA/2J. *Biochem. Genet.* 8:249–57

46. Greenlee WF, Poland A. 1978. An improved assay of 7-ethoxycoumarin O-

deethylase activity: induction of hepatic enzyme activity in C57BL/6J and DBA/2J mice by phenobarbital, 3-methylcholanthrene and 2,3,7,8-tetrachlorodibenzo-p-dioxin. *J. Pharmacol. Exp. Ther.* 205:596–605

47. Harper PA, Golas CL, Okey AB. 1991. Ah receptor in mice genetically "nonresponsive" for cytochrome P4501A1 induction: cytosolic Ah receptor, transformation to the nuclear binding state, and induction of aryl hydrocarbon hydroxylase by halogenated and nonhalogenated aromatic hydrocarbons in embryonic tissues and cells. *Mol. Pharmacol.* 40:818–26

48. Bigelow SW, Nebert DW. 1986. The murine aromatic hydrocarbon responsiveness locus: a comparison of receptor levels and several inducible enzyme activities among recombinant inbred lines. *J. Biochem. Toxicol.* 1:1–14

49. Ema M, Ohe N, Suzuki M, Mimura J, Sogawa K, et al. 1994. Dioxin binding activities of polymorphic forms of mouse and human aryl hydrocarbon receptors. *J. Biol. Chem.* 269:27337–43

50. Bradfield CA, Glover E, Poland A. 1991. Purification and N-terminal amino acid sequence of the Ah receptor from the C57BL/6J mouse. *Mol. Pharmacol.* 39:13–19

51. Poland A, Glover E, Bradfield CA. 1991. Characterization of polyclonal antibodies to the Ah receptor prepared by immunization with a synthetic peptide hapten. *Mol. Pharmacol.* 39:20–26; Erratum. 1991. *Mol. Pharmacol.* 39(4):435

52. Hahn ME, Poland A, Glover E, Stegeman JJ. 1994. Photoaffinity labeling of the Ah receptor: phylogenetic survey of diverse vertebrate and invertebrate species. *Arch. Biochem. Biophys.* 310:218–28

53. Poland A, Glover E. 1987. Variation in the molecular mass of the Ah receptor among vertebrate species and strains of

rats. *Biochem. Biophys. Res. Commun.* 146:1439–49

54. Ema M, Sogawa K, Watanabe N, Chujoh Y, Matsushita N, et al. 1992. cDNA cloning and structure of mouse putative Ah receptor. *Biochem. Biophys. Res. Commun.* 184:246–53

55. Reyes H, Reisz-Porszasz S, Hankinson O. 1992. Identification of the Ah receptor nuclear translocator protein (Arnt) as a component of the DNA binding form of the Ah receptor. *Science* 256:1193–95

56. Carver LA, LaPres JJ, Jain S, Dunham EE, Bradfield CA. 1998. Characterization of the Ah receptor-associated protein, ARA9. *J. Biol. Chem.* 273:33580–87

57. Ma Q, Whitlock JP Jr. 1997. A novel cytoplasmic protein that interacts with the Ah receptor, contains tetratricopeptide repeat motifs, and augments the transcriptional response to 2,3,7,8-tetrachlorodibenzo-p-dioxin. *J. Biol. Chem.* 272:8878–84

58. Meyer BK, Pray-Grant MG, Vanden Heuvel JP, Perdew GH. 1998. Hepatitis B virus X-associated protein 2 is a subunit of the unliganded aryl hydrocarbon receptor core complex and exhibits transcriptional enhancer activity. *Mol. Cell. Biol.* 18:978–88

59. Kazlauskas A, Poellinger L, Pongratz I. 1999. Evidence that the co-chaperone p23 regulates ligand responsiveness of the dioxin (Aryl hydrocarbon) receptor. *J. Biol. Chem.* 274:13519–24

60. Antonsson C, Whitelaw ML, McGuire J, Gustafsson JA, Poellinger L. 1995. Distinct roles of the molecular chaperone hsp90 in modulating dioxin receptor function via the basic helix-loop-helix and PAS domains. *Mol. Cell. Biol.* 15:756–65

61. Pongratz I, Mason GG, Poellinger L. 1992. Dual roles of the 90-kDa heat shock protein hsp90 in modulating functional activities of the dioxin receptor. *J. Biol. Chem.* 267:13728–34

62. Carver LA, Jackiw V, Bradfield CA. 1994. The 90-kDa heat shock protein is essential for Ah receptor signaling in a yeast expression system. *J. Biol. Chem.* 269:30109–12

63. Whitelaw ML, McGuire J, Picard D, Gustafsson JA, Poellinger L. 1995. Heat shock protein hsp90 regulates dioxin receptor function *in vivo*. *Proc. Natl. Acad. Sci. USA* 92:4437–41

64. Carver LA, Bradfield CA. 1997. Ligand dependent interaction of the Ah receptor with a novel immunophilin homolog *in vivo*. *J. Biol. Chem.* 272:11452–56

65. LaPres JJ, Glover E, Dunham EE, Bradfield CA. 1999. ARA9 modifies agonist signaling through an increase in available aryl hydrocarbon receptor. *J. Biol. Chem.* In press

66. Meyer BK, Perdew GH. 1999. Characterization of the AhR-hsp90-XAP2 core complex and the role of the immunophilin-related protein XAP2 in AhR stabilization. *Biochemistry* 38:8907–17

67. Goffeau A, Barrell BG, Bussey H, Davis RW, Dujon B, et al. 1996. Life with 6000 genes. *Science* 274:546, 563–67

68. Ikuta T, Eguchi H, Tachibana T, Yoneda Y, Kawajiri K. 1998. Nuclear localization and export signals of the human aryl hydrocarbon receptor. *J. Biol. Chem.* 273:2895–904

69. Abbott BD, Probst MR, Perdew GH. 1994. Immunohistochemical double-staining for Ah receptor and ARNT in human embryonic palatal shelves. *Teratology* 50:361–66

70. Elferink CJ, Whitlock JP Jr. 1994. Dioxin-dependent, DNA sequence-specific binding of a multiprotein complex containing the Ah receptor. *Receptor* 4:157–73

71. Probst MR, Reisz-Porszasz S, Agbunag RV, Ong MS, Hankinson O. 1993. Role of the aryl hydrocarbon receptor nuclear translocator protein in aryl hydrocarbon (dioxin) receptor action. *Mol. Pharmacol.* 44:511–18

72. Eguchi H, Ikuta T, Tachibana T, Yoneda Y, Kawajiri K. 1997. A nuclear localization signal of human aryl hydrocarbon receptor nuclear translocator/hypoxia-inducible factor 1β is a novel bipartite type recognized by the two components of nuclear pore-targeting complex. *J. Biol. Chem.* 272:17640–47

73. McLane KE, Whitlock JP Jr. 1994. DNA sequence requirements for Ah receptor/Arnt recognition determined by in vitro transcription. *Receptor* 4:209–22

74. Shen ES, Whitlock JP Jr. 1992. Protein-DNA interactions at a dioxin-responsive enhancer. Mutational analysis of the DNA-binding site for the liganded Ah receptor. *J. Biol. Chem.* 267:6815–19

75. Lusska A, Shen E, Whitlock JP Jr. 1993. Protein-DNA interactions at a dioxin-responsive enhancer. Analysis of six bona fide DNA-binding sites for the liganded Ah receptor. *J. Biol. Chem.* 268:6575–80

76. Matsushita N, Sogawa K, Ema M, Yoshida A, Fujii-Kuriyama Y. 1993. A factor binding to the xenobiotic responsive element (XRE) of P-4501A1 gene consists of at least two helix-loop-helix proteins, Ah receptor and Arnt. *J. Biol. Chem.* 28:21002–6

77. Mason GG, Witte AM, Whitelaw ML, Antonsson C, McGuire J, et al. 1994. Purification of the DNA binding form of dioxin receptor. Role of the Arnt cofactor in regulation of dioxin receptor function. *J. Biol. Chem.* 269:4438–49

78. Swanson HI, Tullis K, Denison MS. 1993. Binding of transformed Ah receptor complex to a dioxin responsive transcriptional enhancer: evidence for two distinct heteromeric DNA-binding forms. *Biochemistry* 32:12841–49

79. Swanson HI, Chan WK, Bradfield CA. 1995. DNA binding specificities and pairing rules of the Ah receptor, ARNT, and SIM proteins. *J. Biol. Chem.* 270:26292–302

80. Bacsi SG, Reisz-Porszasz S, Hankinson O. 1995. Orientation of the heterodimeric aryl hydrocarbon (dioxin) receptor complex on its asymmetric DNA recognition sequence. *Mol. Pharmacol.* 47:432–38

81. Sogawa K, Nakano R, Kobayashi A, Kikuchi Y, Ohe N, et al. 1995. Possible function of Ah receptor nuclear translocator (Arnt) homodimer in transcriptional regulation. *Proc. Natl. Acad. Sci. USA* 92:1936–40

82. Denison MS, Phelps CL, Dehoog J, Kim HJ, Bank PA, Yao EF. 1991. Species variation in Ah receptor transformation and DNA binding. In *Biological Basis of Risk Assessment of Dioxins and Related Compounds, Banbury Rep.*, ed. MA Gallo, 35:337–50. Cold Spring Harbor, NY: Cold Spring Harbor Lab

83. Jain S, Dolwick KM, Schmidt JV, Bradfield CA. 1994. Potent transactivation domains of the Ah receptor and the Ah receptor nuclear translocator map to their carboxyl termini. *J. Biol. Chem.* 269:31518–24

84. Li H, Dong L, Whitlock JP Jr. 1994. Transcriptional activation function of the mouse Ah receptor nuclear translocator. *J. Biol. Chem.* 269:28098–105

85. Ma Q, Dong L, Whitlock JP Jr. 1995. Transcriptional activation by the mouse Ah receptor. Interplay between multiple stimulatory and inhibitory functions. *J. Biol. Chem.* 270:12697–703

86. Whitelaw ML, Gustafsson JA, Poellinger L. 1994. Identification of transactivation and repression functions of the dioxin receptor and its basic helix-loop-helix/PAS partner factor Arnt: inducible versus constitutive modes of regulation. *Mol. Cell. Biol.* 14:8343–55

87. Fukunaga BN, Probst MR, Reisz-Porszasz S, Hankinson O. 1995. Identification of functional domains of the aryl hydrocarbon receptor. *J. Biol. Chem.* 270:29270–78

88. Ko HP, Okino ST, Ma Q, Whitlock JP Jr. 1996. Dioxin-induced CYP1A1 transcription in vivo: the aromatic hydrocar-

bon receptor mediates transactivation, enhancer-promoter communication, and changes in chromatin structure. *Mol. Cell. Biol.* 16:430–36

89. Poland A, Knutson J, Glover E. 1985. Studies on the mechanism of action of halogenated aromatic hydrocarbons. *Clin. Physiol. Biochem.* 3:147–54

90. Schmidt JV, Bradfield CA. 1996. Ah receptor signaling pathways. *Annu. Rev. Cell Dev. Biol.* 12:55–89

91. Moos AB, Baecher-Steppan L, Kerkvliet NI. 1994. Acute inflammatory response to sheep red blood cells in mice treated with 2,3,7,8-tetrachlorodibenzo-p-dioxin: the role of proinflammatory cytokines, IL-1 and TNF. *Toxicol. Appl. Pharmacol.* 127:331–35

92. Fan F, Yan B, Wood G, Viluksela M, Rozman KK. 1997. Cytokines (IL-1beta and TNFalpha) in relation to biochemical and immunological effects of 2,3,7,8-tetrachlorodibenzo-p-dioxin (TCDD) in rats. *Toxicology* 116:9–16

93. Lavin AL, Hahn DJ, Gasiewicz TA. 1998. Expression of functional aromatic hydrocarbon receptor and aromatic hydrocarbon nuclear translocator proteins in murine bone marrow stromal cells. *Arch. Biochem. Biophys.* 352:9–18

94. Yamaguchi K, Near RI, Matulka RA, Shneider A, Toselli P, et al. 1997. Activation of the aryl hydrocarbon receptor/transcription factor and bone marrow stromal cell-dependent preB cell apoptosis. *J. Immunol.* 158:2165–73

95. Pratt RM, Dencker L, Diewert VM. 1984. 2,3,7,8-Tetrachlorodibenzo-p-dioxin-induced cleft palate in the mouse: evidence for alterations in palatal shelf fusion. *Teratogen. Carcinogen. Mutagen.* 4:427–36

96. Abbott BD, Birnbaum LS. 1989. TCDD alters medial epithelial cell differentiation during palatogenesis. *Toxicol. Appl. Pharmacol.* 99:276–86

97. Sutter TR, Guzman K, Dold KM, Greenlee WF. 1991. Targets for dioxin: genes for plasminogen activator inhibitor-2 and interleukin-1b. *Science* 254:415–18

98. Zaher H, Fernandez-Salguero PM, Letterio J, Sheikh MS, Fornace AJ, et al. 1998. The involvement of aryl hydrocarbon receptor in the activation of transforming growth factor-beta and apoptosis. *Mol. Pharmacol.* 54:313–21

99. Peterson RE, Theobald HM, Kimmel GL. 1993. Developmental and reproductive toxicity of dioxins and related compounds: cross-species comparisons. *Crit. Rev. Toxicol.* 23:283–35

100. Chan WK, Yao G, Gu YZ, Bradfield CA. 1999. Cross-talk between the aryl hydrocarbon receptor and hypoxia inducible factor signaling pathways. Demonstration of competition and compensation. *J. Biol. Chem.* 274:12115–23

101. Enan E, Matsumura F. 1995. Evidence for a second pathway in the action mechanism of 2,3,7,8-tetrachlorodibenzo-p-dioxin (TCDD). Significance of Ah-receptor mediated activation of protein kinase under cell-free conditions. *Biochem. Pharmacol.* 49:249–61

102. Carrier F, Owens RA, Nebert DW, Puga A. 1992. Dioxin-dependent activation of murine Cyp1a-1 gene transcription requires protein kinase C-dependent phosphorylation. *Mol. Cell. Biol.* 12:1856–63

103. Mimura J, Ema M, Sogawa K, Fujii-Kuriyama Y. 1999. Identification of a novel mechanism of regulation of Ah (dioxin) receptor function. *Genes Dev.* 13:20–25

104. Lees MJ, Whitelaw ML. 1999. Multiple roles of ligand in transforming the dioxin receptor to an active basic helix-loop-helix/PAS transcription factor complex with the nuclear protein Arnt. *Mol. Cell. Biol.* 19:5811–22

105. Swanson HI, Perdew GH. 1993. Half-life of aryl hydrocarbon receptor in Hepa 1 cells: evidence for ligand-dependent alterations in cytosolic receptor levels. *Arch. Biochem. Biophys.* 302:167–74

106. Roman BL, Pollenz RS, Peterson RE. 1998. Responsiveness of the adult male rat reproductive tract to 2,3,7,8-tetrachlorodibenzo-p-dioxin exposure: Ah receptor and ARNT expression, CYP1A1 induction, and Ah receptor down-regulation. *Toxicol. Appl. Pharmacol.* 150:228–39

107. Hirose K, Morita M, Ema M, Mimura J, Hamada H, et al. 1996. cDna cloning and tissue-specific expression of a novel basic helix-loop-helix/Pas factor (arnt2) with close sequence similarity to the aryl hydrocarbon receptor nuclear translocator (arnt). *Mol. Cell. Biol.* 16:1706–13

108. Drutel G, Kathmann M, Heron A, Schwartz JC, Arrang JM. 1996. Cloning and selective expression in brain and kidney of ARNT2 homologous to the Ah receptor nuclear translocator (ARNT). *Biochem. Biophys. Res. Commun.* 225:333–39

109. Jain S, Maltepe E, Lu MM, Simon C, Bradfield CA. 1998. Expression of ARNT, ARNT2, HIF1 alpha, HIF2 alpha, and Ah receptor mRNAs in the developing mouse. *Mech. Dev.* 73:117–23

110. Abbott BD, Probst MR, Perdew GH, Buckalew AR. 1998. AH receptor, ARNT, glucocorticoid receptor, EGF receptor, EGF, TGF alpha, TGF beta 1, TGF beta 2, and TGF beta 3 expression in human embryonic palate, and effects of 2,3,7,8-tetrachlorodibenzo-p-dioxin (TCDD). *Teratology* 58:30–43

111. Hogenesch JB, Chan WC, Jackiw VH, Brown RC, Gu Y-Z, et al. 1997. Characterization of a subset of the basic-helix-loop-helix-PAS superfamily that interact with components of the dioxin signaling pathway. *J. Biol. Chem.* 272:8581–93

112. Ikeda M, Nomura M. 1997. cDNA cloning and tissue-specific expression of a novel basic helix-loop-helix/Pas protein (Bmal1) and identification of alternatively spliced variants with alternative

translation initiation site usage. *Biochem. Biophys. Res. Commun.* 233:258–64

113. Takahata S, Sogawa K, Kobayashi A, Ema M, Mimura J, et al. 1998. Transcriptionally active heterodimer formation of an Arnt-like PAS protein, Arnt3, with HIF-1a, HLF, and clock. *Biochem. Biophys. Res. Commun.* 248:789–94

114. Hogenesch JB, Gu Y-Z, Jain S, Bradfield CA. 1998. The basic-helix-loop-helix-PAS orphan MOP3 forms transcriptionally active complexes with circadian and hypoxia factors. *Proc. Natl. Acad. Sci. USA* 95:5474–79

115. Hahn ME, Karchner SI, Shapiro MA, Perera SA. 1997. Molecular evolution of two vertebrate aryl hydrocarbon (dioxin) receptors (AHR1 and AHR2) and the PAS family. *Proc. Natl. Acad. Sci. USA* 94:13743–48

116. Tanguay RL, Abnet CC, Heideman W, Peterson RE. 1999. Cloning and characterization of the zebrafish (Danio rerio) aryl hydrocarbon receptor. *Biochim. Biophys. Acta* 1444:35–48

117. Pollenz RS, Sullivan HR, Holmes J, Necela B, Peterson RE. 1996. Isolation and expression of cDNAs from rainbow trout (*Oncorhynchus mykiss*) that encode two novel basic helix-loop-Helix/PER-ARNT-SIM (bHLH/PAS) proteins with distinct functions in the presence of the aryl hydrocarbon receptor. Evidence for alternative mRNA splicing and dominant negative activity in the bHLH/PAS family. *J. Biol. Chem.* 271:30886–96

118. Fernandez-Salguero P, Pineau T, Hilbert DM, McPhail T, Lee SS, et al. 1995. Immune system impairment and hepatic fibrosis in mice lacking the dioxin-binding Ah receptor. *Science* 268:722–26

119. Schmidt JV, Su GH-T, Reddy JK, Simon MC, Bradfield CA. 1996. Characterization of a murine *Ahr* null allele: involvement of the Ah receptor in hepatic growth and development. *Proc. Natl. Acad. Sci. USA* 93:6731–36

120. Mimura J, Yamashita K, Nakamura K,

Morita M, Takagi TN, et al. 1997. Loss of teratogenic response to 2,3,7,8-tetrachlorodibenzo-p-dioxin (TCDD) in mice lacking the Ah (dioxin) receptor. *Genes Cells* 2:645–54

121. Lahvis GP, Bradfield CA. 1998. Ahr null alleles: distinctive or different? *Biochem. Pharmacol.* 56:781–87

122. Gonzalez FJ, Fernandez-Salguero P, Lee SS, Pineau T, Ward JM. 1995. Xenobiotic receptor knockout mice. *Toxicol. Lett.* 82–83:117–21

123. Fernandez-Salguero PM, Hilbert DM, Rudikoff S, Ward JM, Gonzalez FJ. 1996. Aryl-hydrocarbon receptor-deficient mice are resistant to 2,3,7,8-tetrachlorodibenzo-p-dioxin-induced toxicity. *Toxicol. Appl. Pharmacol.* 140:173–79

124. Guillemin K, Krasnow MA. 1997. The hypoxic response: huffing and HIFing. *Cell* 89:9–12

125. Goldberg MA, Dunning SP, Bunn HF. 1988. Regulation of the erythropoietin gene: evidence that the oxygen sensor is a heme protein. *Science* 242:1412–15

126. Czyzyk-Krzeska MF, Bayliss DA, Lawson EE, Millhorn DE. 1992. Regulation of tyrosine hydroxylase gene expression in the rat carotid body by hypoxia. *J. Neurochem.* 58:1538–46

127. Forsythe JA, Jiang BH, Iyer NV, Agani F, Leung SW, et al. 1996. Activation of vascular endothelial growth factor gene transcription by hypoxia-inducible factor 1. *Mol. Cell. Biol.* 16:4604–13

128. Levy AP, Levy NS, Wegner S, Goldberg MA. 1995. Transcriptional regulation of the rat vascular endothelial growth factor gene by hypoxia. *J. Biol. Chem.* 270:13333–40

129. Kuwabara K, Ogawa S, Matsumoto M, Koga S, Clauss M, et al. 1995. Hypoxia-mediated induction of acidic/basic fibroblast growth factor and platelet-derived growth factor in mononuclear phagocytes stimulates growth of hypoxic endothelial cells. *Proc. Natl. Acad. Sci. USA* 92:4606–10

130. Archer SL, Freude KA, Shultz PJ. 1995. Effect of graded hypoxia on the induction and function of inducible nitric oxide synthase in rat mesangial cells. *Circ. Res.* 77:21–28

131. Lee PJ, Jiang BH, Chin BY, Iyer NV, Alam J, et al. 1997. Hypoxia-inducible factor-1 mediates transcriptional activation of the heme oxygenase-1 gene in response to hypoxia. *J. Biol. Chem.* 272:5375–81

132. Semenza GL, Roth PH, Fang HM, Wang GL. 1994. Transcriptional regulation of genes encoding glycolytic enzymes by hypoxia-inducible factor 1. *J. Biol. Chem.* 269:23757–63

133. Semenza GL, Jiang BH, Leung SW, Passantino R, Concordet JP, et al. 1996. Hypoxia response elements in the aldolase A, enolase 1, and lactate dehydrogenase A gene promoters contain essential binding sites for hypoxia-inducible factor 1. *J. Biol. Chem.* 271:32529–37

134. Li H, Ko HP, Whitlock JP. 1996. Induction of phosphoglycerate kinase 1 gene expression by hypoxia. Roles of Arnt and HIF1alpha. *J. Biol. Chem.* 271:21262–67

135. Gleadle JM, Ratcliffe PJ. 1997. Induction of hypoxia-inducible factor-1, erythropoietin, vascular endothelial growth factor, and glucose transporter-1 by hypoxia: evidence against a regulatory role for Src kinase. *Blood* 89:503–9

136. Semenza GL, Nejfelt MK, Chi SM, Antonarakis SE. 1991. Hypoxia-inducible nuclear factors bind to an enhancer element located 3' to the human erythropoietin gene. *Proc. Natl. Acad. Sci. USA* 88:5680–84

137. Goldberg MA, Gaut CC, Bunn HF. 1991. Erythropoietin mRNA levels are governed by both the rate of gene transcription and posttranscriptional events. *Blood* 77:271–77

138. Semenza GL, Wang GL. 1992. A nuclear factor induced by hypoxia via de novo protein synthesis binds to the human erythropoietin gene enhancer at a site

required for transcriptional activation. *Mol. Cell. Biol.* 12:5447–54

139. Ho V, Acquaviva A, Duh E, Bunn HF. 1995. Use of a marked erythropoietin gene for investigation of its cis-acting elements. *J. Biol. Chem.* 270:10084–90

140. Wang GL, Jiang BH, Rue EA, Semenza GL. 1995. Hypoxia-inducible factor 1 is a basic-helix-loop-helix-PAS heterodimer regulated by cellular O₂ tension. *Proc. Natl. Acad. Sci. USA* 92:5510–14

141. Wang GL, Semenza GL. 1995. Purification and characterization of hypoxia-inducible factor 1. *J. Biol. Chem.* 270:1230–37

142. Wenger RH, Gassmann M. 1997. Oxygen(es) and the hypoxia-inducible factor-1. *Biol. Chem.* 378:609–16

143. Wang GL, Semenza GL. 1993. Characterization of hypoxia-inducible factor 1 and regulation of DNA binding activity by hypoxia. *J. Biol. Chem.* 268:21513–18

144. Swanson HI, Yang JH. 1996. Mapping the protein/DNA contact sites of the Ah receptor and the Ah receptor nuclear translocator. *J. Biol. Chem.* 271:31657–65

145. Fukunaga BN, Hankinson O. 1996. Identification of a novel domain in the aryl hydrocarbon receptor required for DNA binding. *J. Biol. Chem.* 271:3743–49

146. Gradin K, McGuire J, Wenger RH, Kvietikova I, Whitelaw ML, et al. 1996. Functional interference between hypoxia and dioxin signal transduction pathways: competition for recruitment of the Arnt transcription factor. *Mol. Cell. Biol.* 16:5221–31

147. Kallio PJ, Pongratz I, Gradin K, McGuire J, Poellinger L. 1997. Activation of hypoxia-inducible factor 1alpha: post-transcriptional regulation and conformational change by recruitment of the Arnt transcription factor. *Proc. Natl. Acad. Sci. USA* 94:5667–72

148. Huang LE, Arany Z, Livingston DM, Bunn HF. 1996. Activation of hypoxia-inducible transcription factor depends primarily upon redox-sensitive stabilization of its alpha subunit. *J. Biol. Chem.* 271:32253–59

149. Wenger RH, Kvietikova I, Rolfs A, Gassmann M, Marti HH. 1997. Hypoxia-inducible factor-1 alpha is regulated at the post-mRNA level. *Kidney Int.* 51:560–63

150. Salceda S, Caro J. 1997. Hypoxia-inducible factor 1alpha (HIF-1alpha) protein is rapidly degraded by the ubiquitin-proteasome system under normoxic conditions. Its stabilization by hypoxia depends on redox-induced changes. *J. Biol. Chem.* 272:22642–47

151. Huang LE, Gu J, Schau M, Bunn HF. 1998. Regulation of hypoxia-inducible factor 1alpha is mediated by an O₂-dependent degradation domain via the ubiquitin-proteasome pathway. *Proc. Natl. Acad. Sci. USA* 95:7987–92

152. Kallio PJ, Wilson WJ, O'Brien S, Makino Y, Poellinger L. 1999. Regulation of the hypoxia-inducible transcription factor 1alpha by the ubiquitin-proteasome pathway. *J. Biol. Chem.* 274:6519–25

153. Wang GL, Jiang BH, Semenza GL. 1995. Effect of protein kinase and phosphatase inhibitors on expression of hypoxia-inducible factor 1. *Biochem. Biophys. Res. Commun.* 216:669–75

154. Chandel NS, Maltepe E, Goldwasser E, Mathieu CE, Simon MC, Schumacker PT. 1998. Mitochondrial reactive oxygen species trigger hypoxia-induced transcription. *Proc. Natl. Acad. Sci. USA* 95:11715–20

155. Wang GL, Semenza GL. 1993. Desferrioxamine induces erythropoietin gene expression and hypoxia-inducible factor 1 DNA-binding activity: implications for models of hypoxia signal transduction. *Blood* 82:3610–15

156. Ladoux A, Frelin C. 1997. Cardiac expressions of HIF-1 alpha and HLF/EPAS, two basic loop helix/PAS domain

transcription factors involved in adaptative responses to hypoxic stresses. *Biochem. Biophys. Res. Commun.* 240: 552–56

157. Der SD, Zhou A, Williams BR, Silverman RH. 1998. Identification of genes differentially regulated by interferon alpha, beta, or gamma using oligonucleotide arrays. *Proc. Natl. Acad. Sci. USA* 95:15623–28

158. Jiang BH, Rue E, Wang GL, Roe R, Semenza GL. 1996. Dimerization, DNA binding, and transactivation properties of hypoxia-inducible factor 1. *J. Biol. Chem.* 271:17771–78

159. Pugh CW, O'Rourke JF, Nagao M, Gleadle JM, Ratcliffe PJ. 1997. Activation of hypoxia-inducible factor-1; definition of regulatory domains within the alpha subunit. *J. Biol. Chem.* 272:11205–14

160. Jiang BH, Zheng JZ, Leung SW, Roe R, Semenza GL. 1997. Transactivation and inhibitory domains of hypoxia-inducible factor 1alpha. Modulation of transcriptional activity by oxygen tension. *J. Biol. Chem.* 272:19253–60

161. Arany Z, Huang LE, Eckner R, Bhattacharya S, Jiang C, et al. 1996. An essential role for p300/CBP in the cellular response to hypoxia. *Proc. Natl. Acad. Sci. USA* 93:12969–73

162. Kallio PJ, Okamoto K, O'Brien S, Carrero P, Makino Y, et al. 1998. Signal transduction in hypoxic cells: inducible nuclear translocation and recruitment of the CBP/p300 coactivator by the hypoxia-inducible factor-1alpha. *EMBO J.* 17:6573–86

163. Gu YZ, Moran SM, Hogenesch JB, Wartman L, Bradfield CA. 1998. Molecular characterization and chromosomal localization of a third alpha-class hypoxia inducible factor subunit, HIF3alpha. *Gene Expr.* 7:205–13

164. Ema M, Taya S, Yokotani N, Sogawa K, Matsuda Y, Fujii-Kuriyama Y. 1997. A novel bHLH-PAS factor with close sequence similarity to hypoxia-inducible factor 1alpha regulates the VEGF expression and is potentially involved in lung and vascular development. *Proc. Natl. Acad. Sci. USA* 94:4273–78

165. Tian H, McKnight SL, Russell DW. 1997. Endothelial PAS domain protein 1 (EPAS1), a transcription factor selectively expressed in endothelial cells. *Genes Dev.* 11:72–82

166. Flamme I, Frohlich T, von Reutern M, Kappel A, Damert A, Risau W. 1997. HRF, a putative basic helix-loop-helix-PAS-domain transcription factor is closely related to hypoxia-inducible factor-1 alpha and developmentally expressed in blood vessels. *Mech. Dev.* 63:51–60

167. O'Rourke JF, Tian YM, Ratcliffe PJ, Pugh CW. 1999. Oxygen-regulated and transactivating domains in endothelial PAS protein 1: comparison with hypoxia-inducible factor-1α. *J. Biol. Chem.* 274:2060–71

168. Wiesener MS, Turley H, Allen WE, Willam C, Eckardt KU, et al. 1998. Induction of endothelial PAS domain protein-1 by hypoxia: characterization and comparison with hypoxia-inducible factor-1alpha. *Blood* 92:2260–68

169. Maltepe E, Schmidt JV, Baunoch D, Bradfield CA, Simon MC. 1997. Abnormal angiogenesis and responses to glucose and oxygen deprivation in mice lacking the protein ARNT. *Nature* 386:403–7

170. Kozak KR, Abbott B, Hankinson O. 1997. ARNT-deficient mice and placental differentiation. *Dev. Biol.* 191:297–305

171. Iyer NV, Kotch LE, Agani F, Leung SW, Laughner E, et al. 1998. Cellular and developmental control of O_2 homeostasis by hypoxia-inducible factor 1 alpha. *Genes Dev.* 12:149–62

172. Ryan HE, Lo J, Johnson RS. 1998. HIF-1 alpha is required for solid tumor formation and embryonic vascularization. *EMBO J.* 17:3005–15

173. Carmeliet P, Dor Y, Herbert JM, Fuku-mura D, Brusselmans K, et al. 1998. Role of HIF-1alpha in hypoxia-mediated apoptosis, cell proliferation and tumour angiogenesis. *Nature* 394:485–90
174. Tian H, Hammer RE, Matsumoto AM, Russell DW, McKnight SL. 1998. The hypoxia-responsive transcription factor EPAS1 is essential for catecholamine homeostasis and protection against heart failure during embryonic development. *Genes Dev.* 12:3320–24
175. Minchenko A, Bauer T, Salceda S, Caro J. 1994. Hypoxic stimulation of vascular endothelial growth factor expression in vitro and in vivo. *Lab. Invest.* 71:374–79
176. Eckardt KU, Koury ST, Tan CC, Schuster SJ, Kaissling B, et al. 1993. Distribution of erythropoietin producing cells in rat kidneys during hypoxic hypoxia. *Kidney Int.* 43:815–23
177. Jiang BH, Semenza GL, Bauer C, Marti HH. 1996. Hypoxia-inducible factor 1 levels vary exponentially over a physiologically relevant range of O_2 tension. *Am. J. Physiol.* 271:C1172–80
178. An WG, Kanekal M, Simon MC, Maltepe E, Blagosklonny MV, Neckers LM. 1998. Stabilization of wild-type p53 by hypoxia-inducible factor 1alpha. *Nature* 392:405–8
179. Maxwell PH, Wiesener MS, Chang GW, Clifford SC, Vaux EC, et al. 1999. The tumour suppressor protein VHL targets hypoxia-inducible factors for oxygen-dependent proteolysis. *Nature* 399:271–75
180. Kaelin WG Jr, Maher ER. 1998. The VHL tumour-suppressor gene paradigm. *Trends Genet.* 14:423–26
181. Crosthwaite SK, Dunlap JC, Loros JJ. 1997. Neurospora wc-1 and wc-2: transcription, photoresponses, and the origins of circadian rhythmicity. *Science* 276:763–69
182. Ballario P, Macino G. 1997. White collar proteins: PASsing the light signal in *Neu-

rospora crassa. Trends Microbiol.* 5:458–62
183. Ballario P, Talora C, Galli D, Linden H, Macino G. 1998. Roles in dimerization and blue light photoresponse of the PAS and LOV domains of *Neurospora crassa* white collar proteins. *Mol. Microbiol.* 29:719–29
184. Zehring WA, Wheeler DA, Reddy P, Konopka RJ, Kyriacou CP, et al. 1984. P-element transformation with period locus DNA restores rhythmicity to mutant, arrhythmic Drosophila melanogaster. *Cell* 39:369–76
185. Yu Q, Jacquier AC, Citri Y, Hamblen M, Hall JC, Rosbash M. 1987. Molecular mapping of point mutations in the period gene that stop or speed up biological clocks in *Drosophila melanogaster. Proc. Natl. Acad. Sci. USA* 84:784–88
186. Crews ST, Thomas JB, Goodman CS. 1988. The Drosophila single-minded gene encodes a nuclear protein with sequence similarity to the per gene product. *Cell* 52:143–51
187. Zwiebel LJ, Hardin PE, Hall JC, Rosbash M. 1991. Circadian oscillations in protein and mRNA levels of the period gene of *Drosophila melanogaster. Biochem. Soc. Transact.* 19:533–37
188. Liu X, Zwiebel LJ, Hinton D, Benzer S, Hall JC, Rosbash R. 1992. The period gene encodes a predominantly nuclear protein in adult Drosophila. *J. Neurosci.* 12:2735–44
189. Curtin KD, Huang ZJ, Rosbash M. 1995. Temporally regulated nuclear entry of the Drosophila period protein contributes to the circadian clock. *Neuron* 14:365–72
190. Myers MP, Wager-Smith K, Wesley CS, Young MW, Sehgal A. 1995. Positional cloning and sequence analysis of the Drosophila clock gene, timeless. *Science* 270:805–8
191. Gekakis N, Saez L, Delahaye-Brown AM, Myers MP, Sehgal A, et al. 1995. Isolation of timeless by PER protein interaction: defective   interaction

between timeless protein and long-period mutant PER$_L$. *Science* 270:811–15

192. Huang ZJ, Edery I, Rosbash M. 1993. PAS is a dimerization domain common to Drosophila period and several transcription factors. *Nature* 364:259–62

193. Hardin PE, Hall JC, Rosbash M. 1990. Feedback of the Drosophila period gene product on circadian cycling of its messenger RNA levels. *Nature* 343:536–40

194. Lassar A, Munsterberg A. 1994. Wiring diagrams: regulatory circuits and the control of skeletal myogenesis. *Curr. Opin. Cell Biol.* 6:432–42

195. Darlington TK, Wager-Smith K, Ceriani MF, Staknis D, Gekakis N, et al. 1998. Closing the circadian loop: CLOCK-induced transcription of its own inhibitors per and tim. *Science* 280:1599–603

196. Kume K, Zylka MJ, Sriram S, Shearman LP, Weaver DR, et al. 1999. mCRY1 and mCRY2 are essential components of the negative limb of the circadian clock feedback loop. *Cell* 98:193–205

197. Lee C, Bae K, Edery I. 1999. PER and TIM inhibit the DNA binding activity of a Drosophila CLOCK-CYC/dBMAL1 heterodimer without disrupt formation of the heterodimer: a basis for circadian transcription. *Mol. Cell. Biol.* 19:5316–25

198. Sangoram AM, Saez L, Antoch MP, Gekakis N, Staknis D, et al. 1998. Mammalian circadian autoregulatory loop: a timeless ortholog and mPer1 interact and negatively regulate CLOCK-BMAL1-induced transcription. *Neuron* 21:1101–13

199. King DP, Zhao Y, Sangoram AM, Wilsbacher LD, Tanaka M, et al. 1997. Positional cloning of the mouse circadian clock gene. *Cell* 89:641–53

200. Vitaterna MH, King DP, Chang AM, Kornhauser JM, Lowrey PL, et al. 1994. Mutagenesis and mapping of a mouse gene, Clock, essential for circadian behavior. *Science* 264:719–25

201. Antoch MP, Song EJ, Chang AM, Vita-

terna MH, Zhao Y, et al. 1997. Functional identification of the mouse circadian Clock gene by transgenic BAC rescue. *Cell* 89:655–67

202. Sun ZS, Albrecht U, Zhuchenko O, Bailey J, Eichele G, Lee CC. 1997. RIGUI, a putative mammalian ortholog of the Drosophila period gene. *Cell* 90:1003–11

203. Albrecht U, Sun ZS, Eichele G, Lee CC. 1997. A differential response of two putative mammalian circadian regulators, mper1 and mper2, to light. *Cell* 91:1055–64

204. Tei H, Okamura H, Shigeyoshi Y, Fukuhara C, Ozawa R, et al. 1997. Circadian oscillation of a mammalian homologue of the Drosophila period gene. *Nature* 389:512–16

205. Shearman LP, Zylka MJ, Weaver DR, Kolakowski LF Jr, Reppert SM. 1997. Two period homologs: circadian expression and photic regulation in the suprachiasmatic nuclei. *Neuron* 19:1261–69

206. Hao H, Allen DL, Hardin PE. 1997. A circadian enhancer mediates PER-dependent mRNA cycling in *Drosophila melanogaster. Mol. Cell. Biol.* 17:3687–93

207. Gekakis N, Staknis D, Nguyen HB, Davis FC, Wilsbacher LD, et al. 1998. Role of the CLOCK protein in the mammalian circadian mechanism. *Science* 280:1564–69

208. Allada R, White NE, So WV, Hall JC, Rosbash M. 1998. A mutant Drosophila homolog of mammalian *clock* disrupts circadian rhythms and transcription of *period* and *timeless. Cell* 93:791–804

209. Rutila JE, Suri V, Le M, So WV, Rosbash M, Hall J. 1998. CYCLE is a second bHLH-PAS Clock protein essential for circadian rhythmicity and transcription of *Drosophila period* and *timeless. Cell* 93:805–14

210. Zhou YD, Barnard M, Tian H, Li X, Ring HZ, et al. 1997. Molecular characterization of two mammalian bHLH-PAS

domain proteins selectively expressed in the central nervous system. *Proc. Natl. Acad. Sci. USA* 94:713–18

211. Sehgal A, Rothenfluh-Hilfiker A, Hunter-Ensor M, Chen Y, Myers MP, Young MW. 1995. Rhythmic expression of timeless: a basis for promoting circadian cycles in period gene autoregulation. *Science* 270:808–10

212. Saez L, Young MW. 1996. Regulation of nuclear entry of the Drosophila clock proteins period and timeless. *Neuron* 17:911–20

213. Myers MP, Wager-Smith K, Rothenfluh-Hilfiker A, Young MW. 1996. Light-induced degradation of TIMELESS and entrainment of the Drosophila circadian clock. *Science* 271:1736–40

214. Kloss B, Price JL, Saez L, Blau J, Rothenfluh A, et al. 1998. The Drosophila clock gene double-time encodes a protein closely related to human casein kinase Iepsilon. *Cell* 94:97–107

215. Price JL, Blau J, Rothenfluh A, Abodeely M, Kloss B, Young MW. 1998. *Double-time* is a novel *Drosophila* clock gene that regulates PERIOD protein accumulation. *Cell* 94:83–95

216. Emery P, So WV, Kaneko M, Hall JC, Rosbash M. 1998. CRY, a Drosophila clock and light-regulated cryptochrome, is a major contributor to circadian rhythm resetting and photosensitivity. *Cell* 95:669–79

217. Kobayashi K, Kanno S, Smit B, van der Horst GT, Takao M, Yasui A. 1998. Characterization of photolyase/blue-light receptor homologs in mouse and human cells. *Nucleic Acids Res.* 26:5086–92

218. Stanewsky R, Kaneko M, Emery P, Beretta B, Wager-Smith K, et al. 1998. The cryb mutation identifies cryptochrome as a circadian photoreceptor in Drosophila. *Cell* 95:681–92

219. van der Horst GT, Muijtjens M, Kobayashi K, Takano R, Kanno S, et al. 1999. Mammalian Cry1 and Cry2 are essential for maintenance of circadian rhythms. *Nature* 398:627–30

220. Thresher RJ, Vitaterna MH, Miyamoto Y, Kazantsev A, Hsu DS, et al. 1998. Role of mouse cryptochrome blue-light photoreceptor in circadian photoresponses. *Science* 282:1490–94

221. Ceriani MF, Darlington TK, Staknis D, Mas P, Petti AA, et al. 1999. Light-dependent sequestration of TIMELESS by CRYPTOCHROME. *Science* 285:553–56

222. Cashmore AR, Jarillo JA, Wu YJ, Liu D. 1999. Cryptochromes: blue light receptors for plants and animals. *Science* 284:760–65

223. Whitelam GC, Halliday KJ. 1999. Photomorphogenesis: phytochrome takes a partner. *Curr. Biol.* 9:R225–27

224. Fankhauser C, Chory J. 1999. Photomorphogenesis: light receptor kinase in plants. *Curr. Biol.* 9:R123–26

225. Nambu JR, Franks RG, Hu S, Crews ST. 1990. The single-minded gene of Drosophila is required for the expression of genes important for the development of CNS midline cells. *Cell* 63:63–75

226. Fan CM, Kuwana E, Bulfone A, Fletcher CF, Copeland NG, et al. 1996. Expression patterns of two murine homologs of Drosophila single-minded suggest possible roles in embryonic patterning and in the pathogenesis of Down syndrome. *Mol. Cell. Neurosci.* 7:519

227. Ema M, Suzuki M, Morita M, Hirose K, Sogawa K, et al. 1996. cDNA cloning of a murine homologue of Drosophila single-minded, its mRNA expression in mouse development, and chromosome localization. *Biochem. Biophys. Res. Commun.* 218:588–94

228. Ema M, Morita M, Ikawa S, Tanaka M, Matsuda Y, et al. 1996. Two new members of the murine Sim gene family are transcriptional repressors and show different expression patterns during mouse embryogenesis. *Mol. Cell. Biol.* 16:5865–75

229. Probst MR, Fan CM, Tessier-Lavigne M, Hankinson O. 1997. Two murine homologs of the Drosophila single-minded protein that interact with the mouse aryl hydrocarbon receptor nuclear translocator protein. *J. Biol. Chem.* 272:4451–57

230. Chrast R, Scott HS, Chen H, Kudoh J, Rossier C, et al. 1997. Cloning of two human homologs of the Drosophila single-minded gene SIM1 on chromosome 6q and SIM2 on 21q within the Down syndrome chromosomal region. *Genome Res.* 7:615–24

231. Michaud JL, Rosenquist T, May NR, Fan CM. 1998. Development of neuroendocrine lineages requires the bHLH-PAS transcription factor SIM1. *Genes Dev.* 12:3264–75

232. Wilk R, Weizman I, Shilo BZ. 1996. Trachealess encodes a bHLH-PAS protein that is an inducer of tracheal cell fates in Drosophila. *Genes Dev.* 10:93–102

233. Isaac DD, Andrew DJ. 1996. Tubulogenesis in Drosophila: a requirement for the trachealess gene product. *Genes Dev.* 10:103–17

234. Semenza GL, Agani F, Iyer N, Jiang BH, Leung S, et al. 1998. Hypoxia-inducible factor 1: from molecular biology to cardiopulmonary physiology. *Chest* 114:40–45S

235. Sonnenfeld M, Ward M, Nystrom G, Mosher J, Stahl S, Crews S. 1997. The Drosophila tango gene encodes a bHLH-PAS protein that is orthologous to mammalian Arnt and controls CNS midline and tracheal development. *Development* 124:4571–82

236. Ward MP, Mosher JT, Crews ST. 1998. Regulation of bHLH-PAS protein subcellular localization during Drosophila embryogenesis. *Development* 125:1599–608

237. Nambu JR, Chen W, Hu S, Crews ST. 1996. The *Drosophila melanogaster* similar bHLH-PAS gene encodes a protein related to human hypoxia-inducible factor 1 alpha and *Drosophila* single-minded. *Gene* 172:249–54

238. Bacon NC, Wappner P, O'Rourke JF, Bartlett SM, Shilo B, et al. 1998. Regulation of the Drosophila bHLH-PAS protein Sima by hypoxia: functional evidence for homology with mammalian HIF-1 alpha. *Biochem. Biophys. Res. Commun.* 249:811–16

239. Glass CK, Rose DW, Rosenfeld MG. 1997. Nuclear receptor coactivators. *Curr. Opin. Cell Biol.* 9:222–32

240. Onate SA, Tsai SY, Tsai MJ, O'Malley BW. 1995. Sequence and characterization of a co-activator for the steroid hormone receptor superfamily. *Science* 270:1354–57

241. Kamei Y, Xu L, Heinzel T, Torchia J, Kurokawa R, et al. 1996. A CBP integrator complex mediates transcriptional activation and AP-1 inhibition by nuclear receptors. *Cell* 85:403–14

242. Yao TP, Ku G, Zhou N, Scully R, Livingston DM. 1996. The nuclear hormone receptor coactivator SRC-1 is a specific target of p300. *Proc. Natl. Acad. Sci. USA* 93:10626–31

243. Voegel JJ, Heine MJ, Zechel C, Chambon P, Gronemeyer H. 1996. TIF2, a 160 kDa transcriptional mediator for the ligand-dependent activation function AF-2 of nuclear receptors. *EMBO J.* 15:3667–75

244. Li H, Gomes PJ, Chen JD. 1997. RAC3, a steroid/nuclear receptor-associated coactivator that is related to SRC-1 and TIF2. *Proc. Natl. Acad. Sci. USA* 94:8479–84

245. Onate SA, Boonyaratanakornkit V, Spencer TE, Tsai SY, Tsai MJ, et al. 1998. The steroid receptor coactivator-1 contains multiple receptor interacting and activation domains that cooperatively enhance the activation function 1 (AF1) and AF2 domains of steroid receptors. *J. Biol. Chem.* 273:12101–8

246. Heery DM, Kalkhoven E, Hoare S, Parker MG. 1997. A signature motif in

transcriptional co-activators mediates binding to nuclear receptors. *Nature* 387:733–36

247. Xu L, Glass CK, Rosenfeld MG. 1999. Coactivator and corepressor complexes in nuclear receptor function. *Curr. Opin. Genet. Dev.* 9:140–47

248. Gassmann M, Kvietikova I, Rolfs A, Wenger RH. 1997. Oxygen- and dioxin-regulated gene expression in mouse hepatoma cells. *Kidney Int.* 51:567–74

249. Kuil CW, Brouwer A, van der Saag PT, van der Burg B. 1998. Interference between progesterone and dioxin signal transduction pathways. Different mechanisms are involved in repression by the progesterone receptor A and B isoforms. *J. Biol. Chem.* 273:8829–34

250. Pellequer JL, Brudler R, Getzoff ED. 1999. Biological sensors: more than one way to sense oxygen. *Curr. Biol.* 9:R416–18

251. Taylor BL, Zhulin IB. 1999. PAS domains: internal sensors of oxygen, redox potential, and light. *Microbiol. Mol. Biol. Rev.* 63:479–506

252. Perego M, Cole SP, Burbulys D, Trach K, Hoch JA. 1989. Characterization of the gene for a protein kinase which phosphorylates the sporulation-regulatory proteins SpoOA and SpoOF of *Bacillus subtilis. J. Bacteriol.* 171:6187–96

253. David M, Daveran ML, Batut J, Dedieu A, Domergue O, et al. 1988. Cascade regulation of nif gene expression in *Rhizobium meliloti. Cell* 54:671–83

254. Pellequer JL, Wager-Smith KA, Kay SA, Getzoff ED. 1998. Photoactive yellow protein: a structural prototype for the three-dimensional fold of the PAS domain superfamily. *Proc. Natl. Acad. Sci. USA* 95:5884–90

255. Agron PG, Monson EK, Ditta GS, Helinski DR. 1994. Oxygen regulation of expression of nitrogen fixation genes in Rhizobium meliloti. *Res. Microbiol.* 145:454–59

256. Monson EK, Weinstein M, Ditta GS,

Helinski DR. 1992. The FixL protein of *Rhizobium meliloti* can be separated into a heme-binding oxygen-sensing domain and a functional C-terminal kinase domain. *Proc. Natl. Acad. Sci. USA* 89:4280–84

257. Genick UK, Borgstahl GE, Ng K, Ren Z, Pradervand C, et al. 1997. Structure of a protein photocycle intermediate by millisecond time-resolved crystallography. *Science* 275:1471–75

258. Genick UK, Soltis SM, Kuhn P, Canestrelli IL, Getzoff ED. 1998. Structure at 0.85 A resolution of an early protein photocycle intermediate. *Nature* 392:206–9

259. Gong W, Hao B, Mansy SS, Gonzalez G, Gilles-Gonzalez MA, Chan MK. 1998. Structure of a biological oxygen sensor: a new mechanism for heme-driven signal transduction. *Proc. Natl. Acad. Sci. USA* 95:15177–82

260. Christie JM, Reymond P, Powell GK, Bernasconi P, Raibekas AA, et al. 1998. Arabidopsis NPH1: a flavoprotein with the properties of a photoreceptor for phototropism. *Science* 282:1698–701

261. Christie JM, Salomon M, Nozue K, Wada M, Briggs WR. 1999. LOV (light, oxygen, or voltage) domains of the blue-light photoreceptor phototropin (nph1): binding sites for the chromophore flavin mononucleotide. *Proc. Natl. Acad. Sci. USA* 96:8779–83

262. Ni M, Tepperman JM, Quail PH. 1998. PIF3, a phytochrome-interacting factor necessary for normal photoinduced signal transduction, is a novel basic helix-loop-helix protein. *Cell* 95:657–67

263. Morais Cabral JH, Lee A, Cohen SL, Chait BT, Li M, Mackinnon R. 1998. Crystal structure and functional analysis of the HERG potassium channel N terminus: a eukaryotic PAS domain. *Cell* 95:649–55

264. Sun W, Zhang J, Hankinson O. 1997. A mutation in the aryl hydrocarbon receptor (AHR) in a cultured mammalian cell line identifies a novel region of AHR that

affects DNA binding. *J. Biol. Chem.* 272:31845–54

265. Higgins DG, Sharp PM. 1988. CLUS-TAL: a package for performing multiple sequence alignment on a microcomputer. *Gene* 73:237–44

266. Ashok M, Turner C, Wilson TG. 1998. Insect juvenile hormone resistance gene homology with the bHLH-PAS family of transcriptional regulators. *Proc. Natl. Acad. Sci. USA* 95:2761–66

Annu. Rev. Pharmacol. Toxicol. 2000. 40:563–80

PHARMACOLOGY OF CLONED P2X RECEPTORS

R. Alan North and Annmarie Surprenant

Institute of Molecular Physiology, University of Sheffield, Sheffield, S10 2TN, United Kingdom; e-mail: r.a.north@Sheffield.ac.uk, a.surprenant@sheffield.ac.uk

Key Words   adenosine 5'-triphosphate, ATP, purines, ion channels, antagonists, nucleotide receptors

■ **Abstract**   There are seven P2X receptor cDNAs currently known. Six homomeric ($P2X_1$, $P2X_2$, $P2X_3$, $P2X_4$, $P2X_5$, $P2X_7$) and three heteromeric ($P2X_2$/$P2X_3$, $P2X_4$/$P2X_6$, $P2X_1$/$P2X_5$) P2X receptor channels have been characterized in heterologous expression systems. Homomeric $P2X_1$ and $P2X_3$ receptors are readily distinguishable by their rapid desensitization, the agonist action of αβmethyleneATP, and the block by 2',3'-O-(2,4,6-trinitrophenyl)-ATP. $P2X_2$ receptors are unique among homomeric forms in their potentiation by low pH. Homomeric $P2X_4$ receptors are much less sensitive to antagonism by suramin and pyridoxal 5-phosphate-6-azo-2',4'-disulfonic acid. Homomeric $P2X_7$ receptors are the only form in which 2',3'-O-(4-benzoylbenzoyl)-ATP is more potent than ATP. The heteromeric $P2X_2$/$P2X_3$ receptor resembles $P2X_2$ in slow desensitization kinetics and potentiation by low pH and is similar to $P2X_3$ with respect to agonism by αβmethyleneATP and block by 2',3'-O-(2,4,6-trinitrophenyl)-ATP. Other agonists, antagonists, and ions that can be used to differentiate among the receptors are discussed.

INTRODUCTION

P2X receptors are membrane ion channels activated by the binding of extracellular adenosine 5'-triphosphate (ATP). This action of ATP, the direct gating of a cation selective channel, was first demonstrated some 15 years ago (1–3); since then there have been many additional reports of such actions of exogenous ATP [reviewed elsewhere (4–7)]. Extracellular ATP can also activate P2Y receptors. Because few of the available agonists or antagonists are very selective between P2X and P2Y receptors, the main criteria used to define the involvement of P2X receptors have been the time course of the response and/or the observation of unitary currents in outside-out patches. Thus, the opening of a cation-conducting pathway within a few milliseconds of applying the ATP indicates involvement of a P2X receptor. Such effects have now been described for a wide range of mammalian cells, including neurons, striated, smooth and cardiac muscles, epithelia, bone, and many different leukocytes. The properties of the unitary currents flowing through single ion channels have been described in several cases, and the

0362–1642/00/0415–0563$14.00

range in values suggests considerable receptor heterogeneity [PC12 cells (8), smooth muscle (9, 10), and hippocampal (11) and autonomic (12–14) neurons]. Where it is not possible to obtain such direct kinetic demonstration of the involvement of a ligand-gated ion channel, pharmacological tests become important. Much reliance has been placed on the use of available agonists and antagonists to identify actions mediated by P2X receptors.

The availability of selective antagonists becomes even more critical when addressing the functional role for endogenous ATP at P2X receptors. The initial evidence for a transmitter role for ATP was provided at the autonomic neuro-effector junction, with direct recording of the excitatory junction potential and block by the desensitizing agonist αβmethyleneATP (αβmeATP) or by the antagonist suramin (15–17); similar approaches have been used to imply that ATP mediates synaptic transmission at neuro-neuronal junctions (18, 19).

Seven P2X receptor subunit cDNAs have been cloned; Figure 1 illustrates the relatedness of the deduced amino acid sequences. Several splice variants have also been described, but these are not discussed here because many have not been functionally expressed and most have not been tested with a range of agonists and antagonists. The cDNAs have been expressed in oocytes (DNA or RNA injection), HEK293 cells (transfection or Semliki forest virus infection), or insect cells (baculovirus infection); there seem to be no obvious consistent differences among the expression systems. When expressed singly, $P2X_1$ through $P2X_4$ subunits assemble into ion channels, which provide robust currents when activated with ATP. $P2X_5$ receptors also express, but the currents are much smaller. Expression of homomeric $P2X_6$ receptors has been reported only in a small fraction of transfections (20) and is not considered further.

There are important kinetic differences among the currents evoked by ATP in cells expressing P2X receptors, and these mimic the variability also observed in native cells [reviewed elsewhere (5–7)]. When ATP is applied briefly (1–2 s) to cells expressing $P2X_3$ receptors, lower concentrations (<1 μM) elicit inward currents, which are maintained throughout the application. However, currents decline almost to zero during the application of higher concentrations. Subsequent applications within the next few minutes produce much smaller responses (sometimes called run-down). For the $P2X_1$ receptor, the time constant of desensitization itself is about 300 ms at maximal concentrations; recovery from desensitization occurs over 10–30 min. For the $P2X_3$ receptor, there is also little or no desensitization with low ATP concentrations (100–300 nM), but higher concentrations evoke currents that decline even more quickly than that observed for $P2X_1$ receptors (time constant ≈ 100 ms), and recovery from desensitization requires up to 15 min. In contrast, $P2X_2$ and $P2X_4$ receptors show little or no desensitization on this timescale (1–2 s), even with maximal concentrations. However, when the ATP application is continued for several seconds, the currents decline, and this occurs more rapidly for the $P2X_4$ receptor [reviewed elsewhere (6, 20)].

A further complication is that the permeability of the ionic channel can change during ATP applications that are continued for several seconds [$P2X_2$ and $P2X_4$

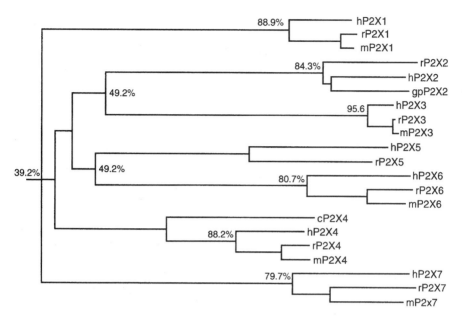

Figure 1 Relatedness of P2X receptor subunits. Amino acid sequences including both transmembrane domains and the extracellular domain were aligned by ClustalW (default parameters) and displayed by Treeview. Percentage of identical amino acids is shown between human and rat receptors for $P2X_1$, $P2X_2$, $P2X_3$, $P2X_4$, $P2X_6$, and $P2X_7$, and between $rP2X_2$ and $rP2X_3$, $rP2X_5$ and $rP2X_6$, and $rP2X_1$ and $rP2X_7$. National Center for Biotechnology Information accession numbers of these sequences are as follows: $hP2X_1$, P51575 (79); $rP2X_1$, P47824 (80); $mP2X_1$, P51576 (79); $hP2X_2$, AAD42947; $gpP2X_2$, O70397 (81); $rP2X_2$, P49653 (82); $hP2X_3$, P56373 (83); $rP2X_3$, P49654 (25, 84); $mP2X_3$ (85); $hP2X_4$, NP002551 (57); $rP2X_4$, S62359 (60); $mP2X_4$, AAC95601 (86); $cP2X_4$, AAD01645; $hP2X_5$, Q93086 (87); $rP2X_5$, CAA63052 (20); $hP2X_6$, O15547 (88); $rP2X_6$, P51579 (20); $mP2X_6$, O54803; $hP2X_7$, Q99572 (64); $rP2X_7$, Q64663 (23); $mP2X_7$, CAA08853 (89). Abbreviations: h, human; r, rat; m, mouse; gp, guinea pig; c, chicken.

receptors (21, 22); $P2X_7$ receptors (23, 24)]. The permeability increases so as to allow the passage of fluorescent cations such as quinolinium,4-[(3-methyl-2-(3H)-benzoxazolylidene)methyl]-1-[3-(triethylammonio)propyl]di-iodide (YOPRO-1) and has proven particularly useful for studies of the $P2X_7$ receptor. Except where stated, the pharmacological properties described in this chapter refer to measurements of membrane currents when agonists are applied briefly (for 1–2 s).

There is both functional and biochemical evidence for P2X receptor formation as heteromultimers; this includes $P2X_2/P2X_3$ (25, 26), $P2X_1/P2X_5$ (27, 28), and $P2X_4/P2X_6$ (22, 29). Agonists, antagonists, or modulators that are selective among these many possible subtypes of P2X receptor are needed for at least three reasons. First, they might be used to identify further physiological roles for endogenous ATP. It is particularly important in this respect to recognize that some of the currently available antagonists block other ion channel receptors at concentrations similar to those that block P2X receptors (30). Second, it may be possible to use them to determine the subunit composition of the native multimeric receptors (31). Third, P2X antagonists have several potential therapeutic applications. In this chapter we review what is currently known of such molecules, with respect to their actions at heterologously expressed P2X receptors.

HOMOMERIC RECEPTORS

P2X$_1$ Receptors

Agonists   The defining features of homomeric P2X$_1$ receptors are high sensitivity to αβmeATP [50% effective concentration (EC$_{50}$) ~1 μM] (Table 1) and the rapid desensitization of the current during agonist applications lasting 1–2 s. αβmeATP is about equally active at P2X$_3$ receptors, whereas βγmeATP shows about 30-fold selectivity for P2X$_1$ compared with P2X$_3$ (25, 32) (Table 1). Diadenosine polyphosphates (Ap$_n$A) allow further distinctions to be made among rat homomeric receptors P2X$_1$ through P2X$_4$ (33, 34). In the case of the rat P2X$_1$ receptor, activity increases with an increasing number of phosphate moieties: Ap$_6$A is a full agonist, whereas Ap$_5$A and Ap$_4$A are partial agonists (EC$_{50}$ is close to that of ATP); Ap$_3$A has a very weak effect, and Ap$_2$A has no effect at 30 μM. A similar result was reported for Ap$_5$A in human P2X$_1$ receptors (32).

Antagonists   Antagonists selective for P2X$_1$ receptors have been reported. MRS2220 (cyclic pyridoxine-α4,5-monophosphate-6-azo-phenyl-2′,5′disulfonate) blocks at a concentration of ~10 μM, whereas similar concentrations of the parent cyclic pyridoxal phosphate analog (cyclic pyridoxine-α4,5-monophosphate) potentiate responses at P2X$_1$ receptors (35). These compounds have no effect on currents evoked at P2X$_2$ or P2X$_4$ receptors (or hP2Y$_2$, hP2Y$_4$, or rP2Y$_6$) (35).

 2′,3′-O-(2′,4′,6′)-trinitrophenyl-ATP (TNP-ATP) is 1000-fold more effective when blocking ATP-induced currents at P2X$_1$ receptors [50% inhibitory concentration (IC$_{50}$) ~1 nM] than at P2X$_2$, P2X$_4$, and P2X$_7$ (36) (Table 2). This action of TNP-ATP is shared by TNP-ADP and TNP-AMP, though not by TNP-adenosine. The nanomolar affinity at P2X$_1$ (and P2X$_3$) receptors has led to its use in characterizing receptors on native tissues (31, 37). In nodose ganglion, TNP-ATP inhibits ATP-evoked currents with a biphasic inhibition curve, implying at least two receptors on a single cell (31). TNP-ATP also antagonizes the action of αβmeATP to induce currents in dissociated mesenteric artery smooth muscle, with an IC$_{50}$ of 2 nM; this is consistent with a P2X$_1$ receptor. On the other hand, it is much less effective to inhibit nerve-evoked contractions of the muscle, indicating either that the synaptic receptors are not P2X$_1$ receptors or perhaps that TNP-ATP is rapidly degraded in intact tissue preparations (37).

TABLE 1   Agonist sensitivities of cloned P2X receptors[a]

Receptor	ATP	ADP	αβmeATP	βγmeATP	2meSATP	BzATP	References
P2X$_1$	1	30	1-3	10	1	3	79, 80
		80%	100%	40%	100%	60%	
P2X$_2$	10	≈300	>100	>300	3	30	82
		100%	<5%	<10%	100%	60%	
P2X$_3$[b]	1	≈50	1	>300	0.3	—	25, 83, 84
		>80%	100%	—	100%	—	
P2X$_4$[c]	10	>>100	>>100	—	10–100	—	53–57, 60
		—	<10%	—	30–80%	—	
P2X$_5$[d]	10	≈300	>>100	—	10	>500	20, 83, 87
		>80%	—	—	—	—	
P2X$_7$[e]	100	>>300	>>300	>100	10	3	23, 64, 89
		—	—	—	80%	300%	
P2X$_2$/P2X$_3$[f]	1	—	1	—	—	—	25
P2X$_1$/P2X$_5$[f]	1	10	5	—	—	—	28, 71
P2X$_4$/P2X$_6$[f,g]	10	—	30	—	—	—	29, 58

[a]The upper of the two values in each cell is the concentration eliciting 50% of maximal response to that agonist (micromolar) [50% effective concentration (EC$_{50}$)]; the lower value is the maximal response evoked by that agonist as a fraction of the maximal response evoked by ATP. There are differences among EC$_{50}$ reported for agonists that range up to 10-fold. These differences occur between laboratories and also at various times from the same laboratory; the reasons for the differences are not known but may include seasonal and other differences in host cells, and the purity and stability of agonists, variable rates of desensitization, and differences in the divalent ion concentrations used (values reported are in presence of 1–2 mM calcium and magnesium) (see Table 3). The values presented here are approximate averages of the published value; they refer to rat receptors because those data are most complete. However, there are often species differences and some of these have been highlighted in the notes.

[b]EC$_{50}$ for CTP of 18 μM at hP2X$_3$ (63) but >100 μM at rP2X$_3$ (84).

[c]EC$_{50}$ for 2MeSATP at rP2X$_4$ varies [≈10 μM (60); 20 μM but only 30% maximum (55); ≈100 μM (56)].

[d]hP2X$_5$ receptors so far described are missing either exon X (P2X$_{5A}$) or both exons III and X (P2X$_{5B}$); these do not form functional channels. A human/rat chimeric receptor has been expressed that would have all the extracellular regions of hP2X$_5$ (87).

[e]Human hP2X$_7$ receptors are 10-fold less sensitive to BzATP and ATP than are rat receptors (64, 68), and mouse receptors are approximately twofold less sensitive than are human receptors (89) when ionic currents are measured.

[f]When a mixture of P2X$_2$ and P2X$_3$ subunits is expressed, the cell might be expected to make homomeric P2X$_2$ and P2X$_3$ channels in addition to heteromeric P2X$_2$/P2X$_3$ channels. ATP would activate all three species of channel, and EC$_{50}$ values are therefore difficult to interpret without further information (e.g. kinetics). Because αβmeATP does not activate P2X$_2$ receptors, and because currents at P2X$_3$ receptors desensitize fully within a second. Any current measured at 2 s after applying αβmeATP is assumed to result from P2X$_2$/P2X$_3$ heteromers. Similar considerations apply for the other heteromers.

[g]In oocytes expressing both P2X$_4$ and P2X$_6$ subunits, αβmeATP evokes a maximum current that is 13% that evoked by ATP; for P2X$_4$ homomers this is 7% (29).

The suramin analog 8,8′-(carbonylbis(imino-3,1-phenylene carbonyli-mino)bis(1,3,5-naphthalenetrisulfonic acid) (NF023) also shows selectivity for P2X$_1$ receptors (38). Both rP2X$_1$ and hP2X$_1$ have an IC$_{50}$ of ~200 nM, which is about 20-fold more sensitive than P2X$_3$ and over 50-fold more sensitive than P2X$_2$ and P2X$_4$ receptors. In summary, NF023 and TNP-ATP are useful tools for iden-

TABLE 2   Antagonist sensitivities of cloned P2X receptors

	Suramin	NF023	PPADS	TNP-ATP	References
P2X$_1$	1 μM	200 nM	1 μM	6 nM	32, 38, 79, 80
P2X$_2$	10 μM	~100 nM	1 μM	1 μM	38, 80
P2X$_3$	3 μM	1 μM	1 μM	1 nM	25, 84
P2X$_4$	>300 μM	>100 μM	>300 μM	15 μM	36, 38, 53–57, 60
P2X$_5$	4 μM	—	3 μM	—	23
P2X$_7$[c]	~500 μM	—	50 μM	>30 μM	23, 39, 68, 89
P2X$_2$/P2X$_3$[c]	—	1 μM	~5 μM	7 nM	25, 38
P2X$_1$/P2X$_5$[a]	—	—	—	~200 nM	28, 71
P2X$_4$/P2X$_6$[b]	—	—	—	—	29

Values are expressed as concentration causing 50% inhibition of current evoked by ATP (IC$_{50}$). Concentrations of ATP vary, but submaximal concentration has been chosen where possible.
[a]Values reported (28) report 200 nM for P2X$_1$ and 64 nM for P2X$_1$/P2X$_5$ but without any preincubation of antagonist; these values are much higher than those found by Virginio et al. for P2X$_1$ (36).
[b]There is no selective way to activate P2X$_4$/P2X$_6$ heteromers separately from P2X$_4$ homomers.
[c]αβmeATP used as agonist to avoid homomeric P2X$_2$ receptors, and currents measured after desensitzation of homomeric P2X$_3$ receptors.

tifying the participation of P2X$_1$ receptors, although in each case care must be taken with the concentrations used, and P2X$_3$ components should be eliminated by further tests.

Ions   The effects of ions have not been systematically studied on expressed P2X$_1$ receptor subunits (Table 3). Calcium has little or no inhibitory effect up to 100 mM, which is in pronounced contrast to the P2X$_2$ receptor (39). The current evoked by ATP at homomeric P2X$_1$ receptors is about 50% inhibited by a 10-fold increase in proton concentration (pH change from 7.3 to 6.3) (40). Gadolinium and lanthanum also inhibit currents at P2X$_1$ receptors (41).

P2X$_2$ Receptors

Agonists and Antagonists   There are no agonists or antagonists that selectively recognize homomeric P2X$_2$ receptors. The EC$_{50}$ for ATP is typically about 10-fold higher than for P2X$_1$ receptors, although there is considerable variability among published values. They are not activated by αβmeATP, at least at concentrations up to 300 μM (Table 1). They are sensitive to suramin and pyridoxal-phosphate-6-azophenyl-2′,4′-disulfonate (PPADS), but not TNP-ATP (Table 2).

Ions   P2X$_2$ receptors have a unique phenotype with respect to ions (Table 3). Thus, they are the only P2X receptor at which the response to ATP is increased by acidification of the extracellular solution (40, 42–44). Low pH does not affect the amplitude of unitary P2X$_2$ receptor currents, but it introduces more brief

TABLE 3   Ion sensitivities of cloned P2X receptors[a]

Receptor	Calcium	Magnesium	Zinc	Copper	Hydrogen	References
P2X$_1$	No effect	—	—	—	Decrease	39, 40
	>100 mM				pK$_a$ ≈6.3	
P2X$_2$	Decrease	—	Increase	Increase	Increase	40, 45, 82
	5 mM		20 μM	16 μM	pK$_a$ ≈7.3	
P2X$_3$	Decrease	—	—	—	Decrease	40, 46
	90 mM				pK$_a$ ≈6.0	
P2X$_4$	—	—	Increase	No effect	Decrease	45, 55, 56, 62
			2 μM	to 50 μM	pK$_a$ ≈7.0	
P2X$_7$	Decrease	Decrease	Decrease	Decrease	Decrease	
	3 mM	500 μM	10 μM	0.5 μM	pK$_a$ ≈6.1	
P2X$_2$/P2X$_3$	Decrease	—	—	—	Increase	46
	15 mM				pK$_a$ ≈7.3	

[a]The effects shown are those of increasing the ion concentration, and the values are the concentrations that decrease by 50% (pKa in the case of hydrogen) or cause 50% of the maximal increase in response to ATP. There are no studies of P2X$_5$ or P2X$_1$/P2X$_5$ receptors. Studies on P2X$_4$/P2X$_6$ are difficult to interpret because it is not possible to separate components of current through homomeric P2X$_4$ receptors.

closings into the channel openings (44). In this way, the potentiation by protons was similar to the effect of increasing the ATP concentration, which suggests that protons increase the affinity of the channel for ATP.

ATP-induced currents are potentiated by both zinc and copper at low micro-molar concentrations; this allows the receptors to be distinguished from P2X$_4$ receptors, which are less sensitive to copper (45). They can also be distinguished from P2X$_4$ receptors by their sensitivity to extracellular calcium (IC$_{50}$ ~5 mM) (39, 46). Single channel recordings indicate that this is in part due to "fast" block; that is, the kinetics of the individual blocking events are too fast to be resolved, leading to an apparent decrease in the unitary current amplitude (8, 47). Extra-cellular calcium also profoundly affects the time course of the currents evoked by ATP. As described above, whole-cell recordings of ATP-induced current show little or no decline during the applications of ATP that continue for several seconds. But in excised outside-out patches, the current declines with a time constant of approximately 100 ms. This decline is critically dependent on extracellular calcium, and it does not occur in calcium-free external solution (48). This inactivation of the current is strongly dependent on the concentrations of ATP and calcium. For ATP (in 1 mM calcium), the EC$_{50}$ is ~20 μM, the Hill coefficient is close to 3, and the fastest time constant of inactivation is ~100 ms. For calcium (using 50 μM ATP), the EC$_{50}$ is 1.3 mM, the Hill coefficient is close to 4, and the fastest time constant of inactivation (at 3 mM calcium) is 28 ms. These results indicate that the maintained activation of the channel is strongly inhibited both by extracellular calcium and by a diffusible messenger that is rapidly lost in outside-out recordings. Other divalents (magnesium, barium, manganese) are considerably less effective than calcium. A splice variant of the $P2X_2$ receptor (or a fully processed mRNA?) that misses 69 amino acids in the intracellular C-terminus region inactivates more rapidly than the wild-type receptor (49–51); the effects of calcium and other ions on this difference have not been systematically studied.

$P2X_3$ Receptors

Homomeric $P2X_3$ receptors have a similar pharmacological profile to $P2X_1$ receptors as far as the agonists ATP and $\alpha\beta$meATP are concerned; Ap_3A is somewhat more effective at $P2X_3$ than $P2X_1$ receptors (33), whereas $\beta\gamma$meATP has the opposite selectivity (Table 1). The most useful discriminating antagonist is NF023, which is approximately 40 times less active at $P2X_3$ receptors than $P2X_1$ receptors (38), but suramin, PPADS, and TNP-ATP do not readily distinguish between these receptors (Table 1). The effects of calcium ions at $P2X_3$ receptors have been studied on HEK293 cells expressing $P2X_3$ receptors (and on rat dissociated trigeminal ganglion neurones, which project to tooth pulp) (52). Increasing the calcium concentration from 1 to 10 mM had no effect on the current elicited by a single application of ATP. However, exposure to a high-calcium solution between ATP applications much accelerated the rate of recovery from desensitization. So long as the rise in calcium concentration was of sufficient duration (>10 s), its presence was "remembered" by the cell for several minutes after washout. Convincing evidence was presented that this effect resulted from a direct action of calcium on the extracellular domain of the $P2X_3$ receptor; 10 μM gadolinium mimicked the effect of 10 mM calcium.

$P2X_4$ Receptors

Agonists   Several groups have reported that 2-methylthioATP (2MeSATP) is 10- to 30-fold less potent than ATP in activating $P2X_4$ receptors [$rP2X_4$ (53–56), $hP2X_4$ (57)], and the receptors have little or no sensitivity to any of the Ap_nA compounds (33) (Table 1). Agonist actions at $P2X_4$ receptors are also unusual in that they are much potentiated by ivermectin (58). Ivermectin activates the glutamate-gated chloride channel of several invertebrates, including the nematode responsible for onchocerciasis, and it also allosterically modulates mammalian $GABA_A$ and nicotinic $\alpha7$ receptors. Khakh et al (58) report that ivermectin (EC_{50} 250 nM) reversibly increases currents evoked by ATP in oocytes expressing $P2X_4$ receptors. The effect is use- and voltage-independent and fully reversible on washing; it is not seen in oocytes expressing homomeric $P2X_2$, $P2X_3$, or $P2X_7$ receptors or heteromeric $P2X_2/P2X_3$ receptors. Cibacron blue (3–30 μM) also increases ATP-evoked currents in HEK293 cells expressing $P2X_4$ receptors, but not in cells expressing $P2X_2$ receptors (59).

Antagonists P2X$_4$ receptors are also unusual with respect to antagonist sensitivity (Table 2). They are much less sensitive to suramin and NF023 than to other P2X receptors (38, 56, 60). The differences in suramin sensitivity between the human and rat P2X$_4$ receptor prompted experiments to determine the regions of the molecule that might be involved (57). Currents elicited by ATP (5 μM) in oocytes expressing hP2X$_4$ receptors are about 50% inhibited by suramin (200 μM). The rP2X$_4$ receptor with a single amino acid substitution (Q78K) has a much increased sensitivity to suramin and to NF023 ($\approx$90% inhibition by 200 μM) (56, 57). PPADS is also a very weak antagonist at the rP2X$_4$ receptor (53, 56, 58, 60); however, a point mutation that provides the receptor with a lysine (E249K) at the equivalent position to that found in the P2X$_1$, P2X$_2$, and P2X$_3$ receptors restores the ability of PPADS to produce slowly reversible inhibition (70% by 10 μM) (60). The human receptor is more sensitive to PPADS than is the rat receptor, and the domain responsible for this difference was mapped to a 22–amino acid sequence beginning at Arg^{82} in hP2X$_4$ (57).

Ions With regard to ions (Table 3), the P2X$_4$ receptor seems to be among the most sensitive to potentiation by zinc (53, 56, 57, 61, 62), but the maximal degree of potentiation seen is less than that observed for the P2X$_2$ receptor (33). P2X$_4$ receptors are not inhibited by copper, and in this respect they differ from P2X$_2$ receptors (45).

P2X$_5$ Receptors

The currents elicited by ATP in cells expressing P2X$_5$ receptors are some 100-fold lower than those observed for P2X$_1$ through P2X$_4$, even when the procedures used for expression are very similar (20, 63). However, the agonist and antagonist profiles at the P2X$_5$ receptor appear to be similar to those reported for the P2X$_2$ receptor (20, 63); the effects of ions have not been systematically tested.

P2X$_7$ Receptors

Agonists The defining agonist pharmacology of P2X$_7$ receptors is that they are remarkably insensitive to ATP, but more sensitive to the analog 2′,3′-O-(4-benzoylbenzoyl)ATP (BzATP). BzATP is not specific for P2X$_7$ receptors; other P2X receptors are activated by BzATP, but at these it is equipotent with or less potent than ATP (e.g. 32). There are serious difficulties in making comparisons of agonist actions among studies, because the effects of agonists (and perhaps antagonists) at P2X$_7$ receptors are sensitive to the extracellular concentration of divalent cations (see below). In "normal" divalent concentrations (2 mM calcium, 1 mM magnesium) ions, the EC$_{50}$s for ATP and BzATP are about 300 μM and 8 μM, respectively, at the rat receptor (23); higher concentrations are required to activate the human P2X$_7$ receptor (64). Other agonists tested are either less effective than ATP (2MeSATP, ATPγS, ADP) or ineffective at 300–1000 μM (αβmeATP, βγmeATP, UTP, adenosine). The need to use such high ATP concentrations to activate the receptor can pose problems (for example, a 1 mM solution of ATP is acidic and can also contain significant concentrations of other nucleotides), and this has led to the extensive use of BzATP as the agonist of choice.

Antagonists   At rat receptors, currents evoked by BzATP (30 μM) are antagonized only poorly by suramin (30% inhibition by 300 μM) and PPADS (IC$_{50}$ ~50 μM) (Table 2) (23). Preincubation with 2'3'-dialdehyde-ATP (oxoATP) (100 μM) for 1–2 h irreversibly blocks currents induced by BzATP; this concentration also blocks ATP-evoked currents at P2X$_1$ and P2X$_2$ receptors by 60%, but at those receptors the inhibition is reversible by washing (32). TNP-ATP is a weak antagonist at rat P2X$_7$ receptors (IC$_{50}$ > 30 μM) (36). Calmidazolium potently inhibits BzATP-activated currents in HEK293 cells expressing P2X$_7$ receptors (IC$_{50}$ ~10 nM) (65). This action of calmidazolium seems unrelated to its more commonly studied use as an inhibitor of calmodulin; the effective concentrations are lower and the compound, which is cationic, acts from the extracellular aspect of the cell. Remarkably, calmidazolium has little or no effect on YOPRO-1 uptake into cells expressing P2X$_7$ receptors (65). This difference might represent the binding of calmidazolium to distinct conformations of the channel (i.e. the small cation permeable vs the large cation permeable states). On the other hand, the maximal inhibition of the current by calmidazolium was never more than 95%, so it is possible that the 5% of channels that remain unblocked provide a route for sufficient YOPRO-1 to enter to make the fluorescence signal appear undiminished.

The final group of compound used as P2X$_7$ receptor blockers are the isoquinolines related to KN-62 (1-[N,O-bis(5-isoquinolinesulfonyl)-N-methyl-L-tyrosyl]-4-phenylpiperazine) and KN-04 (N-[1-[N-methyl-p-(5-isoquinolinesulfonyl)benzyl]-2-(4-phenylpiperazine)ethyl]-5-isoquinolinesulfonamide) (66). KN-62 inhibits currents evoked by BzATP in HEK293 cells expressing human P2X$_7$ receptors (IC$_{50}$ 50 nM), but not those expressing rat receptors (66); a similar species selectivity had been first shown for the native P2Z receptor by Gargett & Wiley (67). It also inhibits currents in cells expressing a rat receptor in which the first 335 amino acids had been replaced with the human sequence (i.e. the entire subunit up to the beginning of the second transmembrane domain), indicating that parts of the large extracellular loop were involved in the KN-62 binding site. KN-04 had a similar effect; this indicates that inhibition of calmodulin-dependent kinase type II, for which these compounds were originally introduced, did not play any role (because KN-04 is inactive toward CaM kinase II). Essentially similar results were observed when ethidium uptake was measured (66).

Ions   The concentrations of extracellular ions have marked effects on responses at P2X$_7$ receptors. In the case of the human receptor, removal of magnesium (from 1 to 0 mM) causes a six- to eightfold increase in the amplitude of the currents evoked by ATP or BzATP, with only a relatively small increase in potency (EC$_{50}$) (23, 64); in the case of the rat receptor, the increase is about fourfold. This potentiation by removal of magnesium (and/or calcium) is a hallmark of ATP actions at the $P2X_7$ receptor and is one of the features that suggests that the receptor corresponds to the P2Z receptor of native cells (23). Because nucleotides bind divalent cations, removal of magnesium (and/or calcium) will change the relative concentrations of the different forms of ATP, particularly increasing the amount of ATP^{4-}. However, several arguments suggest that this is not the major reason for the increased effectiveness of ATP; a direct effect on the receptor of the altered divalent ion concentration is presumably responsible (65).

Systematic studies of the effects of cations at the rat $P2X_7$ receptor show that the concentrations causing half-maximal inhibition of the current evoked by BzATP (30 μM) are calcium 3000 μM, magnesium 500 μM, zinc 11 μM, hydrogen 1 μM (pH 6), and copper 0.5 μM (65). Broadly similar results have been reported for YOPRO-1 uptake (65). These experiments were carried out in normal extracellular sodium and in 2 mM calcium and 1 mM magnesium (except when those ions were being studied). Reducing the extracellular sodium concentration [N-methyl-D-glucamine (NMDG) substitution] increases the rate at which YOPRO-1 enters the cells after adding BzATP, indicating the external sodium is itself inhibitory to $P2X_7$ function (see below).

Because reduction of the divalent ion concentration has such a marked potentiating effect on agonist-induced currents at $P2X_7$ receptors, in some studies this has been used as a baseline condition. For example, the human $P2X_7$ receptor was studied in a magnesium-free, 0.5 mM calcium solution. It is more sensitive to inhibition by PPADS, with 50% inhibition by 1 μM (with 8 min preincubation); inhibition by suramin, KN-62, and calmidazolium are broadly as described above (68). In this low-divalent concentration, current measurements show that BzATP is approximately 30-fold more potent when chloride is replaced by glutamate, indicating a clear effect of the extracellular anion (69). YOPRO-1 uptake measurements showed that BzATP was 10-fold more potent in extracellular choline chloride, as compared with sodium chloride (potassium chloride was intermediate). Such an inhibitory effect of extracellular sodium ions on dye uptake has previously been shown for P2Z receptors in human lymphocytes (70, 71).

HETEROMERIC RECEPTORS

The subunit composition of native heteromeric receptors is not known. However, using epitope-tagged constructs, physical association can be shown between some pairs of P2X subunits in heterologous expression systems (26–29, 72, 73). $P2X_7$ subunits do not coimmunoprecipitate with any others, $P2X_5$ subunits coimmunoprecipitate with all others (except $P2X_7$), and the others have intermediate selectivities (72). Of those pairs that are now known to coimmunoprecipitate, some have also been studied functionally after coexpression.

P2X$_2$/P2X$_3$ Receptors

When P2X$_2$ and P2X$_3$ subunits are coexpressed, one must assume that P2X$_2$ homomers and P2X$_3$ homomers are formed in addition to one or more heteromeric channel species. Currents at homomeric P2X$_2$ receptors are not activated by $\alpha\beta$meATP; currents at homomeric P2X$_3$ recover from desensitization so slowly that they can be eliminated by repeated applications at relatively short intervals (≈ 2 min). These currents are readily antagonized by suramin and PPADS (25) (Table 2). They are also very sensitive to NF023 (38) and to TNP-ATP (36), implying that for both these antagonists, the presence of the P2X$_3$ subunit in the heteromer is sufficient to endow high sensitivity. On the other hand, the effect of pH changes is similar to that seen for homomeric P2X$_2$ receptors; acidification increases the currents at P2X$_2$/P2X$_3$ heteromers (39). In short, the P2X$_2$/P2X$_3$ heteromer (a) is activated by $\alpha\beta$meATP, (b) is blocked by TNP-ATP, (c) is potentiated by low pH, and (d) shows little or no desensitization. The first two properties are contributed by the P2X$_3$ subunit and the latter two by the P2X$_2$ subunit.

P2X$_1$/P2X$_5$ Receptors

There are two kinds of functional evidence for heteromeric channels formed from P2X$_1$ and P2X$_5$ subunits (27, 28), and these are analogous to the situation for P2X$_2$/P2X$_3$ heteromers described above (25). First, $\alpha\beta$meATP induces a sustained current, whereas with homomeric P2X$_1$ receptors the current desensitizes rapidly (<1 s) and with homomeric P2X$_5$ receptors $\alpha\beta$meATP has no effect. Second, currents evoked by $\alpha\beta$meATP at homomeric P2X$_1$ receptors exhibit marked "run-down" when the applications are repeated at intervals of less than several minutes; in the case of the heteromer, there is no such run-down even with applications every 10 s. The sensitivity of the heteromeric receptor to suramin, PPADS, and NF023 has not been reported; the antagonist TNP-ATP has an inhibitory effect similar to that observed at the P2X$_1$ receptor in the same study (28). Sensitivity to ions and protons has not been described.

P2X$_4$/P2X$_6$ Receptors

P2X$_4$ and P2X$_6$ subunits are extensively coexpressed throughout the central nervous system (20), and there is evidence for their heteropolymerization in *Xenopus* oocytes (29). Oocytes expressing the heteromeric channels gave larger currents (after 5 days) than those expressing homomeric P2X$_4$ receptors (P2X$_6$ alone gave no currents). The coinjected oocytes were also slightly more sensitive to 2Me-SATP and $\alpha\beta$meATP than were oocytes injected only with the P2X$_4$ subunit cDNA. In the case of $\alpha\beta$meATP, a maximal concentration (300 µM) elicited a current that was about 13% of the current evoked by ATP (100 µM) in the P2X$_4$/P2X$_6$ oocytes, whereas this value was only about 6% in oocytes expressing P2X$_4$ alone (29, 58). Khakh et al (58) reported that the threshold concentration for $\alpha\beta$meATP was significantly lower (10 µM) in coinjected oocytes than in oocytes expressing only P2X$_4$ receptors (300 μM), and this threshold was even lower (3 μM) in the presence of ivermectin. The coinjected (P2X$_4$/P2X$_6$) oocytes were more sensitive to inhibition by suramin and reactive blue than were singly injected oocytes (P2X$_4$) (29); there was no difference in the effects of zinc (10 μM; 80% potentiation) or protons (pH 6.5; 50% inhibition). One must assume in these experiments that the coinjected oocytes express a mixture of P2X$_4$ homomers and P2X$_4$/P2X$_6$ heteromers; the agonists used would be activating both sets of channels, and this makes experiments on antagonist sensitivity particularly difficult to interpret.

CONCLUDING REMARKS

There are several classes of ligand-gated ion channels. The first is the nicotinic superfamily—this includes both cation- and anion-selective channels, and channels activated by acetylcholine, 5-hydroxytryptamine, γ-aminobutyric acid, and glutamic acid. The molecular cloning of this family began (74) well after we had a thorough understanding of their agonist and antagonist pharmacology; indeed, it was also after the successful therapeutic exploitation of these receptors by drugs exemplified by tubocurare, hexamethonium, benzodiazepines, and ivermectin. The second family is the glutamate receptor family; the discovery of selective receptor agonists and antagonists (75) again predated the isolation of cDNAs and their heterologous expression (76–78); the tools were available with which to characterize the clones. In both these areas, much more highly subtype selective agonists and antagonists continue to be developed by using heterologously expressed receptors. P2X receptors form a third class of ligand-gated channels; it is to be hoped that the expression of cloned receptors will lead to the development of high-affinity and selective compounds, which are urgently required to probe their physiological role and to test for therapeutic potential.

Visit the Annual Reviews home page at www.AnnualReviews.org.

LITERATURE CITED

1. Jahr CE, Jessell TM. 1983. ATP excites a subpopulation of rat dorsal horn neurones. *Nature* 304:730–33
2. Kolb HA, Wakelam MJ. 1983. Transmitter-like action of ATP on patched membranes of cultured myoblasts and myotubes. *Nature* 303:621–23
3. Krishtal OA, Marchenko SM, Pidoplichko VI. 1983. Receptor for ATP in the membrane of mammalian sensory neurones. *Neurosci. Lett.* 35:41–45
4. Bean BP. 1992. Pharmacology and electrophysiology of ATP-activated ion channels. *Trends Pharmacol. Sci.* 13:87–90
5. Surprenant A, Buell G, North RA. 1995. P2X receptors bring new structure to ligand-gated ion channels. *Trends Neurosci.* 18:224–29
6. North RA, Barnard EA. 1997. Nucleotide receptors. *Curr. Opin. Neurobiol.* 7:346–57

7. Ralevic V, Burnstock G. 1998. Receptors for purines and pyrimidines. *Pharmacol. Rev.* 50:413–92

8. Nakazawa K, Hess P. 1993. Block by calcium of ATP-activated channels in pheochromocytoma cells. *J. Gen. Physiol.* 101:377–92

9. Friel DD. 1988. An ATP-sensitive conductance in single smooth muscle cells from the rat vas deferens. *J. Physiol.* 401:361–80

10. Benham CD, Tsien RW. 1987. A novel receptor-operated Ca^{2+}-permeable channel activated by ATP in smooth muscle. *Nature* 328:275–78

11. Wong AYC, Burnstock G, Gibb AJ. 1998. Characterization of P2X ATP receptor single-channel properties in outside-out patches from granule cells in rat hippocampal slices. *J. Physiol.* 511:17P

12. Barajas-Lopez C, Huizinga JD, Collins SM, Gerzanich V, Espinosa-Luna R, Peres AL. 1996. P2x-purinoceptors of myenteric neurones from the guinea-pig ileum and their unusual pharmacological properties. *Br. J. Pharmacol.* 119:1541–48

13. Searl TJ, Redman RS, Silinsky EM. 1998. Mutual occlusion of P2X ATP receptors and nicotinic receptors on sympathetic neurons of the guinea-pig. *J. Physiol.* 510:783–91

14. Cloues R. 1995. Properties of ATP-gated channels recorded from rat sympathetic neurons: voltage dependence and regulation by Zn^{2+} ions. *J. Neurophysiol.* 73:312–19

15. Sneddon P. 1992. Suramin inhibits excitatory junction potentials in guinea-pig isolated vas deferens. *Br. J. Pharmacol.* 107:1010–13

16. Ramme D, Regenold JT, Starke K, Busse R, Illes P. 1997. Identification of the neuroeffector transmitter in jejunal branches of the rabbit mesenteric artery. *Naunyn Schmiedebergs Arch. Pharmacol.* 336:267–73

17. Evans RJ, Surprenant A. 1992. Vasoconstriction of guinea-pig submucosal arterioles following sympathetic nerve stimulation is mediated by the release of ATP. *Br. J. Pharmacol.* 106:2424–29

18. Evans RJ, Derkach V, Surprenant A. 1992. ATP mediates fast synaptic transmission in mammalian neurons. *Nature* 357:503–5

19. Edwards FA, Gibb AJ, Colquhoun D. 1992. ATP receptor-mediated synaptic currents in the central nervous system. *Nature* 359:144–47

20. Collo G, North RA, Kawashima E, Merlo-Pich E, Neidhart S, et al. 1996. Cloning of $P2X_5$ and $P2X_6$ receptors and the distribution and properties of an extended family of ATP-gated ion channels. *J. Neurosci.* 16:2495–507

21. Virginio C, MacKenzie A, Rassendren FA, North RA, Surprenant A. 1999. Pore dilatation of neuronal P2X receptor channels. *Nat. Neurosci.* 2:315–22

22. Khakh BS, Bao XR, Labarca C, Lester HA. 1999. Neuronal P2X transmitter-gated cation channels change their ion selectivity in seconds. *Nat. Neurosci.* 2:322–30

23. Surprenant A, Rassendren F, Kawashima E, North RA, Buell G. 1996. The cytolytic P2Z receptor for extracellular ATP identified as a P2X receptor ($P2X_7$). *Science* 272:735–38

24. Virginio C, MacKenzie A, North RA, Surprenant A. 1999. Kinetics of cell lysis, dye uptake and permeability changes in cells expressing the rat $P2X_7$ receptor. *J. Physiol.* 519:335–46

25. Lewis C, Neidhart S, Holy C, North RA, Buell G, Surprenant A. 1995. Coexpression of P_{2X2} and P_{2X3} receptor subunits can account for ATP-gated currents in sensory neurones. *Nature* 377:432–34

26. Radford KM, Virginio C, Surprenant A, North RA, Kawashima E. 1997. Baculovirus expression provides direct evidence for heteromeric assembly of $P2X_2$ and $P2X_3$ receptors. *J. Neurosci.* 17:6529–33

27. Torres GE, Haines WR, Egan TM, Voigt MM. 1998. Co-expression of P2X$_1$ and P2X$_5$ receptor subunits reveals a novel ATP-gated ion channel. *Mol. Pharmacol.* 54:989–93

28. Lê K-T, Buoé-Grabot E, Archambault V, Séguéla P. 1999. Functional and biochemical evidence for heteromeric ATP-gated channels composed of P2X$_1$ and P2X$_5$ subunits. *J. Biol. Chem.* 274: 15415–59

29. Lê K-T, Babinski K, Séguéla P. 1998. Central P2X$_4$ and P2X$_6$ channel subunits coassemble into a novel heteromeric ATP receptor. *J. Neurosci.* 18:7152–59

30. Nakazawa K, Inoue K, Ito K, Koizumi S, Inoue K. 1995. Inhibition by suramin and reactive blue 2 of GABA and glutamate receptor channels in rat hippocampal neurons. *Naunyn Schmiedebergs Arch. Pharmacol.* 351:202–8

31. Thomas S, Virginio C, North RA, Surprenant A. 1998. The antagonist trinitrophenyl-ATP reveals co-existence of distinct P2X receptor channels in rat nodose neurones. *J. Physiol.* 509:411–17

32. Evans RJ, Lewis C, Buell G, North RA, Surprenant A. 1995. Pharmacological characterization of heterologously expressed ATP-gated cation channels (P$_{2X}$-purinoceptors). *Mol. Pharmacol.* 48:178–83

33. Wildman SS, Brown SG, King BF, Burnstock G. 1999. Selectivity of diadenosine polyphosphates for rat P2X receptor subunits. *Eur. J. Pharmacol.* 367:119–23

34. Pintor J, King BF, Miras-Portugal MT, Burnstock G. 1996. Selectivity and activity of adenine dinucleotides at recombinant P2X$_2$ and P2Y$_1$ purinoceptors. *Br. J. Pharmacol.* 119:1006–12

35. Jacobson KA, Kim YC, Wildman SS, Mohanram A, Harden TK, et al. 1998. A pyridoxine cyclic phosphate and its 6-azoaryl derivative selectively potentiate and antagonize activation of P2X$_1$ receptors. *J. Med. Chem.* 41:2201–6

36. Virginio C, Robertson G, Surprenant A, North RA. 1998. Trinitrophenyl-substituted nucleotides are potent antagonists selective for P2X$_1$, P2X$_3$, and heteromeric P2X$_{2/3}$ receptors. *Mol. Pharmacol.* 53:969–73

37. Lewis CJ, Surprenant A, Evans RJ. 1998. 2',3'(O)-(2,4,6-Trinitrophenyl) adenosine 5'-triphosphate (TNP-ATP)—a nanomolar antagonist at rat mesenteric artery P2X ion channels. *Br. J. Pharmacol.* 124:1463–66

38. Soto F, Lambrecht G, Nickel P, Stuhmer W, Busch AE. 1999. Antagonistic properties of the suramin analogue NF023 at heterologously expressed P2X receptors. *Neuropharmacology* 38:141–49

39. Evans RJ, Lewis C, Virginio C, Lundstrom K, Buell G, et al. 1996. Ionic permeability of, and divalent cation effects on, two ATP-gated cation channels (P2X receptors) expressed in mammalian cells. *J. Physiol.* 497:413–22

40. Stoop R, Surprenant A, North RA. 1997. Different sensitivities to pH of ATP-induced currents at four cloned P2X receptors. *J. Neurophysiol.* 78:1837–40

41. Nakazawa K, Liu M, Inoue K, Ohno Y. 1997. Potent inhibition by trivalent cations of ATP-gated channels. *Eur. J. Pharmacol.* 325:237–43

42. King BF, Wildman SS, Ziganshin LE, Pintor J, Burnstock G. 1997. Effects of extracellular pH on agonism and antagonism at a recombinant P2X$_2$ receptor. *Br. J. Pharmacol.* 121:1445–53

43. Nakazawa K, Liu M, Inoue K, Ohno Y. 1997. pH dependence of facilitation by neurotransmitters and divalent cations of P2X$_2$ purinoceptor/channels. *Eur. J. Pharmacol.* 337:309–14

44. Ding S, Sachs F. 1999. Single channel properties of P2X$_2$ purinoceptors. *J. Gen. Physiol.* 113:695–720

45. Xiong K, Peoples RW, Montgomery JP, Chiang Y, Stewart RR, et al. 1999. Differential modulation by copper and zinc

of $P2X_2$ and $P2X_4$ receptor function. *J. Neurophysiol.* 81:2088–94

46. Virginio C, North RA, Surprenant A. 1998. Calcium permeability and block at homomeric and heteromeric $P2X_2$ and $P2X_3$ receptors, and P2X receptors in rat nodose neurones. *J. Physiol.* 510:27–35

47. Ding S, Sachs F. 1999. Ion permeation and block of $P2x_2$ purinoceptors from single channel recordings. *J. Memb. Biol.* In press

48. Ding S, Sachs F. 2000. Inactivation of $P2X_2$ purinoceptors by divalent cations. *J. Physiol.* 522:190–214

49. Brandle U, Spielmanns P, Osteroth R, Sim J, Surprenant A, et al. 1997. Desensitization of the P2X(2) receptor controlled by alternative splicing. *FEBS Lett.* 404:294–98

50. Simon J, Kidd EJ, Smith FM, Chessell IP, Murrell-Lagnado R, et al. 1997. Localization and functional expression of splice variants of the $P2X_2$ receptor. *Mol. Pharmacol.* 52:237–48

51. Koshimizu T, Tomic M, Van Goor F, Stojilkovic SS. 1998. Functional role of alternative splicing in pituitary $P2X_2$ receptor-channel activation and desensitization. *Mol. Endocrinol.* 12:901–13

52. Cook SP, Rodland KD, McCleskey EW. 1998. A memory for extracellular Ca^{2+} by speeding recovery of P2X receptors from desensitization. *J. Neurosci.* 18: 9238–44

53. Bo X, Zhang Y, Nassar M, Burnstock G, Schoepfer R. 1995. A P2X purinoceptor cDNA conferring a novel pharmacological profile. *FEBS Lett.* 375:129–33

54. Wang CZ, Namba N, Gonoi T, Inagaki N, Seino S. 1996. Cloning and pharmacological characterization of a fourth P2X receptor subtype widely expressed in brain and peripheral tissues including various endocrine tissues. *Biochem. Biophys. Res. Commun.* 220:196–202

55. Seguela P, Haghighi A, Soghomonian J-J, Cooper E. 1996. A novel neuronal P2X

receptor with widespread distribution in the brain. *J. Neurosci.* 16:448–55

56. Soto F, Garcia-Guzman M, Gomez-Hernandez JM, Hollmann M, Karschin C, Stuhmer W. 1996. P2x4: an ATP-gated ionotropic receptor cloned from rat brain. *Proc. Natl. Acad. Sci. USA* 93:3684–88

57. Garcia-Guzman M, Soto F, Gomez-Hernandez JM, Lund PE, Stuhmer W. 1997. Characterization of recombinant human $P2X_4$ receptor reveals pharmacological differences to the rat homologue. *Mol. Pharmacol.* 51:109–18

58. Khakh BS, Proctor WR, Dunwiddie TV, Labarca C, Lester HA. 1999. Allosteric control of gating and kinetics at $P2X_4$ receptor-channels. *J. Neurosci.* 19:7289–99

59. Miller KJ, Michel AD, Chessell IP, Humphrey PPA. 1998. Cibacron blue allosterically modulates the rat $P2X_4$ receptor. *Neuropharmacology* 37:1579–86

60. Buell G, Lewis C, Collo G, North RA, Surprenant A. 1996. An antagonist-insensitive P2X receptor expressed in epithelia and brain. *EMBO J.* 15:55–62

61. Nakazawa K, Ohno Y. 1997. Effects of neuroamines and divalent cations on cloned and mutated ATP-gated channels. *Eur. J. Pharmacol.* 325:101–8

62. Wildman SS, King BF, Burnstock G. 1999. Modulation of ATP-responses at recombinant rP2X4 receptors by extracellular pH and zinc. *Br. J. Pharmacol.* 126:762–68

63. Garcia-Guzman M, Stuhmer W, Soto F. 1997. Molecular characterization and pharmacological properties of the human P2X3 purinoceptor. *Mol. Brain Res.* 47:59–66

64. Rassendren F, Buell GN, Virginio C, Collo G, North RA, Surprenant A. 1997. The permeabilizing ATP receptor, $P2X_7$. Cloning and expression of a human cDNA. *J. Biol. Chem.* 272:5482–86

65. Virginio C, Church D, North RA, Surprenant A. 1997. Effects of divalent cations, protons and calmidazolium at the

rat P2X$_7$ receptor. *Neuropharmacology* 36:1285–94

66. Humphreys BD, Virginio C, Surprenant A, Rice J, Dubyak GR. 1998. Isoquinolines as antagonists of the P2X$_7$ nucleotide receptor: high selectivity for the human versus rat receptor homologues. *Mol. Pharmacol.* 54:22–32

67. Gargett CE, Wiley JS. 1997. The isoquinoline derivative KN-62 a potent antagonist of the P2Z-receptor of human lymphocytes. *Br. J. Pharmacol.* 120: 1483–90

68. Chessell IP, Michel AD, Humphrey PP. 1998. Effects of antagonists at the human recombinant P2X7 receptor. *Br. J. Pharmacol.* 124:1314–20

69. Michel AD, Chessell IP, Humphrey PP. 1999. Ionic effects on human recombinant P2X$_7$ receptor function. *Naunyn Schmiedebergs Arch. Pharmacol.* 359: 102–9

70. Wiley JS, Chen R, Wiley MJ, Jamieson GP. 1992. The ATP^4-receptor-operated ion channel of human lymphocytes: inhibition of ion fluxes by amiloride analogs and by extracellular sodium ions. *Arch. Biochem. Biophys.* 292:411–18

71. Pizzo P, Zanovello P, Brontew V, Di Virgilio F. 1991. Extracellular ATP causes lysis of mouse thymocytes and activates a plasma-membrane ion channel. *Biochem. J.* 274:139–44

72. Torres GE, Egan TM, Voigt MM. 1999. Hetero-oligomeric assembly of P2X receptor subunits. Specificities exist with regard to possible partners. *J. Biol. Chem.* 274:6653–59

73. Torres GE, Egan TM, Voigt MM. 1999. Identification of a domain involved in ATP-gated ionotropic receptor subunit assembly. *J. Biol. Chem.* 274:22359–65

74. Noda M, Takahashi H, Tanabe T, Toyosato M, Furutani Y, et al. 1982. Primary structure of alpha-subunit precursor of *Torpedo californica* acetylcholine receptor deduced from cDNA sequence. *Nature* 299:793–97

75. Watkins JC, Evans RH. 1981. Excitatory amino acid transmitters. *Annu. Rev. Pharmacol. Toxicol.* 21:165–204

76. Moriyoshi K, Masu M, Ishii T, Shigemoto R, Mizuno N, Nakanishi S. 1991. Molecular cloning and characterization of the rat NMDA receptor. *Nature* 354:31–37

77. Hollmann M, O'Shea-Greenfield A, Rogers SW, Heinemann S. 1989. Cloning by functional expression of a member of the glutamate receptor family. *Nature* 342:643–48

78. Keinanen K, Wisden W, Sommer B, Werner P, Herb A, et al. 1990. A family of AMPA-selective glutamate receptors. *Science* 249:556–60

79. Valera S, Talabot F, Evans RJ, Gos A, Antonarakis SE, et al. 1995. Characterization and chromosomal localization of a human P2X receptor from the urinary bladder. *Recept. Channels* 3:283–89

80. Valera S, Hussy N, Evans RJ, Adami N, North RA, et al. 1994. A new class of ligand-gated ion channel defined by P$_{2X}$ receptor for extracellular ATP. *Nature* 371:516–19

81. Parker MS, Larroque ML, Campbell JM, Bobbin RP, Deininger P. 1998. Novel variant of the P2X$_2$ ATP receptor from the guinea pig organ of Corti. *Hear. Res.* 121:62–70

82. Brake AJ, Wagenbach MJ, Julius D. 1994. New structural motif for ligand-gated ion channels defined by an ionotropic ATP receptor. *Nature* 371:519–23

83. Garcia-Guzman M, Soto F, Laube B, Stuhmer W. 1996. Molecular cloning and functional expression of a novel rat heart P2X purinoceptor. *FEBS Lett.* 388:123–27

84. Chen C-C, Akopina AN, Sivilotti L, Colquhoun D, Burnstock G, Wood JN. 1995. A P2X purinoceptor expressed by a subset of sensory neurons. *Nature* 377:428–31

85. Souslova V, Ravenall S, Fox M, Wells D, Wood JN, et al. 1997. Structure and chro-

mosomal mapping of the mouse P2X$_3$ gene. *Gene* 195:101–11

86. Townsend-Nicholson A, King BF, Wildman SS, Burnstock G. 1999. Molecular cloning, functional characterization and possible co-operativity between the murine P2X$_4$ and P2X$_{4a}$ receptors. *Mol. Brain Res.* 64:246–54

87. Lê KT, Paquet M, Nouel D, Babinski K, Séguéla P. 1997. Primary structure and expression of a naturally truncated human P2X ATP receptor subunit from brain and immune system. *FEBS Lett.* 418:195–99

88. Urano T, Nishimori H, Han H, Furuhata T, Kimura Y, et al. 1997. Cloning of P2XM, a novel human P2X receptor gene regulated by p53. *Cancer Res.* 57:3281–87

89. Chessell IP, Simon J, Hibell AD, Michel AD, Barnard EA, et al. 1999. Cloning and functional characterisation of the mouse P2X$_7$ receptor. FEBS Lett. 439:26–30

Annu. Rev. Pharmacol. Toxicol. 2000. 40:581–616

HUMAN UDP-GLUCURONOSYLTRANSFERASES: Metabolism, Expression, and Disease

Robert H. Tukey[1] and Christian P. Strassburg[2]

[1]*Departments of Chemistry & Biochemistry and Pharmacology, Cancer Center, University of California, San Diego, La Jolla, California 92093; e-mail: rtukey@ucsd.edu*
[2]*Department of Gastroenterology and Hepatology, Hannover Medical School, 30625 Hannover, Germany; e-mail: strassburg.christian@mh-hanover.de*

Key Words   glucuronidation, tissue specificity, extrahepatic, cancer, autoimmunity

■ **Abstract**   In vertebrates, the glucuronidation of small lipophilic agents is catalyzed by the endoplasmic reticulum UDP-glucuronosyltransferases (UGTs). This metabolic pathway leads to the formation of water-soluble metabolites originating from normal dietary processes, cellular catabolism, or exposure to drugs and xenobiotics. This classic detoxification process, which led to the discovery nearly 50 years ago of the cosubstrate UDP-glucuronic acid (19), is now known to be carried out by 15 human UGTs. Characterization of the individual gene products using cDNA expression experiments has led to the identification of over 350 individual compounds that serve as substrates for this superfamily of proteins. This data, coupled with the introduction of sophisticated RNA detection techniques designed to elucidate patterns of gene expression of the UGT superfamily in human liver and extrahepatic tissues of the gastrointestinal tract, has aided in understanding the contribution of glucuronidation toward epithelial first-pass metabolism. In addition, characterization of the *UGT1A* locus and genetic studies directed at understanding the role of bilirubin glucuronidation and the biochemical basis of the clinical symptoms found in unconjugated hyperbilirubinemia have uncovered the structural gene polymorphisms associated with Crigler-Najjar's and Gilbert's syndrome. The role of the UGTs in metabolism and different disease states in humans is the topic of this review.

INTRODUCTION

The catalytic reaction that utilizes UDP-glucuronic acid (UDPGlcUA) as a cosubstrate for the formation of lipophilic glucuronides from non–membrane-associated substrates, such as steroids, bile acids, bilirubin, hormones, dietary constituents, and thousands of xenobiotics that include drugs, environmental toxicants, and carcinogens, has evolved as a highly specialized function in higher organisms.

The UDP-glucuronosyltransferases (UGTs) (EC 2.4.1.17) utilize UDPGlcUA as a sugar acceptor and transfer glucuronic acid to available substrates, a process that forms β-glucuronidase–sensitive β-D-glucopyranosiduronic acids (glucuronides). These β-D-glucuronides can be formed through hydroxyl (alcoholic, phenolic), carboxyl, sulfuryl, carbonyl, and amino (primary, secondary, or tertiary) linkages. This type of structural diversity in substrate specificity allows for the acceptance of thousands of agents to be targeted for glucuronidation. Although there are examples of glucuronides possessing biological activity, such as the analgesic action of morphine 6-glucuronide, this pathway is primarily catabolic and is therefore generally regarded as a "detoxification" reaction (1). Thus, glucuronidation serves as an integral step in transforming lipophilic substrates into hydrophilic glucuronides, a process that increases their ability to partition into the aqueous intra- and extracellular compartments of the body, facilitating the transport to excretory organs and subsequent elimination through the bile and urine.

The past decade has seen significant advances in the applications of recombinant methodologies toward the investigation of the genetic multiplicity of the UGT gene families (2). For example, investigations into the specificity of bilirubin glucuronidation have identified the genes (3) involved in the hereditary metabolic errors associated with Crigler-Najjar syndrome type I (4), which is transmitted as an autosomal recessive trait in humans and characterized by an inability to glucuronidate bilirubin (reviewed in 5, 6). The accumulation of unconjugated bilirubin (hyperbilirubinemia) in Crigler-Najjar syndrome type I leads to nonhemolytic icterus within the first few days of life and is followed eventually by the accumulation of bilirubin in nerve terminals and glial cells, a clinical condition termed kerinicterus. The homozygous inheritance of nonfunctional bilirubin UGT and the onset of Crigler-Najjar syndrome type I results in early childhood death. The discovery of the genetic defect and the development of chimeraplasty, a form of gene transplantation, is being evaluated as potential therapy for the deadly disease (6a).

The realization that most vertebrates are capable of generating UGT-directed glucuronides from a virtual plethora of structurally divergent substances fostered the belief that this unique catalytic pathway involved a family of UGTs, with the catalytic potential for a wide range of substrate specificities. From early experiments in protein purification (7–11) that led to the characterization of several animal UGTs, and which were followed by the first cloning of cDNAs encoding rodent UGTs (12, 13), over 50 vertebrate UGT cDNAs (14) have been characterized and deposited in the National Institutes of Health Genbank and European Molecular Biology Laboratory. To further define the substrate specificities of proteins encoded by the cDNAs, stable and transient expression experiments in a variety of cell lines has allowed investigation of the potential substrate specificities of individual UGTs (15). Although there are potential drawbacks in attempting to compare the significance of results generated in different laboratories, because they are defining their own biological tools for protein expression, a good understanding of the role of the UGTs in endogenous and xenobiotic metabolism is starting to occur (16).

For the most part, investigations that have elaborated on human glucuronidation have focused primarily on hepatic tissue, because of the greater availability of this tissue source and the well-understood role of the liver in drug metabolism. However, methodologies sensitive enough to detect RNA transcripts, e.g. polymerase chain reaction (PCR) technology and information garnered from unique DNA sequences obtained from cDNA or gene sequence databases make it possible to identify precisely the potential of different human tissues to carry out glucuronidation (17, 18). In combining the ease of obtaining substrate specificity information for any single UGT through in vivo expression experiments, conclusions about the importance of human tissue in specific glucuronidation patterns can be obtained. These data are important in understanding the role of glucuronidation in metabolism and human disease, particularly when defining the role of glucuronidation in different tissues.

Since the discovery and characterization in 1953 of UDPGlcUA as the donor nucleotide sugar acting as cosubstrate in the generation of o-aminophenol and (−)menthol glucuronides (19), and the localization of the catalytic activity to the microsomal fraction of liver homogenates (20), many outstanding reviews and monographs have been written addressing the regulation and function of the UGTs (e.g. 1, 5, 21–24). Although glucuronidation has been identified in various vertebrates (1), this review addresses the recent advances that have helped to elucidate the regulatory and functional aspects of glucuronidation in man. We have elected to focus primarily on the contributions that have defined the genetics and the multiplicity of the *UGT* gene families, and how this information has helped in advancing a greater understanding of the role these enzymes play in metabolism and disease.

NOMENCLATURE

In this article, we define the UDP-glucuronosyltransferases as UGTs, in contrast to the classification as UDP-glycosyltranferases, as previously recommended (14). This decision to modify the recommended nomenclature is based upon several considerations.

Although the characterization of over 50 vertebrate UGTs has been described, those localized in the endoplasmic reticulum (ER) have been grouped into a gene family that consists of (*a*) several other known vertebrate UTP-sugar acceptor proteins and (*b*) a diverse number of invertebrate proteins that have not been characterized. This grouping relied both on limited homology (as low as 10% identity between some sequences) and on a predicted UDP-glycosyltransferase signature sequence that is conserved among several UTP-sugar glycosyltransfer-

Identity	Accession Number	Identity	Accession Number
C elegans	AAC69026	UGT1A8h	AAB84259
Drosophila	AAD22028	UGT1A8r	Q64634
Felis1	BAA24692	UGT1A9h	AAB19791
Felis2	AAB96667	UGT1B1p	CAA52214
Plaice	CAB51369	UGT2A1b	No Number
UGT18A1	CAA99957	UGT2A1h	CAB41974
UGT18B1	CAA99955	UGT2A1r	P36510
UGT18C1	CAA99956	UGT2B10h	P36537
UGT18D1	CAA94871	UGT2B11h	CAA44961
UGT18D2	CAA94870	UGT2B12r	P36511
UGT18E1	CAA99954	UGT2B13l	P36512
Ugt1a1	Q63886	UGT2B14l	P36513
UGT1A10h	AAB81537	UGT2B15h	AAA83406
UGT1A1h	P22309	UGT2B16l	AAB71494
UGT1A1r	Q64550	UGT2B17h	NP 001068
Ugt1a2	P70691	UGT2B19m	AAD24435
UGT1A2r	P20720	UGT2B1r	P09875
UGT1A3h	P35503	UGT2B2r	P08541
UGT1A3r	Q64637	UGT2B3r	P08542
UGT1A4l	Q28612	UGT2B4h	CAA68415
UGT1A4h	P22310	Ugt2b5	P17717
UGT1A5h	P35504	UGT2B6r	P19488
UGT1A5r	Q64638	UGT2B7h	AAA36793
Ugt1a6	Q64435	UGT2B8r	AAA86833
UGT1A6l	Q28611	UGT2B9m	AAB50249
UGT1A6b	BAA23359	UGT2C11	P36514
UGT1A6h	AAA61251	UGT31B1v	AAB03658
UGT1A6o	BAA77457	UGT74ma	A54739
UGT1A6r	P08430	UGT77A1ma	P16166
Ugt1a7	Q62452	Ugt8	Q64676
UGT1A7h	AAB81536	UGT8h	Q16880
UGT1A7r	Q64633	UGT8r	Q09426

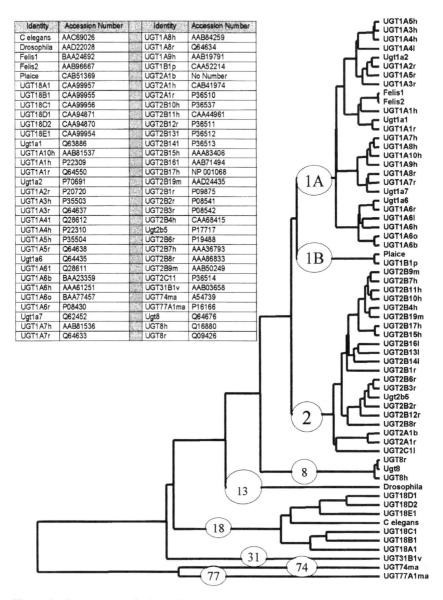

Figure 1   See next page for legend.

ases. Using the predicted prosite sequence (http://www.expasy.ch/cgi-bin/get-prosite-entry?PS00375) and computer algorithms to search protein databases, the mammalian UDP-galactose-ceramide galactosytransferases (EC 2.4.1.45), the plant flavonol O-(3)-glucosyltransferase (EC 2.4.1.91), the baculovirus ecdysteroid UDP-glucosyltransferase (EC 2.4.1.-), the prokaryotic zeaxanthin glucosyl transferase (EC 2.4.1.-), and the streptomyces macrolide glycosyltransferases (EC 2.4.1.-) have been identified. In addition, a host of other putative gene families, most without any known function and identified strictly through limited sequence similarities, have also been included. In combination with the known *UGT1* and *UGT2* gene families, an additional 31 gene families are included. A representative phylogenetic tree generated using UGT1 and UGT2 sequences and representatives of the other UDP-glycosyltransferases is shown in Figure 1. Based upon the homologies and speculated branch distances, there is most likely an evolutionary link between the vertebrate UGTs and the other vertebrate glycosyltransferase gene family (UGT8), because there exists approximately 30% identity between these gene families. However, there exists little structural or functional similarity between the ER-specific UGTs and UGT8. In addition, there is very limited identity with any of the invertebrate sequences (e.g. *Caenorhabditis elegans,* baculovirus, and plant sequences). It should also be noted that the signature sequence is not found in glycosyltransferases with the function of catalyzing the addition of the glycosyl group from UTP-sugar toward the synthesis of proteoglycans. Most important, as we think about the evolution of these genes and the specificity of the proteins to utilize UDPGlcUA as cosubstrate, there is also no similarity in amino acid or prosite sequence with the Golgi-specific UGT I, a type two glycosyltransferase that transfers GlcUA from UDPGlcUA to glycosaminoglycans (25–27).

As outlined by Mackenzie et al (14), it is being recommended that UGT be

← **Figure 1** Phylogenic tree showing divergence patterns of the 50 vertebrate UDP-glucuronosyltransferases (UGTs) (families 1 and 2) with other presumed glycosyltransferases. The table in the middle outlines the accession numbers used to obtain the protein sequences from GenBank and European Molecular Biology Laboratory. The Phylip program that we utilized was downloaded from http://evolution.genetics.washington.edu/phylip/getme.html, and the tree view program was obtained from http://taxonomy.zoology.gla.ac.uk/rod/treeview.html. The sequences were aligned using ClustalX (ftp://ftp.ebi.ac.uk/pub/software/dos/clustalw/clustalx.) and the dendrogram was generated with the average linkage clustering method (UP6MA), which assumes an evolutionary clock. The species represented can be identified as follows: Ugt, mouse; h, human: 1, lagomorph; r, rat; o, sheep; b, bovine; felis, cat; p, flounder; m, monkey; d, drosophila; v, veres; ma, maize; UGT18, *Caenorhabditis elegans.* The sequences for Felis1 -2, Plaice, *Drosophila,* and *C. elegans* have not been assigned to a UGT family but were identified in the databases. With the exception of UGT1 and UGT2, not all families are represented as previously outlined (14).

used as the synonym to reference UDP-glycosyltransferases. This poses potential problems in accurately describing the well-characterized UGTs. (*a*) The utilization of amino acid similarities to predict evolutionary relatedness to all UDP-glycosyltransferases will result in the exclusion of other important UTP-sugar–accepting proteins (and gene families), as indicated above. This has been noted by Mackenzie et al (14). Thus, the use of a defined term such as UGT to link all UDP-glycosyltransferases is not representative of all the gene families of proteins that utilize UTP-sugars as cosubstrates. (*b*) There is no experimental evidence that any of the nonvertebrate-related UDP-glycosyltransferases or those proteins that are distantly related in evolution to the UGTs utilize UDPGlcUA as cosubstrate. The ability to incorporate UDPGlcUA as cosubstrate in a biochemical reaction that catalyzes the formation of small-molecule glucuronides has evolved as a highly selective process in higher organisms, as is evident from the identification and function of these enzymes only in vertebrates.

Although the remnants of some conserved sequences are found in different phyla and species (i.e. families UGT18, UGT31, and UGT77 in Figure 1), evolution has resulted in the formation of the UGT gene family, whose function is unique to other distantly related glycosyltransferases. For these reasons, we propose that the synonym UGT represent UDP-glucuronosyltransferase. The criteria for classification as we would recommend might rely on the following. (*a*) All protein sequences grouped into the UGT supergene family would share at a minimum 45% similarity in sequence identity, a parameter similar to those of the cytochrome P450s (28). In the absence of function, preliminary assignment of nomenclature to a family could be established based upon relative similarity of amino acid sequence to the other UGTs. (*b*) All of the protein sequences within a UGT family would maintain approximately 55% similarity. Based upon this designation, the Plaice (Flounder) sequences (UGT1B), which share less than 50% identity to the other UGT1A sequences, would be assigned to a new UGT family, such as UGT3. (*c*) The sequences within a family could be arbitrarily grouped into subfamilies based upon predictions of phylogenetic divergence. As it now stands, the sequences within the UGT1A and UGT2 subfamilies share 60% similarity in amino acid identity. (*d*) The designated UGTs must utilize UDPGlcUA as cosubstrate. This is appropriate because evolution has naturally selected a large family of proteins to utilize UDPGlcUA for the conjugation of small lipophilic substances. This distinguishing property would separate the family of UGTs from other UTP-sugar–accepting glycosyltransferases. Under these guidelines and what is available in the present protein and DNA sequence databases, only the vertebrate sequences would constitute the present UGT supergene family. Based upon the lack of functional relatedness and the significant divergence in sequence homology to the ER-based UGTs, it may be more appropriate to assign the functional glycosyltransferases (i.e. UDP-galactose-ceramide galactosyltransferase) and the predicted glycosyltransferases (i.e. *C. elegans*) into different families.

HUMAN UDP-GLUCURONOSYLTRANSFERASES

Currently, 15 human UGT cDNAs have been identified (Figure 2), eight UGT1A proteins encoded by the *UGT1A* locus and seven proteins encoded by *UGT2* genes. Structural information from the *UGT2B17* (29) and *UGT2B4* (30) genes demonstrates that these genes consist of six exons spanning approximately 30 kb. Conservation in exon/intron organization is maintained in rodents, as several *UGT2* genes have been characterized and shown to contain the same exon/intron branch points (31, 32). Transcripts encoding UGT2A1 (33), UGT2B4 (34–36), UGT2B7 (36–39), UGT2B10 (35), UGT2B11 (40), UGT2B15 (41, 42), and UGT2B17 (29, 43) have been characterized, and these genes have been mapped to human chromosome 4-q13 (44, 45) and 4q28 (41). Three of the *UGT2* genes are tightly clustered within a 195-kb region and maintain a provisional ordering as *UGT2B7* (previously *UGT2B9*)-*UGT2B4*-*UG2B15* (44). The clustering of gene families on the same chromosome is evidence for gene duplication events. Note in Figure 1 that the UGT2B sequences from primates do not cluster with the rodent or lagomorph forms, which suggests that following speciation, the *UGT2B* genes have evolved from a common ancestrial lineage in each species by independent gene duplication and selective pressure events. This would account for the divergence in function of these proteins in the different species. There is little evidence for truly orthologous UGT2B proteins between the different species. In humans, there is considerable tissue specific regulation with the *UGT2* genes, as evident from the identification of *UGT2A* gene products in olfactory tissue (33), and the differential regulatory patterns of the *UGT2B* genes throughout the gastrointestinal tract (discussed below). Little is known about the mechanisms that contribute to *UGT2* tissue-specific regulation.

The *UGT1A* locus in humans (2) is located on chromosome 2-q37 (46–48) and encodes UGT1A1 (2, 49), UGT1A3 (50), UGT1A4 (2), UGT1A5 (to date, no active transcript), UGT1A6 (51), UGT1A7 (18), UGT1A8 (52–53), UGT1A9 (55), and UGT1A10 (18, 54, 56). Although only eight active gene transcripts have been identified, the *UGT1A* locus evolved with the potential to encode 12 separate UGT RNA transcripts. A representation of the organization of the *UGT1A* locus is shown in Figure 3 (see color insert). The *UGT1A* locus has been estimated to span 160 kb, with four 3' exons flanked 5'-ward by 12 cassette exons, each encoding one of the UGT1A first exon RNAs (5). The 5' flanking region of each first-exon cassette contains appropriate promoter elements that would attract PolII and the transcriptional initiation factors. At the 3' end of each first-exon cassette can be found consensus 5' splice sequences, recognized by the RNA spliceosome. Transcription of each individual first exon leads to a strategy of exon sharing, combining the first exon sequences with common exons 2–5. Thus, all of the UGT1A proteins are identical in the carboxyl 245 amino acids, which is encoded by exons 2–5. This transcriptional mechanism is often mistakenly referred to as alternative splicing. The process of alternative RNA splicing can

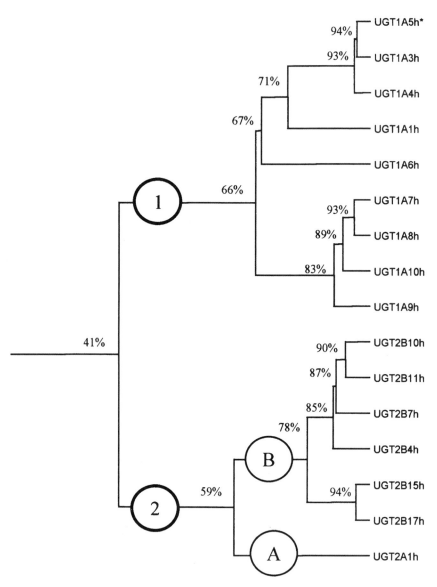

Figure 2 Phylogenetic tree showing the relationships between the human UDP-glucuronosyltransferases (UGTs). The median percentage identity of amino acid sequences between UGTs split by a mode is shown. (*Asterisk*) Indicates the gene product has not been identified.

only occur if mature or cryptic 5′ and 3′ consensus splice sites are transcribed as RNA and recognized in a regulated fashion to serve as substrates for splicing reactions catalyzed in spliceosomes (57). This most likely does not occur with the UGT1A RNA transcripts. Based upon the structure of the *UGT1A* locus, each of the UGT1 transcripts are produced independently following transcriptional initiation. Note, 3′ consensus splice sites do not exist until the presence of exon 2. Thus, during transcriptional elongation, the spliceosome must wait until the sequence encoding exon 2 is transcribed, at which time the process of RNA splicing begins. For example, if transcription commences at the *UGT1A7* gene, the sequences encoding *UGT1A6-UGT1A1* is simply considered intronic. The RNA encoding UGT1A6–1A1 is processed by normal RNA splicing mechanisms. Thus, the regulatory sequences flanking each of the exon 1 regions dictate the unique aspects of expression of the *UGT1A* genes.

The human UGTs range from 529 amino acids to 534 amino acids in length, with several highly conserved domains that are important for membrane targeting and activity (reviewed in 58). Although the UGT1 proteins are encoded by five exons and UGT2 proteins are encoded by six exons, the UGTs share a high degree of similarity in the carboxyl end, which spans the last 250 amino amino acids. The amino terminal 280 amino acids are divergent. With the exception of UGT1A10, all of the UGTs contain an N-terminal signal peptide (18), which is removed following insertion of the proteins into the ER (59). Although anchorage of the UGTs to the ER is predicted to be facilitated by a membrane retention signal at the carboxyl end of the proteins (60), Meech & Mackenzie recently demonstrated that other regions of the UGTs participate in securing the protein to the membrane (61). Studies carried out using chimeric constructs of different UGT cDNAs followed by expression studies indicate that the amino terminal may be important in substrate specificity of the different UGTs (62), whereas other studies have clearly shown that the carboxyl region of the UGTs are also critical for activity (36, 63, 64). As a result of the high degree of similarity in the carboxyl portion of the UGTs, it has been proposed that this region controls the conformational properties that underlie the binding of the cosubstrate UDPGlcUA, but this remains to be conclusively demonstrated. Under this type of model, it is presumed that a substrate or aglycone binding pocket and a separate UDPGlcUA domain interact to coordinate transfer of glucuronic acid to the facilitating substrate. Such a model would indicate that the UDPGlcUA binding domain and possibly the secondary structure responsible for forming this region is closely related in all of the UGTs.

Functional Diversity of the Human UDP-Glucuronosyltransferases

In the absence of modern molecular biology, it had been known that there existed a variety of chemically divergent agents that were conjugated in humans. These range from the many hundreds of endogenous substrates and xenobiotics to many clinically relevant drugs (23, 24, 65). Glucuronides contain glucopyranuronosyl linked to -O.R, -S.R, -N.R'R", or -C.R groups (for review see 1). A significant advantage of the utilization of recombinant DNA methodologies is the ability to express the different UGT cDNAs in cell lines that express minimal levels of the respective proteins. All the human UGT cDNAs shown in Figure 2 have been expressed to evaluate their potential to metabolize endogenous and xenobiotic substances. Examination of classes of compounds known to be glucuronidated by expressed UGTs are shown in Table 1, with several examples of their structure presented in Figure 4. Methods of choice include standard transient transfections of recombinant DNA where the cells are harvested approximately 48 h after transfection, or following the stable introduction of the DNA into the genome following selection of the cells with an appropriate antibiotic (15, 58). Other laboratories have utilized the expression of UGTs in insect *Spodoptera frugiperda* cells following infection with UGT-recombinant AcMNPV viruses (53, 66–68).

As discussed by Remmel & Burchell (15), estimations of the catalytic activity attributed to any single enzyme is dependent on a number of critical factors, such as the method of choice used for transfection (i.e. transient or stable), the type of cell line, or the choice of membrane preparation (i.e. microsomes or whole cell extracts). Even when different laboratories use the same cell line for stable expression experiments, the concentration of expressed protein can vary considerably.

TABLE 1   Xenobiotic substrates glucuronidated by expressed human UDP-glucuronosyltransferases (UGTs)

Human glucuronides	Substrates[a]
Linkage through -O-	
Aryl hydroxy (ether)	Simple and complex phenols, anthraquinones and flavones, opioids and steroids, hydroxylated coumarins
Aryl or alkyl enolic	Coumarins, steroid-dione structures
Alkyl hydroxy	Primary, secondary, tertiary alcohols
Acyl hydroxy (carboxylic esters)	Bilirubin, carboxylic acids
Linkage through -S-	
Aryl and Alkyl thiols	No examples reported
Linkage through -C-	No examples reported
Linkage through -O-	
Sulfonamides	No examples reported
Nonquaternary	Primary and secondary amines, arylamine N-OH, tetrazoles
Quarternary	Cyclic tertiary, alicyclic tertiary, imidazoles, pyridines, triazoles

[a]Examples of chemical classes used by different laboratories to demonstrate specificity toward expressed human UGTs.

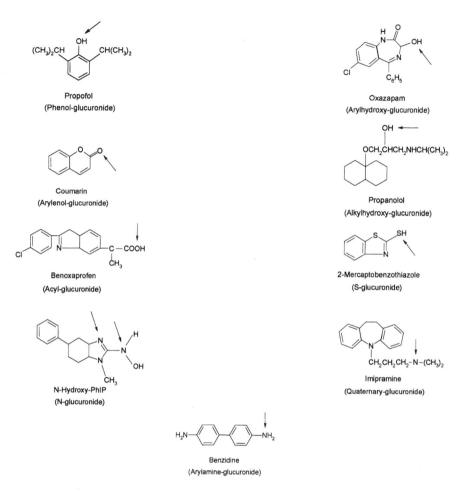

Figure 4 Chemical structures of compounds that form glucuronides. (*Arrows*) The position on each molecule where glucuronidation occurs.

Coupled with the fact that expression experiments are performed with variations in assay conditions, concentrations of substrates, and concentrations of the cosubstrate UDPGlcUA, estimations of substrate UGT activity can vary significantly. However, a picture is emerging that defines the ability of the different enzymes to glucuronidate the many different classes of substrates. To evaluate the specificity and diversity of the UGTs, we have assembled a database of human UGT activities compiled from expression experiments. Our database, assembled in Microsoft Access, covers over 350 substrates and is available on the Web (www.AnnualReviews.org). For evaluation purposes, we have taken the highest reported activities within the different classes of chemical substrates and condensed this information into Table 2. Based upon the predicted substrate specificities, several unique patterns of expression can be observed.

O-Linked Glucuronidation   As outlined in the historic monograph on glucurondiation by Dutton (1), the different classes of O-glucuronides predominate those compounds that serve as substrates for the UGTs. The predominant substrates in this list are those that form the aryl-O-(phenolic)-glucuronides, whereas substrates susceptible to acyl-O-glucuronidation (carboxylic acids) as well as aryl- and alkyl-O-(enolic)-glucuronidation (coumarins) have been extensively investigated. Glucuronidation through O-linked moieties (acyl, phenolic, hydroxy) predominates the diversity in substrate recognition, and all of the UGTs are capable of forming O-linked glucuronides, albeit with different efficiencies and turnover rates. The small molecules that form such phenolic-hydroxy glucuronides as 4-nitrophenol and 1-napthol and the coumarin derivative 4-methylumbelliferone serve as substrates for most of the UGT proteins but are catalyzed most efficiently by the UGT1 proteins, with the exception of UGT1A4. The simple and complex phenols are also efficiently glucuronidated by the nasal mucosa-specific UGT2A1 (33), but overall they are glucuronidated at reduced rates by UGT2B4 (35), UGT2B7 (39, 69), and UGT2B15 (70). Small phenolic substrates such as p-nitrophenol and 4-methylumbelliferone are often used for analysis of total UGT activity in tissue microsomes, but when compared with the catalytic activities of the UGT1 proteins, these substrates are glucuronidated at rates that are 10- to 20-fold lower by UGT2B4 (35), UGT2B7 (39, 41), and UGT2B15 (70). There is considerable substrate-specific redundancy in phenolic glucuronidation between UGT1A1, UGT1A3, UGT1A7, UGT1A8, UGT1A9, and UGT1A10, as evident from the glucuronidation activities observed with small and bulky phenols as well as the hydroxy-glucuronide forming polynuclear hydrocarbons, anthraquinones, flavones, and coumarins. The slightly larger bulky phenols (i.e. 4-tert-butyl phenol) and those that include the naturally occurring anthraquinones and flavanoids, although excellent substrates for most of the UGT1 proteins, are not readily glucuronidated by UGT1A6 (71). Because the *UGT1A* locus is highly conserved in other mammals and the individual UGT1 proteins are differentially expressed throughout the gastrointestinal tract, we can predict that these proteins have evolved to facilitate the metabolism of digested matter, much of which exists as simple and complex phenols.

Phenanthrene Glucuronidation   The glucuronidation of morphine and other structurally similar opioids are metabolized at relatively low rates by UGT1A1 (72), UGT1A8 (73), and UGT2A1 (33). However, Coffman et al (38, 69) indicate that UGT2B7 is the major isoform responsible for the glucuronidation of opioids of the morphinan and oripavine class. Morphine, a phenanthrene alkaloid, is glucuronidated at the phenolic 3-hydroxyl as well as the alcoholic 6-hydroxyl group,

TABLE 2 UDP-glucuronosyltransferases (UGT) glucuronidation activity with selected substrate classes[a]

Chemical class	1A1	1A3	1A4	1A6	1A7	1A8	1A9	1A10	2A1	2B4	2B7	2B15	2B17
Simple phenols	1900	239	30	2400	175	1346	5300	88	735	0.4	5	167	38
Complex phenols	420	299	11	13300	480	2217	1200	85	2440	0.2	3	176	7
Aliphatic alcohols	ND	0	75	ND	ND	0	270	ND	1290	0	388	41	ND
Anthraquinones/flavones	1720	1072	0	0	57	1534	2500	35	320	ND	ND	103	ND
Coumarins	800	1970	0	1100	220	4970	1500	11	898	0	4	170	0
Bilirubin	400	0	2	0	0	ND	0	ND	ND	0	0	0	0
Bile acids	0	10[b]	0	0	ND	ND	0	0	ND	1.8	20	0	0
Carboxylic acids	0	121	0	ND	0	0	170	0	68	0	1.8	0	ND
Primary amines	0.3	84	540	10600	0	42	1800	0	22	ND	2.5	0	ND
Secondary amines	0	12	240	ND	ND	15	ND	20	ND	ND	ND	0	ND
Tertiary amines	0	87	165	1	0	0	0	0	ND	0	0	0	0
Heterocyclic amines	0	49	ND	50	3	71	91	156	ND	ND	ND	ND	ND
Opioids	0	130	0	0	ND	126	0	ND	73	0	3462	0	ND
C_{18} steroids	350	313	25	0	6	711	450	48	40	0.3	980	14	0
C_{19} steroids	0	0	110	0	0	43	0	4	207	0	2	73	15
C_{21} steroids	0	ND	130	ND	ND	0	ND	ND	53	0	0	ND	8
Sapogenins	0	0	330	ND	ND	0	ND	ND	ND	ND	ND	ND	ND

[a]Represented are maximal specific activities (in picomoles per minute per milligram of protein) using substrates that can be defined for each of the different chemical classes. ND, Not determined; 0, enzyme preparations that have been tested with no detectable activity. Table generated from the following reports for expressed UGT: UGT1A1 (49, 67, 82, 84a, 86, 109, 139, 156, 157); UGT1A3 (67, 79, 84, 86, 88, 139); 1A4 (67, 81, 83, 84a, 86, 139); UGT1A6 (51, 67, 74, 84a–87, 138, 139, 158–160); UGT1A7 (53, 68, 86); UGT1A8 (52, 73, 139); UGT1A9 (55, 55, 67, 71, 84a, 86, 99, 109, 139, 156, 161); UGT1A10 (52, 53, 67, 139, 139); UGT2A1 (33); UGT2B4 (34, 35, 41, 67, 78, 80, 86, 162); UGT2B7 (36–39, 67, 69, 80, 84a, 86, 139); UGT2B11 (40); UGT2B15 (41, 67, 70, 139); UGT2B17 (29, 43).

[b]Value for hyodeoxycholic acid conducted in the authors laboratory.

593

at a ratio of approximately 7:1 (38). It is interesting to note that the 6-O-glucu-ronide is a more potent analgesic than the parent compound, whereas the 3-O-glucuronide contains no biological activity. It is significant that UGT2B7 has been found recently also in the brain, where metabolism to the 6-O-glucuronide may facilitate analgesic activity (74).

Steroid Glucuronidation   Steroid glucuronidation is an important pathway for removing biologically active endogenous ligands, such as the androgens (C_{19} steroids), estrogens (C_{18} steroids), progestins (C_{21} steroids), and bile acids (C_{24} steroids), and both the UGT1 and UGT2 family of proteins participate in these reactions (75–77). Hyodeoxycholic acid, one of the bile acids that is actively glucuronidated, was first demonstrated to serve as a substrate for UGT2B4 (34, 78) and was later found to be more efficiently conjugated by UGT2B7 (36). These are the only UGTs known to conjugate hyodeoxycholic acid. Human UGT2B7 (37, 39, 79) and to a lesser degree UGT2B4 and UGT2B15 (35, 36, 70) are also capable of glucuronidating through the hydroxylated A-ring of the steroid a num-ber of estrogenic derivatives, including catechol-estrogens. A comprehensive sur-vey of the regional and stereo-selectivity of UGT2B4 and UGT2B7 to glucuronidate C_{19} and C_{21} steroids has recently been conducted (80), and it is evident that UGT2B7 is 10- to 20-fold more active in conjugating hydroxyan-drogens and pregnanes. UGT2B15 and UGT2B17 are also active toward a number of androgens and are the only two UGTs to glucuronidate testosterone (43, 70). Glucuronidation of C_{19} and C_{21} steroids has also been observed with expressed UGT1A4 (81), and all of the UGT1 (49, 53, 73, 79) proteins with the exception of UGT1A6 are capable of glucuronidating some of the C_{18} estrogenic steroids. On the other hand, UGT1A3 (50) and UGT1A10 (53) are the only two proteins known to glucuronidate estrone. Although the UGT2B proteins are often per-ceived to play the central role in steroid-like glucuronidation, it is clear that steroid metabolism by the UGTs is an extremely diversified process, and substrate spec-ificities of the many different steroid metabolites cannot be considered exclusive to any one or group of proteins.

Carboxylic Acid Glucuronidation   One of the first characterized aglycone-GlcUA linkages was the carboxylic acid (ester) linkage of anthranilic acid. Many therapeutic agents, such as aglycones that are aryl, primary, secondary, tertiary aliphatic, or heterocyclic (1), are metabolized to acyl-O-glucuronides (carboxylic esters). As shown in Table 2, the majority of these substrates are glucuronidated principally by UGT1A3 and UGT1A9, although valproic acid is subject to glu-curonidation by the nasal-specific UGT2A1 (33). Bilirubin, which is also metab-olized to an acyl-O-glucuronide, is selectively glucuronidated by UGT1A1. However, bilirubin glucuronidation by UGT1A1 is a rare example of the ability of this enzyme to form carboxylic ester glucuronides, because other carboxylic acids are not glucuronidated by this protein (82). Although UGT1A7 and

UGT1A10 have not been examined extensively for their ability to glucuronidate carboxylic acids, UGT1A8 is not active toward these substrates (73). UGT1A4, which is active in the N-glucuronidation of tertiary amines, also possesses no activity toward carboxylic acids. It is interesting to note that cynomologous monkey UGT2B9, which is 89% identical in amino acid sequence to human UGT2B7, catalyzes the glucuronidation of a number of nonsteroidal anti-inflammatory agents at the carboxylic acid moiety. An allelic variant of UGT2B7 (37) has been shown to possess a minimal amount of catalytic activity toward several carboxylic acid–containing nonsteroidal anti-inflammatory agents.

N-Glucuronidation   The UGT1 family of proteins are primarily responsible for N-glucuronide formation. The formation of N-glucuronides can be classified into two groups: those compounds that form nonquaternary N-conjugates (heterocyclic aromatic amines, primary and secondary amines), and those that form quaternary glucuronides (cyclic tertiary amines, alicyclic tertiary amines, aromatic heterocyclic amines) (65). Many clinically useful drugs, such as antihistiminics (i.e. tripelenamine), antipsychotic (chlorpromazine), and tricyclic antidepressants (i.e. amitryptyline), contain aliphatic tertiary amine moieties that are substrates for UGT quaternary N-glucuronidation, whereas secondary amines such as desipramine and nortriptyline form nonquaternary glucuronides. A host of primary aromatic amines that have been shown to be carcinogenic, such as benzidine and 1/2-naphthylamine, are also glucuronidated through the primary amine. In examining the UGT1 proteins to form N-glucuronides, there have been no reported activities for UGT1A7 and UGT1A10 (53). Primary and/or secondary amine glucuronidation is seen with UGT1A1 (84a), UGT1A3 and UGT1A4 (83, 84, 84a), UGT1A6 (84a, 85), UGT1A8 (73), and UGT1A9 (71, 84a). Glucuronidation of a new anticonvulsant, retigabine, at the primary amino group has been demonstrated with UGT1A1, UGT1A3, UGT1A4, and UGT1A9 (86). UGT1A6 is also capable of forming direct N-glucuronides from N-containing heterocylic compounds, such as methylbiphenyl-tetrazole (87). Benzidine is also metabolized by UGT2B7 (84a). However, the formation of quaternary ammonium glucuronides is selective and has only been observed when tertiary amines serve as substrates for UGT1A3 (84) and UGT1A4 (83). Several excellent discussions on the role of amine glucuronidation have recently been published (65, 88).

EXTRAHEPATIC UDP-GLUCURONOSYLTRANSFERASES GENE EXPRESSION

Until recently, glucuronidation has been considered to represent a metabolic pathway performed mainly by the liver (1). However, multiple studies have indicated that UGT activity toward bile acids, phenols, and bilirubin was resident in human intestinal (89–93), kidney (91, 92, 94–96), and colon tissue (89, 97). Although the liver is the organ with the most diverse metabolic capabilities and a central locus of catabolic metabolism, contact with xenobiotic material is first established in surface epithelia of the gastrointestinal tract and respiratory system prior to resorption. Thus, glucuronidation is likely to represent an important mechanism of moving lipophilic nutrients out of the digestive tract membranes. In addition, it is well known that enterohepatic circulation requires gastrointestinal means of glucuronidation to counteract the activities of bacterial β-glucuronidases. An appreciation of the multiplicity and genetics of extrahepatic UGTs has made it possible to define the role of glucuronidation in extrahepatic tissues.

UGT1A Locus

The development of specific reverse transcriptase (RT)-PCR–based methodology made it possible to distinguish single base pair differences between highly homologous sequences, as evident between the *UGT1A* gene products (18). This has made it possible to identify the precise expression patterns in liver as well as in other extrahepatic tissues (Figure 5, see color insert). The *UGT1A* locus in human liver is defined by UGT1A1, UGT1A3, UGT1A4, UGT1A6, and UGT1A9 mRNA expression (54). Of significance, UGT1A7 and UGT1A10 (18) were discovered and cloned from gastric tissue and UGT1A10 in biliary tissue (18, 53, 54), indicating these RNAs are exclusively extrahepatic *UGT1A* gene products (54). The detection of UGT1A10 also in human colon (53, 56) confirmed that UGT1A10 is expressed in multiple extrahepatic organs of the gastrointestinal tract. We now know that UGT1A10 appears to be expressed in all tissues of the gastrointestinal tract except liver. This is significant because UGT1A10 has one of the widest range of substrate specificities of any of the UGTs, encompassing the small phenolics to steroids, an indication that it may play a vital role in most extrahepatic tissues for the glucuronidation of endogenous and xenobiotic substrates.

The analysis of human esophagus demonstrated a pattern of expression that focused exclusively on the UGT1A7–10 cluster of gene products (67). It is interesting to note that UGT1A7 is expressed only in the proximal tissues of the gastrointestinal tract, such as the esophagus and stomach (18, 53, 98). Analysis of extrahepatic tissues outside the gastrointestinal tract have documented the expression of UGT1A9 mRNA in kidney (99), and following the identification of UGT1A6 in rat brain (100), UGT1A6 mRNA was also detected in human brain (74). Expression of the *UGT1A* locus in colon represents one of the more diverse patterns of expression, with RNA detected for UGT1A1, UGT1A3, UGT1A4, UGT1A6, UGT1A8, UGT1A9, and UGT1A10 (53). In addition, UGT1A8 (53) was expressed in human jejunum and ileum (52, 73). These recent findings demonstrate tissue-specific patterns of expression of *UGT1A* gene products and support the hypothesis that glucuronidation requirements of different metabolically active tissues are tightly regulated (17).

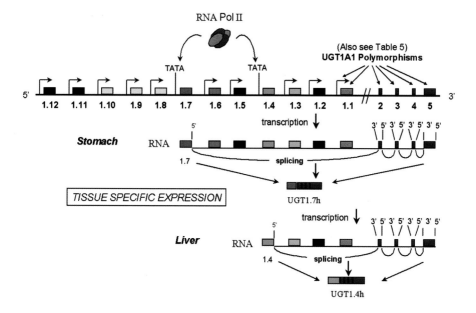

Figure 3 Representation of the organization of the *UGT1A* locus and an example of how different UGT1A RNAs are processed. Four common exons, 2-5, are shown in all the the UGT1A RNAs. The 5′ portion of the locus contains sequences encoding the divergent portion of each UGT1A protein, represented by exons 1.1 through 1.12. Following the initiation of transcription at promotors that flank each of the exon-1 sequences, the 5′ and 3′ consensus splice sites are recognized by the spliceosome and the intervening sequences are removed. In the example show, the tissue specific expression of *UGT1A7* is regulated in gastric epithelium, and UGT1A4 is expressed in hepatic tissue. Also shown by arrows are the different exon sequences that contain mutations and that have been linked clinically to unconjugated hyperbilirubinemia (see also Table 5).

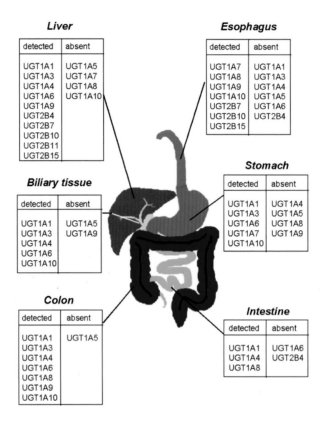

Figure 5 Representation of the tissues of the gastrointestinal tract that express the different UGTs. The majority of the data obtained for this figure was acquired by cloning the respective cDNAs from the different tissues, or gene transcripts quantitated by RT-PCR methodologies.

UGT2 Gene Products

The expression of *UGT2* genes also follows a tissue-specific pattern (Table 3, Figure 5). The human olfactory UGT2A1, which has been shown to be one of the more versatile of the UGTs by recognizing all of the major classes of substrates, is restricted in expression to olfactory tissue, although RT-PCR experiments detected minimal levels also in brain and fetal lung (33). One could predict that UGT2A1 has evolved for the need to serve as a first line of metabolic defense for many substances that enter the body through the nasal mucosa, and possibly to terminate olfactory signals efficient to ensure a rapid adaptation to changing olfactory stimuli and signals. In human liver, cDNAs have been identified for UGT2B4, UGT2B7, UGT2B10, UGT2B11, and UGT2B15 (35, 40, 67, 70, 101, 102). A significant observation is that UGT2B transcripts are abundantly expressed in steroid-sensitive target tissues such as prostate and mammary gland. For example, UGT2B10, UGT2B11, UGT2B15, and UGT2B17 gene transcripts have been identified in human prostate, and UGT2B11 is also expressed in mammary gland tissue. A wide expression pattern including liver, kidney, breast, prostate, skin, adipose tissue, adrenal tissue, and lung has been shown for UGT2B11

TABLE 3 Expression of human UDP-glucuronosyltransferases (UGTs) mRNA in the human body

UGT	Tissues	References
UGT1A1	Liver, bile ducts, stomach, colon	53, 98, 109
UGT1A3	Liver, bile ducts, stomach, colon	2, 18, 50, 53, 98
UGT1A4	Liver, bile ducts, colon	18, 53, 109
UGT1A5	Not detected	53, 67
UGT1A6	Liver, bile ducts, stomach, colon, brain	18, 51, 53, 74
UGT1A7	Esophagus, stomach	67, 98
UGT1A8	Esophagus, ileum, jejunum, colon	53, 67, 73
UGT1A9	Liver, colon, kidney	53, 55, 99
UGT1A10	Esophagus, stomach, bile ducts, intestine, colon	53, 54, 56
UGT2A1	Olfactory epithelium, brain, fetal lung	33
UGT2B4	Liver	67, 101
UGT2B7	Esophagus, liver, intestine, colon, brain, kidney, pancreas	39, 67, 74, 103, 104, 163
UGT2B10	Esophagus, liver, mammary gland, prostate	35, 67, 103
UGT2B11	Liver, kidney, mammary gland, prostate, adrenal, skin, adipose tissue, lung	40
UGT2B15	Esophagus, liver, prostate	40, 67, 69, 102
UGT2B17	Prostate	29, 45

(40). The presence of UGT2B17 may have a significant impact on cancer of the prostate gland by glucuronidating androgens and thus protecting this tissue from the carcinogenic actions of these steroids. Similarly, UGT2B7 transcripts are found in liver, intestine, esophagus, brain, kidney, and pancreas (74, 103, 104). In the gastrointestinal tract, a differential expression pattern is also evident with UGT2B4 and UGT2B7. Although UGT2B7 is expressed in intestine, esophagus, and pancreas (67, 74, 104), no UGT2B4 transcripts have been identified in intestine or esophagus (67, 104).

Glucuronidation in the Gastrointestinal Tract

It is apparent that the human digestive tract is capable of significant glucuronidation activity, as evident from detection of gene products (Figure 5) and the analysis of catalytic activities, which appear to function complementary to hepatic glucuronidation. What is the role of glucuronidation in the physiological functions of the gastrointestinal tract? Glucuronidation most likely represents a metabolic barrier function of the gastrointestinal mucosa. Lipophilic compounds enter the body as components of our diet and are likely to diffuse into the membranes of resorptive tissues. UGTs can fulfill a dual role at this critical localization of the resorption process. First, digestive material can be transformed into water-soluble glucuronides and remain in the lumen of the digestive tract, or second, it can be resorbed and transported to the kidney for excretion or ultimately targeted to the biliary tract for elimination. There is no conclusive experimental evidence measuring endoluminal nonbile glucuronide formation to determine which of the illustrated pathways is more significant in humans. However, the presence of bacterial β-glucuronidases in the lumen of the colon suggests that epithelial UGT proteins may serve to protect against deconjugation of compounds designated to exit the body. These considerations would assign a critical role to the human colon. Immunofluorescence analysis has confirmed that UGT protein is expressed selectively in the epithelial cell layer of the human colon (17), where the resorbed compounds would be available as substrates for the large pool of UGTs. In addition, UGT1A protein detected by Western blot has been found to be expressed at levels comparable to the human liver. The colon may therefore exert a "scavenger function" at the distal end of the digestive system. For compounds that are reabsorbed in the colon, the battery of UGTs would assure the formation of glucuronides as a final detoxification step, with the water-soluble metabolites targeted for biliary or renal excretion. A yet-unexplained observation is the significantly lower glucuronidation rates in colon compared with liver (17, 89, 93, 97).

The discovered regulation of the *UGT* genes provides first insight in the potential role of first pass kinetics of orally administered drugs. Given the diversity of glucuronidation enzymes in the gastrointestinal tract, prehepatic metabolism may be significantly underestimated and may be the biochemical basis of differences in resorption rates between individuals frequently observed in standardized clinical drug treatment regiments. For example, in human stomach, the polymorphic expression of the UGT1A isoforms UGT1A1, UGT1A3, and UGT1A6 has been demonstrated (98). These variations correlate with a fourfold interindividual variation of glucuronidation activities for a number of phenolic compounds between individuals. It could be predicted that a UGT1A6 polymorphism may be related to the interidividual variations seen in acetaminophen toxicity (105). Acetaminophen toxicity at doses as low as 6000 mg is observed to lead to acute liver failure. In some individuals, extremely high doses are tolerated without liver failure. In our experience, the highest dose survived was 20,000 mg, which suggests that polymorphisms in drug metabolism may have a significant impact on acetaminophen tolerance and metabolism. Also observed in gastric mucosa was a qualitative variation in the hyodeoxycholic acid glucuronidation (98), which corresponds to polymorphic alleles identified for UGT2B7 (69). The biochemical and physiological basis of these phenomena are emerging as the glucuronidation capabilities of the human digestive system and other tissues are elucidated.

UDP-GLUCURONOSYLTRANSFERASES IN HUMAN DISEASES

Inherited Unconjugated Hyperbilirubinemia

Jaundice is one of the most striking and stigmatizing symptoms of human disease. Hyperbilirubinemia becomes clinically evident when serum bilirubin levels exceed 35 μM/liter. Given a daily production rate of about 500 μM in a 70-kg adult, the necessity of effective means of bilirubin transport and quantitative elimination from the body are obvious (106). Bilirubin is a breakdown product of heme containing proteins, 80% of which originates from the catalysis of circulating hemoglobin, and 20% of which originates from hepatic heme-containing proteins such as cytochrome P450s, tryptophan pyrrolase, and catalase as well as from the body's pool of free heme. Bilirubin is highly hydrophobic and mainly exists bound reversibly to albumin. Its hydrophobicity is the reason why elimination from the body requires additional metabolic steps (107). The failure of either transport or conjugation leads to the saturation of albumin and consequently to tissue accumulation of bilirubin. When serum levels exceed 300 μm/liter, bilirubin can pass the blood brain barrier and lead to a fatal necrosis of neurons and glial tissue (kernicterus). Only 5% of the bilirubin pool exists as water-soluble bilirubin diglucuronide. This metabolite is key to the elimination of bilirubin from the body, and therefore, the glucuronidation of bilirubin by UGT1A1 is an essential metabolic pathway of human metabolism.

The symptoms of hyperbilirubinemia can have multiple etiologies, including viral, toxic, or autoimmune liver disease (108) as well as biliary obstruction and hemolysis. However, the observation of physiological hyperbilirubinemia in neo-nates and the hereditary unconjugated hyperbilirubinemias in children and adults have led to the investigation of bilirubin metabolism and have ultimately proved to be the driving force of the discovery of the human *UGT1A* gene locus (2, 109, 110). Although the human *UGT1A* locus potentially encompasses nine functional transferase genes, only one isoform, UGT1A1, is involved in inherited diseases of bilirubin metabolism (2, 109, 111). With the exception of minor bilirubin UGT activity detected in vitro with expressed UGT1A4 (109), only UGT1A1 is capable of forming bilirubin glucuronides. Because a number of patients suffering from a complete loss of bilirubin glucuronidation exhibit homozygous mutations of the *UGT1A1* first exon only, it is not likely that additional bilirubin UGTs exist in humans (112). Mutations of the *UGT1A1* first exon (113–119) lead to a selective effect on the *UGT1A1* gene product. Because bilirubin glucuronidation can be completely abrogated by such a mutational event (117), there appears to be no substitute isoform capable of bilirubin glucuronidation and the reported bilirubin activity of UGT1A4 by in vitro experiments does not appear to have any bio-logical significance.

In humans, three forms of inheritable unconjugated hyperbilirubinemic dis-eases exist: Crigler-Najjar syndrome type I, Crigler-Najjar syndrome type II, and Gilbert's syndrome (Table 4). Crigler-Najjar syndrome type I is diagnosed as a complete lack of bilirubin glucuronidation, and therefore, no conjugated bilirubin is clinically detectable in duodenal biliary secretions. Crigler-Najjar syndrome type II is diagnostically differentiated by the presence of low amounts of bilirubin diglucuronides and monoglucuronides in duodenal biliary secretions and a response to induction therapy with phenobarbital (106). The biochemical basis of this disease variant is UGT1A1 deficiency with at least 10% of normal activity remaining. The therapeutic approach for Crigler-Najjar syndrome type I and type II is different (Table 4). Crigler-Najjar syndrome type I patients invariably require immediate orthotopic liver transplantation as a surgical means of gene therapy capable of replacing the defective UGT1A1 alleles, whereas Crigler-Najjar syn-drome type II patients can frequently be treated by induction therapy or photo-therapy for prolonged periods of time. The third condition with jaundice and UGT involvement was described by Gilbert and Lereboullet in 1901 (120). This benign condition of young adults does not require therapy and is characterized by fluc-tuating unconjugated hyperbilirubinemia in response to psychological stress, infection, fasting, or physical activity. The levels of unconjugated serum bilirubin are lower than in Crigler-Najjar's syndrome, and the hepatic bilirubin UGT activ-ity is reduced to 60–70% of an unaffected individual.

The inheritable unconjugated hyperbilirubinemias are all the result of either mutant *UGT1A1* alleles (112–115, 117, 119) or *UGT1A1* promoter polymor-phisms (121, 122). To date, 33 mutant *UGT1A1* alleles have been identified (14, 117, 123) (Table 5, Figure 3). Nine of these mutations have been located within the unique first exon of the UGT1A1 gene (113, 119). All the other polymorphic

TABLE 4 The clinical classification of unconjugated hyperbilirubinemia[a]

Determinants	Crigler-Najjar type 1	Crigler-Najjar type 2	Gilbert (meulengracht) disease
Incidence	Rare	Very rare	7% of population
Bilirubin	Unconjugated	Unconjugated (conjugated)	Unconjugated (conjugated)
Serum liver function tests	Normal	Normal	Normal
Liver histology	Normal	Normal	Normal
Inheritance	Autosomal recessive	Autosomal recessive	Autosomal recessive
Hemolysis	Absent	Absent	Absent
Affected gene	*UGTIA* coding region and/or promoter	*UGTIA* coding region and/or promoter	*UGTIA* coding region and/or promoter
Effect of mutation	Absence of activity	10% of activity	60% of activity
Clinical response to induction	No induction	Induction with phenobarbital	Induction with phenobarbital, self-limiting, stress induced
Therapy	Blood exchange, transfusion, liver transplantation	Phototherapy, sometime liver transplantation	Not necessary
Prognosis	Untreated: death	Variable	Excellent

[a]Listed are the pertinent clinical and genetic findings that discriminate between the three known syndromes that lead to unconjugated hyperbilirubinemia.

TABLE 5 Allelic polymorphism of the human UGT1A1 gene and association with unconjugated hyperbilirubinemia[a]

Allele	Nucleotide changes	Protein changes	Type	Exon	Disease	Reference
UGT1A1*1	Wild type	—	—	—	—	109
UGT1A1*2	879 del 13	Truncation	Deletion	2	CN1	3
UGT1A1*3	1124 C→T	S375F	Missense	4	CN1	124
UGT1A1*4	1069 C→T	Q357X	Nonsense	3	CN1	126
UGT1A1*5	991 C→T	Q331 del 44	132 nt deletion	2	CN1	124
UGT1A1*6	221G→A	G71R	Missense	1	Gilbert	113
UGT1A1*7	145 T→G	Y486D	Missense	5	CN2	130
UGT1A1*8	625 C→T	R209W	Missense	1	CN2	114
UGT1A1*9	992 A→G	Q331R	Missense	2	CN2	128
UGT1A1*10	1021 C→T	R341X	Nonsense	3	CN1	129
UGT1A1*11	923 G→A	G308E	Missense	2	CN1	125, 127
UGT1A1*12	524 T→A	L175Q	Missense	1	CN2	115
UGT1A1*13	508 del 3	F170del	Deletion	1	CN1	116
UGT1A1*14	826 G→C	G276R	Missense	1	CN1	115
UGT1A1*15	529 T→C	C177R	Missense	1	CN2	115
UGT1A1*16	1070 A→G	O357R	Missense	3	CN1	127
UGT1A1*17	1143 C→G	S381R	Missense	4	CN1	127
UGT1A1*18	1201 G→C	A401P	Missense	4	CN1	127
UGT1A1*19	1005 G→A	W335X	Missense	3	CN1	127
UGT1A1*20	1102 G→A	A368T	Missense	4	CN1	127
UGT1A1*21	1223 ins G	Frameshift	Frameshift	4	CN2	127
UGT1A1*22	875 C→T	A292V	Missense	2	CN1	127
UGT1A1*23	1282 A→G	K426E	Missense	4	CN1	127
UGT1A1*24	1309 A→T	K437X	Missense	5	CN1	127
UGT1A1*25	840 C→A	C280X	Missense	1	CN1	112
UGT1A1*26	973 del G	Frameshift	Frameshift	2	CN2	115
UGT1A1*27	686 C→A	P229Q	Missense	1	Gilbert	119
UGT1A1*28	TAATA7	Transcription	Insertion	Promotor	Gilbert	121
UGT1A1*29	1099 C→G	R367G	Missense	4	Gilbert	119
UGT1A1*30	44 T→G	L15R	Missense	1	CN2	118
UGT1A1*31	11609 CC→GT	P387R	2 nt missense	4	CN1	105
UGT1A1*32	1006 C→T	R336W	Missense	3	CN1	123
UGT1A1*33	881 T→C	I294T	Missense	2	CN2	123

Footnotes on facing page

alleles have differences located in exons 2–5 (3, 115, 124–131). It is debatable whether the distinction of Crigler-Najjar syndrome type I and type II and of Gilbert's disease, which is based on serum bilirubin levels and the clinical course of the metabolic error, should be regarded as a single disease entity with a combination of functionally relevant or silent allelic polymorphisms of the *UGT1A1* gene. Studies have shown that homozygous or compound heterozygous mutations can lead to Crigler-Najjar syndrome type I (112) and type II (130). Promoter polymorphisms plus mutant coding region alleles can lead to Crigler-Najjar syndrome type I and type II (123) and to Gilbert's disease (121) as well as to no detectable disease at all (121, 123, 132). Given the theoretically unpredictable impact of an individual mutant allele or of the combination of itself with a different mutant allele or a promoter polymorphism, a database of all identified allelic variants is likely to serve as a decision tool to predict the course and management of patients with unconjugated hyperbilirubinemia, in addition to gaining insight into the functional properties of the UGT1A1 protein. However, for a clinically apparent hyperbilirubinemic state, homozygous or compound heterozygous mutant alleles are required. The presence of a single mutant allele without other abnormalities does not result in clinically detectable disease.

UDP-Glucuronosyltransferases in Carcinogenesis

Chemical carcinogenesis is considered to be one of the most prevalent mechanisms of neoplastic transformation and is linked to cancer of the esophagus, stomach, bladder, liver, colon, lung, and pleura (133–135). In addition, steroid metabolism is implicated as a factor of neoplastic transformation for prostate and breast cancer development (29, 136, 137). A potential model for neoplastic transformation predicts that enzymes involved in normal detoxification of potential mutagens and gene modulators such as sulphation, acetylation, and glucuronidation may be modified in diseased tissues. This has been demonstrated in Gunn rats, where a mutation in the *UGT1A* allele renders the entire locus inactive. The production of benzo(a)pyrene glucuronides is dramatically reduced, leading to elevated levels of DNA adducts. The ability to alter the mutagenic actions of polycyclic aromatic hydrocarbons through glucuronidation is good evidence that the UGTs may represent a metabolic defense against environmental carcinogens. One approach to examine the actions of the UGTs in diseased tissues is to identify the cancer and quantitatively identify expression patterns in normal and cancer tissue.

---

[a]List of all identified polymorphic alleles of the human *UGT1A1* gene and their association with different forms of unconjugated hyperbilirubinemias. Note that although an individual allele may have been identified in a specific disease, e.g. Crigler-Najjar disease type 1, different combinations of alleles as compound heterozygous traits may result in a differing clinical picture. CN1, Crigler-Najjar type 1 disease; CN2, Crigler-Najjar type 2 disease; Gilbert, Gilbert's disease; del, deletion; ins, insertion; nu, nucleotide.

The human gastrointestinal tract represents one of the largest external surface organs involved in immediate contact and the metabolism of xenobiotic material. The five most frequent sites of carcinogen-associated cancer development are esophagus, stomach, liver, biliary tree, and distal colon. Comparisons of surrounding healthy tissue with the *UGT1A* locus has led to the identification of a pattern of down-regulation of UGT1A mRNA and microsomal UGT catalytic activity in gastrointestinal tumors of the esophagus (67), stomach (98), liver (54), and bile ducts (54). The *UGT1A* genes are regulated individually. Although some are up-regulated (98) and some are not regulated at all (54), in malignant tissues the majority of gene expression is reflected in dramatic down-regulation of specific gene transcripts (54). For example, differential down-regulation of UGT1A mRNA is observed in the early stages of cancer, as represented by expression in pre-malignant adenomatous hyperplasia of the liver, as well as in the more advanced malignant hepatocellular carcinoma (54). In contrast, no such regulation was seen in benign tumorgenesis, represented by focal nodular hyperplasia of the liver. In addition, down-regulation of UGT transcripts in malignant tissue coincides with a reduction in UGT1A-specific protein, as identified by Western blot analysis, as well as differences in microsomal catalytic activity when assayed with polycyclic aromatic hydrocarbons. It should be noted, however, that although there is clearly a pattern of expression, which supports the hypothesis that the UGTs may be involved in genoprotection, it remains to be determined whether these events are an early marker in cancer development or a result of neoplastic events that lead to tissue transformation.

The availability of catalytically active preparations of the UGTs makes it possible to examine the ability of these proteins to participate in the glucuronidation of potential carcinogens. For example, analysis of recombinant UGTs has confirmed that primary amines, which are known environmental mutagens, are glucuronidated by UGT1A3 (84), UGT1A4 (81, 83), UGT1A6 (85), UGT1A8 (73), UGT1A9 (71, 85), and UGT2A1 (33) (see Table 2), whereas several of the benzo(a)pyrenes have been identified as substrates for UGT1A6 (138), UGT1A7 (53), UGT1A8 (52), UGT1A9 (138), UGT1A10 (52, 53), and UGT2B7 (138). We demonstrated that 2-hydroxyamino-1-methyl-6-phenylimidazo-(4,5-β) pyridine (N-hydroxy PhIP), a heterocyclic amine and mutagen found in food as well as in tobacco smoke, was glucuronidated in human esophagus by UGT1A7, UGT1A9, and UGT1A10 (67), but that additional forms of UGTs were most likely involved in other human tissues. This is supported by recent findings demonstrating that N-hydroxy PhIP is also subject to glucuronidation by UGT1A3 and UGT1A8 (139). Clearly, these findings underline the hypothesis that multiple UGT isoforms participate in the metabolism and elimination of potential direct or indirect human carcinogens.

Other clues that suggest the UGTs may play a significant role in genoprotection come from results of gene expression and catalytic activity recorded in colonic mucosa. Colon cancer accounts for 9.7% of all newly diagnosed cancers and is the second most common cancer site in humans (140). The majority of malignant digestive system tumors develop in the distal portions of the colon, whereas the intestine is virtually free of cancer development. It is interesting to note that analysis of gastrointestinal UGT activities in humans has demonstrated a sharp decrease of catalytic UGT activity from intestinal tissue to colon tissue (93), a pattern that is inversely proportional to tumor formation. The low UGT activity levels in colon may therefore represent an example of diminished genoprotection in this tissue. It is interesting to note that colon tissue displays an abundance of *UGT1A* gene expression represented by UGT1A1, UGT1A3, UGT1A4, UGT1A6, UGT1A8, UGT1A9, and UGT1A10 gene transcripts that correspond to similar levels of UGT protein, as detected by Western blot analysis (17). However, the high levels of *UGT1A* gene expression are not concordant with the dramatic reduction in many of the substrate-specific UGT activities in human colon, which suggests that this tissue is subject to a novel mechanism that abruptly diminishes the glucuronidation potential and conversely may predispose this tissue to the proneoplasitic effects of potential mutagens.

Although environmental carcinogens that enter the body through the lungs or gastrointestinal tract mainly act as direct carcinogens with genotoxic capablilities, other tumors are stimulated by nongenotoxic carcinogens, which directly affect growth control. Among these are the steroid hormone–sensitive neoplasms, including prostate and breast cancer. Standard treatment in prostate carcinoma involves the removal of androgen production by orchiectomy, or the administration of lutenizing hormone releasing hormone agonists with androgen blockers such as flutamide (29, 136). This strategy limits the proneoplastic effects of androgens on prostate carcinoma tissue. Steroid hormone UGT activity was detected in typically steroid-sensitive tissues, including prostate, mammary gland, and ovary. The analysis of human prostatic cell lines and prostate tissue has led to the cloning and characterization of UGT2B15 and UGT2B17 (43, 103). Humans have measurable levels of circulating C19 androgen glucuronides. It has been proposed that these circulating conjugates reflect the peripheral conversion of adrenal and gonadal C19 steroids to potent androgens, in particular to dihydrotestosterone. Catalytic UGT activity with C19 steroid hormones has been demonstrated for UGT2B15 and UGT2B17 (Table 2) (29). These findings suggest that steroid UGT activity functions to terminate activation of steroid-sensitive tissues by generating water-soluble hormone glucuronides. For the etiology and progression of prostate cancer, this may be an important mechanism, because the reduced elimination of androgens from prostatic tissue would enhance the growth signal and promote neoplastic transformation or lead to progression of cancer. Recent analyses have demonstrated that in the steroid-sensitive prostate carcinoma cell line LNCaP, the administration of interleukin 1 was capable of down-regulating UGT2B17 expression and protein levels, as well as dihydrotestosterone glucuronide formation (141). The regulation of UGT proteins, therefore, appears to play a critical role in steroid-sensitive tissues and their neoplasms.

UDP-Glucuronosyltransferases in Autoimmunity

Autoimmune hepatitis was first described in 1950 (142) and represents a chronic inflammatory disease of the liver characterized by a loss of self tolerance toward the liver. The etiology of this life-threatening condition is not known, and the diagnosis is reached by exclusion of viral, toxic, metabolic, or inherited errors of metabolism, as well as by the detection of circulating autoantibodies and additional markers of immune-mediated pathophysiology (108). In autoimmune hepatitis as well as viral hepatitis C and D, drug metabolizing enzymes have been identified as human hepatocellular autoantigens. Among these are autoantibodies directed against proteins of the ER, which are identified by immunofluorescence detection of antigens expressed in liver and the distal renal tubules and are, therefore, termed liver/kidney microsomal antibodies (LKM) (143). LKM autoantibodies have been characterized to target cytochromes CYP2D6 (LKM1) (143–147), CYP2C9 (LKM2) (148), and CYP1A2 (LM, for staining of the liver tissue only) (148–151). A third group of LKM autoantibodies (LKM3) was identified as targeting UGT1A proteins (68, 152, 153). These autoantibodies serve as diagnostic markers for autoimmune hepatitis type II (143–145), the autoimmune polyendrocrine syndrome type I (APS1) (150, 151), and drug induced hepatitis (148, 149), and they also serve as markers to discriminate between viral hepatitis C and D and idiopathic autoimmune hepatitis (154). In humans, LKM3 autoantibodies have been identified as targeting UGT1A1, UGT1A6, UGT1A4, and rabbit UGT1A6, as well as targeting a minor reactivity with UGT2B isoforms (68, 153). It has been suggested that in drug-induced hepatitis, the formation of drug adducts with CYP proteins and their subsequent recognition by the immune system, generation of a B-cell response, and production of autoantibodies is a pathophysiological mechanism (155). However, in genuine autoimmune hepatitis, the reasons why drug metabolizing enzymes serve as hepatocellular autoantigens remain unclear.

ACKNOWLEDGMENTS

This work was supported in part by NIH grants GM49138 and CA79834 (RHT) and grant STR493/3–1 from the Deutsche Forschungsgemeinschaft (CPS). We wish to thank Amanda Brown for preparing the phylogenetic trees and Don Geske for assembling the UGT activity database.

Visit the Annual Reviews home page at www.AnnualReviews.org.

LITERATURE CITED

1. Dutton GJ. 1980. *Glucuronidation of Drugs and Other Compounds.* Boca Raton, FL: CRC. 268 pp.
2. Ritter JK, Chen F, Sheen YY, Tran HM, Kimura S, et al. 1992. A novel complex locus *UGT1* encodes human bilirubin, phenol, and other UDP-glucuronosyltransferase isozymes with identical carboxyl termini. *J. Biol. Chem.* 267:3257–61
3. Ritter JK, Yeatman MT, Ferreira P, Owens IS. 1992. Identification of a genetic alteration in the code for bilirubin UDP-glucuronosyltransferase in the *UGT1* gene complex of a Crigler-Najjar type I patient. *J. Clin. Invest.* 90:150–55
4. Crigler JF, Najjar VA. 1952. Congenital familial nonhemolytic jaundice and kernicterus. *Pediatrics* 10:169–79
5. Owens IS, Ritter JK. 1995. Gene structure at the human *UGT1* locus creates diversity in isozyme structure, substrate specificity, and regulation. *Prog. Nucleic Acid Res.* 51:306–38
6. Jansen PL, Bosma PJ, Chowdhury JR. 1995. Molecular biology of bilirubin metabolism. *Prog. Liver Dis.* 13:125–50
6a. Gura T. 1999. Repairing the genomes splicing mistakes. *Science* 285:316–18
7. Burchell B. 1977. Studies on the purification of rat liver uridine diphosphate glucuronyltransferase. *Biochem. J.* 161:543–49
8. Burchell B. 1978. Substrate specificity and properties of uridine diphosphate glucuronyltransferase purified to apparent homogeneity from phenobarbital-treated rat liver. *Biochem. J.* 173:749–57
9. Gorski JP, Kasper CB. 1977. Purification and properties of microsomal UDP-glucuronosyltransferase from rat liver. *J. Biol. Chem.* 252:1336–43
10. Bock KW, von Clausbruch UC, Josting D, Ottenwalder H. 1977. Separation and partial purification of two differentially inducible UDP-glucuronyltransferases from rat liver. *Biochem. Pharmacol.* 26:1097–100
11. Tukey RH, Billings RE, Tephly TR. 1978. Separation of oestrone UDP-glucuronyltransferase and p-nitrophenol UDP-glucuronyltransferase activities. *Biochem. J.* 171:659–63
12. Mackenzie PI, Gonzalez FJ, Owens IS. 1984. Cloning and characterization of DNA complementary to rat liver UDP-glucuronosyltransferase mRNA. *J. Biol. Chem.* 259:12153–60
13. Jackson MR, McCarthy LR, Corser RB, Barr GC, Burchell B. 1984. Cloning of cDNAs coding for rat hepatic microsomal UDP-glucuronyltransferases. *Gene* 34:147–53
14. Mackenzie PI, Owens IS, Burchell B, Bock KW, Bairoch A, et al. 1997. The UDP glycosyltransferase gene superfamily: recommended nomenclature update based on evolutionary divergence. *Pharmacogenetics* 7:255–69
15. Remmel RP, Burchell B. 1993. Validation and use of cloned, expressed human drug-metabolizing enzymes in heterologous cells for analysis of drug metabolism and drug-drug interactions. *Biochem. Pharmacol.* 46:559–66
16. Guengerich FP, Parikh A, Johnson EF, Richardson TH, Von Wachenfeldt C, et al. 1997. Heterologous expression of human drug-metabolizing enzymes. *Drug Metab. Dispos.* 25:1234–41
17. Strassburg CP, Nguyen N, Manns MP, Tukey RH. 1999. UDP-glucuronosyltransferase activity in human liver and colon. *Gastroenterology* 116:149–60
18. Strassburg CP, Oldhafer K, Manns MP, Tukey RH. 1997. Differential expression of the *UGT1A* locus in human liver, biliary and gastric tissue. Identification of UGT1A7 and UGT1A10 transcripts in

extrahepatic tissue. *Mol. Pharmacol.* 52:212–20

19. Dutton GJ, Storey IDE. 1953. The isolation of a compound of uridine diphosphate and glucuronic acid from liver. *Biochem. J.* 53:37–x38

20. Isselbacher KJ. 1956. Enzymatic mechanisms of hormone metabolism. II. Mechanism of hormonal glucuronide formation. *Recent Prog. Hormone Res.* 12:134–51

21. Iyanagi T, Emi Y, Ikushiro S. 1998. Biochemical and molecular aspects of genetic disorders of bilirubin metabolism. *Biochim. Biophys. Acta* 1407:173–84

22. Coughtrie MWH. 1992. Role of molecular biology in the structural and functional characterization of the UDP-glucuronosyltransferase. In *Progress in Drug Metabolism,* ed. GG Gibson, 13:35–72. Bristol, UK: Taylor & Francis. 13th ed.

23. Burchell B, Brierley CH, Clarke DJ. 1995. Cloning and expression of human UDP-glucuronosyltransferase genes. In *Advances in Drug Metabolism in Man,* ed. GM Pacifici, GN Fracchia, pp. 608–57. Luxembourg, Netherelands: Eur. Comm.

24. Miners JO, Mackenzie PI. 1991. Drug glucuronidation in humans. *Pharmacol. Ther.* 51:347–69

25. Wei G, Bai X, Sarkar AK, Esko JD. 1999. Formation of HNK-1 determinants and the glycosaminoglycan tetrasaccharide linkage region by UDP-GlcUA:Galactose β1,3-glucuronosyltransferases. *J. Biol. Chem.* 274:7857–64

26. Bai X, Wei G, Sinha A, Esko JD. 1999. Chinese hamster ovary cell mutants defective in glycosaminoglycan assembly and glucuronosyltransferase I. *J. Biol. Chem.* 274:13017–24

27. Shimoda Y, Tajima Y, Nagase T, Harii K, Osumi N, Sanai Y. 1999. Cloning and

expression of a novel galactoside β1,3-glucuronyltransferase involved in the biosynthesis of HNK-1 epitope. *J. Biol. Chem.* 274:17115–22

28. Nelson DR, Koymans L, Kamataki T, Stegeman JJ, Feyereisen R, et al. 1996. P450 superfamily: update on new sequences, gene mapping, accession numbers and nomenclature. *Pharmacogenetics* 6:1–42

29. Belanger A, Hum DW, Beaulieu M, Levesque E, Guillemette C, et al. 1998. Characterization and regulation of UDP-glucuronosyltransferases in steroid target tissues. *J. Steroid. Biochem. Mol. Biol.* 65:301–10

30. Monaghan G, Burchell B, Boxer M. 1997. Structure of the human *UGT2B4* gene encoding a bile acid UDP-glucuronosyltransferase. *Mamm. Genome* 9:692–94

31. Haque SJ, Peterson DD, Nebert DW, Mackenzie PI. 1991. Isolation, sequence, and developmental expression of rat UGT2B2: the gene encoding a constitutive UDP glucuronosyltransferase that metabolizes etiocholanolone and androsterone. *DNA Cell Biol.* 10:515–24

32. Mackenzie PI, Rodbourn L. 1990. Organization of the rat UDP-glucuronosyltransferase, UDPGTr-2, gene and characterization of its promoter. *J. Biol. Chem.* 265:11328–32

33. Jedlitschky G, Cassidy AJ, Sales M, Pratt N, Burchell B. 1999. Cloning and characterization of a novel human olfactory UDP-glucuronosyltransferase. *Biochem. J.* 340:837–43

34. Fournel Gigleux S, Jackson MR, Wooster R, Burchell B. 1989. Expression of a human liver cDNA encoding a UDP-glucuronosyltransferase catalysing the glucuronidation of hyodeoxycholic acid in cell culture. *FEBS Lett.* 243:119–22

35. Jin C-J, Miners JO, Lillywhite KJ, Mackenzie PI. 1993. cDNA cloning and

expression of two new members of the human liver UDP-glucuronosyltransferase 2B subfamily. *Biochem. Biophys. Res. Commun.* 194:496–503

36. Ritter JK, Chen F, Sheen YY, Lubet RA, Owens IS. 1992. Two human liver cDNAs encode UDP-glucuronosyltransferases with 2 log differences in activity toward parallel substrates including hyodeoxycholic acid and certain estrogen derivatives. *Biochemistry* 31:3409–14

37. Jin C, Miners JO, Lillywhite KJ, Mackenzie PI. 1993. Complementary deoxyribonucleic acid cloning and expression of a human liver uridine diphosphate-glucuronosyltransferase glucuronidating carboxylic acid-containing drugs. *J. Pharm. Exp. Ther.* 264:475–79

38. Coffman BL, Rios GR, King CD, Tephly TR. 1997. Human UGT2B7 catalyzes morphine glucuronidation. *Drug Metab. Dispos.* 25:1–4

39. Ritter JK, Sheen YY, Owens IS. 1990. Cloning and expression of human liver UDP-glucuronosyltransferase in COS-1 cells. 3,4-Catechol estrogens and estriol as primary substrates. *J. Biol. Chem.* 265:7900–6

40. Beaulieu M, Levesque E, Hum DW, Belanger A. 1998. Isolation and characterization of a human orphan UDP-glucuronosyltransferase, UGT2B11. *Biochem. Biophys. Res. Commun.* 248:44–50

41. Chen F, Ritter JK, Wang MG, McBride OW, Lubet RA, Owens IS. 1993. Characterization of a cloned human dihydrotestosterone/androstanediol UDP-glucuronosyltransferase and its comparison to other steroid isoforms. *Biochemistry* 32:10648–57

42. Shepherd SR, Baird SJ, Hallinan T, Burchell B. 1989. An investigation of the transverse topology of bilirubin UDP-glucuronosyltransferase in rat hepatic

endoplasmic reticulum. *Biochem. J.* 259:617–20

43. Beaulieu M, Levesque E, Hum DW, Belanger A. 1996. Isolation and characterization of a novel cDNA encoding a human UDP-glucuronosyltransferase active on C19 steroids. *J. Biol. Chem.* 271:22855–62

44. Monaghan G, Clarke DJ, Povey S, See CG, Boxer M, Burchell B. 1994. Isolation of a human YAC contig encompassing a cluster of *UGT2* genes and its regional localization to chromosome 4q13. *Genomics* 23:496–99

45. Beaulieu M, Levesque E, Tchernof A, Beatty BG, Belanger A, Hum DW. 1997. Chromosomal localization, structure, and regulation of the *UGT2B17* gene, encoding a C19 steroid metabolizing enzyme. *DNA Cell Biol.* 16:1143–54

46. Harding D, Jeremiah SJ, Povey S, Burchell B. 1990. Chromosomal mapping of a human phenol UDP-glucuronosyltransferase, *GNT1. Ann. Hum. Genet.* 54:17–21

47. Clarke DJ, Cassidy AJ, See CG, Povey S, Burchell B. 1997. Cloning of the human *UGT1* gene complex in yeast artificial chromosomes: novel aspects of gene structure and subchromosomal mapping to 2q37. *Biochem. Soc. Trans.* 25:S562

48. Van Es HHG, Bout A, Liu J, Anderson L, Duncan AMV, et al. 1993. Assignment of the human UDP glucuronosyltransferase gene (*UGT1A1*) to chromosome region 2q37. *Cytogenet. Cell Genet.* 63:114–16

49. Ebner T, Remmel RP, Burchell B. 1993. Human bilirubin UDP-glucuronosyltransferase catalyzes the glucuronidation of ethinylestradiol. *Mol. Pharmacol.* 43:649–54

50. Mojarrabi B, Butler R, Mackenzie PI. 1996. cDNA cloning and characterization of the human UDP glucuronosyl-

transferase, UGT1A3. *Biochem. Biophys. Res. Commun.* 225:785–90

51. Harding D, Fournel-Gigleux S, Jackson MR, Burchell B. 1988. Cloning and substrate specificity of a human phenol UDP-glucuronosyltransferase expressed in COS-7 cells. *Proc. Natl. Acad. Sci. USA* 85:8381–85

52. Mojarrabi B, Mackenzie PI. 1998. Characterization of two UDP glucuronosyltransferases that are predominantly expressed in human colon. *Biochem. Biophys. Res. Commun.* 247:704–9

53. Strassburg CP, Manns MP, Tukey RH. 1998. Expression of the *UDP-glucuronosyltransferase 1A* locus in human colon. Identification and characterization of the novel extrahepatic UGT1A8. *J. Biol. Chem.* 273:8719–26

54. Strassburg CP, Manns MP, Tukey RH. 1997. Differential down regulation of the *UDP-glucuronosyltransferase 1A* locus is an early event in human liver and biliary cancer. *Cancer Res.* 57:2979–85

55. Wooster R, Sutherland L, Ebner T, Clarke D, Da Cruz e Silva O, Burchell B. 1991. Cloning and stable expression of a new member of the human liver phenol/bilirubin: UDP-glucuronosyltransferase cDNA family. *Biochem. J.* 278:465–69

56. Mojarrabi B, Mackenzie PI. 1997. The human UDP glucuronosyltransferase, UGT1A10, glucuronidates mycophenolic acid. *Biochem. Biophys. Res. Commun.* 238:775–78

57. Hodges D, Bernstein SI. 1994. Genetic and biochemical analysis of alternative RNA splicing. *Adv. Genet.* 31:207–81

58. Wooster R, Ebner T, Sutherland L, Clarke D, Burchell B. 1993. Drug and xenobiotic glucuronidation catalysed by cloned human liver UDP-glucuronosyltransferases stably expressed in tissue culture cell lines. *Toxicology* 82:119–29

59. Mackenzie PI, Owens IS. 1984. Cleav-

age of nascent UDP glucuronosyltransferase from rat liver by dog pancreatic microsomes. *Biochem. Biophys. Res. Commun.* 122:1441–49

60. Iyanagi T, Haniu M, Sogawa K, Fujii-Kuriyama Y, Watanabe S, et al. 1986. Cloning and characterization of cDNA encoding 3-methylcholanthrene inducible rat mRNA for UDP-glucuronosylatransferase. *J. Biol. Chem.* 261:15607–14

61. Meech R, Mackenzie PI. 1998. Determinants of UDP glucuronosyltransferase membrane association and residency in the endoplasmic reticulum. *Arch. Biochem. Biophys.* 356:77–85

62. Mackenzie PI. 1990. Expression of chimeric cDNAs in cell culture defines a region of UDP glucuronosyltransferase involved in substrate selection. *J. Biol. Chem.* 265:3432–35

63. Meech R, Yogalingam G, Mackenzie PI. 1996. Mutational analysis of the carboxy-terminal region of UDP-glucuronosyltransferase 2B1. *DNA Cell Biol.* 15:489–94

64. Li Q, Lou X, Peyronneau M-A, Straub PO, Tukey RH. 1997. Expression and functional domains of rabbit liver UDP-glucuronosyltranferase 2B16 and 2B13. *J. Biol. Chem.* 272:3272–79

65. Chiu S-HL, Huskey S-EW. 1998. Species differences in *N*-glucuronidation. *Drug Metab. Dispos.* 26:838–47

66. Nguyen N, Tukey RH. 1997. Baculovirus-directed expression of rabbit UDP-glucuronosyltransferases in *Spodoptera frugiperda* cells. *Drug Metab. Dispos.* 25:745–49

67. Strassburg CP, Strassburg A, Nguyen N, Li Q, Manns MP, Tukey RH. 1999. Regulation and function of family 1 and family 2 UDP-glucuronosyltransferase genes (*UGT1A, UGT2B*) in human oesophagus. *Biochem. J.* 338(2):489–98

68. Strassburg CP, Obermayer-Straub P, Alex B, Durazzo M, Rizzetto M, et al.

1996. Autoantibodies against glucuronosyltransferases differ between viral and autoimmune hepatitis. *Gastroenterology* 111:1576–86

69. Coffman BL, King CD, Rios GR, Tephly TR. 1998. The glucuronidation of opioids, other xenobiotics, and androgens by human UGT2B7Y(268) and UGT2B7H(268). *Drug Metab. Dispos.* 26:73–77

70. Green MD, Oturu EM, Tephly TR. 1994. Stable expression of a human liver UDP-glucuronosyltransferase (UGT2B15) with activity toward steroid and xenobiotic substrates. *Drug Metab. Dispos.* 22:799–805

71. Ebner T, Burchell B. 1993. Substrate specificities of two stably expressed human liver UDP-glucuronosyltransferases of the *UGT1* gene family. *Drug Metab. Dispos.* 21:50–55

72. Coffman BL, Green MD, King CD, Tephly TR. 1995. Cloning and stable expression of a cDNA encoding a rat liver UDP-glucuronosyltransferase (UDP-glucuronosyltransferase 1.1) that catalyzes the glucuronidation of opioids and bilirubin. *Mol. Pharmacol.* 47:1101–5

73. Cheng Z, Radominska-Pandya A, Tephly TR. 1998. Cloning and expression of human UDP-glucuronosyltransferase (UGT) 1A8. *Arch. Biochem. Biophys.* 356:301–5

74. King CD, Rios GR, Assouline JA, Tephly TR. 1999. Expression of UDP-glucuronosyltransferases (UGTs) 2B7 and 1A6 in the human brain and identification of 5-hydroxytryptamine as a substrate. *Arch. Biochem. Biophys.* 365:156–62

75. Hum DW, Belanger A, Levesque E, Barbier O, Beaulieu M, et al. 1999. Characterization of UDP-glucuronosyltransferases active on steroid hormones. *J. Steroid. Biochem. Mol. Biol.* 69:413–23

76. Mackenzie PI, Rodbourne L, Stranks S.

1992. Steroid UDP glucuronosyltransferases. *J. Steroid. Biochem. Mol. Biol.* 43:1099–105

77. Mackenzie PI, Mojarrabi B, Meech R, Hansen A. 1996. Steriod UDP glucuronosyltransferases: characterization and regulation. *J. Endocrinol.* 150(Suppl.): S79–86

78. Fournel-Gigleux S, Sutherland L, Sabolovic N, Burchell B, Siest G. 1991. Stable expression of two human UDP-glucuronosyltransferase cDNAs in V79 cell cultures. *J. Pharmacol. Exp. Ther.* 39:177–83

79. Cheng Z, Rios GR, King CD, Coffman BL, Green MD, et al. 1998. Glucuronidation of catechol estrogens by expressed human UDP-glucuronosyltransferases (UGTs) 1A1, 1A3, and 2B7. *Toxicol. Sci.* 45:52–57

80. Jin CJ, Mackenzie PI, Miners JO. 1997. The regio- and stereo-selectivity of C19 and C21 hydroxysteroid glucuronidation by UGT2B7 and UGT2B11. *Arch. Biochem. Biophys.* 341:207–11

81. Green MD, Tephly TR. 1996. Glucuronidation of amines and hydroxylated xenobiotics and endobiotics catalyzed by expressed human UGT1.4 protein. *Drug Metab. Dispos.* 24:356–63

82. King CD, Green MD, Rios GR, Coffman BL, Owens IS, et al. 1996. The glucuronidation of exogenous and endogenous compounds by stably expressed rat and human UDP-glucuronosyltransferase 1.1. *Arch. Biochem. Biophys.* 332:92–100

83. Green MD, Bishop WP, Tephly TR. 1995. Expressed human UGT1.4 protein catalyzes the formation of quaternary ammonium-linked glucuronides. *Drug Metab. Dispos.* 23:299–302

84. Green MD, King CD, Mojarrabi B, Mackenzie PI, Tephly TR. 1998. Glucuronidation of amines and other xenobiotics catalyzed by expressed human UDP-glu-

curonosyltransferase 1A3. *Drug Metab. Dispos.* 26:507–12

84a. Ciotti M, Lakshmi VM, Basu N, Davis BB, Owens IS, Zenser TV. 1999. Glucuronidation of benzidine and its metabolites by cDNA-expressed human UDP-glucuronosyltransferases and pH stability of glucuronides. *Carcinogenesis* 20:1963–69

85. Orzechowski A, Schrenk D, Bock-Hennig BS, Bock KW. 1994. Glucuronidation of carcinogenic arylamines and their *N*-hydroxy derivatives by rat and human phenol UDP-glucuronosyltransferases of the *UGT1* gene complex. *Carcinogenesis* 15:1549–54

86. Hiller A, Nguyen N, Strassburg CP, Li Q, Jainta H, et al. 1999. Retigabine N-glucuronidation and its potential role in enterohepatic circulation. *Drug Metab. Dispos.* 27:605–12

87. Huskey S-EW, Magdalou J, Ouzzine M, Siest G, Chiu S-HL. 1994. N-glucuronidation reactions. III. Regioselectivity of N-glucuronidation of methylbiphenyl tetrazole, methylbiphenyl triazole, and methylbiphenyl imidazole using human and rat recombinant UDP-glucuronosyltransferases stably expressed in V79 cells. *Drug Metab. Dispos.* 22:659–62

88. Green MD, Tephly TR. 1998. Glucuronidation of amine substrates by purified and expressed UDP-glucuronosyltransferase proteins. *Drug Metab. Dispos.* 26:860–67

89. Matern S, Matern H, Farthmann EH, Gerok W. 1984. Hepatic and extrahepatic glucuronidation of bile acids in man. Characterization of bile acid uridine 5′-diphosphate-glucuronosyltransferase in hepatic, renal, and intestinal microsomes. *J. Clin. Invest.* 74:402–10

90. Pacifici GM, Giuliani L, Calcaprina R. 1986. Glucuronodation of 1-napthol in nuclear and microsomal fractions of the human intestine. *Pharmacology* 33:103–9

91. Parquet M, Pessah M, Sacquet E, Salvat C, Raizman A, Infante R. 1985. Glucuronidation of bile acids in human liver, intestine and kidney. An in vitro study on hyodeoxycholic acid. *FEBS Lett.* 189:183–87

92. Peters WH, Nagengast FM, van Tongeren JH. 1989. Glutathione S-transferase, cytochrome P450, and uridine 5′-diphosphate-glucuronosyltransferase in human small intestine and liver. *Gastroenterology* 96:783–89

93. Peters WH, Kock L, Nagengast FM, Kremers PG. 1991. Biotransformation enzymes in human intestine: critical low levels in the colon? *Gut* 32:408–12

94. Pacifici GM, Franchi M, Bencini C, Repetti F, Di Lascio N, Muraro GB. 1988. Tissue distribution of drug-metabolizing enzymes in humans. *Xenobiotica* 18:849–56

95. Peters WH, Allebes WA, Jansen PL, Poels LG, Capel PJ. 1987. Characterization and tissue specificity of a monoclonal antibody against human uridine 5′-diphosphate-glucuronosyltransferase. *Gastroenterology* 93:162–69

96. Peters WH, Jansen PL. 1988. Immunocharacterization of UDP-glucuronyltransferase isoenzymes in human liver, intestine and kidney. *Biochem. Pharmacol.* 37:564–67

97. McDonnell WM, Hitomi E, Askari FK. 1996. Identification of bilirubin UDP-GTs in the human alimentary tract in accordance with the gut as a putative metabolic organ. *Biochem. Pharmacol.* 51:483–88

98. Strassburg CP, Nguyen N, Manns MP, Tukey RH. 1998. Polymorphic expression of the UDP-glucuronosyltransferase *UGT1A* gene locus in human gastric epithelium. *Mol. Pharmacol.* 54:647–54

99. McGurk KA, Brierley CH, Burchell B. 1998. Drug glucuronidation by human renal UDP-glucuronosyltransferases. *Biochem. Pharmacol.* 55:1005–12

100. Suleman FG, Abid A, Gradinaru D, Daval JL, Magdalou J, Minn A. 1998. Identification of the uridine diphosphate glucuronosyltransferase isoform UGT1A6 in rat brain and in primary cultures of neurons and astrocytes. *Arch. Biochem. Biophys.* 358:63–67

101. Jackson MR, McCarthy LR, Harding D, Wilson S, Coughtrie MWH, Burchell B. 1987. Cloning of a human liver microsomal UDP-glucuronosyltransferase cDNA. *Biochem. J.* 242:581–88

102. Chen F, Ritter JK, Wang MG, McBride OW, Lubet RA, Owens IS. 1993. Characterization of a cloned human dihydrotestosterone/androstanediol UDP-glucuronosyltransferase and its comparison to other steroid isoforms. *Biochemistry* 32:10648–57

103. Belanger G, Beaulieu M, Marcotte B, Levesque E, Guillemette C, et al. 1995. Expression of transcripts encoding steroid UDP-glucuronosyltransferases in human prostate hyperplastic tissue and the LNCaP cell line. *Mol. Cell. Endocrinol.* 113:165–73

104. Radominska-Pandya A, Little JM, Pandya JT, Tephly TR, King CD, et al. 1998. UDP-glucuronosyltransferases in human intestinal mucosa. *Biochim. Biophys. Acta* 1394:199–208

105. Ciotti M, Marrone A, Potter B, Owens IS. 1997. Genetic polymorphism in the human UGT1A6 (planar phenol) UDP-glucuronosyltransferase: pharmacological implications. *Pharmacogenetics* 7:485–95

106. Berk PD, Noyer C. 1994. Bilirubin metabolism and the hereditary hyperbilirubinemias. *Sem. Liver Dis.* 14:323–94

107. Bissel DM. 1986. Heme catabolism and bilirubin formation. In *Bile Pigments and Jaundice*, ed. JD Ostrow, pp. 133–56. New York: Dekker

108. Manns MP, Strassburg CP. 1996. Chronic hepatitis. In *Current Therapy in Allergy Immunology and Rheumatology*, ed. LM Lichtenstein, AS Fauci, pp. 301–9. Philadelphia, PA: Mosby

109. Ritter JK, Crawford JM, Owens IS. 1991. Cloning of two human liver bilirubin UDP-glucuronosyltransferase cDNAs with expression in COS-1 cells. *J. Biol. Chem.* 266:1043–47

110. Burchell B, Nebert DW, Nelson DR, Bock KW, Iyanagi T, et al. 1991. The UDP glucuronosyltransferase gene superfamily. Suggested nomenclature based on evolutionary divergence. *DNA Cell Biol.* 10:487–94

111. Bosma PJ, Seppen J, Goldhoorn B, Bakker C, Oude ER, et al. 1994. Bilirubin UDP-glucuronosyltransferase 1 is the only relevant bilirubin glucuronidating isoform in man. *J. Biol. Chem.* 269:17960–64

112. Aono S, Yamada Y, Keino H, Sasaoka Y, Nakagawa T, et al. 1994. A new type of defect in the gene for bilirubin uridine 5′-diphosphate-glucuronosyltransferase in a patient with Crigler-Najjar syndrome type I. *Pediatr. Res.* 35:629–32

113. Aono S, Adachi Y, Uyama E, Yamada Y, Keino H, et al. 1995. Analysis of genes for bilirubin UDP-glucuronosyltransferase in Gilbert's syndrome. *Lancet* 345:958–59

114. Bosma PJ, Goldhoorn B, Oude ER, Sinaasappel M, Oostra BA, Jansen PL. 1993. A mutation in bilirubin uridine 5′-diphosphate-glucuronosyltransferase isoform 1 causing Crigler-Najjar syndrome type II. *Gastroenterology* 105: 216–20

115. Seppen J, Bosma PJ, Goldhoorn BG, Bakker CT, Chowdhury JR, et al. 1994. Discrimination between Crigler-Najjar syndrome type I and II by expression of mutant bilirubin uridine diphosphate-glucuronosyltransferase. *J. Clin. Invest.* 94:2385–91

116. Ritter JK, Yeatman MT, Kaiser C, Gri-

delli B, Owens IS. 1993. A phenylalanine codon deletion at the *UGT1* gene complex locus of a Crigler-Najjar type I patient generates a pH-sensitive bilirubin UDP-glucuronosyltransferase. *J. Biol. Chem.* 268:23573–79

117. Ciotti M, Yeatman MT, Sokol RJ, Owens IS. 1995. Altered coding for a strictly conserved di-glycine in the major bilirubin UDP-glucuronosyltransferase of a Crigler-Najjar type I patient. *J. Biol. Chem.* 270:3284–91

118. Seppen J, Steenken E, Lindhout D, Bosma PJ, Elferink RPJO. 1996. A mutation which disrupts the hydrophobic core of the signal peptide of bilirubin UDP-glucuronosyltransferase, an endoplasmic reticulum membrane protein, causes Crigler-Najjar type II. *FEBS Lett.* 390:294–98

119. Koiwai O, Nishizawa M, Hasada K, Aono S, Adachi Y, et al. 1995. Gilbert's syndrome is caused by a heterozygous missense mutation in the gene for bilirubin UDP-glucuronosyltransferase. *Hum. Mol. Genet.* 4:1183–86

120. Gilbert A, Lereboullet P. 1901. La cholamae simple familiale. *Sem. Med.* 21:241–48

121. Bosma PJ, Chowdhury JR, Bakker C, Gantla S, De Boer A, et al. 1995. The genetic basis of the reduced expression of bilirubin UDP-glucuronosyltransferase 1 in Gilbert's syndrome. *N. Engl. J. Med.* 333:1171–75

122. Monaghan G, Ryan M, Seddon R, Hume R, Burchell B. 1996. Genetic variation in bilirubin UDP-glucuronosyltransferase gene promoter and Gilbert's syndrome. *Lancet* 347:578–81

123. Ciotti M, Chen F, Rubaltelli FF, Owens IS. 1998. Coding defect and a TATA box mutation at the bilirubin UDP-glucuronosyltransferase gene cause Crigler-Najjar type I disease. *Biochim. Biophys. Acta* 1407:40–50

124. Bosma PJ, Chowdhury JR, Huang T-J, Lahiri P, Oude Elferink RPJ, et al. 1992. Mechanisms of inherited deficiencies of multiple UDP-glucuronosyltransferase isoforms in two patients with Crigler-Najjar syndrome, type I. *FASEB J.* 6:2859–63

125. Erps LT, Ritter JK, Hersh JH, Blossom D, Martin NC, Owens IS. 1994. Identification of two single base substitutions in the *UGT1* gene locus which abolish bilirubin uridine diphosphate glucuronosyltransferase activity in vitro. *J. Clin. Invest.* 93:564–70

126. Bosma PJ, Chowdhury NR, Goldhoorn BG, Hofker MH, Oude Elferink RP, et al. 1992. Sequence of exons and the flanking regions of human bilirubin-UDP-glucuronosyltransferase gene complex and identification of a genetic mutation in a patient with Crigler-Najjar syndrome, type I. *Hepatology* 15:941–47

127. Labrune P, Myara A, Hadchouel M, Ronchi F, Bernard O, et al. 1994. Genetic heterogeneity of Crigler-Najjar syndrome type I: a study of 14 cases. *Hum. Genet.* 94:693–97

128. Moghrabi N, Clarke DJ, Boxer M, Burchell B. 1993. Identification of an A-to-G missense mutation in exon 2 of the *UGT1* gene complex that causes Crigler-Najjar syndrome type II. *Genomics* 18:171–73

129. Moghrabi N, Clarke DJ, Burchell B, Boxer M. 1993. Cosegregation of intragenic markers with a novel mutation that causes Crigler-Najjar syndrome type I: implication in carrier detection and prenatal diagnosis. *Am. J. Hum. Genet.* 53:722–29

130. Aono S, Yamada Y, Keino H, Hanada N, Nakagawa T, et al. 1993. Identification of defect in the genes for bilirubin UDP-glucuronosyl-transferase in a patient with Crigler-Najjar syndrome type II.

Biochem. Biophys. Res. Commun. 197: 1239–44

131. Ciotti M, Obaray R, Martin MG, Owens IS. 1997. Genetic defects at the *UGT1* locus associated with Crigler-Najjar type I disease, including a prenatal diagnosis. *Am. J. Med. Genet.* 68:173–78

132. Jansen PL. 1996. Genetic diseases of bilirubin metabolism: the inherited unconjugated hyperbilirubinemias. *J. Hepatol.* 25:398–404

133. Lutz WK. 1999. Carcinogens in the diet vs. overnutrition. Individual dietary habits, malnutrition, and genetic susceptibility modify carcinogenic potency and cancer risk. *Mutat. Res.* 443:251–58

134. Lai C, Shields PG. 1999. The role of interindividual variation in human carcinogenesis. *J. Nutr.* 129:552–55

135. Bock KW. 1991. Roles of UDP-glucuronosyltransferases in chemical carcinogenesis. *Crit. Rev. Biochem. Mol. Biol.* 26:129–50

136. Rambeaud JJ. 1999. Intermittent complete androgen blockade in metastatic prostate cancer. *Eur. Urol.* 35(Suppl. 1):32–36

137. Schroder FH. 1998. Antiandrogens as monotherapy for prostate cancer. *Eur. Urol.* 34(Suppl. 3):12–17

138. Jin C-J, Miners JO, Burchell B, Mackenzie PI. 1993. The glucuronidation of hydroxylated metabolites of benzo[*a*]pyrene and 2-acetylaminofluorene by cDNA-expressed human UDP-glucuronosyltransferases. *Carcinogenesis* 14: 2637–39

139. Nowell SA, Massengill JS, Williams S, Radominska-Pandya A, Tephly TR, et al. 1999. Glucuronidation of 2-hydroxyamino-1-methyl-6-phenylimidazo[4,5-β]pyridine by human microsomal UDP-glucuronosyltransferases: identification of specific UGT1A family isoforms involved. *Carcinogenesis* 20: 1107–14

140. Parkin DM, Pisani P, Ferlay J. 1999. Global cancer statistics. *CA. Cancer J. Clin.* 49:33–64

141. Levesque E, Beaulieu M, Guillemette C, Hum DW, Belanger A. 1998. Effect of interleukins on UGT2B15 and UGT2B17 steroid uridine diphosphate-glucuronosyltransferase expression and activity in the LNCaP cell line. *Endocrinology* 139:2375–81

142. Waldenström JL. 1950. Blutproteine und Nahrungseiweiss. *Dtsch. Ges. Verd. Soffw.* 15:113–19

143. Rizzetto M, Swana G, Doniach D. 1973. Microsomal antibodies in active chronic hepatitis and other disorders. *Clin. Exp. Immunol.* 15:331–44

144. Manns MP, Johnson EF, Griffin KJ, Tan EM, Sullivan KF. 1989. Major antigen of liver kidney microsomal autoantibodies in idiopathic autoimmune hepatitis is cytochrome P450db1. *J. Clin. Invest.* 83:1066–72

145. Homberg JC, Abuaf N, Bernard O, Islam S, Alvarez F, et al. 1987. Chronic active hepatitis associated with antiliver/kidney microsome antibody type I: a second type of "autoimmune" hepatitis. *Hepatology* 7:1333–39

146. Gueguen M, Yamamoto AM, Bernard O, Alvarez F. 1989. Anti-liver kidney microsome antibody type I recognizes human cytochrome P450 dbl. *Biochem. Biophys. Res. Commun.* 159:542–47

147. Zanger UM, Hauri H-P, Loeper J, Homberg J-C, Meyer UA. 1988. Antibodies against human cytochrome P-450db1 in autoimmune hepatitis type II. *Proc. Natl. Acad. Sci. USA* 85:8256–60

148. Beaune P, Dansette PM, Mansuy D, Kiffel L, Finck M, et al. 1987. Human anti-endoplasmic reticulum autoantibodies appearing in a drug-induced hepatitis are directed against a human liver cytochrome P-450 that hydroxylates the drug. *Proc. Natl. Acad. Sci. USA* 84:551–55

149. Bourdi M, Larrey D, Nataf J, Bernuau J,

Pessayre D, et al. 1990. Anti-liver endoplasmic reticulum autoantibodies are directed against human cytochrome P-450IA2. A specific marker of dihydralazine-induced hepatitis. *J. Clin. Invest.* 85:1967–73

150. Manns MP, Griffin KJ, Quattrochi LC, Sacher M, Thaler H, et al. 1990. Identification of cytochrome P450IA2 as a human autoantigen. *Arch. Biochem. Biophys.* 280:229–32

151. Clemente MG, Obermayer-Straub P, Meloni A, Strassburg CP, Arangino V, et al. 1997. Cytochrome P450 1A2 is a hepatic autoantigen in autoimmune polyglandular syndrome type I. *J. Clin. Endocrinol. Metab.* 82:1353–61

152. Hellmold H, Övervik E, Strömstedt M, Gustafsson J-Å. 1993. Cytochrome P450 forms in the rodent lung involved in the metabolic activation of food-derived heterocyclic amines. *Carcinogenesis* 14:1751–57

153. Philipp T, Durazzo M, Trautwein C, Alex B, Straub P, et al. 1994. Recognition of uridine diphosphate glucuronosyltransferases by LKM-3 antibodies in chronic hepatitis D. *Lancet* 344:578–81

154. Strassburg CP, Obermayer-Straub P, Manns MP. 1996. Autoimmunity in hepatitis C and D virus infection. *J. Viral. Hepat.* 3:49–59

155. Beaune PH, Lecoeur S, Bourdi M, Gauffre A, Belloc C, et al. 1996. Anticytochrome P450 autoantibodies in drug-induced disease. *Eur. J. Haematol.* 57(Suppl. 60):89–92

156. Visser TJ, Kaptein E, Gijzel AL, de Herder WW, Ebner T, Burchell B. 1993. Glucuronidation of thyroid hormone by human bilirubin and phenol UDP-glucuronyltrasferase isoenzymes. *FEBS Lett.* 324:358–60

157. Senafi SB, Clarke DJ, Burchell B. 1994.

Investigation of the substrate specificity of a cloned expressed human bilirubin UDP-glucuronosyltransferase: UDP-sugar specificity and involvement in steroid and xenobiotic glucuronidation. *Biochem. J.* 303:233–40

158. Gschaidmeier H, Seidel A, Burchell B, Bock KW. 1995. Formation of mono- and diglucuronides and other glycosides of benzo(*a*)pyrene-3,6-quinol by V79 cell-expressed human phenol UDP-glucuronosyltransferases of the *UGT1* gene complex. *Biochem. Pharmacol.* 49: 1601–6

159. Bock KW, Forster A, Gschaidmeier H, Bruck M, Munzel P, et al. 1993. Paracetamol glucuronidation by recombinant rat and human phenol UDP-glucuronosyltransferases. *Biochem. Pharmacol.* 45: 1809–14

160. Jackson MR, Fournel-Gigleux S, Harding D, Burchell B. 1988. Examination of the substrate specificity of cloned rat kidney phenol UDP-glucuronyltransferase expressed in COS-7 cells. *Mol. Pharmacol.* 34:638–42

161. Sutherland L, Bin Senafi S, Ebner T, Clarke DJ, Burchell B. 1992. Characterization of a human bilirubin UDP-glucuronosyltransferase stably expressed in hamster lung fibroblast cell cultures. *FEBS Lett.* 308:161–64

162. Roy-Chowdhury J, Huang T, Kesari K, Lederstein M, Arias IM, Roy-Chowdhury N. 1991. Molecular basis for the lack of bilirubin-specific and 3-methylcholanthrene-inducible UDP-glucuronosyltransferase activities in gunn rats. *J. Biol. Chem.* 266:18294–98

163. Iyanagi T. 1991. Molecular basis of multiple UDP-glucuronosyltransferase isoenzyme deficiencies in the hyperbilirubinemic rat (Gunn rat). *J. Biol. Chem.* 266:24048–52

Annu. Rev. Pharmacol. Toxicol. 2000. 40:617–47

14-3-3 PROTEINS: Structure, Function, and Regulation

Haian Fu, Romesh R. Subramanian, and Shane C. Masters

Department of Pharmacology, Emory University School of Medicine, Atlanta, Georgia 30322; e-mail: hfu@pharm.emory.edu, rsubram@emory.edu, smast01@emory.edu

Key Words   signal transduction, phosphoserine, protein-protein interaction, apoptosis, cell cycle

■ **Abstract**   The 14-3-3 proteins are a family of conserved regulatory molecules expressed in all eukaryotic cells. A striking feature of the 14-3-3 proteins is their ability to bind a multitude of functionally diverse signaling proteins, including kinases, phosphatases, and transmembrane receptors. This plethora of interacting proteins allows 14-3-3 to play important roles in a wide range of vital regulatory processes, such as mitogenic signal transduction, apoptotic cell death, and cell cycle control. In this review, we examine the structural basis for 14-3-3–ligand interactions, proposed functions of 14-3-3 in various signaling pathways, and emerging views of mechanisms that regulate 14-3-3 actions.

INTRODUCTION

The 14-3-3 protein was initially described as an acidic, abundant brain protein by Moore & Perez in 1967 (1). The name is derived from the combination of its fraction number on DEAE-cellulose chromatography and its migration position in the subsequent starch–gel electrophoresis. The unique terminology remains while the concept of 14-3-3 has evolved from a brain-specific protein to a family of ubiquitously expressed regulatory molecules of eukaryotic organisms. 14-3-3 has emerged as a group of multifunctional proteins that bind to and modulate the function of a wide array of cellular proteins. More than 50 signaling proteins have been reported as 14-3-3 ligands (see Annual Reviews' web site, www.AnnualReviews.org, Supplementary Table: 14-3-3–associated proteins, for a detailed list and references). This broad range of partners suggests for 14-3-3 a role as a general biochemical regulator, reminiscent of the well-defined regulatory protein calmodulin. Through interaction with its effector proteins, 14-3-3 participates in the regulation of diverse biological processes, including neuronal development, cell growth control, and viral and bacterial pathogenesis. This review focuses on recent developments in the understanding of the structural basis

0362–1642/00/0415–0617$14.00

of 14-3-3–ligand interactions and on roles for 14-3-3 in three model systems. The functions of 14-3-3 in neuronal development (2), signal transduction (3–5), and plant biology (6, 7) have recently been reviewed elsewhere.

General Properties

14-3-3 is a family of highly homologous proteins encoded by separate genes. There are seven known mammalian 14-3-3 isoforms, named with Greek letters (β, ε, γ, η, σ, τ, ζ) after their elution profile on reversed phase high-performance liquid chromatography (8, 9). The species initially designated α and δ are actually the phosphorylated forms of β and ζ (10). The 14-3-3 proteins exist mainly as dimers with a monomeric molecular mass of approximately 30,000 and an acidic isoelectric point of 4–5.

14-3-3 proteins exhibit a remarkable degree of sequence conservation between species (11). For example, the *Saccharomyces cerevisiae* BMH1 and human ε isoforms are approximately 70% similar at the amino acid level. 14-3-3 proteins also share some basic biochemical properties, such as activation of the ExoS ADP-ribosyltransferase (12, 13) and of tryptophan hydroxylase (14). These similarities argue strongly for a high degree of functional conservation.

14-3-3 is abundant in the brain, comprising approximately 1% of its total soluble protein (15). It is now clear that 14-3-3 is also present in almost all tissues, including testes, liver, and heart (16). Within a eukaryotic cell, 14-3-3 is largely found in the cytoplasmic compartment. However, 14-3-3 proteins can also be detected at the plasma membrane and in intracellular organelles such as the nucleus and the Golgi apparatus (16–21). Like their high degree of conservation, the ubiquitous nature of 14-3-3 proteins may reflect their fundamental importance in eukaryotic biology. Indeed, recent research on 14-3-3 supports this view.

Rediscoveries

Since the initial discovery of 14-3-3, the history of 14-3-3 proteins has been full of rediscoveries. Characterization of a protein cofactor that activates tryptophan and tyrosine hydroxylases uncovered 14-3-3 (22) and led to the cloning of the first 14-3-3 gene (8). The availability of a 14-3-3 sequence set the stage for a flood of rediscoveries by investigators interested in a wide range of biological questions.

The initial introduction of 14-3-3 into some biological systems was based on functional studies aimed at identifying regulatory proteins. For instance, the isolation of inhibitors of protein kinase C (PKC) (23), the identification of stimulators of calcium-dependent exocytosis (24), and the cloning of a eukaryotic activator of the *Pseudomonas aeruginosa* ExoS ADP-ribosyltransferase (12) each resulted in the rediscovery of the 14-3-3 proteins. Similarly, 14-3-3 has been found as an activator of the 43-kDa inositol polyphosphate 5-phosphatase (5-phosphatase)

(25). It seems that 14-3-3 functions as an allosteric cofactor to affect the catalytic activity of some of its ligands.

Another major avenue of rediscovery of 14-3-3 accompanied technological advances in detecting protein-protein interactions, such as the yeast two-hybrid system. In recent years, many signal transduction pathways have been unveiled that control cell proliferation, differentiation, and apoptosis, but understanding the intricate mechanisms that regulate these pathways remains a daunting challenge (26). Many investigators search for clues by identifying proteins that interact with key signaling components. 14-3-3 proteins are easy prey for a variety of bait proteins in a large array of these screens. Such 14-3-3–associated proteins include receptors [e.g. glucocorticoid receptor (27) and insulin-like growth factor I receptor (IGFIR) (28, 29)], kinases [e.g. Raf-1 (17, 30–34), Bcr (35), and phosphatidylinositol 3 kinase (36)], phosphatases [e.g. Cdc25 (37) and PTPH1 (38)], docking molecules [e.g. insulin receptor substrate I (39) and p130^{Cas} (18)], death regulators [e.g. Bad (40) and A20 (41)], and oncogene products [e.g. polyomavirus middle tumor antigen (MT) (42) and Bcr-Abl (35)]. These protein-protein interaction-based studies have dramatically expanded the range of 14-3-3–regulated events.

A third road to the rediscovery of 14-3-3 has been via genetic suppressor analysis. For instance, the 14-3-3 proteins Rad24 and Rad25 were isolated as suppressors that complement the radiation sensitivity of a *rad24* mutant in *Schizosaccharomyces pombe* (43). The *rad24* mutant is defective in the DNA damage checkpoint, linking 14-3-3 function to cell cycle control. In *S. cerevisiae*, expression of 14-3-3 homologs BMH1 or BMH2 complements the phenotype of the *CHC1* clathrin heavy-chain gene deletion, which supports a potential role for 14-3-3 in vesicular transport (44). Golgi localization and interaction with invariant chain p35 (Iip35) in the endoplasmic reticulum suggest a related purpose for 14-3-3 in mammalian cells (45). It is intriguing to note that BMH1 and BMH2 can also prevent rapamycin-mediated lethality in *S. cerevisiae* (46). Rapamycin, when combined with its immunophilin receptor FKBP12, interacts with Tor (target of rapamycin) to induce cell growth arrest, primarily via an effect on protein synthesis machinery. Although the role of 14-3-3 in this system is not clear, it stands as further proof that 14-3-3 is a significant component of many complex cellular processes.

The frequent isolation of 14-3-3 from many biochemical and genetic screens for different targets must reflect the physiological importance of 14-3-3 in diverse cellular pathways. Depending on its interaction with specific effectors, 14-3-3 participates in many vital regulatory processes, such as cell cycle control, survival signaling, cell adhesion, and neuronal plasticity. The trend of rediscovery of 14-3-3 proteins shows no sign of diminishing and in fact will likely become more common because of an increased understanding of the regulation of 14-3-3–ligand interactions.

14-3-3–LIGAND INTERACTIONS

The heterogeneity and sheer number of binding partners for 14-3-3 allows the prediction of some properties of the interaction. A natural conclusion that can be drawn is that 14-3-3 ligands share a common binding determinant that mediates their contact with 14-3-3. One such determinant is a specifically phosphorylated residue in 14-3-3 ligands. Several early observations guided the realization that phosphorylation of target proteins is the primary mechanism that controls 14-3-3 binding (47–49). In particular, S259 of Raf-1, a conserved phosphorylation site, was shown to be required for 14-3-3–Raf-1 interaction (48). Detailed dissection of the residues surrounding phosphorylated S259 led Muslin et al (49) to define a consensus 14-3-3 recognition motif, RSxpSxP, where x represents any amino acid and pS stands for phosphorylated serine. Screening degenerate phosphoserine-oriented peptide libraries against 14-3-3 revealed a similar sequence, in strong support of the above consensus motif (50). Indeed, numerous 14-3-3–associated proteins bind 14-3-3 through a phosphorylated serine site and contain this motif (Table 1).

The definition of 14-3-3 as a phosphoserine binding protein represents a major conceptual advancement in the study of 14-3-3 function. More important, it defines a novel paradigm by which phosphorylated serine, like phosphorylated tyrosine, can serve as a recognition signal for protein-protein interactions. Analogous to SH2 and PTB domain–containing proteins that bind phosphotyrosine motifs, 14-3-3 proteins represent a novel class of protein modules that recognize phosphoserine motifs (5). Thus, understanding the mechanisms that control 14-3-3–ligand interactions will provide insight into more general questions concerning the control of intracellular signal transduction.

14-3-3 Recognition Sequences

Phosphoserine-Mediated Interactions   The prototype phosphorylated serine recognition motif, RSxpSxP, was deduced from a 15-mer Raf-1 peptide containing RQRS^{257}TS^{259}TP (49). This peptide, when phosphorylated on S259, directly binds 14-3-3ζ with an apparent K_d of 122 nM. The binding is site specific because the same peptide cannot interact efficiently with 14-3-3 when it is unphosphorylated or when phosphorylated at S257 or at S257 and S259 together. An Arg residue in the –3 or –4 position relative to the phosphoserine is also crucial for 14-3-3 association. The proline residue at +2 is important, but this position can tolerate other residues (51). Extensive screening of phosphoserine-oriented peptide libraries identified two alternative consensus motifs with one (mode 1) closely related to the RSxpSxP motif (50). However, the peptide library approach revealed some preference for certain amino acids in the –1, –2, and +1 positions. Accordingly, the 14-3-3 recognition motif is refined to R[S/Ar][+/Ar]pS[L/E/A/M]P, where Ar represents an aromatic residue and + indicates a basic residue. The second identified motif (mode 2) uses the optimal sequence Rx[Ar][+]pS[L/

TABLE 1 Ligands of 14-3-3 that are known to contain defined interaction motifs[a]

Ligand	Property	Sequence[b]	Effect of 14-3-3 binding[c]	References
RSxpSxP and related motifs				
Raf-1[d]	S/T kinase	RSTS^{259} TP, RSAS^{621} EP	Dual role: maintain both inactive and active conformations	49, 81
Bad[e]	Bcl-2 homolog	RHSS^{112} YP, RSRS^{136} AP	Cytoplasmic retention; inhibit proapoptotic function	40, 100
Cdc25C	Y/T phosphatase	RSPS^{216} MP	Cytoplasmic retention; block entry into M phase	53, 112, 113, 115, 118
ASK1	S/T kinase	RSIS^{967} LP	Inhibit proapoptotic function	78
Middle T antigen	Oncoprotein	RSHS^{257} YP	Promote tumors in certain tissues	135, 151
KSR[d]	S/T kinase	RSKS^{297} HE, RTES^{392} VP	—	152, 154
PTPH1	Y phosphatase	RSLS^{359} VE, RVDS^{853} EP	—	38
IRS-1	Docking protein	RSKS^{270} QS, HSRS^{374} IP, KSVS^{641} AP	—	39
Iip35	MHC-associated protein	RSRS^8CR	Allows exit from ER	45
FKHRL1	Transcription factor	RSCT^{32} WP, RAVS^{253} MD	Cytoplasmic retention; inhibit proapoptotic function	54
Slob	K^+ channel binding protein	RSNS^{54} AI, RSAS^{79} SE	Modulate voltage sensitivity of associated Slowpoke K^+ channels	153

(continued)

TABLE 1 (continued) Ligands of 14-3-3 that are known to contain defined interaction motifs[a]

Ligand	Property	Sequence[b]	Effect of 14-3-3 binding[c]	References
$Rx_{1-2}Sx_{2-3}S$ motifs				
Cbl	Adaptor protein	RHS^{619} $LPFS^{623}$, $RLGS^{639}$ TFS^{642}	—	55
Keratin 18	Cytoskeletal component	$RPVSSAAS^{33}$	—	57
PKCμ	S/T kinase	RLS^{205} NVS^{208}, $RTSS^{219}$ $AELS^{223}$	Inhibit kinase activity	56
Other phosphoserine motifs				
IGF-I receptor	Y kinase	$SVPLDPSA$ $SSSS^{1283}$ LP	—	28, 29
GP1bβ	Adhesion receptor	RLS^{166} $LTDP$	—	155–157
p53	Transcription factor	$KGQSTS^{378}$ RH	Increase DNA binding	58
Nonphosphorylated motifs				
43 kDa 5-phosphatase	Lipid phosphatase	$ELVLRSESEEKVV^{371}$	Stimulate phosphatase activity	25
R18	Synthetic peptide	$WLDLE^{14}$		65, 71

[a]ASK1, apoptosis signal-regulating kinase 1; KSR, kinase suppressor of Ras; IRS-1, insulin receptor substrate I; MHC, major histocompatibility complex; ER, endoplasmic reticulum; PKC, protein kinase C.

[b]Residues implicated by mutation to be important for 14-3-3 binding are italicized.

[c]The effects of phosphorylation and 14-3-3 binding are not clearly distinguished for most of these ligands.

[d]Raf-1 and KSR also bind 14-3-3 via their cysteine rich domains.

[e]The role of Bad S^{112} in 14-3-3 binding is not clear.

E/A/M]P. It is important to note that synthetic peptides containing these motifs bind 14-3-3 with high affinities (50), which suggests that they may reflect the 14-3-3 binding determinant in proteins.

The prototype 14-3-3 recognition motif has been found in a number of 14-3-3–associated proteins, and its role in mediating 14-3-3 binding has been well established in several biological systems (Table 1). For instance, Raf-1 contains two such phosphoserine motifs encompassing S259 and S621 (49, 52). These Ser residues are phosphorylated in vivo, indicating their physiological significance (52). Unphosphorylatable mutants of Raf-1 that convert S259 and S621 to Ala exhibit diminished association with 14-3-3, which underscores the importance of these motifs for 14-3-3 binding (48). It is interesting to note that the defined 14-3-3 consensus motifs can have some predictive value, as several proteins that were anticipated to bind 14-3-3 based on these recognition sequences have now been experimentally verified, including Cdc25 (53) and Bad (40). However, the broad range of substitutions allowed in these motifs (Table 1), such as the use of phosphothreonine instead of phosphoserine in FKHRL1 (54), makes it clear that more work will be necessary to fully understand this mode of interaction between 14-3-3 and phosphoproteins.

Studies on the proto-oncogene product Cbl revealed another variation of the 14-3-3 binding motif, the Ser-rich motif (55). A consensus sequence was postulated: $Rx_{1-2}Sx_{2-3}S$, where x denotes any amino acid and where at least one of the Ser is phosphorylated. The Cbl protein contains two such motifs. Two Cbl-like motifs have also been identified in PKCμ (56). In contrast to Cbl, which requires both of its motifs to be intact for 14-3-3 binding, either one alone is sufficient for the 14-3-3 association with PKCμ. Depending on which Ser residue is phosphorylated, these motifs may be analogous to the RSxpSxP motif. On the other hand, a well-defined 14-3-3 binding site in keratin 18 appears to be novel (57). It is similar to the Cbl-like motif, but only S33 is required for 14-3-3 binding (Table 1). Another atypical phosphoserine epitope can be seen in the tumor suppressor p53. This is an interesting example because double phosphorylation in the 14-3-3 binding motif inhibits 14-3-3 association (58). Dephosphorylation of pS376 of p53 generates a functional motif at pS378 for 14-3-3 association (Table 1). In general, the necessity of phosphorylation for 14-3-3–ligand interaction permits control of these binding events by intracellular kinase/phosphatase signaling networks. The example provided by p53 should serve notice that this control can be a complex process.

Binding of Unphosphorylated Ligands   It is clear that 14-3-3 primarily binds phosphorylated ligands. However, several observations have led to the notion that 14-3-3 is also capable of interacting with unphosphorylated ligands. For example, Raf-1 contains a third 14-3-3 binding site, the cysteine-rich domain (CRD) (residues 139–184) (48, 59). The CRD can directly bind 14-3-3 in vitro, although it is uncertain how the CRD participates in 14-3-3 binding in intact Raf-1 (60, 61). Other examples of unphosphorylated 14-3-3 ligands include mitochondrial targeting signal sequences (62), the platelet GPIbα (63), the ExoS ADP-ribosyl-transferase (12, 64), and 5-phosphatase (25). The interactions of 14-3-3 with unphosphorylated ligands are of high affinity, similar to those with phosphorylated proteins. Indeed, there are structural homologies between the two classes of ligands in some cases, such as 5-phosphatase, which displays an RSxSxP-like motif, RSESEE (25). However, unlike typical phosphoserine motifs, where phosphorylation is required for high-affinity binding, a nonphosphorylated 13-mer peptide containing the RSESEE motif interacts with 14-3-3 with a K_d of 92 nM (25). It is likely that the necessity of phosphorylation is overcome by the presence of multiple negatively charged Glu residues. In support of this notion, random selection of 14-3-3 binding peptides using phage display libraries has resulted in the isolation of several sequences with RSx_{1-3} E-like motifs (65). Because the interaction of 14-3-3 with unphosphorylated ligands can be inhibited by phosphoserine containing peptides (64), it is likely that both types of ligands employ a similar ligand binding site on 14-3-3.

Structural Basis

The 14-3-3 Monomer Contains a Conserved Amphipathic Groove   The drive to comprehend the molecular mechanisms by which 14-3-3 interacts with its ligands led to the solution of the crystal structures of 14-3-3ζ (66) and 14-3-3τ (67), revealing strikingly similar dimeric structures. Each monomer consists of a bundle of nine α-helices organized in an antiparallel fashion [Figure 1a (see color insert)]. The molecule has a cup-like shape with a highly conserved, inner, concave surface and a variable outer surface. A striking feature of the concave surface is an amphipathic groove in each monomer [Figure 1b (see color insert)]. As revealed from the ζ structure (66), on one side of the groove, helices 3 and 5 present a cluster of charged and polar residues. On the other side of the groove, helices 7 and 9 present a patch of hydrophobic residues. It is interesting to note that these residues lining the concave surface of the groove are mostly conserved among different isoforms of the 14-3-3 family (50, 66, 67, 71). Because many 14-3-3 ligands bind well to all isoforms, it was thought that this conserved amphipathic groove could mediate the binding of 14-3-3 to its target proteins (66). It was further postulated that a basic cluster in the groove, consisting of K49, R56, and R127, may mediate the interaction of 14-3-3 with the phosphoamino acid in its ligands. This model has been unequivocally confirmed by both mutational analysis (68–70) and co-crystallization studies (50, 51, 71).

14-3-3ζ has been co-crystallized in complex with several peptide ligands, providing critical insights into the structural details of 14-3-3–ligand interactions (50, 51, 71). In the complexes, both phosphorylated and unphosphorylated 14-3-3 binding peptides lie in the conserved amphipathic groove [Figure 1c,e (see color insert)]. Instead of the α-helical structure originally proposed, 14-3-3 binding peptides adopt an extended conformation. These extended structures may have fewer steric constraints and greater conformational flexibility to sample different residues in the groove for optimal association. This gives 14-3-3 great versatility in the recognition of a diverse range of ligand sequences.

The high-resolution model of 14-3-3ζ in complex with a mode 1 phosphoserine peptide derived from MT (MA*RSH*p*SYP*AKK) provides a structural explanation for the 14-3-3–phosphoserine motif interaction (50, 51). The phosphoserine contacts 14-3-3 by salt bridges to the side chains of K49, R56, and R127 in the basic cluster and a hydrogen bond to the hydroxyl group of Y128 (Figure 1*e*). In support of this interpretation, charge-reversal mutations K49E, R56E, and R127E drastically disrupt the interaction of 14-3-3ζ with Raf-1 and Bcr (68, 70; H Wang & H Fu, unpublished data). K120 in the charged face of the groove, together with N173 and N224, stabilize an extended ligand conformation by contacting backbone groups of the +1 and –1 residues, which may be important for positioning the phosphoserine to interact with the basic cluster of 14-3-3. All of these interactions were similar for a synthetic peptide based on the mode 2 binding motif (51), which suggests that diverse ligands use the basic cluster and its accessory residues to bind to 14-3-3. Outside of this cluster, there is considerable variability in 14-3-3–ligand connections, as assessed by comparison of the MT co-crystal structure with that of the mode 2 peptide. For example, E180 forms a hydrogen bond with the –2 Ser in the MT peptide but bonds with the –4 Arg in the mode 2 peptide (51). Similarly, several hydrophobic residues, including L172, L216, I217, and L220, are consistently involved in binding, but they interact with different parts of the two ligands. This type of flexible interaction may explain the diversity among 14-3-3 binding sequences from various ligands.

The conserved ligand binding groove is also involved in binding unphosphorylated ligands, such as R18 (Figure 1*c,e*). R18 is a peptide selected from a phage display library for its high affinity for 14-3-3 proteins (65). In the 14-3-3ζ–R18 complex, R18 assumes an extended conformation in the amphipathic groove, similar to phosphorylated peptides (71). Its core WLDLE sequence is located in the phosphoserine binding site with its two acidic residues, Asp and Glu, next to the basic cluster of 14-3-3. Two Leu of R18 interact with amino acids on the hydrophobic side of the 14-3-3 groove, including L172 and L220. Thus, R18 assumes a true amphipathic structure.

It has been reported that C-terminal fragments of 14-3-3 are capable of ligand binding (33, 72, 73). For example, the "box-1" region, which spans residues 171–213 of 14-3-3η, efficiently binds tryptophan hydroxylase, Raf-1, and Bcr (72, 74). Although several hydrophobic and polar residues that contribute to the ligand binding groove of 14-3-3 are located in these regions, the exact nature of the stable interaction of these regions with different proteins remains to be clarified.

The 14-3-3 Dimer Can Simultaneously Bind Two Ligands   As seen in the various crystal structures, the N-terminal portion of 14-3-3 is involved in dimer formation (Figure 1) (66, 67). The dimer interface is formed by the packing of helix α1 from one monomer against α3 and α4 from the other, leaving a 6- to 8-Å hole in the center. Several hydrophobic and polar residues are buried in the dimer interface, including L12, A16, V62, I65, and Y82. These residues are largely conserved among mammalian 14-3-3 isoforms, which raises the possibility that 14-3-3 proteins can form heterodimers between different isoforms (75).

The dimeric structure of the 14-3-3 protein allows it to bind two ligands simultaneously (Figure 1c,d). In the co-crystal structures of 14-3-3 with peptides, the ligand binding sites are located within the same concave surface, and each site is occupied (50, 71). The dimer is arranged such that the ligand binding groove runs in opposite directions in each monomer of the molecule (Figure 1d). Simultaneous binding of a 14-3-3 dimer to two protein ligands would have significant implications. In this regard, it is interesting to note that many 14-3-3 ligands, such as Raf-1 and Cbl, have multiple recognition motifs (Table 1). Dual recognition by 14-3-3 of two weakly interacting motifs, such as those found in Cbl, may promote a more stable interaction. In contrast, 14-3-3 may bind to two high-affinity sites, such as those found in Raf-1, perhaps to promote a regulatory conformational change in Raf-1. Alternatively, 14-3-3 may bring together two different signaling molecules to modulate each other's activity. Some evidence has been provided that 14-3-3 can mediate the association of Raf-1 with Bcr (76) or A20 (41), but the physiological significance of these complexes is unclear. It is plausible that this adaptor function of 14-3-3 exists only for specific ligand pairs. Yet another possible role for dimerization of 14-3-3 is in subcellular localization. For example, one monomer could function as a targeting unit by binding an anchored ligand while the other binds a cargo protein. Depending on the site of the anchored ligand, 14-3-3 may localize the cargo protein to distinct intracelluar compartments. The recently reported binding of 14-3-3 to CRM1 may serve such a purpose (51).

Although the exact function of 14-3-3 dimerization is not clear, the importance of this phenomenon is supported by data showing that several ligand binding–defective mutants of 14-3-3 act as dominant negative inhibitors in vivo (70, 77–79). The dimeric nature of 14-3-3 may hold the key to many critical roles of 14-3-3 in cells.

REGULATION OF INTRACELLULAR SIGNALING BY 14-3-3

By interacting with various regulatory proteins, 14-3-3 participates in diverse signal transduction pathways. Although the role of 14-3-3 in many cases remains elusive, some insights have been gained from recent investigations involving three 14-3-3 ligands, Raf-1, Bad, and Cdc25.

Raf-1–Mediated Signal Transduction

Raf-1 is a Ser/Thr kinase that plays a pivotal role in the signal transduction pathway induced by growth factors (80, 81, and references therein). On activation, the small GTP binding protein Ras interacts directly with Raf-1 and recruits

Raf-1 to the plasma membrane. There, Raf-1 is activated by a poorly understood mechanism. Raf-1 then phosphorylates the kinase MEK, leading to stimulation of the mitogen-activated protein kinases, and ultimately to transcription of genes involved in cell division. How Raf-1 is activated is a question of central importance in the field of signal transduction. The identification of 14-3-3 as a Raf-1 binding protein added a new element to the regulatory machinery of Raf-1. Genetic analysis in yeast and *Drosophila* has now convincingly demonstrated a critical regulatory role of 14-3-3 in the Ras-Raf signaling pathway (2, 77, 82–84). Taken together, the available data support a dual role for 14-3-3 in Raf-1 activation: 14-3-3 maintains Raf-1 in an inactive state in the absence of activation signals but promotes Raf-1 activation and stabilizes its active conformation when such signals are received (48, 59, 81). This complex behavior may be explained in part by the existence of three regulated 14-3-3 interaction sites on Raf-1.

Raf-1 can be separated into two functional domains, an N-terminal inhibitory fragment and a C-terminal catalytic fragment (Figure 2). The N-terminal portion contains RBD (a Ras binding domain); CRD (a cysteine-rich domain), which can also bind Ras; and the phosphoserine-259 site for 14-3-3 interaction. Raf-CRD can bind 14-3-3 in addition to Ras and phosphatidylserine (85). The third site for

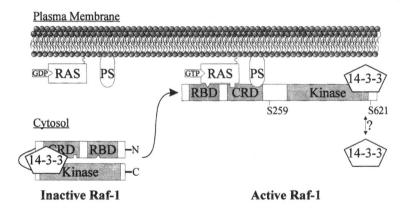

Figure 2 Dual role model of 14-3-3 in Raf-1 activation. In quiescent cells, 14-3-3 may function to keep Raf-1 in an inactive state by binding to pS259 and the cysteine-rich domain (CRD) (81, 85). pS621 may also be associated with 14-3-3. This 14-3-3-bound conformation of Raf-1 is inactive, but permissive for activation. In response to mitogenic signals, GTP-Ras associates with the Ras binding domain (RBD) and recruits Raf-1 to the plasma membrane. This event may lead to the contact of phosphatidylserine (PS) with the CRD and displacement of 14-3-3 from the CRD and pS259 sites of Raf-1. Removal of the inhibitory effect of 14-3-3 partially activates Raf-1, which can be further stimulated by other mechanisms. During activation, 14-3-3 may bind the pS621 site, maintaining its active conformation. An alternative model (90) is that on Ras binding, 14-3-3 is completely displaced from Raf-1. 14-3-3 is required for generating a Raf-1 conformation that is competent for activation, but it is no longer needed after Raf-1 is activated at the membrane.

14-3-3 binding, pS621, is located C-terminal to the kinase domain. Binding of 14-3-3 to CRD and pS259 sites in the N-terminal domain may negatively regulate Raf-1 function. (*a*) Mutations in Raf-1 that block the interaction of 14-3-3 with S259 stimulate Raf-1 kinase activity (48), potentiate mitogenic signal-induced Raf-1 activation (86), and activate Raf-mediated biological functions (48, 87). (*b*) Mutations in Raf-CRD that selectively decrease 14-3-3 binding enhance Raf-1 function (48, 59, 60). (*c*) 14-3-3 is displaced from the N-terminal domain by activated Ras, implying a requirement of 14-3-3 dissociation for Raf-1 activation (87, 88). These observations are the basis for the model that 14-3-3 is required to maintain an inactive conformation of Raf-1.

In contrast to the pS259 and CRD sites, the interaction of 14-3-3 with Raf-1 at the pS621 site may be required for Raf-1 activation (52, 70, 86). Tzivion et al (86) used a phosphoserine peptide to strip 14-3-3 away from epidermal growth factor–activated Raf-1 in vitro. Removing 14-3-3 from the Raf-1 complex leads to its inactivation, which suggests a strict requirement of 14-3-3 for Raf-1 activity. It is important to note that addition of recombinant 14-3-3ζ protein to the phosphopeptide-treated Raf-1 preparations significantly reactivates Raf-1. Thus, 14-3-3 may function as an essential cofactor for Raf-1 kinase activity (86). This conclusion was independently reached by Thorson et al (70) using a constitutively active, C-terminal fragment of Raf-1, CT-Raf. CT-Raf contains only one 14-3-3 binding site, pS621. They found that displacement of 14-3-3 from the CT-Raf complex with the detergent Empigen-BB reversibly abolishes CT-Raf kinase activity. These experiments suggest a requirement for the continuous presence of 14-3-3 for Raf-1 activity. Thorson et al (70) also postulate that 14-3-3 may be necessary for maintaining the phosphorylation state of S621 in vivo. This is consistent with an earlier demonstration that 14-3-3 protects Raf-1 from phosphatase treatment in vitro (89). These results together suggest that S621 is a site for positive regulation by phosphorylation and 14-3-3 binding.

A requirement of 14-3-3 for Raf-1 kinase activity is challenged by other reports (48, 61, 90). Subcellular fractionation studies show that 14-3-3 is bound to inactive Raf-1 in the cytosol but is totally displaced when Raf-1 is recruited to the plasma membrane, which suggests that activated Raf-1 does not bind 14-3-3 (90). This is consistent with the ability to isolate 14-3-3–Raf-1 complexes from extracts of quiescent, but not mitogen-stimulated, NIH 3T3 cells (34). However, such data do not preclude a positive role of 14-3-3 in Raf-1 activation. Roy et al (90) found that 14-3-3 potentiates the kinase activity of membrane-recruited Raf-1, even though such membrane-localized Raf-1 is not bound to 14-3-3. It is possible that 14-3-3 is required for Raf-1 recruitment to the plasma membrane and for inducing a conformation of Raf-1 competent for activation (90).

A major discrepancy has emerged from recent reports, concerning whether 14-3-3 must be continuously associated with Raf-1 for its catalytic activity. The different results reported may reflect the complexity of this biological system as well as experimental limitations to the faithful recapitulation in vitro of the activation mechanism of Raf-1. A critical examination of the phosphorylation status

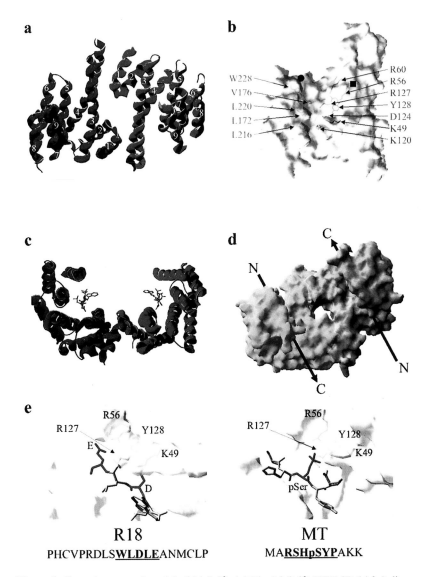

a

b

W228
V176
L220
L172
L216

R60
R56
R127
Y128
D124
K49
K120

c

d

C

N

N

C

e

R127
R56
Y128
E
K49
D

R18

PHCVPRDLS**WLDLE**ANMCLP

R127
R56
Y128
K49
pSer

MT

MA**RSHpSYP**AKK

Figure 1 Crystal structural model of 14-3-3ζ. (*a*) The 14-3-3ζ (PDB ID 1A3o) dimer. Each monomer (*red* or *blue*) is composed of nine α-helices (*numbered*). (*b*) A surface representation of a 14-3-3ζ monomer. Selected hydrophobic (*green*), acidic (*red*), and basic (*blue*) residues are displayed to illustrate the amphipathic nature of the groove. Phosphorylation sites are marked (S58, *square*; S184, *circle*). (*c*) 14-3-3ζ crystallized with R18 (PDB ID 1A38), rotated 90° relative to (*a*). This peptide is localized in the amphipathic groove of 14-3-3. In this view, its position is indistinguishable from that of phosphoserine peptides. (d) Solvent accessible surface of 14-3-3ζ with bound peptides (*represented by arrows*). Dimerization forces bound ligands to adopt opposite orientations. (*Continued on next page.*)

(e) Surface representation of 14-3-3ζ crystallized with R18 or a phosphopeptide derived from middle tumor antigen (MT) (PDB ID 14PS). The peptide sequences are listed and a segment is visible in the crystal structure (*bold underline*). R18 and MT occupy similar positions in the 14-3-3 groove, and the two acidic residues of R18 (*red*) act in a homologous fashion as the phosphoserine of MT to contact the basic cluster. This figure was created using Swiss-PdbViewer 3.5β4 (149), POV-Ray 3.1, and Corel Draw 8.

of Raf-1 at S259 and S621 under different activation states will be essential for resolving the conflicting data, by clarifying which sites 14-3-3 binds in each state.

The dual role model of 14-3-3 in Raf-1 activation remains an attractive choice because this model explains most of the data in the literature (Figure 2) (48, 59, 81). 14-3-3 plays a negative role because it needs to be displaced at least from the N-terminal regulatory domain during Raf-1 activation. In a positive role, 14-3-3 may function as an allosteric cofactor to induce and maintain a conformation of Raf-1 competent for activation or required for activity. It is also possible that 14-3-3 may promote Raf-1 function through efficient coupling of Raf-1 to its downstream effectors. It is clear that more research must be done to clarify the detailed mechanism of how 14-3-3 regulates Raf-1 activation.

Bad and Cell Death Pathways

Apoptosis is a process of cell death that plays a critical role in normal development as well as in the pathophysiology of a variety of diseases, such as cancer (reviewed in 91). It is tightly regulated, and a pivotal component of this regulation is the Bcl-2 family of pro- and antiapoptotic proteins. 14-3-3 has been found to interact with a proapoptotic member of the Bcl-2 family, Bad, in a phosphoserine-dependent manner (40). 14-3-3 binding antagonizes the proapoptotic activity of Bad, providing a novel signal integration point for control of cell death.

Bad, like other Bcl-2 homologs, is capable of dimerizing with some of its family members, and it was discovered in a search for Bcl-2 binding proteins (92). The importance of Bad as a mediator of cell death has since become well established for several reasons. It is broadly expressed in human tissues (93), and its levels are dynamically regulated by apoptotic stimuli (94). Forced expression of Bad in the T cells of Bad transgenic mice leads to a dramatic reduction in the T cell population (94). Bad causes cell death by binding to and inhibiting the antiapoptotic effects of $Bcl-X_L$ and Bcl-2 (92, 94, 95, 107, 108). 14-3-3 is involved in preventing the interaction of Bad with $Bcl-X_L$ and Bcl-2 and, thus, Bad-induced cell death (40). Put briefly, when the binding of 14-3-3 to Bad is induced by phosphorylation, Bad is complexed with 14-3-3 in the cytosol, seques-tered from mitochondrially localized $Bcl-X_L$/Bcl-2 and unable to induce apoptosis (Figure 3a). In this way, Bad is under the strict control of survival and death signal–driven kinases and phosphatases (40, 96–99).

Sequence analysis of murine Bad reveals two potential 14-3-3 phosphoserine motifs, $RHSpS^{112}YP$ and $RSRpS^{136}AP$. It was suggestive when mapping of the in vivo phosphorylation sites of Bad showed only two residues: S112 and S136 (40). That S136 of Bad has an important role in 14-3-3 binding has been sub-stantiated, whereas the role of S112 remains uncertain (40, 99, 100; H Yang, SC Masters & H Fu, unpublished results). The issue of which sites mediate 14-3-3–Bad complex formation is important because the phosphorylation of S112 and S136 is regulated by different signaling pathways.

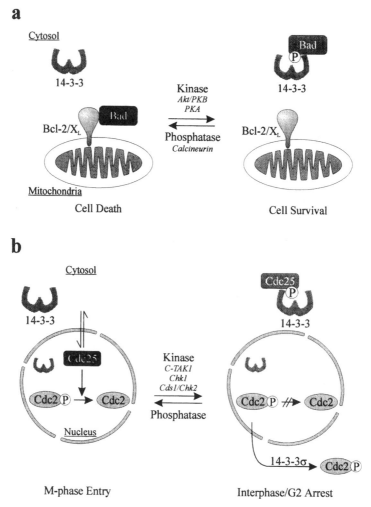

Figure 3 Parallel models for 14-3-3 effects on Bad and Cdc25. (*a*) 14-3-3 sequesters Bad from mitochondrial Bcl-X$_L$/Bcl-2. In its default state, Bad binds Bcl-X$_L$/Bcl-2 in the mitochondria, favoring the induction of apoptosis. Survival signals stimulate kinases, such as Akt/protein kinase B (PKB), leading to phosphorylation of Bad. Phosphorylated Bad is found in the cytosol bound to 14-3-3, where it is unable to induce death. Phosphatases such as calcineurin reverse this process. (*b*) 14-3-3 retains Cdc25 in the cytosol. During interphase or in response to DNA damage, Cdc25 can be phosphorylated by several kinases to create a 14-3-3 binding site. 14-3-3–bound Cdc25 is found in the cytosol where it cannot act on Cdc2, thus preventing mitosis. An unknown phosphatase is presumably involved in disrupting the Cdc25–14-3-3 interaction when mitosis is to be initiated. By an unknown mechanism, 14-3-3σ may sequester the Cdc2/cyclin B1 complex in the cytosol on DNA damage (110, 122a). PKA, Protein kinase A.

At least four kinases are capable of phosphorylating Bad in vitro, including protein kinase A (PKA) (40, 98), Akt/protein kinase B (96, 99), PKC (40), and Raf-1 (40, 101). However, of these, only PKA and Akt phosphorylate Bad at the S112 or S136 sites relevant to 14-3-3 interaction. Akt is a Ser/Thr kinase that is broadly involved in cell survival and differentiation signaling (reviewed in 102). It is located in a pathway downstream of phosphatidylinositol 3'-kinase and thus is activated in response to a multitude of prosurvival signals, including IGF-I, interleukin-3, and nerve growth factor. Akt signaling can also be stimulated in other ways, such as via Ca^{2+}/calmodulin-dependent protein kinase kinase (103). In any case, active Akt leads to the phosphorylation of S136 of Bad, to association of 14-3-3 with Bad, and to inhibition of Bad-induced cell death (99; SC Masters, SR Datta, ME Greenberg & H Fu, unpublished data). Phosphorylation of Bad by Akt at S136 directly links a general survival signaling pathway to a death promoter, one way that survival factors can inhibit cell death. The Akt effect on Bad may be cell-type specific, as several reports have raised questions regarding the relative importance of Akt as a Bad S136 kinase (98, 104–106). Bad S112 is phosphorylated by the mitochondrially localized pool of PKA (98). Phosphorylation of S112 by PKA appears to inhibit Bad proapoptotic activity. Whether or not the PKA/Bad system involves 14-3-3 awaits further testing.

Bad is the target for both anti- and proapoptotic signals. It can be dephosphorylated at S112 and S136 by the phosphatase calcineurin in response to Ca^{2+} influx (97). This dephosphorylation has been correlated with the dissociation of 14-3-3 from Bad, mitochondrial localization of Bad, and enhanced apoptotic cell death. Calcineurin completes a reversible regulatory system for Bad, and it emphasizes the importance of removing 14-3-3 for Bad proapoptotic activity. This work also highlights the necessity of determining the inactivating phosphatases for other 14-3-3 ligands.

Bad is thought to induce apoptosis by binding and inactivating $Bcl-X_L$/Bcl-2 (92, 107, 108). Thus, active, death-inducing Bad is found localized to the mitochondria. Because 14-3-3–bound, inactive Bad is found in the cytosol, it was proposed that 14-3-3 acts to sequester Bad away from its death effectors (Figure 3a) (40). Specific kinases and phosphatases thus dynamically regulate the phosphorylation of and 14-3-3 binding to Bad, which determines its proapoptotic function. Several other possible mechanisms can be devised. For example, phosphorylated Bad may be inactive, and binding of 14-3-3 could serve to protect Bad from the action of phosphatases, such as calcineurin (97). Alternately, 14-3-3 may block the $Bcl-X_L$/Bcl-2 interaction site on Bad, forcefully separating Bad from its effectors rather than stabilizing the cytosolic localization of free Bad protein. It should be noted that these mechanisms are not mutually exclusive. Dissecting the role of 14-3-3 in Bad-induced apoptosis may provide a model system for 14-3-3–ligand interactions in general.

Bad is not the only 14-3-3 ligand involved in apoptosis. Indeed, a large fraction of the known 14-3-3 binding proteins can directly or indirectly modulate cell-death pathways. For example, apoptosis signal-regulating kinase 1 (ASK1) is a component of multiple death signaling pathways, including those activated by tumor necrosis factor α, Fas, and oxidative stress (109). 14-3-3 binding to ASK1 can suppress its proapoptotic activity, and an ASK1 mutant that cannot bind 14-3-3 has dramatically enhanced ability to kill (78). Besides Bad, Akt has several other substrates that are involved in apoptosis, and 14-3-3 also targets some of these, such as the Forkhead transcription factor FKHRL1 (54). When phosphorylated by Akt, FKHRL1 becomes a 14-3-3 ligand and is no longer able to induce cell death. A few of the other 14-3-3 ligands that are involved in the cell death or survival process include MEKK1 (19), A20 (41), IGFIR (28, 29), phosphatidylinositol 3'-kinase (36), and Raf-1 (101). The hypothesis that 14-3-3 plays a key role in the regulation of cell fate determination is strongly supported by this large list of ligands. It is possible that 14-3-3 serves as a general survival factor by enhancing prosurvival signaling while suppressing proapoptotic pathways.

Cdc25 and Cell Cycle Control

The requirement of Rad24 and Rad25 for G2-checkpoint control in *S. pombe* links 14-3-3 to the cell cycle machinery (43). Genetic and biochemical studies in yeast, frog, and human cells have now defined a specific 14-3-3 role in cell cycle control. Mounting evidence has indicated that one major effector of 14-3-3 in this system is the phosphatase Cdc25.

Cdc25 is a major cell cycle regulator that dephosphorylates and activates the protein kinase Cdc2 to trigger entry into mitosis (reviewed in 111). Inhibition of Cdc2 dephosphorylation is pivotal for blocking mitosis in response to damaged or unreplicated DNA. Thus it is not surprising that Cdc25, a key activator of Cdc2, is highly regulated. During interphase, human Cdc25C is predominantly phosphorylated at S216 (53). Conversely, this site is not phosphorylated during mitosis, which suggests that phosphorylation of S216 negatively regulates Cdc25C function. Peng et al (53) have found that phosphorylation of S216 generates a 14-3-3 binding motif (Table 1) and leads to Cdc25–14-3-3 association. As expected, substitution of S216 with Ala abrogates the Cdc25C–14-3-3 interaction. 14-3-3 may be required to maintain an inactive state of Cdc25 because expression of S216A Cdc25 accelerates mitotic entry and allows cells to escape the G2-checkpoint arrest induced by DNA damage signals (53). An analogous mechanism may operate in *Xenopus* oocytes (112, 113) and in fission yeast (114, 115, 115a). Thus, it is conceivable that the regulation of Cdc25–14-3-3 complex formation is a critical, conserved part of the cell cycle machinery. However, 14-3-3 binding does not affect the catalytic activity of Cdc25 (37, 53), which suggests that 14-3-3 plays an indirect role in the inhibition of Cdc25 function.

The mitosis-inducing function of Cdc25 requires its entry into the nucleus where its substrate Cdc2 is located. Notably, Cdc25 contains a putative bipartite nuclear localization sequence near S216 (116) as well as a nuclear export sequence (NES) (113, 117). It is possible that 14-3-3 binding regulates the shuttling of Cdc25 between the cytosol and nucleus (Figure 3b). Recent data support this hypothesis. Elimination of a 14-3-3 homologue, Rad24, in *S. pombe* causes nuclear accumulation of Cdc25 (115). Expression of 14-3-3ε in a *Xenopus* tissue culture system causes the localization of Cdc25 in the cytosol whereas a mutant Cdc25 that cannot bind 14-3-3 is exclusively nuclear (117). Similarly, human Cdc25C is retained in the cytoplasm during interphase, under the control of 14-3-3 (118). Thus, 14-3-3 binding correlates well with cytoplasmic localization of Cdc25 (Figure 3*b*). To explain the role of 14-3-3 in Cdc25 localization, two alternative models have been proposed. Lopez-Girona et al (115) suggested that 14-3-3 is actively excluded from the nucleus. Mutations in a putative NES in Rad24, equivalent to residues I217 and L221 in helix 9 of 14-3-3ζ, impair nuclear export of Rad24 as well as the DNA damage-induced nuclear depletion of Cdc25. Thus, Rad24 may function as "an attachable nuclear export signal" that promotes the nuclear export of associated Cdc25 (115). In support of the NES model, Rittinger et al (51) report the interaction of 14-3-3ζ with CRM1, a component of the nuclear export machinery, in vitro and suggest that hydrophobic residues in helix 9 of 14-3-3ζ play a role in both ligand binding and nuclear export. Another possible explanation is that mutations in the putative NES sequence of Rad24 disrupted the 14-3-3 interaction with Cdc25, rendering 14-3-3 inactive (69, 115a, 117). Examination in the *Xenopus* system suggests an alternative model: 14-3-3 inhibits Cdc25 function primarily by attenuating its nuclear import, in part through blockage of the Cdc25-importin α interaction (113, 117). In contrast to fission yeast, 14-3-3 binding is neither necessary nor sufficient for Cdc25 nuclear export in *Xenopus*. However, the above models may not be mutually exclusive because 14-3-3 may cooperate with the NES and nuclear localization sequence of Cdc25 in controlling the dynamic shuttling of Cdc25.

The Cdc25–14-3-3 interaction is regulated by specific phosphorylation in response to cellular signals. Several kinases that phosphorylate S216 of Cdc25C have been described, including C-TAK1 (119), Chk1 (53, 120, 121, 121a), and Cds1/Chk2 (121a, 150). Chk1 is activated in response to DNA damage (122). Both Chk1 and Cds1/Chk2 are found in the nucleus and may induce Cdc25 phosphorylation and 14-3-3 binding in response to activation signals, such as DNA damage. Therefore, these kinases can indirectly act to localize Cdc25 in the cytoplasm, preventing entry into mitosis.

Another major event during mitotic entry is the accumulation of activated Cdc2 in the nucleus. In addition to its importance in the control of Cdc25, 14-3-3 may play a critical role in Cdc2 localization (110, 122a). Following DNA damage signals, 14-3-3σ is dramatically up-regulated by a p53-dependent mechanism (125). The induction of 14-3-3σ appears to enhance the cytoplasmic localization of Cdc2, thus preventing Cdc2 from entering the nucleus and initiating mitosis (122a). 14-3-3σ–deficient cells exhibited nuclear localization of Cdc2 and failed to maintain G2 arrest on DNA damage. Thus, using analogous mechanisms, 14-3-3 isoforms may ensure DNA damage-induced cell cycle arrest by simultaneously sequestering Cdc25 and Cdc2 in the cytoplasm.

14-3-3 has been found to interact with other proteins involved in the control of the cell cycle, such as Chk1 (123), Wee1 (122a, 124), and p53 (58). Interaction of 14-3-3 with multiple cell cycle regulators suggests that 14-3-3 may help coordinate cell cycle progression.

REGULATION OF 14-3-3

The interaction of 14-3-3 with its ligands is under tight control. Besides phosphorylation of target proteins, the status of 14-3-3 itself is also a critical determinant of this control. Mechanisms that regulate 14-3-3 may include isoform specificity, posttranslational modifications, and expression levels in cells.

The presence of seven 14-3-3 isoforms in mammalian cells suggests a possible role for isoform-specific interactions with different targets. However, structural studies have not supported this conclusion. The key residues of 14-3-3 involved in ligand binding are conserved among different isoforms (50, 51, 66, 71), which suggests a lack of isoform selectivity for ligands that dock in this binding groove (i.e. most 14-3-3 ligands). In support of this notion, different 14-3-3 isoforms bind phosphoserine peptides with similar affinities and select similar phosphoserine motifs from oriented peptide libraries (49, 50). Also, distinct 14-3-3 isoforms interact equally well with the intact proteins Raf-1, Bad, and ExoS (13, 51; RR Subramanian & H Fu, unpublished data). On the other hand, it is possible that variable residues in and near the ligand binding groove of 14-3-3 may contribute to certain ligand preferences. The selective interaction of A20 with 14-3-3η suggests that 14-3-3 isoforms may bind differentially to some ligands (41). Among the mammalian isoforms, 14-3-3σ has been shown to bind the least well to p130^{Cas} and B-Raf in vitro (18, 51). Further, 14-3-3σ is capable of inducing an isoform-specific biological effect. Overexpression of 14-3-3σ caused a G2 cell cycle arrest in human colorectal cancer cells, whereas 14-3-3β expression did not (125). The 14-3-3σ effect may be a consequence of its preferential interaction with the Cdc2/cyclin B1 complex (122a). One difficulty in assessing isoform specificity is the lack of knowledge of how dramatic a difference in affinity is necessary to create a biologically relevant effect. Thus, the small differences between isoforms observed in vitro may indeed be biologically relevant.

It seems most likely that isoform-specific cellular effects are determined by different posttranslational modifications of 14-3-3 isoforms and by isoform-specific 14-3-3 levels in various subcellular compartments. One intriguing possibility is that 14-3-3 isoforms interact in vivo to form heterodimers. Such molecules would amplify dramatically the implications of any isoform specificity, either intrinsic or due to external regulation.

Phosphorylation of 14-3-3 appears to modulate the function of 14-3-3 isoforms. Three phosphorylation sites have been determined in 14-3-3ζ: S58 (126), S184 (10), and T232 (127). S184 lies within a proline-directed kinase consensus sequence, S^{184}PEK, and is phosphorylated in 14-3-3ζ as well as in β in brain tissues. Such phosphorylation gives rise to the species initially designated as the δ and α isoforms, respectively (10). In the crystal structure of ζ, S184 is a surface residue located at the N terminus of helix 8, near the top of the ligand binding groove (Figure 1*b*) (66). This position implies a possible role of phosphorylation in regulating ligand binding. Consistent with this idea, the phosphorylated forms of β and ζ show increased potency in the inhibition of PKC in vitro (128). The kinase that phosphorylates S184 has not been identified (127). 14-3-3ζ, but not 14-3-3β, is also phosphorylated at T232 in HEK293 cells (127). T232 resides in the C-terminal loop of 14-3-3, which has been implicated in regulating ligand binding (66). In fact, 14-3-3ζ phosphorylated at T232 is devoid of Raf-1 association, which suggests that this modification negatively affects ligand binding (127). Dubois et al (127) have identified casein kinase Iα as a T232 kinase. Among mammalian isoforms, only 14-3-3τ and 14-3-3ζ have a phosphorylation site at the corresponding 232 position, and casein kinase Iα can indeed phosphorylate S232 of 14-3-3τ in vitro. Thus, 14-3-3ζ– and 14-3-3τ–induced ligand interactions may in part be controlled by casein kinase Iα activity. The third site, S58 of 14-3-3ζ, is phosphorylated by sphingosine-dependent protein kinase 1 (SDK1) (126, 129). SDK1 phosphorylates 14-3-3ζ as well as 14-3-3β (S60) and 14-3-3η (S59), but not 14-3-3τ or 14-3-3σ. This phosphorylation is stimulated in response to sphingosine, which is generated after treatment of cells with mitogens such as platelet-derived growth factor and IGF-I (130). S58 is facing away from the ligand binding groove, buried in the dimer interface (Figure 1*b*). Such positioning implies a potential role of S58 phosphorylation in dimer formation or dissociation. Because dimerization of 14-3-3 is thought to be important for its function, modulation of 14-3-3 dimerization by SDK1 may be a key target of sphingosine in cells. In addition to Ser/Thr phosphorylation, 14-3-3 isoforms can be phosphorylated on tyrosine residues, for example by Bcr-Abl (35) and by IGFIR (29).

The interaction of 14-3-3 with ligands can be influenced not only by its modification but also by fluctuation of 14-3-3 levels in cells. It appears that the amount of 14-3-3, or at least of specific isoforms, is limiting in cells despite the relative abundance of 14-3-3. For instance, overexpression of 14-3-3 isoforms enhances the specific activity of Raf-1 in HeLa and COS cells (70, 90) and inhibits PKC activity in Jurkat T cells (56, 131). One role of the multiple isoforms of 14-3-3 may be to allow regulation of the total 14-3-3 pool via unique transcriptional controls for each isoform. Thus, regulation of 14-3-3 expression can serve as an effective mechanism for controlling 14-3-3 functions. In human colorectal cancer cells, 14-3-3σ is dramatically induced by DNA damaging agents in a p53-dependent manner, leading to G2 arrest (125). 14-3-3γ is induced by serum and platelet-derived growth factor in vascular smooth muscle cells (132) whereas 14-3-3ε is down-regulated during differentiation of mesenchyme cells (133). The dynamic expression patterns of various 14-3-3 isoforms during mouse embryogenesis and neuronal development underscore the importance of each 14-3-3 in mediating cellular processes (133, 134). Perhaps the temporal and spatial expression patterns of 14-3-3 isoforms control the interaction of 14-3-3 with its specific effectors, enabling the activation or suppression of particular signaling pathways.

14-3-3 AND DISEASES

Although 14-3-3 has not been directly linked to a specific disease, it has been implicated in a variety of pathological processes. A large number of 14-3-3 ligands are proto-oncogene or oncogene products, which suggests the participation of 14-3-3 in mitogenic signal transduction as well as neoplastic transformation. Indeed, the tumor profile of mice infected with polyomavirus expressing a 14-3-3 binding–defective mutant MT showed a striking deficiency in the induction of salivary gland tumors (135). Another possible connection of 14-3-3 to tumorigenesis is its involvement in regulating cell survival, for example through its interaction with IGFIR. The IGFIR plays an important role in controlling normal cell survival as well as in tumorigenesis (136). The major site for 14-3-3 interaction is located within a Ser quartet critical for IGFIR-mediated cell transformation (28, 29, 137), implying that 14-3-3 participates in this process. Significantly elevated levels of both the IGFIR (138) and 14-3-3 proteins (139) have been detected in all major types of lung cancer. On the other hand, the 14-3-3ε gene is found in a region with frequent loss of heterozygosity in several cancers, which suggests that some 14-3-3 isoforms may be important for suppression of tumorigenesis (140). Taken together, these data argue that 14-3-3 may be involved in the development of human cancer.

The abundance of 14-3-3 proteins in brain tissues points to a critical role of 14-3-3 in neuronal function. There are some indications that 14-3-3 is involved in several neurological disorders. 14-3-3ε is located in a chromosomal region, 17p13.3, that contains genes implicated in isolated lissencephaly sequence (ILS) and Miller-Dieker syndrome (MDS) (141, 142, and references therein). ILS is a brain malformation malady marked by disorganization of the cortical layers. MDS causes malformations similar to those of ILS, as well as additional abnormalities, and is associated with larger deletions of 17p13.3. The 14-3-3ε sequence is deleted in some MDS patients, and this loss may contribute to the development of MDS phenotypes (141). 14-3-3 proteins are also found in the neurofibrillary tangles seen in patients with Alzheimer's disease (143). A possible genetic association of a 14-3-3η polymorphism with early onset schizophrenia has been reported (144). Hsich et al (145) noted that 14-3-3 proteins are specifically detected in cerebrospinal fluid from patients with Creutzfeldt-Jakob disease (CJD) and related transmissible spongiform encephalopathies. This observation has allowed the use of 14-3-3 as a biochemical marker for a premortem diagnostic test for CJD and related diseases (145, 146). It is not known whether 14-3-3 is involved in the pathogenesis of CJD, or whether the presence of 14-3-3 in cerebrospinal fluid is simply the consequence of neuronal cell death in CJD brains.

14-3-3 ANTAGONISTS

Development of 14-3-3 antagonists is important not only for functional analysis of 14-3-3 proteins but also for potential therapeutic interventions against diseases involving 14-3-3 malfunction. Two types of 14-3-3 antagonists have been described, phosphoserine-motif based and nonphosphorylated peptides.

Several phosphoserine-motif–containing peptides have been characterized by kinetic studies and crystallographic analysis. The pS-Raf-259 peptide exhibits high affinity for multiple isoforms of 14-3-3 with K_d values of 120–140 nM (49). This phosphopeptide has been used in a number of systems for probing the function of 14-3-3 association. In particular, it has been extensively used in the establishment of a role of 14-3-3 in Raf-1–mediated functions. This peptide is broadly capable of abolishing 14-3-3–ligand interactions in vitro, including those with ASK1 (78) and the α2 adrenergic receptor i3 loop (147). pS-Raf-259 specifically docks in the conserved amphipathic groove of 14-3-3ζ, which explains the potent inhibitory effect of this peptide on the interaction of 14-3-3 with various ligands. It is expected that the vast majority of phosphopeptides derived from the 14-3-3 binding motifs of natural ligands will be effective 14-3-3 antagonists. Phospho-peptides from insulin receptor substrate-1 and IGFIR can disrupt the interaction of 14-3-3 with these two ligands (28, 39). An interesting enhancement for phos-phopeptide antagonists was described by Yaffe et al (50), where coupling two 14-3-3 binding sequences via a flexible linker led to a ∼30-fold increase in affinity for 14-3-3.

The development of unphosphorylated 14-3-3 antagonists may permit efficient delivery or expression in cells. The R18 peptide is such an antagonist. R18 is one of a set of peptides isolated from phage display libraries (65). This peptide exhib-its a high affinity for many isoforms of 14-3-3 with estimated K_d values of 70–90 nM, similar to those of the 14-3-3 binding phosphopeptides. The binding of R18 to 14-3-3 appears to be specific because R18 recognizes only 14-3-3 proteins in total cell lysates despite the presence of many other proteins. Functionally, the R18 peptide can abolish the association of 14-3-3 with both phosphorylated and unphosphorylated protein ligands, including Raf-1, ASK1, and ExoS (64, 65, 78). The potent inhibitory effect of R18 on 14-3-3–ligand interactions can be explained by the localization of R18 in the conserved amphipathic groove of 14-3-3 (71). Thus, R18 is likely able to block the interaction of 14-3-3 with most or all of its ligands and may serve as a general antagonist of 14-3-3 proteins. Peptides from phosphorylation-independent 14-3-3 ligands, such as the RSESEE-containing sequence of 5-phosphatase (25), may also prove to be effective 14-3-3 antagonists.

CONCLUDING REMARKS

Through protein-protein interactions, 14-3-3 carries out multiple functions. (*a*) In a broad sense, it can act as an allosteric cofactor to modulate the catalytic activity or conformational state of its effectors, such as PKCμ, ExoS, and 5-phosphatase. (*b*) 14-3-3 may function as steric regulator to prevent the interaction of its ligands with other cellular components, leading to altered intracellular localization or complex formation. Disruption of Bad/Bcl-X$_L$ interaction by 14-3-3 could offer such an example. (*c*) The 14-3-3 dimer can simultaneously bind two ligands, which may allow 14-3-3 to operate as an adaptor/scaffold protein to induce protein-protein associations. 14-3-3 has been reported to bring Bcr and Raf-1 together (76). Any of these molecular mechanisms could be used to derive the most notable common effect of 14-3-3 binding: sequestration of effector proteins in the cytosol. 14-3-3 maintains a cytosolic localization of Bad, Cdc25, and inactive Raf-1 to achieve its inhibitory function, although the biochemical details may differ in each case. Given the broad participation of 14-3-3 in diverse physiological processes, dissection of the biochemical mechanisms by which 14-3-3 governs its effector pathways is of central importance for understanding intracellular signal transduction.

14-3-3 may represent a novel class of phosphoserine binding modules, which is reminiscent of the docking of phosphorylated Tyr by SH2 and PTB domains. The presence of a 14-3-3–like tertiary structure in protein phosphatase 5 (148) lends hope that proteins containing a "14-3-3 module" may yet be discovered. Such molecules would expand dramatically the scope of Ser/Thr kinase-regulated events.

The requirement of phosphorylation for 14-3-3 binding subjects 14-3-3–ligand interactions to the control of specific kinases and phosphatases, and thus to specific signaling pathways. Therefore, phosphorylation of a particular 14-3-3 recognition motif on a target protein often serves as a point of cross talk between different pathways. For example, Akt-mediated survival signals and calcineurin-mediated death signals compete to control the phosphorylation of S136 of Bad, and the resulting 14-3-3 inhibition of Bad proapoptotic activity (96, 97, 99). Thus, identifying upstream kinases and phosphatases that modify 14-3-3 recognition sites will be necessary for understanding the dynamic regulation of 14-3-3 actions.

The concept that 14-3-3 lies at points of cross talk between different cell signaling pathways takes on a new life when combined with the knowledge that the amount of 14-3-3 in the cell can be limiting. There is a multitude of 14-3-3 targets in cells that are modified by environmental signals through the actions of kinases and phosphatases. However, it is possible that not all phosphorylated 14-3-3 ligands will be bound, depending on the amount of 14-3-3 present and the relative strength of the signals. Therefore, 14-3-3 could act as a signal integrator, amplifying strong signals and filtering out weaker conflicting ones to achieve a meaningful, coordinated biological output, such as cell death or survival. When other factors such as heterodimerization, subcellular localization, and differential expression of 14-3-3 isoforms are taken into account, it is apparent that this model could produce rich, complex behaviors. As additional proteins and pathways become identified as 14-3-3 targets, a new challenge will emerge, that of determining an integrated model of 14-3-3–mediated signaling.

ACKNOWLEDGMENTS

We thank Drs. Thomas Roberts, Andrey Shaw, Sharon Campbell, Michael Yaffe, Sally Kornbluth, and Richard Kahn for helpful discussions and comments. Work in our laboratory was supported by grants from the NIH (GM53165) and AHA (9950226N). HF is a recipient of the Burroughs Wellcome Fund New Investigator Award and SCM is a predoctoral fellow of the Pharmaceutical Research and Manufacturers of America Foundation.

Visit the Annual Reviews home page at www.AnnualReviews.org.

LITERATURE CITED

1. Moore BW, Perez VJ. 1967. Specific acidic proteins of the nervous system. In *Physiological and Biochemical Aspects of Nervous Integration,* ed. FD Carlson, pp. 343–59. Englewood Cliffs, NJ: Prentice-Hall

2. Skoulakis EM, Davis RL. 1998. 14-3-3 proteins in neuronal development and function. *Mol. Neurobiol.* 16:269–84

3. Aitken A. 1996. 14-3-3 and its possible role in co-ordinating multiple signalling pathways. *Trends Cell Biol.* 6:341–47

4. Morrison D. 1994. 14-3-3: modulators of signaling proteins? *Science* 266:56–57

5. Pawson T, Scott JD. 1997. Signaling through scaffold, anchoring, and adaptor proteins. *Science* 278:2075–80

6. Ferl R. 1996. 14-3-3 proteins and signal transduction. *Annu. Rev. Plant Physiol. Plant Mol. Biol.* 47:49–73

7. Finnie C, Borch J, Collinge DB. 1999. 14-3-3 proteins: eukaryotic regulatory proteins with many functions. *Plant Mol. Biol.* 40:545–54

8. Ichimura T, Isobe T, Okuyama T, Takahashi N, Araki K, et al. 1988. Molecular cloning of cDNA coding for brain-specific 14-3-3 protein, a protein kinase-dependent activator of tyrosine and tryptophan hydroxylases. *Proc. Natl. Acad. Sci. USA* 85:7084–88

9. Martin H, Patel Y, Jones D, Howell S, Robinson K, et al. 1993. Antibodies against the major brain isoforms of 14-3-3 protein: an antibody specific for the N-acetylated amino-terminus of a protein. *FEBS Lett.* 331:296–303

10. Aitken A, Howell S, Jones D, Madrazo J, Patel Y. 1995. 14-3-3 alpha and delta are the phosphorylated forms of Raf-activating 14-3-3 beta and zeta. *J. Biol. Chem.* 270:5706–9

11. Wang W, Shakes DC. 1996. Molecular evolution of the 14-3-3 protein family. *J. Mol. Evol.* 43:384–98

12. Fu H, Coburn J, Collier RJ. 1993. The eukaryotic host factor that activates exoenzyme S of *Pseudomonas aeruginosa* is a member of the 14-3-3 protein family. *Proc. Natl. Acad. Sci. USA* 90:2320–24

13. Zhang L, Wang H, Masters SC, Wang B, Barbieri JT, et al. 1999. Residues of 14-3-3zeta required for activation of exoenzyme S of *Pseudomonas aeruginosa. Biochemistry* 38:12159–64

14. Isobe T, Ichimura T, Sunaya T, Okuyama T, Takahashi N, et al. 1991. Distinct forms of the protein kinase-dependent activator of tyrosine and tryptophan hydroxylases. *J. Mol. Biol.* 217:125–32

15. Boston PF, Jackson P, Thompson RJ. 1982. Human 14-3-3 protein: radioimmunoassay, tissue distribution, and cerebrospinal fluid levels in patients with neurological disorders. *J. Neurochem.* 38:1475–82

16. Celis JE, Gesser B, Rasmussen HH, Madsen P, Leffers H, et al. 1990. Comprehensive two-dimensional gel protein databases offer a global approach to the analysis of human cells: the transformed amnion cells (AMA) master database and its link to genome DNA sequence data. *Electrophoresis* 11:989–1071

17. Freed E, Symons M, Macdonald SG, McCormick F, Ruggieri R. 1994. Binding of 14-3-3 proteins to the protein kinase Raf and effects on its activation. *Science* 265:1713–16

18. Garcia-Guzman M, Dolfi F, Russello M, Vuori K. 1999. Cell adhesion regulates the interaction between the docking protein p130(Cas) and the 14-3-3 proteins. *J. Biol. Chem.* 274:5762–68

19. Fanger GR, Widmann C, Porter AC, Sather S, Johnson GL, et al. 1998. 14-3-3 proteins interact with specific MEK kinases. *J. Biol. Chem.* 273:3476–83

20. Leffers H, Madsen P, Rasmussen HH, Honore B, Andersen AH, et al. 1993. Molecular cloning and expression of the transformation sensitive epithelial marker stratifin. A member of a protein family that has been involved in the protein kinase C signalling pathway. *J. Mol. Biol.* 231:982–98

21. Tang SJ, Suen TC, McInnes RR, Buchwald M. 1998. Association of the TLX-2 homeodomain and 14-3-3eta signaling proteins. *J. Biol. Chem.* 273:25356–63

22. Ichimura T, Isobe T, Okuyama T, Yamauchi T, Fujisawa H. 1987. Brain 14-3-3 protein is an activator protein that activates tryptophan 5-monooxygenase and tyrosine 3-monooxygenase in the presence of Ca^{2+}, calmodulin-dependent protein kinase II. *FEBS Lett.* 219:79–82

23. Toker A, Ellis CA, Sellers LA, Aitken A. 1990. Protein kinase C inhibitor proteins. Purification from sheep brain and sequence similarity to lipocortins and 14-3-3 protein. *Eur. J. Biochem.* 191:421–29

24. Morgan A, Burgoyne RD. 1992. Exo1 and Exo2 proteins stimulate calcium-dependent exocytosis in permeabilized adrenal chromaffin cells. *Nature* 355:833–36

25. Campbell JK, Gurung R, Romero S, Speed CJ, Andrews RK, et al. 1997. Activation of the 43 kDa inositol polyphosphate 5-phosphatase by 14-3-3zeta. *Biochemistry* 36:15363–70

26. Hunter T. 1997. Oncoprotein networks. *Cell* 88:333–46

27. Wakui H, Wright AP, Gustafsson J, Zilliacus J. 1997. Interaction of the ligand-activated glucocorticoid receptor with the 14-3-3 eta protein. *J. Biol. Chem.* 272:8153–56

28. Craparo A, Freund R, Gustafson TA. 1997. 14-3-3 (epsilon) interacts with the insulin-like growth factor I receptor and insulin receptor substrate I in a phosphoserine-dependent manner. *J. Biol. Chem.* 272:11663–69

29. Furlanetto RW, Dey BR, Lopaczynski W, Nissley SP. 1997. 14-3-3 proteins interact with the insulin-like growth factor receptor but not the insulin receptor. *Biochem. J.* 327:765–71

30. Fantl WJ, Muslin AJ, Kikuchi A, Martin JA, MacNicol AM, et al. 1994. Activation of Raf-1 by 14-3-3 proteins. *Nature* 371:612–14

31. Fu H, Xia K, Pallas DC, Cui C, Conroy K, et al. 1994. Interaction of the protein kinase Raf-1 with 14-3-3 proteins. *Science* 266:126–29

32. Irie K, Gotoh Y, Yashar BM, Errede B, Nishida E, et al. 1994. Stimulatory effects of yeast and mammalian 14-3-3 proteins on the Raf protein kinase. *Science* 265:1716–19

33. Luo ZJ, Zhang XF, Rapp U, Avruch J. 1995. Identification of the 14.3.3 zeta domains important for self-association and Raf binding. *J. Biol. Chem.* 270:23681–87

34. Li S, Janosch P, Tanji M, Rosenfeld GC, Waymire JC, et al. 1995. Regulation of Raf-1 kinase activity by the 14-3-3 family of proteins. *EMBO J.* 14:685–96

35. Reuther GW, Fu H, Cripe LD, Collier RJ, Pendergast AM. 1994. Association of the protein kinases c-Bcr and Bcr-Abl with proteins of the 14-3-3 family. *Science* 266:129–33

36. Bonnefoy-Berard N, Liu YC, von Willebrand M, Sung A, Elly C, et al. 1995. Inhibition of phosphatidylinositol 3-kinase activity by association with 14-3-3 proteins in T cells. *Proc. Natl. Acad. Sci. USA* 92:10142–46

37. Conklin DS, Galaktionov K, Beach D. 1995. 14-3-3 proteins associate with cdc25 phosphatases. *Proc. Natl. Acad. Sci. USA* 92:7892–96

38. Zhang SH, Kobayashi R, Graves PR, Piwnica-Worms H, Tonks NK. 1997. Serine phosphorylation-dependent association of the band 4.1-related protein-tyrosine phosphatase PTPH1 with 14-3-3beta protein. *J. Biol. Chem.* 272:27281–87

39. Ogihara T, Isobe T, Ichimura T, Taoka M, Funaki M, et al. 1997. 14-3-3 protein binds to insulin receptor substrate-1, one of the binding sites of which is in the phosphotyrosine binding domain. *J. Biol. Chem.* 272:25267–74

40. Zha J, Harada H, Yang E, Jockel J, Korsmeyer SJ. 1996. Serine phosphorylation of death agonist BAD in response to survival factor results in binding to 14-3-3 not BCL-X(L). *Cell* 87:619–28

41. Vincenz C, Dixit VM. 1996. 14-3-3 proteins associate with A20 in an isoform-specific manner and function both as chaperone and adapter molecules. *J. Biol. Chem.* 271:20029–34

42. Pallas DC, Fu H, Haehnel LC, Weller W, Collier RJ, et al. 1994. Association of polyomavirus middle tumor antigen with 14-3-3 proteins. *Science* 265:535–37

43. Ford JC, al-Khodairy F, Fotou E, Sheldrick KS, Griffiths DJ, et al. 1994. 14-3-3 protein homologs required for the DNA damage checkpoint in fission yeast. *Science* 265:533–35

44. Gelperin D, Weigle J, Nelson K, Roseboom P, Irie K, et al. 1995. 14-3-3 proteins: potential roles in vesicular transport and Ras signaling in *Saccharomyces cerevisiae*. *Proc. Natl. Acad. Sci. USA* 92:11539–43

45. Kuwana T, Peterson PA, Karlsson L. 1998. Exit of major histocompatibility complex class II-invariant chain p35 complexes from the endoplasmic reticulum is modulated by phosphorylation. *Proc. Natl. Acad. Sci. USA* 95:1056–61

46. Bertram PG, Zeng C, Thorson J, Shaw AS, Zheng XF. 1998. The 14-3-3 proteins positively regulate rapamycin-sensitive signaling. *Curr. Biol.* 8:1259–67

47. Furukawa Y, Ikuta N, Omata S, Yamauchi T, Isobe T, et al. 1993. Demonstration of the phosphorylation-dependent interaction of tryptophan hydroxylase with the 14-3-3 protein. *Biochem. Biophys. Res. Commun.* 194:144–49

48. Michaud NR, Fabian JR, Mathes KD, Morrison DK. 1995. 14-3-3 is not essential for Raf-1 function: identification of Raf-1 proteins that are biologically activated in a 14-3-3- and Ras-independent manner. *Mol. Cell Biol.* 15:3390–97

49. Muslin AJ, Tanner JW, Allen PM, Shaw AS. 1996. Interaction of 14-3-3 with signaling proteins is mediated by the recognition of phosphoserine. *Cell* 84:889–97

50. Yaffe MB, Rittinger K, Volinia S, Caron PR, Aitken A, et al. 1997. The structural basis for 14-3-3:phosphopeptide binding specificity. *Cell* 91:961–71

51. Rittinger K, Budman J, Xu J, Volinia S, Cantley LC, et al. 1999. Structural analysis of 14-3-3 phosphopeptide complexes identifies a dual role for the nuclear export signal of 14-3-3 in ligand binding. *Mol. Cell* 4:153–66

52. Morrison DK, Heidecker G, Rapp UR, Copeland TD. 1993. Identification of the major phosphorylation sites of the Raf-1 kinase. *J. Biol. Chem.* 268:17309–16

53. Peng CY, Graves PR, Thoma RS, Wu Z,

Shaw AS, et al. 1997. Mitotic and G2 checkpoint control: regulation of 14-3-3 protein binding by phosphorylation of Cdc25C on serine-216. *Science* 277: 1501–5

54. Brunet A, Bonni A, Zigmond MJ, Lin MZ, Juo P, et al. 1999. Akt promotes cell survival by phosphorylating and inhibiting a Forkhead transcription factor. *Cell* 96:857–68

55. Liu YC, Liu Y, Elly C, Yoshida H, Lipkowitz S, et al. 1997. Serine phosphorylation of Cbl induced by phorbol ester enhances its association with 14-3-3 proteins in T cells via a novel serine-rich 14-3-3-binding motif. *J. Biol. Chem.* 272:9979–85

56. Hausser A, Storz P, Link G, Stoll H, Liu YC, et al. 1999. Protein kinase C mu is negatively regulated by 14-3-3 signal transduction proteins. *J. Biol. Chem.* 274:9258–64

57. Ku NO, Liao J, Omary MB. 1998. Phosphorylation of human keratin 18 serine 33 regulates binding to 14-3-3 proteins. *EMBO J.* 17:1892–906

58. Waterman MJ, Stavridi ES, Waterman JL, Halazonetis TD. 1998. ATM-dependent activation of p53 involves dephosphorylation and association with 14-3-3 proteins. *Nat. Genet.* 19:175–78

59. Clark GJ, Drugan JK, Rossman KL, Carpenter JW, Rogers-Graham K, et al. 1997. 14-3-3 zeta negatively regulates Raf-1 activity by interactions with the Raf-1 cysteine-rich domain. *J. Biol. Chem.* 272:20990–93

60. Winkler DG, Cutler RE Jr, Drugan JK, Campbell S, Morrison DK, et al. 1998. Identification of residues in the cysteine-rich domain of Raf-1 that control Ras binding and Raf-1 activity. *J. Biol. Chem.* 273:21578–84

61. McPherson RA, Harding A, Roy S, Lane A, Hancock JF. 1999. Interactions of c-Raf-1 with phosphatidylserine and 14-3-3. *Oncogene* 18:3862–69

62. Alam R, Hachiya N, Sakaguchi M, Kawabata S, Iwanaga S, et al. 1994. cDNA cloning and characterization of mitochondrial import stimulation factor (MSF) purified from rat liver cytosol. *J. Biochem.* 116:416–25

63. Du X, Fox JE, Pei S. 1996. Identification of a binding sequence for the 14-3-3 protein within the cytoplasmic domain of the adhesion receptor, platelet glycoprotein Ib alpha. *J. Biol. Chem.* 271:7362–67

64. Masters SC, Pederson KJ, Zhang L, Barbieri JT, Fu H. 1999. Interaction of 14-3-3 with a nonphosphorylated protein ligand, exoenzyme S of *Pseudomonas aeruginosa*. *Biochemistry* 38:5216–21

65. Wang B, Yang H, Liu Y, Jelinek T, Zhang L, et al. 1999. Isolation of high-affinity peptide antagonists of 14-3-3 proteins by phage display. *Biochemistry* 38:12499–504

66. Liu D, Bienkowska J, Petosa C, Collier RJ, Fu H, et al. 1995. Crystal structure of the zeta isoform of the 14-3-3 protein. *Nature* 376:191–94

67. Xiao B, Smerdon SJ, Jones DH, Dodson GG, Soneji Y, et al. 1995. Structure of a 14-3-3 protein and implications for coordination of multiple signalling pathways. *Nature* 376:188–91

68. Zhang L, Wang H, Liu D, Liddington R, Fu H. 1997. Raf-1 kinase and exoenzyme S interact with 14-3-3zeta through a common site involving lysine 49. *J. Biol. Chem.* 272:13717–24

69. Wang H, Zhang L, Liddington R, Fu H. 1998. Mutations in the hydrophobic surface of an amphipathic groove of 14-3-3zeta disrupt its interaction with Raf-1 kinase. *J. Biol. Chem.* 273:16297–304

70. Thorson JA, Yu LW, Hsu AL, Shih NY, Graves PR, et al. 1998. 14-3-3 proteins are required for maintenance of Raf-1 phosphorylation and kinase activity. *Mol. Cell Biol.* 18:5229–38

71. Petosa C, Masters SC, Bankston LA, Pohl J, Wang B, et al. 1998. 14-3-3zeta binds a phosphorylated Raf peptide and an unphosphorylated peptide via its con-

served amphipathic groove. *J. Biol. Chem.* 273:16305–10

72. Ichimura T, Uchiyama J, Kunihiro O, Ito M, Horigome T, et al. 1995. Identification of the site of interaction of the 14-3-3 protein with phosphorylated tryptophan hydroxylase. *J. Biol. Chem.* 270:28515–18

73. Gu M, Du X. 1998. A novel ligand-binding site in the zeta-form 14-3-3 protein recognizing the platelet glycoprotein Ibalpha and distinct from the c-Raf-binding site. *J. Biol. Chem.* 273:33465–71

74. Ichimura T, Ito M, Itagaki C, Takahashi M, Horigome T, et al. 1997. The 14-3-3 protein binds its target proteins with a common site located towards the C-terminus. *FEBS Lett.* 413:273–76

75. Jones DH, Ley S, Aitken A. 1995. Isoforms of 14-3-3 protein can form homo- and heterodimers in vivo and in vitro: implications for function as adapter proteins. *FEBS Lett.* 368:55–58

76. Braselmann S, McCormick F. 1995. Bcr and Raf form a complex in vivo via 14-3-3-3 proteins. *EMBO J.* 14:4839–48

77. Chang HC, Rubin GM. 1997. 14-3-3 epsilon positively regulates Ras-mediated signaling in *Drosophila. Genes Dev.* 11:1132–39

78. Zhang L, Chen J, Fu H. 1999. Suppression of apoptosis signal-regulating kinase 1-induced cell death by 14-3-3 proteins. *Proc. Natl. Acad. Sci. USA* 96:8511–15

79. Zhang S, Xing H, Muslin AJ. 1999. Nuclear localization of protein kinase U-alpha is regulated by 14-3-3. *J. Biol. Chem.* 274:24865–72

80. Williams NG, Roberts TM. 1994. Signal transduction pathways involving the Raf proto-oncogene. *Cancer Metastasis Rev.* 13:105–16

81. Morrison DK, Cutler RE. 1997. The complexity of Raf-1 regulation. *Curr. Opin. Cell Biol.* 9:174–79

82. Roberts RL, Mosch HU, Fink GR. 1997.

14-3-3 proteins are essential for RAS/MAPK cascade signaling during pseudohyphal development in *S. cerevisiae. Cell* 89:1055–65

83. Kockel L, Vorbruggen G, Jackle H, Mlodzik M, Bohmann D. 1997. Requirement for *Drosophila* 14-3-3 zeta in Raf-dependent photoreceptor development. *Genes Dev.* 11:1140–47

84. Li W, Skoulakis EM, Davis RL, Perrimon N. 1997. The *Drosophila* 14-3-3 protein Leonardo enhances Torso signaling through D-Raf in a Ras 1-dependent manner. *Development* 124:4163–71

85. Campbell SL, Khosravi-Far R, Rossman KL, Clark GJ, Der CJ. 1998. Increasing complexity of Ras signaling. *Oncogene* 17:1395–413

86. Tzivion G, Luo Z, Avruch J. 1998. A dimeric 14-3-3 protein is an essential cofactor for Raf kinase activity. *Nature* 394:88–92

87. Rommel C, Radziwill G, Moelling K, Hafen E. 1997. Negative regulation of Raf activity by binding of 14-3-3 to the amino terminus of Raf in vivo. *Mech. Dev.* 64:95–104

88. Rommel C, Radziwill G, Lovric J, Noeldeke J, Heinicke T, et al. 1996. Activated Ras displaces 14-3-3 protein from the amino terminus of c-Raf-1. *Oncogene* 12:609–19

89. Dent P, Jelinek T, Morrison DK, Weber MJ, Sturgill TW. 1995. Reversal of Raf-1 activation by purified and membrane-associated protein phosphatases. *Science* 268:1902–6

90. Roy S, McPherson RA, Apolloni A, Yan J, Lane A, et al. 1998. 14-3-3 facilitates Ras-dependent Raf-1 activation in vitro and in vivo. *Mol. Cell Biol.* 18:3947–55

91. Vaux DL, Korsmeyer SJ. 1999. Cell death in development. *Cell* 96:245–54

92. Yang E, Zha J, Jockel J, Boise LH, Thompson CB, et al. 1995. Bad, a heterodimeric partner for Bcl-X_L and Bcl-2, displaces Bax and promotes cell death. *Cell* 80:285–91

93. Kitada S, Krajewska M, Zhang X, Scudiero D, Zapata JM, et al. 1998. Expression and location of pro-apoptotic Bcl-2 family protein BAD in normal human tissues and tumor cell lines. *Am. J. Pathol.* 152:51–61

94. Mok CL, Gil-Gomez G, Williams O, Coles M, Taga S, et al. 1999. Bad can act as a key regulator of T cell apoptosis and T cell development. *J. Exp. Med.* 189:575–86

95. Ottilie S, Diaz JL, Horne W, Chang J, Wang Y, et al. 1997. Dimerization properties of human BAD. Identification of a BH-3 domain and analysis of its binding to mutant BCL-2 and BCL-X$_L$ proteins. *J. Biol. Chem.* 272:30866–72

96. del Peso L, Gonzalez-Garcia M, Page C, Herrera R, Nunez G. 1997. Interleukin-3-induced phosphorylation of BAD through the protein kinase Akt. *Science* 278:687–89

97. Wang HG, Pathan N, Ethell IM, Krajewski S, Yamaguchi Y, et al. 1999. Ca^{2+}-induced apoptosis through calcineurin dephosphorylation of BAD. *Science* 284:339–43

98. Harada H, Becknell B, Wilm M, Mann M, Huang LJ, et al. 1999. Phosphorylation and inactivation of BAD by mitochondria-anchored protein kinase A. *Mol. Cell* 3:413–22

99. Datta SR, Dudek H, Tao X, Masters S, Fu H, et al. 1997. Akt phosphorylation of BAD couples survival signals to the cell-intrinsic death machinery. *Cell* 91:231–41

100. Hsu SY, Kaipia A, Zhu L, Hsueh AJ. 1997. Interference of BAD (Bcl-xL/Bcl-2-associated death promoter)-induced apoptosis in mammalian cells by 14-3-3 isoforms and P11. *Mol. Endocrinol.* 11:1858–67

101. Wang HG, Rapp UR, Reed JC. 1996. Bcl-2 targets the protein kinase Raf-1 to mitochondria. *Cell* 87:629–38

102. Downward J. 1998. Mechanisms and consequences of activation of protein kinase B/Akt. *Curr. Opin. Cell Biol.* 10:262–67

103. Yano S, Tokumitsu H, Soderling TR. 1998. Calcium promotes cell survival through CaM-K kinase activation of the protein-kinase-B pathway. *Nature* 396:584–87

104. Hinton HJ, Welham MJ. 1999. Cytokine-induced protein kinase B activation and Bad phosphorylation do not correlate with cell survival of hemopoietic cells. *J. Immunol.* 162:7002–9

105. Scheid MP, Duronio V. 1998. Dissociation of cytokine-induced phosphorylation of Bad and activation of PKB/akt: involvement of MEK upstream of Bad phosphorylation. *Proc. Natl. Acad. Sci. USA* 95:7439–44

106. Majewski M, Nieborowska-Skorska M, Salomoni P, Slupianek A, Reiss K, et al. 1999. Activation of mitochondrial Raf-1 is involved in the antiapoptotic effects of Akt. *Cancer Res.* 59:2815–19

107. Zha J, Harada H, Osipov K, Jockel J, Waksman G, et al. 1997. BH3 domain of BAD is required for heterodimerization with BCL-X$_L$ and pro-apoptotic activity. *J. Biol. Chem.* 272:24101–4

108. Kelekar A, Chang BS, Harlan JE, Fesik SW, Thompson CB. 1997. Bad is a BH3 domain-containing protein that forms an inactivating dimer with Bcl-X$_L$. *Mol. Cell Biol.* 17:7040–46

109. Ichijo H, Nishida E, Irie K, ten Dijke P, Saitoh M, et al. 1997. Induction of apoptosis by ASK1, a mammalian MAPKKK that activates SAPK/JNK and p38 signaling pathways. *Science* 275:90–94

110. Piwnica-Worms H. 1999. Fools rush in. *Nature.* 401:535–37

111. Russell P. 1998. Checkpoints on the road to mitosis. *Trends Biochem. Sci.* 23:399–402

112. Kumagai A, Yakowec PS, Dunphy WG. 1998. 14-3-3 proteins act as negative regulators of the mitotic inducer Cdc25 in *Xenopus* egg extracts. *Mol. Biol. Cell* 9:345–54

113. Yang J, Winkler K, Yoshida M, Kornbluth S. 1999. Maintenance of G2 arrest in the *Xenopus* oocyte: a role for 14-3-3-mediated inhibition of Cdc25 nuclear import. *EMBO J.* 18:2174–83

114. Zeng Y, Forbes KC, Wu Z, Moreno S, Piwnica-Worms H, et al. 1998. Replication checkpoint requires phosphorylation of the phosphatase Cdc25 by Cds1 or Chk1. *Nature* 395:507–10

115. Lopez-Girona A, Furnari B, Mondesert O, Russell P. 1999. Nuclear localization of Cdc25 is regulated by DNA damage and a 14-3-3 protein. *Nature* 397:172–75

115a. Zeng Y, Piwnica-Worms H. 1999. DNA damage and replication checkpoints in fission yeast require nuclear exclusion of the Cdc25 phosphatase via 14-3-3 binding. *Mol. Cell Biol.* 19:7410–19

116. Ogg S, Gabrielli B, Piwnica-Worms H. 1994. Purification of a serine kinase that associates with and phosphorylates human Cdc25C on serine 216. *J. Biol. Chem.* 269:30461–69

117. Kumagai A, Dunphy WG. 1999. Binding of 14-3-3 proteins and nuclear export control the intracellular localization of the mitotic inducer Cdc25. *Genes Dev.* 13:1067–72

118. Dalal SN, Schweitzer CM, Gan J, DeCaprio JA. 1999. Cytoplasmic localization of human cdc25C during interphase requires an intact 14-3-3 binding site. *Mol. Cell Biol.* 19:4465–79

119. Peng CY, Graves PR, Ogg S, Thoma RS, Byrnes MJ III, et al. 1998. C-TAK1 protein kinase phosphorylates human Cdc25C on serine 216 and promotes 14-3-3 protein binding. *Cell Growth Differ.* 9:197–208

120. Furnari B, Rhind N, Russell P. 1997. Cdc25 mitotic inducer targeted by chk1 DNA damage checkpoint kinase. *Science* 277:1495–97

121. Sanchez Y, Wong C, Thoma RS, Richman R, Wu Z, et al. 1997. Conservation of the Chk1 checkpoint pathway in mammals: linkage of DNA damage to Cdk regulation through Cdc25. *Science* 277:1497–501

121a. Blasina A, de Weyer IV, Laus MC, Luyten WH, Parker AE, McGowan CH. 1999. A human homologue of the checkpoint kinase Cds1 directly inhibits Cdc25 phosphatase. *Curr. Biol.* 9:1–10

122. Walworth N, Davey S, Beach D. 1993. Fission yeast chk1 protein kinase links the rad checkpoint pathway to cdc2. *Nature* 363:368–71

122a. Chan TA, Hermeking H, Lengauer C, Kinzler KW, Vogelstein B. 1999. 14-3-3σ is required to prevent mitotic catastrophe after DNA damage. *Nature* 401:616–20

123. Chen L, Liu TH, Walworth NC. 1999. Association of Chk1 with 14-3-3 proteins is stimulated by DNA damage. *Genes Dev.* 13:675–85

124. Honda R, Ohba Y, Yasuda H. 1997. 14-3-3 zeta protein binds to the carboxyl half of mouse wee1 kinase. *Biochem. Biophys. Res. Commun.* 230:262–65

125. Hermeking H, Lengauer C, Polyak K, He TC, Zhang L, et al. 1997. 14-3-3 sigma is a p53-regulated inhibitor of G2/M progression. *Mol. Cell* 1:3–11

126. Megidish T, Cooper J, Zhang L, Fu H, Hakomori S. 1998. A novel sphingosine-dependent protein kinase (SDK1) specifically phosphorylates certain isoforms of 14-3-3 protein. *J. Biol. Chem.* 273:21834–45

127. Dubois T, Rommel C, Howell S, Steinhussen U, Soneji Y, et al. 1997. 14-3-3 is phosphorylated by casein kinase I on residue 233. Phosphorylation at this site in vivo regulates Raf/14-3-3 interaction. *J. Biol. Chem.* 272:28882–88

128. Aitken A, Howell S, Jones D, Madrazo J, Martin H, et al. 1995. Post-translationally modified 14-3-3 isoforms and inhibition of protein kinase C. *Mol. Cell Biochem.* 149–150:41–49

129. Megidish T, White T, Takio K, Titani K, Igarashi Y, et al. 1995. The signal modulator protein 14-3-3 is a target of sphin-

gosine- or N,N-dimethylsphingosine-dependent kinase in 3T3(A31) cells. *Biochem. Biophys. Res. Commun.* 216:739–47

130. Spiegel S, Milstien S. 1995. Sphingolipid metabolites: members of a new class of lipid second messengers. *J. Membr. Biol.* 146:225–37

131. Meller N, Liu YC, Collins TL, Bonnefoy-Berard N, Baier G, et al. 1996. Direct interaction between protein kinase C theta (PKC theta) and 14-3-3 tau in T cells: 14-3-3 overexpression results in inhibition of PKC theta translocation and function. *Mol. Cell Biol.* 16:5782–91

132. Autieri MV, Haines DS, Romanic AM, Ohlstein EH. 1996. Expression of 14-3-3 gamma in injured arteries and growth factor- and cytokine-stimulated human vascular smooth muscle cells. *Cell Growth Differ.* 7:1453–60

133. McConnell JE, Armstrong JF, Hodges PE, Bard JB. 1995. The mouse 14-3-3 epsilon isoform, a kinase regulator whose expression pattern is modulated in mesenchyme and neuronal differentiation. *Dev. Biol.* 169:218–28

134. Watanabe M, Isobe T, Ichimura T, Kuwano R, Takahashi Y, et al. 1993. Molecular cloning of rat cDNAs for beta and gamma subtypes of 14-3-3 protein and developmental changes in expression of their mRNAs in the nervous system. *Brain Res. Mol. Brain Res.* 17:135–46

135. Cullere X, Rose P, Thathamangalam U, Chatterjee A, Mullane KP, et al. 1998. Serine 257 phosphorylation regulates association of polyomavirus middle T antigen with 14-3-3 proteins. *J. Virol.* 72:558–63

136. Baserga R, Hongo A, Rubini M, Prisco M, Valentinis B. 1997. The IGF-I receptor in cell growth, transformation and apoptosis. *Biochim. Biophys. Acta* 1332:F105–26

137. Li S, Resnicoff M, Baserga R. 1996. Effect of mutations at serines 1280–1283

on the mitogenic and transforming activities of the insulin-like growth factor I receptor. *J. Biol. Chem.* 271:12254–60

138. Kaiser U, Schardt C, Brandscheidt D, Wollmer E, Havemann K. 1993. Expression of insulin-like growth factor receptors I and II in normal human lung and in lung cancer. *J. Cancer Res. Clin. Oncol.* 119:665–68

139. Nakanishi K, Hashizume S, Kato M, Honjoh T, Setoguchi Y, et al. 1997. Elevated expression levels of the 14-3-3 family of proteins in lung cancer tissues. *Hum. Antib.* 8:189–94

140. McDonald JD, Daneshvar L, Willert JR, Matsumura K, Waldman F, et al. 1994. Physical mapping of chromosome 17p13.3 in the region of a putative tumor suppressor gene important in medulloblastoma. *Genomics* 23:229–32

141. Chong SS, Pack SD, Roschke AV, Tanigami A, Carrozzo R, et al. 1997. A revision of the lissencephaly and Miller-Dieker syndrome critical regions in chromosome 17p13.3. *Hum. Mol. Genet.* 6:147–55

142. Hirotsune S, Pack SD, Chong SS, Robbins CM, Pavan WJ, et al. 1997. Genomic organization of the murine Miller-Dieker/lissencephaly region: conservation of linkage with the human region. *Genome Res.* 7:625–34

143. Layfield R, Fergusson J, Aitken A, Lowe J, Landon M, et al. 1996. Neurofibrillary tangles of Alzheimer's disease brains contain 14-3-3 proteins. *Neurosci. Lett.* 209:57–60

144. Toyooka K, Muratake T, Tanaka T, Igarashi S, Watanabe H, et al. 1999. 14-3-3 protein eta chain gene (YWHAH) polymorphism and its genetic association with schizophrenia. *Am. J. Med. Genet.* 88:164–67

145. Hsich G, Kenney K, Gibbs CJ, Lee KH, Harrington MG. 1996. The 14-3-3 brain protein in cerebrospinal fluid as a marker for transmissible spongiform encephalopathies. *N. Engl. J. Med.* 335:924–30

146. Moussavian M, Potolicchio S, Jones R. 1997. The 14-3-3 brain protein and transmissible spongiform encephalopathy. *N. Engl. J. Med.* 336:873–74

147. Prezeau L, Richman JG, Edwards SW, Limbird LE. 1999. The zeta isoform of 14-3-3 proteins interacts with the third intracellular loop of different alpha2-adrenergic receptor subtypes. *J. Biol. Chem.* 274:13462–69

148. Das AK, Cohen PW, Barford D. 1998. The structure of the tetratricopeptide repeats of protein phosphatase 5: implications for TPR-mediated protein-protein interactions. *EMBO J.* 17:1192–99

149. Guex N, Peitsch MC. 1997. SWISS-MODEL and the Swiss-PdbViewer: an environment for comparative protein modeling. *Electrophoresis* 18:2714–23

150. Matsuoka S, Huang M, Elledge SJ. 1998. Linkage of ATM to cell cycle regulation by the Chk2 protein kinase. *Science* 282:1893–17

151. Senften M, Dilworth S, Ballmer-Hofer K. 1997. Multimerization of polyomavirus middle-T antigen. *J. Virol.* 71:6990–95

152. Cacace AM, Michaud NR, Therrien M, Mathes K, Copeland T, et al. 1999. Identification of constitutive and ras-inducible phosphorylation sites of KSR: implications for 14-3-3 binding, mitogen-activated protein kinase binding, and KSR overexpression. *Mol. Cell Biol.* 19:229–40

153. Zhou Y, Schopperle WM, Murrey H, Jaramillo A, Dagan D, et al. 1999. A dynamically regulated 14-3-3, Slob, and Slowpoke potassium channel complex in *Drosophila* presynaptic nerve terminals. *Neuron* 22:809–18

154. Xing H, Kornfeld K, Muslin AJ. 1997. The protein kinase KSR interacts with 14-3-3 protein and Raf. *Curr. Biol.* 7:294–300

155. Andrews RK, Harris SJ, McNally T, Berndt MC. 1998. Binding of purified 14-3-3 zeta signaling protein to discrete amino acid sequences within the cytoplasmic domain of the platelet membrane glycoprotein Ib-IX-V complex. *Biochemistry* 37:638–47

156. Calverley DC, Kavanagh TJ, Roth GJ. 1998. Human signaling protein 14-3-3zeta interacts with platelet glycoprotein Ib subunits Ibalpha and Ibbeta. *Blood* 91:1295–303

157. Wardell MR, Reynolds CC, Berndt MC, Wallace RW, Fox JE. 1989. Platelet glycoprotein Ib beta is phosphorylated on serine 166 by cyclic AMP-dependent protein kinase. *J. Biol. Chem.* 264:15656–61

Annu. Rev. Pharmacol. Toxicol. 2000. 40:649–74

DUAL PROTEASE INHIBITOR THERAPY IN HIV-INFECTED PATIENTS: Pharmacologic Rationale and Clinical Benefits

Charles Flexner

Division of Clinical Pharmacology, Departments of Medicine and Pharmacology and Molecular Sciences, The Johns Hopkins University School of Medicine, Baltimore, Maryland 21287–5554; e-mail: flex@erols.com

Key Words   drug interactions, cytochrome P450, P-glycoprotein, pharmacokinetics, pharmacodynamics

■ **Abstract**   HIV protease inhibitors, as components of combination antiretroviral drug regimens, have substantially reduced the morbidity and mortality associated with HIV infection. They selectively block the action of the virus-encoded protease and stop the virus from replicating. In general, these drugs have poor systemic bioavailability and must be dosed with respect to meals for optimal absorption. Protease inhibitor–containing regimens require ingestion of a large number of capsules, are costly, and produce or are susceptible to metabolic drug interactions. Simultaneous administration of two protease inhibitors takes advantage of beneficial pharmacokinetic interactions and may circumvent many of the drugs' undesirable pharmacologic properties. For example, ritonavir increases saquinavir concentrations at steady state by up to 30-fold, allowing reduction of saquinavir dose and dosing frequency. Ritonavir decreases the systemic clearance of indinavir and overcomes the deleterious effect of food on indinavir bioavailability. These benefits reflect inhibition of presystemic clearance and first-pass metabolism, as well as inhibition of systemic clearance mediated by hepatic cytochrome P450 3A4. Several dual protease inhibitor combination regimens have shown great promise in clinical trials and are now recommended as components of salvage therapy for HIV-infected patients.

HIV PROTEASE INHIBITORS

Peptidic inhibitors of the HIV-encoded protease have had a major impact on the AIDS epidemic, by increasing patient survival and decreasing disease progression (1). Unfortunately, these agents must be given in combination with other active antiretroviral drugs, and regimens associated with clinical benefit have a number of disadvantages and much room for improvement.

The history of the development of these drugs is instructive. The protease gene was recognized within the sequence of the first HIV-1 genome, published in 1985

0362–1642/00/0415–0649$14.00

(2), prior to identification of a functional protein. The biological activity of this enzyme was elucidated the following year (3). The HIV protease is encoded in the 5' end of the *pol* gene and is expressed as part of the *gag-pol* polyprotein. This gene encodes a 99–amino acid aspartyl protease, which functions as a homodimer and is typical of retroviral proteases (4). The enzyme targets HIV-specific amino acid sequences in the *gag* and *gag/pol* polyproteins whose cleavage is essential for the maturation of the nascent virion (5). *Gag* polyprotein cleavage by protease produces four smaller functional proteins (p17, p24, p9, p6), which contribute to virion structure and RNA packaging (6). Although mammalian cells contain a number of aspartyl proteases, none appear to efficiently cleave the *gag* polyprotein, and conversely the HIV-encoded protease is not known to cleave any host cell–encoded proteins (7).

HIV protease was crystallized and its structure resolved at the atomic level in 1987 by two groups working independently at Merck Laboratories and the National Cancer Institute (8, 9). The first reports of inhibitors of this enzyme appeared in 1988 (10); the X-ray crystal structure of HIV protease complexed with peptidic inhibitors was resolved at about the same time (11). Although these initial inhibitors were of low potency, the first selective and potent inhibitors appeared within a few months (12).

One of these compounds, saquinavir, became the first protease inhibitor approved for prescription use in the United States. Saquinavir entered phase I trials in 1992, and just 3 years later, in December of 1995, this drug received accelerated approval from the US Food and Drug Administration (FDA) for use in combination with antiretroviral nucleosides (13). This was one of the most rapidly developed and approved drugs in modern times. However, an even shorter timeline was completed just a few months later, in March of 1996, when ritonavir received full approval for the treatment of patients with advanced AIDS; phase I studies of this agent had begun in late 1993. Indinavir, whose clinical development paralleled that of ritonavir, received FDA approval a few weeks later. A fourth peptidic protease inhibitor, nelfinavir, was approved in 1997, and a fifth, amprenavir, was approved in 1999.

The currently approved HIV protease inhibitors are based on modifications of virus-specific substrate peptides, for example the phenylalanine-proline scissile bond at position 167–168 of the *gag-pol* precursor (1). These compounds contain three or more chiral centers, which must be preserved to retain activity (Figure 1). Available drugs are active against clinical and laboratory isolates of both HIV-1 and HIV-2, with in vitro IC_{50}s (the concentration required to inhibit virus production by 50%) ranging from 2 to 60 nM (1). Antiviral activity parallels the K_i (drug concentration required to reduce enzyme activity by 50%) for purified HIV-1 encoded protease enzyme, which ranges from 0.1 to 2.0 nM (1). These compounds are inactive or weakly active against other human aspartyl proteases, with K_is of >10,000 nM for human renin, pepsin, and gastricin, and have little or no toxicity in tissue culture cell lines (minimal toxic concentrations >10,000 nM) (1).

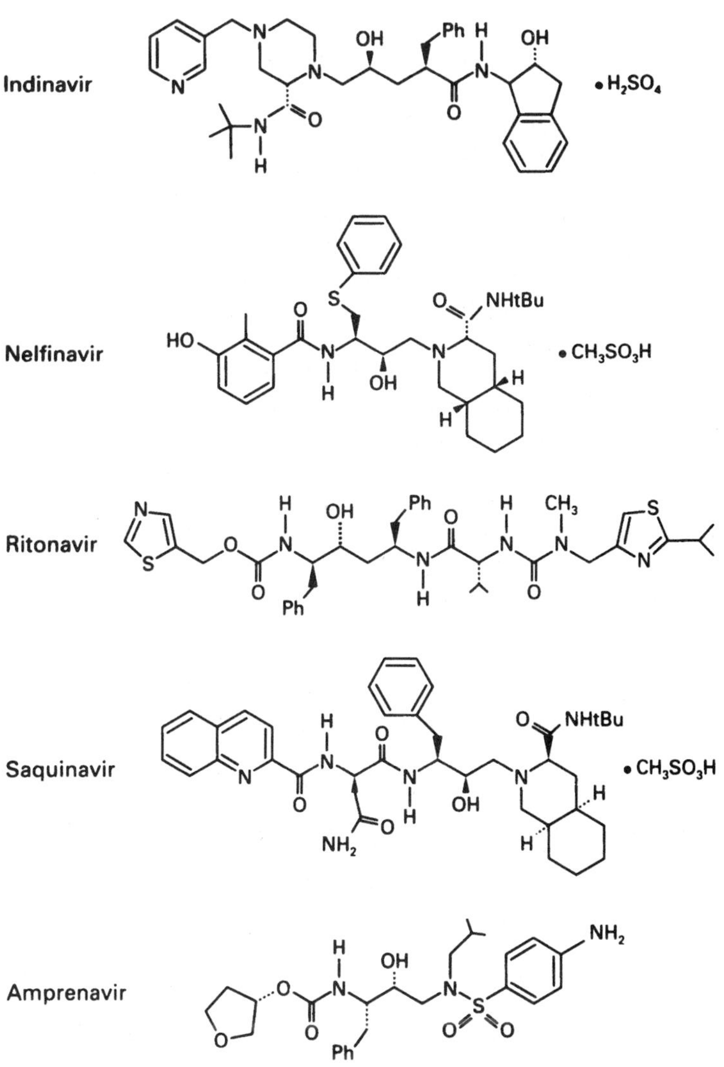

Figure 1 Structures of the five HIV protease inhibitors approved by the US Food and Drug Administration. (Reprinted from Reference 1, with permission.)

All approved HIV protease inhibitors cause a rapid and profound decline in plasma HIV viral loads in patients, as measured by quantitative polymerse chain reaction or branched-chain DNA assays of HIV RNA copies per milliliter of plasma. Protease inhibitor monotherapy produces a 100- to 1000-fold decrease in plasma HIV RNA, with peak effects 4–12 weeks after starting therapy (14, 15). In clinical trials, reductions in viral loads are paralleled by increases in CD4 lymphocyte counts, which average 100–150 cells/mm^3 (14–16). The addition of other antiretroviral drugs has little effect on the magnitude of initial viral load decline, but it improves the durability of response by preventing drug resistance (1).

The magnitude and duration of suppression of viral loads are directly related to drug dose and dosing regimen. With indinavir, regimens employing <2400 mg per day of drug were associated with a rebound in viral loads within 3 months of starting monotherapy (17). With ritonavir, regimens of 300, 400, 500, or 600 mg every 12 h produced in the first weeks of therapy equivalent reductions in viral loads, but sustained reductions in plasma HIV and a sustained increase in CD4 count were associated only with the 600-mg/12-h regimen (14, 15). A similar dose-response has been reported for nelfinavir (18) and amprenavir (19).

In three large randomized and blinded clinical trials, HIV protease inhibitor therapy increased patient survival and decreased morbidity. In a randomized, double-blind, placebo-controlled clinical trial involving 1090 patients, ritonavir, added to existing nucleoside analog therapy in patients with baseline CD4 counts of <100/mm^3, produced a 53% reduction in disease progression or death compared with placebo, and a 43% reduction in mortality (20). In a randomized, placebo-controlled trial involving 978 patients, combination therapy with saquinavir and zalcitabine (ddC) produced a 40% reduction in all clinical endpoints (death or disease progression) and a 68% reduction in death compared with monotherapy arms (21). A three-drug regimen of indinavir plus zidovudine and lamivudine reduced clinical progression and death by 50% compared with the two-drug regimen of zidovudine and lamivudine, and it reduced mortality by 57% (22).

Although combination chemotherapy with protease inhibitors has had a major impact on the morbidity and mortality of HIV infection, these new drug regimens are associated with a number of problems. First, many patients cannot manage the large number of pills and strict dietary requirements and have difficulty adhering to the prescribed regimen. For this reason, in some settings, treatment failure with initial combination regimens may be as high as 50% (23).

The use of HIV protease inhibitors has been associated with a significant number of clinical toxicities. Prominent drug-specific toxicities include circumoral and peripheral parasthesias with ritonavir, and hyperbilirubinemia and nephrolithiasis with indinavir. Class-wide toxicities include nausea, vomiting, diarrhea (with all drugs except indinavir), glucose intolerance, elevated lipids, and fat redistribution (1).

The latter three side effects constitute a cluster of symptoms know as HIV lipodystrophy syndrome. The mechanism of these toxicities is poorly understood. Because HIV infection per se is associated with a number of metabolic abnormalities (24), this may be the consequence of reversing underlying problems mediated by the virus. Proposed drug-specific mechanisms include downregulation of insulin receptor expression, inhibition of adipogenesis, accelerated lipolysis, and interference with retinoic acid receptor pathways (25). Because this syndrome has been reported in individuals taking classes of antiretrovirals other than protease inhibitors (26), it could be induced by or associated with other classes of drugs.

Improving the convenience, tolerability, and cost of available regimens and promoting long-term adherence to effective regimens are priorities for clinical and preclinical drug development.

PHARMACOKINETIC PROPERTIES OF HIV PROTEASE INHIBITORS

The pharmacokinetic properties of five approved protease inhibitors are summarized in Table 1. All of these compounds are primarily metabolized by cytochrome P450 enzymes, four by the 3A4 isoform and one (nelfinavir) by 2C19 (1, 27). Data from in vitro studies suggest that both intestinal and hepatic enzymes contribute to metabolism of orally administered drugs; saquinavir is metabolized as extensively by CYP3A4 from human intestine as by the corresponding enzyme in liver (28). First-pass metabolism accounts for the limited oral bioavailability of several of these drugs. For example, saquinavir's fractional bioavailability ranges from <4% to ~12% (see Table 1). Peak absorption for all these drugs occurs within 3 h of oral administration, and elimination half-lives range from 1.8 to 10 h.

Interindividual variability in pharmacokinetics is large, as indicated by a coefficient of variation for the mean area under the concentration-time curve (AUC) of >30% in all cases (Table 1). Several factors contribute to pharmacokinetic variability, including the effects of first-past metabolism and food (29). A high-fat meal substantially increases the bioavailability of saquinavir and nelfinavir but reduces the bioavailability of indinavir and amprenavir (Table 1). The same high-fat meal increases the bioavailability of ritonavir capsules but decreases the bioavailability of ritonavir liquid formulation (Table 1). It is currently recommended that nelfinavir and saquinavir be given with a moderate-fat meal, and that indinavir be given in the fasted state or with a light, low-fat snack. Amprenavir and ritonavir may be taken with or without food, but amprenavir should not be given with a high-fat meal.

All the approved HIV protease inhibitors are highly protein bound, with the exception of indinavir (Table 1). Amprenavir, nelfinavir, and ritonavir bind extensively to alpha$_1$-acid glycoprotein (AAG); the estimated association constant (K_a) for nelfinavir and saquinavir is close to 1 μM (30). The addition of physiologic concentrations of AAG increases the IC$_{90}$ (that is, reduces the anti-HIV potency) of several peptidic protease inhibitors by a factor of 10 or more (31, 32). Binding affinities for albumin are generally much lower than for AAG, and this protein has less effect on drug activity in vitro (33).

Fractional penetration of HIV protease inhibitors into the central nervous system is low. However, this may be an artifact of protein binding. The reported

TABLE 1 Pharmacokinetics of approved HIV protease inhibitors[a]

Drug	Dose (mg)	Bioavailability (approx. oral F) %	Food effect (%)	C_{max} (µg/ml)	T_{max} (h)	$T_{1/2}$ (h)	Variability (CV%, AUC)	Protein binding (%)	V_d (L/kg)	CSF (%)	Clearance route	P450 induction	P450 inhibition
Amprenavir	1200 BID	NR	−21	5.4	1.9	7.1–10.6	63	90	6.1	2	Hepatic (75%) 3A4	No	Yes (3A4)
Indinavir	800 Q8H	60–65	−77	7.7	0.8	1.8	22–47	60–65	NR	2.2–76	Hepatic (88%–90%)	No	Yes (3A4)
Nelfinavir	750 TID	>78	+200–300	3.0–4.0	2.0–4.0	3.5–5.0	NR	>98	2.0–7.0	<1	Hepatic (>78%) 2C19	Yes	Yes (3A4)
Ritonavir	600 BID	66–75	−7/+15	11.2	2.0–4.0	3.0–5.0	30–36	98–99	0.4	1	Hepatic (>95%) 3A4	Yes	Yes (3A4>>2D6)
Saquinavir	600–1200 TID[b]	<4–12	+670	0.2	NR	NR	46–84	98	10.0	<1	Hepatic (>97%) 3A4	No	Yes (3A4)

[a]Published mean values and ranges from studies in adults without hepatic or renal dysfunction from References 1 and 77. AUC, Area under the concentration–time curve during an average dosing interval; BID, twice daily; C_{max}, maximal concentration during a dosing interval; CSF, cerebrospinal fluid; CV, coefficient of variation; F, bioavailability; L, liters; NR, not reported; P450, cytochrome P450 drug-metabolizing enzymes; Q8H, every 8 h; TID, thrice daily; T_{max}, time to maximal concentration; $T_{1/2}$, half-life of the principal elimination (β) phase; V_d, volume of distribution.
[b]Dose of saquinvir depends on formulation: 600 mg TID for the hard-gel and 1200 mg TID for the soft-gel formation.

ratio of cerebrospinal fluid to plasma concentrations is ≤1% for amprenavir, nelfinavir, ritonavir, and saquinavir, whereas the comparable ratio for indinavir is at least 12%. This roughly parallels the free fraction of each drug available in human plasma (Table 1). Whether this has a bearing on clinical drug activity is controversial; in most studies, reductions in HIV RNA in the plasma are accompanied by similar reductions in the cerebrospinal fluid (34).

METABOLIC DRUG INTERACTIONS AND HIV PROTEASE INHIBITORS

Because available peptidic protease inhibitors are all substrates for cytochrome P450 (CYP450) metabolism, they are susceptible to drug interactions involving P450 inhibitors or inducers (35). All five approved protease inhibitors can inhibit the metabolism of CYP450 3A at clinically achieved concentrations; ritonavir is also a weak inhibitor of CYP 2D6 (36). Nelfinavir and ritonavir are moderately potent inducers of hepatic drug metabolizing enzymes, including various CYP450 isoforms and glucuronyl transferases(1, 35).

Ritonavir is by far the most potent inhibitor of cytochrome P450. Although ritonavir's P450 inhibition has mixed competitive and noncompetitive features in vitro (36), it can be considered a reversible inhibitor in vivo because of the rapid turnover of these enzymes in the liver. Amprenavir, indinavir, and nelfinavir are less potent inhibitors (35), and saquinavir is the least potent (1). For example, the K_i for inhibition of terfenadine metabolism in vitro is 0.017 µM for ritonavir (36) but 0.7 µM for saquinavir (28), a 40-fold difference in potency.

Ritonavir induces its own metabolism; during the first 2 weeks of monotherapy using a fixed dose, steady state trough concentrations fall two- to threefold (37). Ritonavir and nelfinavir can accelerate the clearance of other metabolized drugs through enzyme induction. For example, concurrent nelfinavir reduces the zidovudine area under the concentration time curve (AUC) by 35%, and ritonavir by 25%, presumably as a consequence of induction of glucuronyl transferases (1). Nelfinavir decreases the ethinyl estradiol AUC by 47% and ritonavir by 40%; these protease inhibitors are contraindicated in women taking oral contraceptives that contain the combination of norethindrone and ethinyl estradiol (1).

The p-glycoprotein drug transporter (P-gp), which is the product of the multidrug resistance *mdr1* gene originally described in cells resistant to certain cancer chemotherapies, has recently been shown to play a role in the cellular transport of several antiretroviral drugs. HIV protease inhibitors were shown to be substrates (38, 39) and, in some cases, inhibitors of this transporter (40, 41). Transgenic mice deficient in P-gp had cerebrospinal fluid concentrations of these drugs up to 30-fold higher than those in control animals (42). However, the in vitro anti-HIV activity of indinavir, nelfinavir, saquinavir, and ritonavir was not affected by P-gp expression (43). Drug transport mediated by P-gp may represent an additional pathway for drug interactions, especially those occurring in the intestinal tract. Selective P-gp blockade could reduce first-pass metabolism of drugs like saquinavir and could also be used to increase central nervous system penetration of these drugs.

DRUG RESISTANCE AND THE NEED FOR COMBINATION THERAPY

Drug resistance is the major obstacle to successful long-term suppression of HIV with protease inhibitor–containing regimens. Resistance is associated with specific, well-characterized mutations in the HIV protease gene (44). Resistance is a staged process wherein the virus acquires a single primary amino acid change that produces only a slight (generally less than fivefold) change in drug sensitivity. Thereafter, additional secondary mutations accumulate that confer ever-increasing resistance. Amino acid changes associated with primary resistance generally reside in the enzyme's catalytic site, whereas secondary mutations may be distant from the catalytic site. It is thought that many secondary mutations are compensatory, allowing improved proteolytic activity in the presence of primary active site mutations (44).

HIV protease tolerates a substantial amount of mutation, and catalysis is robust in the presence of altered amino acid sequences. One third or more of the 99 amino acids in the enzyme can deviate from wild-type consensus sequences without altering enzyme function (1, 44). Accumulation of protease inhibitor resistance mutations may reduce virulence in vitro and in animal models (45), but the clinical significance of this is debated.

Cross-resistance among peptidic protease inhibitors is substantial, especially once a virus acquires a number of secondary resistance mutations. Exposure to one protease inhibitor may select virus that is resistant to all other drugs in the class, even those the patient has not yet received. Indinavir monotherapy for a year, for example, can select virus resistant not only to indinavir, but also to all other approved and to several investigational protease inhibitors (46).

Once a patient develops resistant virus, that virus appears to be retained for long periods of time even after treatment stops. Patients with protease inhibitor–resistant virus who are taken off therapy may show initial response when that drug is reintroduced, but fail therapy within a few weeks with a rapid rebound in viral loads (47).

Risk of developing drug resistance is related quantitatively to plasma drug concentrations. Higher doses of drug produce higher plasma concentrations and are associated with greater duration of antiviral response and a decreased risk of genotypic or phenotypic resistance (1). Data from a study of ritonavir monotherapy suggest that the rate of accumulation of resistance mutations is inversely proportional to trough concentration of drug (C_{min}) during an average dosing interval (48). Dosing regimens maintaining plasma drug concentrations above some resistance threshold might therefore suppress emergence of resistant virus.

The current recommended dosing regimens for amprenavir, nelfinavir, indinavir, and ritonavir produce plasma drug concentrations that are equal to or greater than the in vitro IC_{90} throughout an average dosing interval (1, 29). This seems a reasonable target, although the beneficial clinical activity of saquinavir in combination with zalcitabine came with a dosing regimen that produced drug concentrations far below the IC_{90} (21).

Noncompliance appears to play an important role in the development of drug resistance. Compliance monitoring in patients taking high-dose saquinavir suggests that an increased frequency of genotypic resistance is associated with sporadic drug-taking behavior (49). Under the assumptions of current models, combination therapy with three or more drugs should suppress resistance as long as the drugs are properly taken. These models assume that single mutations are common, but that any virus resistant to one drug in a regimen is suppressed by other drugs in the regimen. Selected, highly motivated patient populations can maintain suppression of HIV replication to below detectable limits for more than 3 years with indinavir-lamivudine-zidovudine triple therapy (50).

The most likely scenario for selecting resistant viruses, then, is one in which the patient does not have three or more active drugs present all of the time, because of either inadequate pharmacokinetics or inadequate adherence to the prescribed regimen. Noncompliance, then, becomes the major cause of treatment failure and resistance, as is the case with other chronic infectious diseases, such as tuberculosis (51). These models, as well as clinical experience, dictate that the best way to reduce the risk of resistance and treatment failure is to develop regimens that are simpler to take, better tolerated, and more forgiving of individual problems with drug absorption, drug metabolism, or schedule adherence.

RITONAVIR-SAQUINAVIR PHARMACOKINETIC INTERACTIONS

In April, 1995, investigators at Abbott Laboratories discovered that ritonavir was an extraordinarily potent inhibitor of the in vitro metabolism of saquinavir and other peptidic HIV protease inhibitors. In hepatic microsomes, ritonavir inhibited the metabolism of 3.8 µg/ml of saquinavir with an IC_{50} of 0.029 µg/ml (52). At the same time, saquinavir had no effect on the in vitro metabolism of ritonavir. Animal studies showed that 10 mg/kg of ritonavir increased the saquinavir AUC by up to 38-fold (53).

Further impetus to develop this combination includes the fact that the primary resistance mutations seen in patients treated with either of these drugs (Val→Phe at position 82 of the HIV protease for ritonavir; mutations at position 48 and 90 for saquinavir) do not overlap (44). This suggests that one drug may be used to suppress the emergence of resistance to the other. A complete list of possible benefits from dual protease inhibitor regimens is provided in Table 2.

In a single-dose crossover study using healthy volunteers, ritonavir increased the saquinavir AUC by 50- to 132-fold and increased the saquinavir C_{max} by 23- to 35-fold (52) (Figure 2). For a fixed dose of ritonavir, saquinavir concentrations were proportional to saquinavir dose. However, when the saquinavir dose was held fixed, the relationship between ritonavir dose and saquinavir pharmacokinetics was nonlinear; saquinavir AUC increased in proportion to ritonavir AUC until the ritonavir AUC exceeded 100 µg-hr/ml, at which point the increase in saquinavir AUC became less than proportional (52). Saquinavir had a small but statistically significant effect on the ritonavir AUC (6.4% mean increase) in this study (52).

The authors point out that systemic clearance of saquinavir may be at least 10 times higher than hepatic blood flow. This could be attributed to its administration with food, or to significant prehepatic clearance via intestinal cytochrome P450 or P-glycoprotein. These results suggest that the poor oral bioavailability of saquinavir (1%–12%, depending on formulation and conditions) reflects extensive first-pass metabolism rather than poor absorption. The increase in saquinavir concentrations with ritonavir is the result of improved bioavailability, perhaps to as much as 100%, with little effect on postabsorptive systemic clearance. Estimates that ritonavir reduces saquinavir's first-pass metabolism by 33-fold (52) correspond remarkably well with the increase in saquinavir C_{max} seen in single-dose studies. The fact that the saquinavir AUC ratio, with or without ritonavir,

TABLE 2   Potential clinical advantages of dual protease inhibitor therapy[a]

Pharamacokinetic effects	Clinical consequences	Other potential benefits
Increased bioavailability	Reduced dose	Decreased pill burden
Decreased systemic clearance	Reduced cost of therapy	Decrease cost of therapy
Increased AUC	Increased antiretroviral activity	Improved convenience
Increased trough (C_{min})	Less likelihood of resistance	Dual agents lacking cross-resistance
Decreased peak (C_{max})	Reduced drug toxicity	Improved adherence
Reduced pharmacokinetic variability	More predictable drug concentrations	
Increased formation of active metabolites		
Decreased clearance of active metabolites		

[a]AUC, Area under the concentration-time curve; Cmax, peak concentration; Cmin, trough concentration.

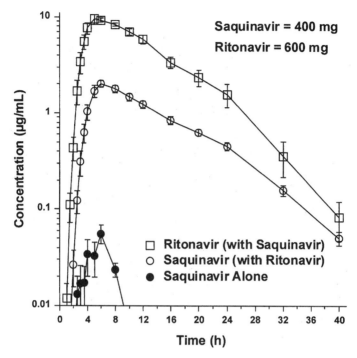

Figure 2 Impact of ritonavir on the pharmacokinetics of saquinavir. Shown are plasma concentration-time profiles in human subjects (mean ± standard error of the mean) for oral saquinavir at 400 mg alone (*closed circles*), 400 mg of saquinavir plus 600 mg of ritonavir (*open circles*), and 600 mg of ritonavir alone (*open squares*). (Reprinted from Reference 52, with permission.)

was 50–400 suggests that the postabsorptive contribution of ritonavir (presumably due to inhibition of P450 3A4) was only a four- to fivefold further increase in the AUC.

Because a high-fat meal increases saquinavir plasma concentrations by three- to fourfold, and because these studies imply that saquinavir's poor bioavailability is a consequence of presystemic clearance rather than poor absorption, one must wonder how a fatty meal enhances saquinavir bioavailability. These data suggest that a high-fat meal may contain substances that (*a*) specifically interfere with saquinavir metabolism by CYP3A, (*b*) block intestinal drug transporters such as P-glycoprotein, or (*c*) do both.

In 1997, the manufacturer of saquinavir made available a new oral formulation that had a two- to threefold improvement in bioavailability. This decreases the relative pharmacokinetic benefit of ritonavir but does not alter the pharmacokinetic profile produced per dose of saquinavir. That is because the presystemic effect of ritonavir is the same regardless of formulation, making the apparent bioavailability of a given oral dose of saquinavir 100% whether its inherent bioavailability is 4% or 12%.

An added pharmacokinetic benefit of combining ritonavir with saquinavir is a reduction in intersubject variance. Ritonavir reduced the percent coefficient of variability for saquinavir pharmacokinetic parameters from about 70% to about 30% (52). Differential expression of intestinal CYP 3A contributes to high intersubject variability in the pharmacokinetics of drugs like saquinavir that undergo extensive first-pass metabolism (54). Eliminating this pathway as a significant contributor to saquinavir clearance would be expected to reduce pharmacokinetic variance, as is the case. This makes drug concentrations more predictable in the clinical setting.

Other known inhibitors of cytochrome P450 3A4 increase the steady state AUC of saquinavir by no more than fivefold, and inhibitors of intestinal cytochrome P450, such as grapefruit juice, increase the saquinavir AUC by no more than threefold (1, 52). Ritonavir does not affect the pharmacokinetics of other P450 substrates, even those with extensive first-pass metabolism—increasing the AUC by no more than fivefold—to nearly the same extent as it affects saquinavir (1). This suggests a unique chemical specificity for the interaction between ritonavir and saquinavir. It is likely that ritonavir inhibits intestinal P450 3A4, and recent data suggest that ritonavir may also be a potent inhibitor of P-glycoprotein (40, 41). Selective interaction with one or both of these pathways may account for the surprising magnitude of ritonavir's effect on saquinavir oral bioavailability.

Because ritonavir is also a P450 inducer and undergoes autoinduction during the first 10–14 days of therapy (37), steady state concentrations of saquinavir should be lower when these two drugs are combined. Multiple-dose pharmacokinetic interaction studies found that the steady state saquinavir AUC was increased only 20- to 30-fold (55). This is still a substantial increase, but lower than that seen in single-dose studies.

The current clinical recommendation is to combine 400 mg of ritonavir with 400 mg of saquinavir twice daily. Although ritonavir's approved dose is 600 mg twice daily (BID), the lower dose was chosen to account for the plateau in ritonavir's pharmacokinetic benefit with increasing doses, and to compensate for gastrointestinal toxicity seen with the 600-mg dose. This regimen has proven to be well tolerated and highly effective in long-term clinical trials.

An interesting question is whether lower doses of ritonavir will have as much pharmacokinetic benefit as the 400-mg dose. One single-dose study using healthy volunteers found that combining 200 mg of ritonavir with 600 mg of saquinavir increased the saquinavir AUC by an average of 74-fold (56), an effect similar to that seen with 400 mg of ritonavir. Combining 100 mg of ritonavir with 600 mg of saquinavir increased the saquinavir AUC by an average of nearly 30-fold (56). Thus, lower doses of ritonavir may provide as much, or nearly as much, pharmacokinetic benefit.

RITONAVIR-INDINAVIR PHARMACOKINETIC INTERACTIONS

The magnitude of the pharmacokinetic interaction between ritonavir and indinavir is not as great as that seen with ritonavir and saquinavir. The estimated K_i for inhibition of indinavir metabolism in human hepatic microsomes is 0.085 µg/ml (57). When rats were given a single dose of 10 mg of each drug per kg, ritonavir increased the indinavir AUC by eightfold (53). Still, there are several features of indinavir pharmacokinetics that would benefit from ritonavir coadministration. These include indinavir's rapid hepatic metabolism with a half-life of 1.8 h, a dosing regimen of every 8 h, food restrictions, hydration requirements, and large interindividual pharmacokinetic variability (see Table 1).

In a steady-state pharmacokinetic interaction study using healthy volunteers on ritonavir for 14 days, the combination of 200 or 400 mg of ritonavir with 400 or 600 mg of indinavir increased the indinavir AUC by three- to sixfold compared with 800 mg of indinavir alone (57). Ritonavir increased the indinavir $C_{\max}$ up to twofold and increased the indinavir concentration 8 h after dosing by 11- to 33-fold (see Figure 3). The estimated K_i for inhibition of indinavir metabolism in vivo, 0.10 µg/ml, was very close to the in vitro K_i in human hepatic microsomes (57). Because ritonavir is a P450 inducer, and baseline indinavir pharmacokinetics were assessed under noninduced conditions, the actual magnitude of metabolic inhibition would be underestimated under these circumstances. In this study indinavir did not appear to have a significant effect on ritonavir pharmacokinetics compared with historical control subjects (57).

Ritonavir coadministration significantly reduced the pharmacokinetic variability of indinavir. The coefficient of variation for indinavir AUC fell from 30% to 16%, and for $C_{\min}$ (concentration after 8 h) from 50% to 39% (57).

Unlike saquinavir, the oral bioavailability of indinavir is at least 60%. The estimated contribution of intestinal CYP450 3A4 to indinavir metabolism is less than 4% (57). Therefore, the pharmacokinetic benefit of ritonavir should be due mainly to decreased systemic clearance rather than to increased bioavailability. Ritonavir decreased the postabsorptive clearance of indinavir by at least two- to threefold compared with baseline, noninduced kinetics (57). This suggests that inhibition of hepatic CYP 3A4 is the main source for pharmacokinetic enhancement of indinavir by ritonavir, with reduced first-pass metabolism making a minor contribution.

For a fixed indinavir dose, increasing ritonavir from 200 to 400 mg produced relatively little increase in the indinavir AUC (57). This could be due to the increasing importance of clearance mechanisms other than CYP3A4 for indinavir as the ritonavir dose increases. As the ritonavir AUC increased, indinavir clearance asymptotically approached the non-CYP3A4 clearance, which was thought to represent the combined contributions of renal clearance, glucuronidation, and

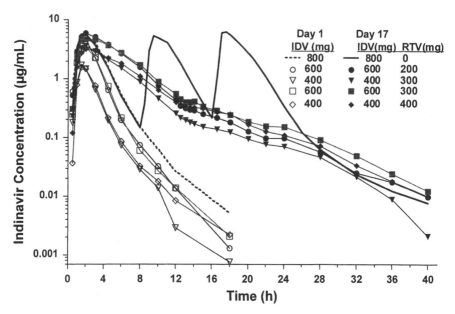

Figure 3 Impact of ritonavir (RTV) on the pharmacokinetics of indinavir (IDV). Shown are mean plasma concentration-time profiles in human subjects at day 1 for oral indinavir alone at a dose of 800 mg (*dashed line*), 600 mg (*open circles* and *open squares*), and 400 mg (*open triangles* and *open diamonds*), and at day 17 for 800 mg of indinavir alone (*solid line*), 600 mg of indinavir plus 200 mg of ritonavir (*closed circles*), 400 mg of indinavir plus 300 mg of ritonavir (*closed triangles*), 600 mg of indinavir plus 300 mg of ritonavir (*closed squares*), and 400 mg of indinavir plus 400 mg of ritonavir (*closed diamonds*). (Reprinted from Reference 57, with permission.)

CYP isoforms other than 3A4. Of note, ritonavir might induce glucuronidation more effectively at higher doses.

The effect of decreasing ritonavir dose and increasing indinavir dose was the subject of a separate study (58). In healthy volunteers administered ritonavir for 14 days, the 24-h indinavir AUC with a regimen of 100 mg BID of ritonavir/800 mg BID of indinavir was fourfold higher than with 800 mg every 8 h of indinavir alone (see Figure 4). In the same study, the 24-h AUC of indinavir with a regimen of 400 mg BID of both ritonavir and indinavir was 40% lower than with the BID regimen of 100 mg of ritonavir/800 mg of indinavir and 55% lower than with the BID regimen of 200 mg of ritonavir/800 mg of indinavir (58). However, the mean 12-h trough concentrations of the 400/400 regimen and the 100/800 regimen were nearly the same (Figure 4).

In two studies, coadministration of ritonavir and indinavir abolished the effect of food on indinavir bioavailability. A high-fat meal reduces the bioavailability of oral indinavir by up to 85% (57). Doses of 100, 200, or 400 mg of ritonavir BID reversed the effect of a high- or low-fat meal on indinavir pharmacokinetics,

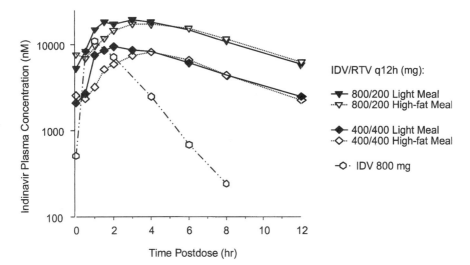

Figure 4   Effect of increasing ritonavir (RTV) dose with high- or low-fat meals on indinavir (IDV) pharmacokinetics. Shown are mean plasma concentration-time profiles from human subjects receiving oral indinavir alone at a dose of 800 mg fasting (*open hexagons*), 400 mg of indinavir plus 400 mg of ritonavir with a high-fat (*open diamonds*) or low-fat (*closed diamonds*) meal, and 800 mg of indinavir plus 200 mg of ritonavir with a high-fat (*open triangles*) or low-fat (*closed triangles*) meal. (Data taken from Reference 58; figure kindly provided by Al Saah, Merck Laboratories.)

compared with 800 mg of indinavir given in the fasted state (58, 59). Ritonavir should be enhancing indinavir oral bioavailability and pharmacokinetics through inhibition of cytochrome P450 and/or drug transporters such as P-glycoprotein. This finding suggests that the deleterious effects of food on indinavir may be mediated by interaction with intestinal epithelial drug transporters or P450 complexes, processes blocked by ritonavir.

PHARMACOKINETIC INTERACTIONS INVOLVING OTHER DUAL PROTEASE INHIBITOR COMBINATIONS

Ritonavir-Nelfinavir

Nelfinavir was originally marketed as a 750-mg thrice-daily (TID) regimen, and combination with ritonavir provided a way to reduce dose and dosing frequency. A single-dose drug interaction study using healthy volunteers showed that ritonavir increased the nelfinavir AUC by 152%, whereas nelfinavir increased ritonavir's AUC by only 9% (1). A steady state pharmacokinetic interaction study using HIV-infected volunteers evaluated the combination of 400 mg of ritonavir BID with 500 or 750 mg of nelfinavir BID. After 5 weeks of dosing, ritonavir use was associated with a 162% median increase in the 24-h AUC after 500 mg of nelfinavir BID (dose normalized), and a 62% increase in the 24-h AUC after 750-mg BID, compared with historical control subjects taking only 750 mg of nelfinavir TID (60). At the same time, the median change in ritonavir's dose-normalized 24-h AUC was +3% with 500 mg of nelfinavir BID, and –21% with the 750-mg BID regimen (not statistically significant, see Figure 5).

This pharmacokinetic interaction is more complicated than others, because both drugs are CYP450 inducers as well as inhibitors. The fact that when the dose was increased from 500 to 750 mg BID, the AUC of nelfinavir did not increase significantly may reflect increased autoinduction with the higher dose. In addition, there was a trend for nelfinavir to reduce ritonavir's trough concentrations at the higher (750 mg) nelfinavir dose. This may have decreased the magnitude of ritonavir's beneficial impact on nelfinavir pharmacokinetics.

Nelfinavir is the only HIV protease inhibitor known to produce an active metabolite, the hydroxy-butylamide M8 (AG1402), which is the major metabolite of nelfinavir in humans and has equipotent anti-HIV activity in vitro (61). Ritonavir had a more significant impact on the pharmacokinetics of the M8 metabolite than on nelfinavir itself. After 5 weeks of dosing, ritonavir use was associated with a 430% median increase in the 24-h AUC of M8 in patients taking nelfinavir (500 mg BID), and a 370% increase in the 750-mg BID M8 AUC, compared with historical control subjects taking 750 mg of nelfinavir TID alone (60) (see Figure 5).

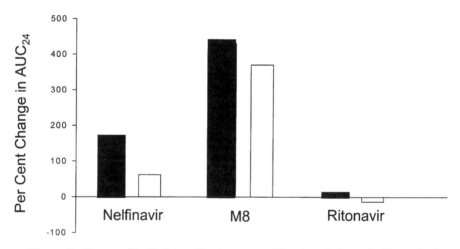

Figure 5   Pharmacokinetic interaction between nelfinavir and ritonavir. Shown is the median percent change in the 24-h AUC (area under the concentration-time curve) of nelfinavir, the nelfinavir hydroxy-butylamide metabolite M8 (AG1402), and ritonavir, normalized for drug dose in milligrams, after 5 weeks of ritonavir at a dose of 400 mg BID plus nelfinavir at 500 mg BID (*closed bars*) or 750 mg BID (*open bars*), compared with historical control subjects taking nelfinavir at 750 mg TID or ritonavir at 400 mg BID. (Data taken from Reference 60.)

M8 formation appears to be mediated mainly by CYP2C19 (27). Thus nelfinavir is the only currently approved HIV protease inhibitor whose major metabolite is not formed predominately by CYP3A4. M8 clearance, however, is mediated mainly by 3A4 (27). The discrepancy between ritonavir's effect on the pharmacokinetics of M8 and nelfinavir parent drug may reflect (*a*) induction of CYP2C19, thus increasing M8 formation, and (*b*) inhibition of CYP3A4, thus decreasing M8 clearance.

Ritonavir is an inducer of CYP2C19 activity and a potent inhibitor of 3A4, but it is a weak inhibitor of 2C19 in vitro (1, 36). Therefore, it is unlikely that the increase in nelfinavir's AUC produced by ritonavir is a consequence of inhibition of systemic clearance; this may, however, reflect improved oral bioavailability, perhaps through inhibition of P-glycoprotein, plus the inhibition of minor metabolic pathways. Alternatively, the M8 metabolite could be an inhibitor of 2C19.

Nelfinavir-Saquinavir

In single-dose pharmacokinetic interaction studies, nelfinavir increased the saquinavir AUC by up to fivefold, without affecting nelfinavir concentrations (1). However, nelfinavir is an inducer of CYP450 3A, and at steady state, the magnitude of this interaction was substantially reduced. Combining 750 mg TID of nelfinavir with 800 mg TID of the soft-gel formulation of saquinavir produced a saquinavir AUC equivalent to 1200 mg TID at steady state (62). This combination was well tolerated and was highly active against HIV in patients who were also taking two nucleoside analogs (63). However, this combination lacks many of the pharmacologic and clinical benefits of other dual protease inhibitor combinations.

Nelfinavir-Indinavir

Combining nelfinavir with indinavir produced a 50% increase in the indinavir AUC and an 80% increase in the nelfinavir AUC in single-dose studies using healthy volunteers (1). However, when these two drugs were administered to patients in a BID regimen, there was little pharmacokinetic enhancement and a disappointing anti-HIV effect, with only 10 of 21 patients suppressing their plasma HIV RNA to <400 copies/ml (the lower limit of quantification) after 32 weeks (64). Presumably hepatic enzyme induction by nelfinavir resulted in reduced concentrations of both drugs, and no real pharmacokinetic benefits.

Indinavir-Saquinavir

The combination of indinavir-saquinavir was reported to be antagonistic when used to inhibit HIV replication in vitro (65). Although the clinical relevance of this finding is unknown, this combination has not been pursued further in vivo, even though indinavir increased saquinavir concentrations by fivefold in single dose studies (1). Theoretical disadvantages of dual protease inhibitor therapy (see Table 3) may discourage clinical development of some combinations.

IMPACT ON CLINICAL TREATMENT OF HIV

Ritonavir-Saquinavir

Dual protease inhibitor combinations have proven to be highly active in clinical trials. When given to antiretroviral-naïve patients as sole therapy, ritonavir plus saquinavir suppressed HIV viral loads to <400 copies/ml in most subjects after 48 weeks of treatment; overall dropout rates were 10%–15%, often due to elevated liver enzymes in subjects with preexisting hepatitis virus infections (66). Of subjects continuing on this regimen, some of whom added nucleoside analogs, 90% had viral loads suppressed to <400 copies/ml (the lower limit of quantification when this study was conducted) after 60 weeks of therapy (66). Success rates in treatment-experienced patients have not been as good (67–69), presumably because of cross-resistance from prior protease inhibitor use. However, adding ritonavir plus saquinavir to zidovudine-lamivudine therapy was associated with a durable suppression of HIV viral loads to <200 copies/ml in 10 of 16 patients taking these four drugs for 48 weeks (70). Further, 10 of 16 patients who had failed nelfinavir- or indinavir-containing regimens had viral loads suppressed to <400 copies/ml 24 weeks after switching to ritonavir plus saquinavir plus nucleoside analogs (71).

Whether ritonavir should be used as a pharmacokinetic crutch for saquinavir and other HIV protease inhibitors, or whether the drug is providing important virologic benefit in its own right, remains controversial. The pharmacokinetic benefits of lower ritonavir doses were nearly as good as those seen with the 400-mg BID regimen (56, 58). Further, a lower ritonavir dose (100 or 200 mg BID) is being used to enhance the pharmacokinetics of the investigational protease inhibitor ABT-378 (lopinavir) (72).

TABLE 3   Potential clinical disadvantages of dual protease inhibitor therapy

Increased number of agents in the regimen

Increased number of potential toxicities

Increased potential for pharmacokinetic drug interactions

Increased formation of toxic metabolites

Decreased clearance of toxic metabolites

Overlapping toxicities

Same viral target for both drugs

Cross-resistance between drugs

Pharmacologic antagonism between drugs

It is likely that 400 mg BID of ritonavir is providing virologic benefit when combined with saquinavir, because the long-term success of the 400/400 ritonavir-saquinavir BID regimen is much greater than that of high-dose saquinavir mono-therapy with regimens producing similar AUCs (73). The virologic benefit of ritonavir doses lower than 400 mg BID is unknown and would have to be addressed in clinical trials. Therefore, if the patient's care provider decides that the antiretroviral regimen needs an additional active agent, the higher dose of ritonavir should probably be used. For example, a regimen of standard doses of zidovudine and lamivudine and 400 mg BID of ritonavir and saquinavir could be viewed as four active drugs; standard-dose zidovudine and lamivudine plus 400 mg BID of saquinavir and 100 mg BID of ritonavir could be viewed as three active drugs.

Ritonavir-Indinavir

Combining ritonavir with indinavir allows a significant reduction in indinavir dose. The 24-h AUC of indinavir administered as 400 mg BID with 400 mg BID of ritonavir is nearly the same as that of the standard indinavir dose of 800 mg given every 8 h (57). The reduced dosing frequency and reduced number of indinavir capsules make this regimen substantially more convenient. The indi-navir trough concentration at the end of a 12-h interval with this regimen is actually higher than the trough with 800 mg of indinavir every 8 h (see Figures 3 and 4). This trough is 2.5-fold higher than the protein-corrected IC_{90} of indi-navir, lengthening the duration of therapeutic coverage and possibly making the regimen more suppressive in patients who occasionally take their doses late (57).

This combination appears to be well tolerated and is highly active in the clinic. In one trial, 67 antiretroviral-naïve patients taking ritonavir and indinavir plus two nucleosides lowered mean plasma viral loads by 3.4 logs after 24 weeks of therapy, and 67% of these subjects had viral loads of <80 copies/ml (74).

The 400/400 ritonavir-indinavir regimen produced a lower C_{max} without affect-ing indinavir's renal clearance. Both of these factors could theoretically contribute to reduction of the risk for indinavir nephrolithiasis, which is thought to be both pH and concentration dependent (57, 75). Reduced indinavir peak concentrations should reduce the risk for formation of indinavir crystals in the urine, which presumably serve as the nidus for indinavir renal stones. Of 79 patients treated for a mean of 34 weeks with the 400/400 ritonavir-indinavir combination, none developed nephrolithiasis (76).

Other potential clinical benefits include elimination of the deleterious effect of food on indinavir bioavailability (58, 59), allowing the drug to be taken regardless of meals. It is also possible, though speculative, that ritonavir could reduce or eliminate the need for extra hydration with indinavir, because the C_{max} is sub-stantially reduced (57).

One theoretical disadvantage of the ritonavir-indinavir combination is that the primary resistance mutations for these drugs (Val $\rightarrow$ Phe at position 82 of the HIV protease) are shared (44). This could make these two agents more prone than other dual protease inhibitor combinations to select resistant mutants. Initial clinical studies in treatment-experienced patients have reported few early treatment failures (76), which suggests that this complication may be largely theoretical.

Amprenavir Combinations

Amprenavir, the most recently approved HIV protease inhibitor, has the longest elimination half-life of this drug class (7–10 h), but it has suboptimal oral bioavailability and must be dosed as eight large 150-mg capsules twice daily (77). Amprenavir is a modest P4503A4 inhibitor but is not a P450 inducer. In single-dose pharmacokinetic interaction studies, indinavir increased the amprenavir AUC by 33%, saquinavir decreased the AUC by 32%, and nelfinavir did not change the AUC compared with historical control subjects (77, 78). Amprenavir decreased the indinavir AUC by 38%, decreased the saquinavir AUC by 19%, and increased the nelfinavir AUC by 15% (77, 78).

Despite these modest pharmacokinetic interactions, combination studies were conducted with amprenavir at a dose of 800 mg TID and indinavir at 800 mg every 8 h, nelfinavir at 750 mg TID, or saquinavir at 800 mg TID. Although most patients achieved HIV viral loads <400 copies/ml at week 16, only 10 out of 17 achieved viral loads <20 copies/ml (79). Gastrointestinal toxicities such as diarrhea and nausea were common in this study.

An interesting recent observation is that ritonavir at a dose of 200 mg BID increased the amprenavir 12-h AUC up to threefold and increased the C_{min} about seven- to eightfold (S Piscitelli, personal communication). This should allow a significant reduction in the amprenavir dose (currently 1200 mg BID), but it should also make possible the exploration of once-daily dosing of amprenavir in combination with ritonavir. An additional problem with amprenavir occurs in combination with the nonnucleoside reverse transcriptase inhibitor efavirenz, which is a P450 inducer and diminishes amprenavir's AUC by up to 40% (77, 78). In the same study, low-dose ritonavir abolished the impact of efavirenz on amprenavir clearance, creating the possibility of a once-a-day antiretroviral combination including amprenavir and ritonavir and once-daily reverse transcriptase inhibitors such as efavirenz and didanosine.

Other Regimens

Other dual protease inhibitor regimens have been less widely studied, and in some cases have proven less useful, than the ritonavir-saquinavir and ritonavir-indinavir regimens. The combination of ritonavir at 400 mg BID with nelfinavir at 500 or 750 mg BID lowered viral loads by a mean of 2.8 and 2.2 logs, respectively, and increased CD4 cells counts by a mean of 236 and 120 cells/mm^3 after 48 weeks (80). However, 5 of 20 patients experienced virologic failure in this study, and all but one subject added nucleoside analogs to this regimen after 12 weeks. This regimen also produced moderate or severe diarrhea in 9 of 20 subjects.

IMPACT ON NEW DRUG DEVELOPMENT

Pharmacokinetic enhancement of one drug by another can improve the pharmacokinetic profile of investigational drugs in development. Clinical trials of ABT-378 (lopinavir), an investigational peptidic HIV protease inhibitor, have principally involved coadministration with ritonavir. Lopinavir is a peptidic analog of ritonavir with more potent anti-HIV activity in vitro (81). In drug interaction studies in hepatic microsomes and in laboratory animals, ritonavir greatly enhanced the pharmacokinetic profile of lopinavir, presumably by improving bioavailability and slowing systemic clearance. Ritonavir's effect on the lopinavir AUC was severalfold greater than ritonavir's effect on the saquinavir AUC in the same in vitro study (72, 81).

This beneficial pharmacokinetic interaction was confirmed in human volunteers; when dosed at 12-h intervals with ritonavir, mean trough concentrations of lopinavir were approximately 50-fold higher than the in vitro IC_{50} for HIV (72). In 101 HIV-infected patients taking lopinavir at 200 or 400 mg BID with ritonavir at 100 or 200 mg BID plus two nucleoside analogs for 24 weeks, HIV viral load was suppressed to <400 copies/ml in 93%–95% of patients and to <50 copies/ml in 89% (72). Mean CD4 cell counts increased by 160 cells/mm^3, a result comparable to that of other highly active antiretroviral combinations. Lopinavir-ritonavir was very well tolerated: No patients dropped out of this study because of toxicity, and mild adverse reactions were seen in only a small number of patients (72).

The availability of ritonavir to enhance the pharmacokinetic profile of lopinavir probably motivated the clinical development of this investigational protease inhibitor. A similar strategy could be employed for other promising investigational drugs in this class.

CONCLUSION

Combining drugs to take advantage of beneficial pharmacokinetic interactions dates back to coadministration of probenecid and penicillin. Additional examples include imipenem-cilastatin and cyclosporine-ketoconazole. These regimens use an inhibitor of drug clearance to allow reduced dose and reduced dosing frequency, with substantial improvement in cost and convenience for the patient. Dual protease inhibitor regimens are unique in that both drugs are active for the disease being treated and both attack the same pharmacologic target. The magnitude of the pharmacokinetic interaction between ritonavir and saquinavir is one of the largest ever described in human subjects. Combining low doses of ritonavir with ABT-378 (lopinavir) takes advantage of a similar interaction to develop a novel antiretroviral regimen. Dual protease inhibitor combinations with a lesser pharmacokinetic impact have been developed to improve concentration-time profiles and reduce the risk of treatment failure. Several of these regimens are now recommended as part of salvage therapy for HIV-infected patients.

ACKNOWLEDGMENTS

I wish to thank Laura Rocco and Nicole Staalesen for assistance in manuscript preparation.

Visit the Annual Reviews home page at www.AnnualReviews.org.

LITERATURE CITED

1. Flexner C. 1998. HIV protease inhibitors. *New Engl. J. Med.* 338:1281–92
2. Ratner L, Haseltine W, Patarca R, Livak KJ, Starcich B, et al. 1985. Complete nucleotide sequence of the AIDS virus, HITV-III. *Nature* 313:277–84
3. Kramer RA, Schaber MD, Skalka AM, Ganguly K, Wong-Staal F, Reddy EP. 1986. HTLV-III *gag* protein is processed in yeast cells by the virus *pol*-protease. *Science* 231:1580–84
4. Pearly LH, Taylor WR. 1987. A structural model for the retroviral proteases. *Nature* 329:351–54
5. Kohl NE, Emini EA, Schleif WA, Davis LJ, Heimbach JC, et al. 1988. Active human immunodeficiency virus protease is required for viral infectivity. *Proc. Natl. Acad. Sci. USA* 85:4686–90
6. Greene WC. 1991. The molecular biology of human immunodeficiency virus type 1 infection. *N. Engl. J. Med.* 324:308–17
7. Flexner C, Broyles SS, Earl P, Chakrabarti S, Moss B. 1988. Characterization of human immunodeficiency virus gag/pol gene products expressed by recombinant vaccinia viruses. *Virology* 166:339–49
8. Navia MA, Fitzgerald PMD, McKeever BM, Leu CT, Heimbach JC, et al. 1989. Three-dimensional structure of aspartyl protease from human immunodeficiency virus HIV-1. *Nature* 337:615–20
9. Wlodawer A, Miller M, Jaskolski M, Sathyanarayana BK, Baldwin E, et al. 1989. Conserved folding in retroviral proteinases: crystal structure of a synthetic HIV-1 protease. *Science* 245:616–21
10. Billich S, Knoop MT, Hansen J, Strop P, Sedlacek J, et al. 1988. Synthetic peptides as substrates and inhibitors of human immune deficiency virus-1 protease. *J. Biol. Chem.* 263:17905–8
11. Erickson JW, Neidhart DJ, VanDrie J, Kempf DJ, Wang XC, et al. 1990. Design, activity, and 2.8 Å crystal structure of a C_2 symmetric inhibitor complexed to HIV-1 protease. *Science* 249:527–33
12. Roberts NA, Martin JA, Kinchington D, Broadhurst AV, Craig JC, et al. 1990. Rational design of peptide-based HIV proteinase inhibitors. *Science* 248:358–61
13. Kitchen VS, Skinner C, Ariyoshi K, Lane EA, Duncan IB, et al. 1995. Safety and activity of saquinavir in HIV infection. *Lancet* 345:952–55
14. Danner SA, Carr A, Leonard JM, Lehman LM, Gudiol F, et al. 1995. A short-term study of the safety, pharmacokinetics and efficacy of ritonavir, an inhibitor of HIV-1 protease. *N. Engl. J. Med.* 333:1528–33
15. Markowitz M, Saag M, Powderly W, Hurley A, Hsu A, et al. 1995. A prelim-

inary study of ritonavir, an inhibitor of HIV-1 protease, to treat HIV-1 infection. *N. Engl. J. Med.* 333:1534–39

16. Gulick RM, Mellors JW, Havlir D, Eron JJ, Gonzalez C, et al. 1997. Treatment with indinavir, zidovudine, and lamivudine in adults with human immunodeficiency virus infection and prior antiretroviral therapy. *New Engl. J. Med.* 337:734–39

17. Steigbigel RT, Berry P, Mellors J, McMahon D, Teppler H, et al. 1996. Efficacy and safety of the HIV protease inhibitor indinavir sulfate (MK 639) at escaling doses. In *Progr. Abstr. 3rd Conf. Retroviruses,* Washington, DC, p 80. Washington, DC: Am. Soc. Microbiol.

18. Moyle GJ, Youle M, Higgs C, Monaghan J, Peterkin J, et al. 1996. Extended follow-up of the safety and activity of Agouron's HIV protease inhibitor AG1343 (Viracept) in virological responders from the UK phase I/II dose finding study. See Ref. 82, p 18

19. Schooley RT. 1996. Preliminary data on the safety and antiviral efficacy of the novel protease inhibitor 141W94 in HIV-infected patients with 150 to 400 CD4 + cells/mm^3. In *Progr. Abstr. 36th Int. Conf. Antimicrob. Agents Chemother.,* New Orleans, LA. Washington, DC: Am. Soc. Microbiol.

20. Cameron B, Heath-Chiozzi M, Danner S, Cohen C, Kravcik S, et al. 1998. Randomized placebo-controlled trial of ritonavir in advanced HIV disease. *Lancet* 351:543–49

21. Noble S, Faulds D. 1996. Saquinavir: a review of its pharmacology and clinical potential in the management of HIV infection. *Drugs* 52:93–112

22. Hammer SM, Squires KE, Hughes MD, Grimes JM, Demeter LM, et al. 1997. A controlled trial of two nucleoside analogues plus indinavir in persons with human immunodeficiency virus infection and CD4 counts of 200 per cubic milli-

meter or less. *New Engl. J. Med.* 337:725–33

23. Volberding PA, Deeks SG. 1998. Antiretroviral therapy for HIV infection: promises and problems. *JAMA* 279: 1343–44

24. Shikuma CM, Waslien C, McKeague J, Baker N, Arakaki M, et al. 1999. Fasting hyperinsulinemia and increased waist-to-hip ratios in non-wasting individuals with AIDS. *AIDS* 13:1359–65

25. Lenhard JM, Weiel JE, Paulik MA, Miller L, Ittoop O, et al. 1999. HIV protease inhibitors block adipogenesis and increase lipolysis in vitro. See Ref. 83, p 666

26. Walli RK, Michl GM, Segerer S, Herfort O, Dieterle C, et al. 1999. Dyslipidemia and insulin resistance in HIV-infected patients treated with reverse transcriptase inhibitors alone and in combination with protease inhibitors. See Ref. 83, p 645

27. Lillibridge JH, Kerr BM, Shetty BV, and Lee CA. 1998. Prediction and interpretation of P450 isoform selective drug interactions for the hydroxy-t-butylamide metabolite of the HIV protease inhibitor nelfinavir mesylate. In *Progr. Abstr. 5th Int. ISSX Meet.,* Cairns, Australia, p. 111. Cairns, Australia: ISSX

28. Fitzsimmons ME, Collins JM. 1997. Selective biotransformation of the human immunodeficiency virus protease inhibitor saquinavir by human small-intestinal cytochrome P4503A4. *Drug Metab. Dispos.* 25:256–66

29. Flexner C. 1996. Pharmacokinetics and pharmacodynamics of HIV protease inhibitors. *Infect. Med.* 13(Suppl. F):16–23

30. Bakker J, Tazartes D, Flexner C. 1998. A fluorescence quenching assay for determining the binding affinity (Ka) of HIV protease inhibitors to alpha-1 acid glycoprotein. See Ref. 84, p. 197

31. Flexner C, Richman DD, Bryant M, Karim A, Yeramian P, et al. 1995. Effect of protein binding on the pharmacody-

namics of an HIV protease inhibitor. *Antiviral Res.* 26:A282 (Abstr.)

32. Lazdins JK, Mestan J, Goutte G, Walker MR, Bold G, Capraro HG. 1997. In vitro effect of a_1-acid glycoprotein on the anti-human immunodeficiency virus activity of the protease inhibitor CGP 61755: a comparative study with other relevant HIV protease inhibitors. *J. Infect. Dis.* 175:1063–70

33. Molla A, Chernyavskiy T, Vasavanonda S, Praestgaard J, Lin T, et al. 1998. Synergistic anti-HIV activity of ritonavir and other protease inhibitors in the presence of human serum. See Ref. 84, p. 76

34. Letendre SL, Caparelli E, Ellis RJ, Dur D, Mccutchan JA. 1999. Levels of serum and cerebrospinal fluid (CSF) indinavir (IDV) and HIV RNA in HIV-infected individuals. See Ref. 83, p. 407

35. Piscitelli SC, Flexner C, Minor JR, Polis MA, Masur H. 1996. Drug interactions in patients infected with human immunodeficiency virus. *Clin. Infect. Dis.* 23:685–93

36. Kumar GN, Rodrigues AD, Buko AM, Denissen JF. 1996. Cytochrome P450-mediated metabolism of the HIV-1 protease inhibitor ritonavir (ABT-538) in human liver microsomes. *J. Pharmacol. Exp. Ther.* 277:423–31

37. Hsu A, Granneman GR, Witt G, Locke C, Denissen J, et al. 1997. Multiple-dose pharmacokinetics of ritonavir in human immunodeficiency virus-infected subjects. *Antimicrob. Agents Chemother.* 41:898–905

38. Alsenz J, Steffen H, Alex R. 1998. Active apical secretory efflux of the HIV protease inhibitors saquinavir and ritonavir in Caco-2 Cell monolayers. *Pharmaceut. Res.* 15:423–28

39. Kim AE, Dintaman JM, Waddell DS, Silverman JA. 1998. Saquinavir, an HIV protease inhibitor, is transported by P-glycoprotein. *J. Pharmacol. Exp. Ther.* 286:1439–45

40. Drewe J, Gutmann H, Fricker G, Torok M, Beglinger C, Huwyler J. 1999. HIV protease inhibitor ritonavir: a more potent inhibitor of P-glycoprotein than the cyclosporine analog SDZ PSC 833. *Biochem. Pharmacol.* 57:1147–52

41. Washington CB, Duran GE, Man MC, Sikic BI, Blaschke T. 1998. Interaction of anti-HIV protease inhibitors with the multidrug transporter P-glycoprotein (P-gp) in human cultured cells. *J. Acquired Immune Defic. Syndr.* 19:203–9

42. Kim RB, Fromm MF, Wandell C, Leake B, Wood AJ, et al. 1998. The drug transporter P-glycoprotein limits oral absorption and brain entry of HIV-1 protease inhibitors. *J. Clin. Invest.* 101:289–94

43. Srinivas RV, Middlemas D, Flynn P, Fridland A. 1998. Human immunodeficiency virus protease inhibitors serve as substrates for multidrug transporter proteins MDR1 and MRP1 but retain antiviral efficacy in cell lines expressing these transporters. *Antimicrob. Agents Chemother.* 42:3157–62

44. Boden D, Markowitz M. 1998. Resistance to human immunodeficiency virus type 1 protease inhibitors. *Antimicrob. Agents Chemother.* 42:2775–83

45. Stoddart C, Mammano F, Moreno M, Linquist-Stepps V, Bare C, et al. 1999. Lack of fitness of protease inhibitor-resistant HIV-1 in vivo. See Ref. 83, p. 4

46. Condra JH, Schleif WA, Blahy OM, Gabryelski LJ, Graham DJ, et al. 1995. In vivo emergence of HIV-1 variants resistant to multiple protease inhibitors. *Nature* 374:569–71

47. Condra J, Schleif WA, Blahy OM, Gabryelski LJ, Graham DJ, et al. 1995. Evidence for the existence of long lived genetic reservoirs of HIV-1 in infected patients. In *Progr. Abstr. 4th Int. Workshop HIV Drug Resist.,* Sardinia, Italy, p. 82. Sardinia, Italy: Int. Drug Resist. Workshop

48. Molla M, Korneyeva M, Gao Q, Vasavanonda S, Schipper PJ, et al. 1996.

Ordered accumulation of mutations in HIV protease confers resistance to ritonavir. *Nat. Med.* 2:760–66

49. Vanhove GF, Schapiro JM, Winters MA, Merigan TC, Blaschke TF. 1996. Patient compliance and drug failure in protease inhibitor monotherapy. *JAMA* 276:1955–56

50. Gulick R, Mellors J, Havlir D, Eron J, Valentine F, et al. 1999. Treatment with indinavir (IDV), zidovudine (ZDV) and lamivudine (3TC): three-year follow-up. See Ref. 83, p. 388

51. Bonhoeffer S. 1998. Models of viral kinetics and drug resistance in HIV-1 infection. *AIDS Patient Care Stand.* 12:769–74

52. Hsu A, Granneman GR, Cao G, Carothers L, El-Shourbagy T, et al. 1998. Pharmacokinetic interactions between two human immunodeficiency virus protease inhibitors, ritonavir and saquinavir. *Clin. Pharmacol. Ther.* 63:453–63

53. Kempf DJ, Marsh KC, Kumar G, Rodrigues AD, Denissen JF, et al. 1997. Pharmacokinetic enhancement of inhibitors of the human immunodeficiency virus protease by coadministration with ritonavir. *Antimicrob. Agents Chemother.* 41:654–60

54. Kolars JC, Lown KS, Schmeidlin-Ren P, Ghosh M, Wrighton SA, et al. 1994. CYP 3A gene expression in human gut epithelium. *Pharmacogenetics* 4:247–59

55. Hsu A, Granneman GR, Sun E, Chen P, El-Shourbagy T, et al. 1996. Assessment of single and multiple-dose interactions between ritonavir and saquinavir. See Ref. 82, p. 30

56. Peytavin G, Bergmann JF, Leibowtich J, Landman R, Dohin E, et al. 1998. Invirase® bioavailability is dramatically increased by ritonavir (RTV) "baby"-doses in healthy volunteers (HV). See Ref. 84, p. 34

57. Hsu A, Granneman GR, Cao G, Carothers L, Japour A, et al. 1998. Pharmacokinetic interaction between ritonavir and indinavir in healthy volunteers. *Antimicrob. Agents. Chemother.* 42:2784–91

58. Saah A, Winchell G, Seniuk M, Mehrotra D, Deutsch P. 1999. Multiple-dose pharmacokinetics (PK) and tolerability of indinavir (IDV)-ritonavir (RTV) combinations in healthy volunteers (Merck 078). See Ref. 83, p. 362

59. Hsu A, Granneman GR, Heath-Chiozzi M, Wong C, Japour A, et al. 1998. Indinavir can be taken with regular meals when taken with ritonavir. See Ref. 84, p. 92

60. Flexner C, Hsu A, Kerr B, Gallant J, Heath-Chiozzi M, Anderson R. 1998. Steady-state pharmacokinetic interactions between ritonavir (RTV), nelfinavir (NFV), and the nelfinavir active metabolite M8 (AG1402). See Ref. 84, p. 197

61. Zhang KE, Wu E, Patick A, Kerr BM, Shetty BV, et al. 1997. Plasma metabolites of nelfinavir, a potent HIV protease inhibitor, in HIV positive patients: quantitation by LC-MS/MS and antiviral activities. In *Progr. Abstr. 6th Eur. ISSX Meet.* Gothenburg, Sweden: ISSX

62. Kravcik S, Farnsworth A, Patick A, Duncan I, Hawley-Foss N, et al. 1998. Long term follow-up of combination protease inhibitor therapy with nelfinavir and saquinavir (soft gel) in HIV infection. See Ref. 85, p. 153

63. Opravil M, SPICE Study Team. 1998. Study of protease inhibitor combination in Europe (SPICE): saquinavir soft gelatin capsule and nelfinavir in HIV-infected individuals. See Ref. 85, p. 153

64. Havlir DV, Riddler S, Squires K, Winslow D, Kerr B, et al. 1998. Coadministration of indinavir (IDV) and nelfinavir (NFV) in a twice daily regimen: preliminary safety, pharmacokinetic and antiviral activity results. See Ref. 85, p. 152

65. Merrill DP, Manion DJ, Chou TC, Hirsch MS. 1997. Antagonism between human immunodeficiency virus type 1 protease inhibitors indinavir and saquinavir in vitro. *J. Infect. Dis.* 176:265–68

66. Cameron DW, Japour A, Mellors J, Farthing C, Cohen C, et al. 1998. Antiretroviral safety & durability of ritonavir (RIT)-saquinavir (SQV) in protease inhibitor-naïve patients in year two of follow-up. See Ref. 85, p. 152

67. Cassano P, Hermans P, Sommereijns B, de Wit S, Kabeya K, et al. 1998. Combined quadruple therapy with ritonavir-saquinavir (RTV-SQV) + nucleosides in patients (p) who failed in triple therapy with RTV, SQV or indinavir (IDV). See Ref. 85, p. 159

68. De Truchis P, Force G, Zucman D, LeClerc V, Rouviex E, et al. 1998. Effects of salvage combination therapy with ritonavir + saquinavir in HIV-infected patients previously treated with protease inhibitors (PI). See Ref. 85, p. 159

69. Tebas P, Kane E, Klebert M, Simpson J, Powderly WG, Henry K. 1998. Virologic responses to a ritonavir/saquinavir containing regimen in patients who have previously failed nelfinavir. See Ref. 85, p. 510

70. Michelet C, Bellissant E, Ruffault A, Arvieux C, Delfraissy JF, et al. 1999. Safety and efficacy of ritonavir and saquinavir in combination with zidovudine and lamivudine. Clin. Pharmacol. Ther. 65:661–71

71. Gallant JE, Hall C, Barnett S, Raines C. 1998. Ritonavir/saquinavir (RTV/SQV) as salvage therapy after failure of initial protease inhibitor (PI) regimen. See Ref. 85, p. 159

72. Murphy R, King M, Brun S, Orth K, Hicks C, et al. 1999. ABT-378/ritonavir therapy in antiretroviral-naive HIV-1 infected patients for 24 weeks. See Ref. 83, p. 15

73. Schapiro JM, Winters MA, Stewart F, Efron B, Norris J, et al. 1996. The effect of high-dose saquinavir on viral load and CD4+ T-cell counts in HIV-infected patients. Ann. Intern. Med. 124:1039–50

74. Rockstroh JK, Bergmann F, Wiesel W, Rieke A, Nadler M, Knechten H. 1999.

Efficacy and safety of BID firstline ritonavir/indinavir plus double nucleoside combination therapy in HIV-infected individuals. See Ref. 83, p. 631

75. Kopp JB, Miller KD, Mican JA, Feverstein IM, Vaughan E, et al. 1997. Crystalluria and urinary tract abnormalities associated with indinavir. Ann. Intern. Med. 127:119–25

76. Workman C, Musson R, Dyer W, Sullivan J. 1998. Novel double protease combinations combining indinavir (IDV) with ritonavir (RTV): results from the first study. See Ref. 84, p. 92

77. Glaxo Wellcome, Inc. 1999. Agenerase^TM (Amprenavir) Capsules Product Monograph. Research Triangle Park, NC: Glaxo Wellcome

78. Sadler BM, Gillotin C, Chittick GE, Symonds WT. 1998. Pharmacokinetic drug interactions with amprenavir. See Ref. 84, p. 37

79. Eron J, Haubrich R, Richman D, Lang W, Tisdale M, et al. 1998. Preliminary assessment of 141W94 in combination with other protease inhibitors. See Ref. 85, p. 80

80. Gallant JE, Raines C, Sun E, Lewis R, Apuzzo L, et al. 1999. Phase II study of ritonavir-nelfinavir combination therapy: 48 week data. See Ref. 83, p. 393

81. Sham HL, Kempf DJ, Molla A, Marsh KC, Kumar GN, et al. 1998. ABT-378, a highly potent inhibitor of the human immunodeficiency virus protease. Antimicrob. Agents Chemother. 42:3218–24

82. 1996. Progr. Abstr. 11th Int. Conf. AIDS, Vancouver, BC. Stockholm, Sweden: Int. AIDS Soc.

83. 1999. Progr. Abstr. 6th Conf. Hum. Retroviruses Opportun. Infect., Chicago, IL. Alexandria, VA: Found. Retrovirol. Human Health

84. 1998. Progr. Abstr. 12th World AIDS Conf., Geneva, Switzerland. Stockholm, Sweden: Int. AIDS Soc.

85. 1998. Progr. Abstr. 5th Conf. Retroviruses Opportun. Infect., Chicago, IL. Alexandria, VA: Found. Retrovirol. Human Health

Subject Index

comparative genomics,
97, 120–23
evolution and, 124
synteny and, 121–23
limits of, 124–25
Gilbert's syndrome, 581
Glucuronidation, 581–606
carboxylic acid, 595–96
gastrointestinal tract, 600–1
O-linked, 593
N–, 596
phenanthrene, 593, 595
steroid, 595
Glycine receptors, 431, 435,
442
P-Glycoprotein, 649
Glycoprotein adhesion molecules
selectins, 283–91
P-Glycoprotein (PGP) efflux
pump, 139–41
G protein–adenylate cyclase
pathway, 390–93
G protein–coupled inwardly
rectifying K⁺ channels,
240
G protein–coupled receptor
kinases (GRKs), 235–36
G protein–coupled receptors
(GPCRs)
agonists
lysophosphatidic acid
(LPA), 459, 463, 465,
467–69, 473
thrombin, 459, 465,
468–69, 471
cross-reactivity of ligands,
201–2
drug discovery targets,
178, 180, 183–85
gene superfamily, 199–202
melanin-concentrating hormone, 200–1
opioid receptors, 389–415
orexins, 200–1
receptor genes, 405–12
receptor phosphorylation,
399–405

receptor structure, 389–99
See also Opioid receptors
G protein–coupled receptor
signaling pathways,
235–62
regulator of G protein signaling (RGS) proteins
and, 235–62
cell types, 240–43
mechanisms of action,
243–44
G protein–coupled signal
transduction, 459–78
Rho-dependent pathways
and, 459–78
apoptosis and, 472–73
bacterial toxins and,
462–64
cell migration and, 468–
69
cell proliferation and,
471
cytoskeleton and, 459,
464–66, 474
effectors, 464
gene transcription and,
469–71, 474
hypertrophic cell
growth, 472
MAP kinase activation
and, 469–71
phospholipid metabo-
lism, 462, 466–67
regulators, 460–64
RhoA, 459–60, 465,
470, 472–74
RhoGAPs, 460
RhoGDI, 460, 462
RhoGEF, 459–61
smooth muscle contrac-
tion, 467–68, 474
tumor cell invasion and,
467–69
G proteins, 389–415
G protein–adenylate
cyclase pathway, 390–93
heterotrimeric, 459, 467

opioid receptor signaling
and, 389–415
small, 459
See also G protein–cou-
pled receptors; Opioid
receptors
Growth suppression, 491,
507–8
GTPase activating proteins
(GAPs), 235–37, 249–
62, 460
mechanism of activity,
252–55
mutagenesis, 254–55
Guanine exchange factors,
236
Guanine nucleotide dissociation inhibitors (GDIs),
460, 462
Guanine nucleotide exchange
factors, 460

H

Halothane, 48, 55
Hemophilia B, 302
Hepatocarcinogenesis
oxidative-stress hypothe-
sis, 504
peroxisome proliferator-
induced, 495, 497, 504–7
Hepatocytes
drug screening and, 133,
148
Hepatotoxicity
biotransformation, 48
chlorinated methanes and,
43–56
free radicals and, 48–50,
55
hepatocellular regeneration
and, 43, 53–55
lipid peroxidation and, 49–
50, 55
oxidative stress leading to,
50, 55
High-throughput screening
(HTS), 133–51, 177,

CUMULATIVE INDEXES

CONTRIBUTING AUTHORS, VOLUMES 36–40

CHAPTER TITLES, VOLUMES 36–40